THE PSYCHIATRIC INTERVIEW IN CLINICAL PRACTICE

THIRD EDITION

THE PSYCHIATRIC INTERVIEW IN CLINICAL PRACTICE

THIRD EDITION

ROGER A. MACKINNON, M.D.

Professor Emeritus of Clinical Psychiatry
College of Physicians and Surgeons of Columbia University
New York, New York

ROBERT MICHELS, M.D.

Walsh McDermott University Professor of Medicine and Psychiatry
Weill Medical College of Cornell University
New York, New York

PETER J. BUCKLEY, M.D.

Professor of Psychiatry and Behavioral Sciences
Albert Einstein College of Medicine of Yeshiva University
Bronx, New York

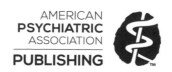

AMERICAN
PSYCHIATRIC
ASSOCIATION
PUBLISHING

If you wish to buy 50 or more copies of the same title, please go to www.appi.org/specialdiscounts for more information.

Copyright © 2016 American Psychiatric Association
ALL RIGHTS RESERVED

Manufactured in the United States of America on acid-free paper
23 22 21 20 19   6 5 4 3 2
Third Edition

Typeset in Palatino and GillSans

American Psychiatric Association Publishing
800 Maine Avenue SW
Suite 900
Washington, DC 20024-2812
www.appi.org

Library of Congress Cataloging-in-Publication Data
MacKinnon, Roger A., author.
    The psychiatric interview in clinical practice / Roger A. Mackinnon, Robert Michels, Peter J. Buckley ; with contributions by John W. Barnhill, Brad Foote, Alessandra Scalmati. — Third edition.
        p. ; cm.
    Includes bibliographical references and index.
    ISBN 978-1-61537-034-4 (hardcover : alk. paper)
    I. Michels, Robert, author. II. Buckley, Peter, author. III. Title.
    [DNLM: 1. Interview, Psychological—methods. 2. Mental Disorders—diagnosis. 3. Physician-Patient Relations. 4. Psychotherapy—methods. WM 143]
    RC480.7
    616.89'14—dc23

                                                                    2015029338

British Library Cataloguing in Publication Data
A CIP record is available from the British Library.

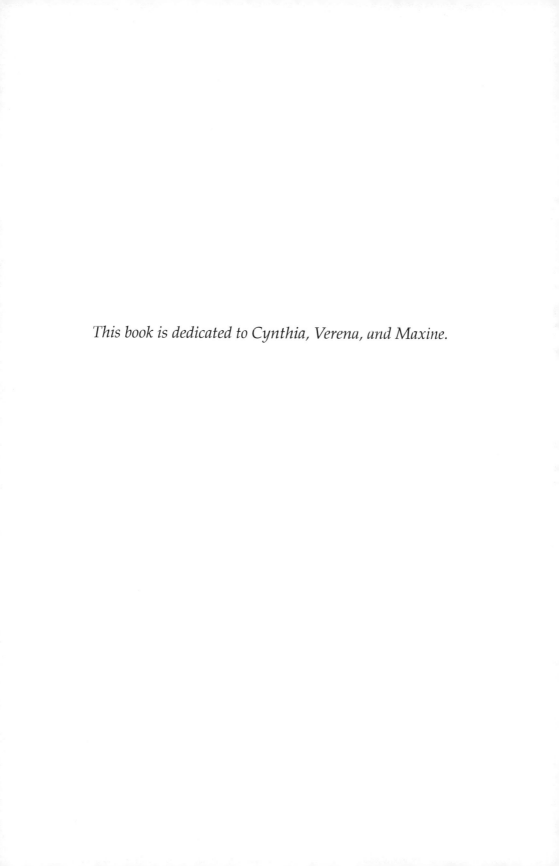

This book is dedicated to Cynthia, Verena, and Maxine.

CONTENTS

P A R T   I

General Principles

P A R T   II

Major Clinical Syndromes

PART III

Special Clinical Situations

PART IV

Technical Factors Affecting the Interview

ABOUT THE AUTHORS

Roger A. MacKinnon, M.D., is Professor Emeritus of Clinical Psychiatry in the College of Physicians and Surgeons of Columbia University, and Training and Supervising Analyst at the Columbia University Center for Psychoanalytic Training and Research, in New York, New York.

Robert Michels, M.D., is Walsh McDermott University Professor of Medicine and Psychiatry at Weill Medical College of Cornell University, and Training and Supervising Analyst at the Columbia University Center for Psychoanalytic Training and Research, in New York, New York.

Peter J. Buckley, M.D., is Professor of Psychiatry and Behavioral Sciences at Albert Einstein College of Medicine of Yeshiva University in Bronx, New York; and Training and Supervising Analyst at the Columbia University Center for Psychoanalytic Training and Research in New York, New York.

Contributors

John W. Barnhill, M.D., is Professor of Clinical Psychiatry, DeWitt Wallace Senior Scholar, and Vice Chair for Psychosomatic Medicine in the Department of Psychiatry at Weill Medical College of Cornell University; and Chief of the Consultation-Liaison Service at New York-Presbyterian Hospital/Weill Cornell Medical Center Hospital for Special Surgery in New York, New York.

Brad Foote, M.D., is Associate Professor of Clinical Psychiatry and Behavioral Sciences at Albert Einstein College of Medicine/Montefiore Medical Center in Bronx, New York.

Alessandra Scalmati, M.D., Ph.D., is Associate Professor of Clinical Psychiatry and Behavioral Sciences at Albert Einstein College of Medicine/Montefiore Medical Center in Bronx, New York.

The authors and contributors have no competing interests to report.

PREFACE

The third edition of this book builds on the second, which was published in 2006. Unlike the second edition, written 35 years after the first, the changes in psychiatry, in the intervening 9 years, have been less enormous or revolutionary. In an editorial in the *American Journal of Psychiatry* in 2006, we delineated and critiqued the radical developments that had occurred in the psychiatric landscape between the publication of the first and second editions. These included the refinement of phenomenological psychiatric diagnosis in DSM-III and subsequent revisions, an increasing biological knowledge base for understanding the somatic origins of mental illness and effective pharmacological treatments, the expansion of psychodynamic thinking beyond ego psychology to incorporate differing theoretical perspectives, and a dramatic shift in sociocultural attitudes toward the clinician-patient relationship. The last-mentioned development remains especially relevant and continues to inform the psychiatric interview. The social relationship between patient and clinician is no longer asymmetric. Patients are now better informed, correctly believe that their bodies and minds belong to them, and wish to be involved in treatment decisions. The therapeutic alliance between doctor and patient has become the foundation of treatment efforts in all of medicine. The assertion of the intrinsic rights of patients has its origins in the cultural changes that began in the 1960s. The civil rights movement, the feminist movement, and the gay liberation movement all provided catalysts for the questioning of authoritarian and paternalistic dogma and for the assertion of individual identities. In the past 9 years we note that this progressive development has extended to transgender patients.

We now know that the subjective experience of being "different" is universal and that psychiatry is enriched by recognizing and exploring that experience, validating its existence and its universality, and attempting to understand how it influences the patient's life. This democratization was anticipated over half a century ago when Anna Freud, commenting on the psychoanalytic situation, wrote:

> But—and this seems important to me—so far as the patient has a healthy part of his personality, his real relationship to the analyst is never wholly submerged. With due respect for the necessary strictest handling and interpretation of the transference, I feel still that we should leave room somewhere for the realization that analyst and patient are also two real people, of equal adult status, in a real personal relationship to each other.

We strongly believe that this credo applies to the psychiatric interview and the interchange between patient and clinician in all its manifestations and vicissitudes.

Alterations in the psychiatric landscape in the past 9 years have been incremental. We have brought this new edition of our book into alignment with DSM-5, which was published in 2013, although we retain some of the criticism of DSM classification that we expressed in our previous edition. As we noted in our second edition, DSM, in its successive editions, has emphasized descriptive phenomenological approaches to psychopathology and, unfortunately, continues to encourage psychiatric interviewing that is overly focused on describing symptoms and establishing diagnoses rather than on learning about the patient, his problems, his illnesses, and his life. As an example, while advances in biological psychiatry have definitively established that schizophrenia is a "brain disease" and neurodevelopmental disorder, there persists an unfortunate diminution in the attention given to the subjective experience of individual psychotic patients. Since psychosis can be expressed only through the personality of the individual patient, that person's personal history and character structure determine many aspects of the psychotic "experience" and should be recognized and addressed in the clinical engagement.

DSM-5 acknowledged controversy in the conceptualization of *personality disorders* by providing an essentially unchanged version of the criteria found in DSM-IV-TR in Section II of the text and an alternative model in Section III that emphasizes impairments in personality functioning and pathological personality *traits.* Personality disorders are a central part of the *major clinical syndromes* component of our book, and we find the original model in Section II more compatible with our clinical approach. Hence, we have maintained these definitions in our current text. Basically we concur with an editorial in the *American Journal of Psychiatry* published in 2010, which argued that the primary unit of diagnosis should be a personality *syndrome* that encompasses cognition, affectivity, interpersonal functioning, behavior, coping, and the defenses and that trait-based systems are less useful in clinical practice.

The advances in biological psychiatry—genetics, cognitive neuroscience, psychopharmacology, brain imaging, and the neurosciences in general—continue apace, inform the culture of psychiatry, and provide growing insight into the provenance of mental illnesses. We continue to subscribe to the view enunciated by Glen Gabbard that "virtually all major psychiatric disorders are complex amalgams of genetic diatheses and environmental influences. Genes and environment are inextricably connected in shaping human behavior."

The psychiatric interview engages the clinician in a spoken dialogue with the patient. In that sense it is about "voice" and its interplay—the vocalist and the response and interpretation of the listener. We hope that in this current edition we have maintained an appreciation for the reader of the complex music involved.

Peter J. Buckley, M.D.
Robert Michels, M.D.
Roger A. MacKinnon, M.D.

ACKNOWLEDGMENTS

As always, we are grateful to our students, colleagues, and patients, all of whom continue to teach and enlighten us. More specifically, we wish to thank John Barnhill, M.D., Brad Foote, M.D., and Alessandra Scalmati, M.D., Ph.D., for their original contributions to this edition.

John McDuffie, Greg Kuny, and Tammy Cordova at American Psychiatric Association Publishing have been superb facilitators for the creation of this new edition. Bessie Jones has provided critical administrative support. Bob Hales is the gentle accoucheur who brought this new edition to life.

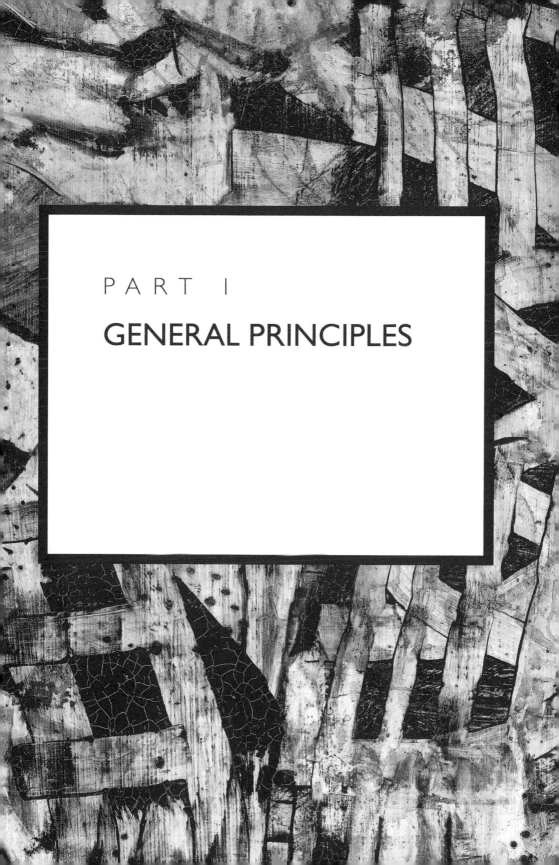

P A R T   I

GENERAL PRINCIPLES

CHAPTER 1

GENERAL PRINCIPLES OF THE INTERVIEW

This book is concerned with psychiatric interviews for the purpose of understanding and treating people with emotional problems or psychiatric illnesses. It does not consider principles or techniques that are designed for research, court procedure, or assessment of suitability for employment, which often involve third parties or a nontherapeutic motivation. Such interviews have little in common with those described here, except that they may be conducted by a mental health professional.

We believe that it takes years for a beginning student to become a skilled interviewer. However, time in itself does not create an experienced psychiatric interviewer. Training in the basic sciences of psychodynamics and psychopathology is essential, along with skillful clinical teachers who themselves interview patients in the presence of the students and also observe and discuss interviews conducted by the students.

Freud provided a foundation for our current knowledge of psychodynamics, although others have broadened and extended his concepts. We have included contributions from ego psychology, object relations theory, behavioral psychology, self psychology, relational psychology, and intersubjective psychology, although not always identified as such. Any systematic attempt to integrate these theories is well beyond the scope of this book. They are addressed briefly in Chapter 2, "General Principles of Psychodynamics," along with biological influences on behavior. We favor an eclectic or pluralistic theoretical orientation.

After the two introductory chapters, the next part addresses major clinical syndromes and personality types. These syndromes and personality styles are major determinants of the unfolding of the interview and of later problems in treatment. Each of these clinical chapters be-

3

gins with a discussion of the psychopathology, clinical findings, and a psychodynamic formulation. They then discuss characteristic interview behavior and offer advice concerning the management of the interview with each type of patient. Clinical vignettes throughout the book have been drawn largely from our clinical practice or teaching experience.

This approach is not meant to imply that these are the "correct" techniques or that one can learn to interview by memorizing them. Our interviewing style will neither appeal to nor be equally suited to all readers. However, there are students who have little opportunity to observe the interviews of experienced clinicians or to be observed themselves. Although this book cannot substitute for good clinical teaching, it can provide some useful glimpses of how experienced clinicians conduct interviews.

A second reason for providing specific clinical responses stems from the common misinterpretations of abstract principles of interviewing. For example, one supervisor, who suggested that a student "interpret the patient's resistance," later learned that the inexperienced therapist had told his patient, "You are being resistant." It was only after the patient reacted negatively and the student shared this with his supervisor that the student recognized his error. After the supervisor pointed out the patient's sensitivity to criticism and the need for tact, the resident rephrased his interpretation and instead said, "You seem to feel that this is not a problem for a psychiatrist" or "Have some of my questions seemed irrelevant?"

Part III concerns interview situations that offer special problems of their own. These can involve patients with any syndrome or illness. Here the emphasis shifts from the specific type of psychopathology to factors inherent in the clinical setting that may take precedence in determining the conduct of the interview. The consultation on the ward of a general hospital or the patient of different background are examples.

The final part is reserved for special technical issues that influence the psychiatric interview, such as note taking and e-mail, the role of the telephone, including the patient's cellular phone or pager, and issues related to other digital media.

THE CLINICAL INTERVIEW

A professional interview differs from other types of interviews in that one individual is consulting another who has been defined as an expert. The "professional" is expected to provide some form of help, whether he is a lawyer, accountant, architect, psychologist, social worker, or physician. In the medical interview, typically, one person is suffering and desires relief; the other is expected to provide this relief. The hope of obtaining help to alleviate his suffering motivates the patient to expose himself and to "tell all." This process is facilitated by the confidentiality of the clinician–patient relationship. As long as the patient views the clinician as a potential source of help, he will communicate more or less freely any material that he feels may be pertinent to his difficulty. Therefore, it is frequently possible to obtain a considerable amount of information about the patient and his suffering merely by listening.

The Psychiatric Interview

The psychiatric interview differs from the general clinical interview in a number of respects. As Sullivan pointed out, the psychiatrist is considered an expert in the field of interpersonal relations, and accordingly the patient expects to find more than a sympathetic listener. Any person seeking psychological help justifiably expects expert handling in the interview. The clinician demonstrates his expertise by the questions he both asks and does not ask and by certain other activities, which are elaborated later. The usual clinical interview is sought voluntarily, and the patient's cooperation is generally assumed. Although this is also the case in many psychiatric interviews, there are occasions when the person being interviewed has not voluntarily consulted the mental health specialist. These interviews are discussed separately later in this book (see Chapter 14, "The Psychotic Patient"; Chapter 15, "The Psychosomatic Patient"; and Chapter 18, "The Hospitalized Patient").

Interviews in nonpsychiatric branches of medicine generally emphasize medical history taking, the purpose of which is to obtain facts that will facilitate the establishment of a correct diagnosis and the institution of appropriate treatment. That interview is organized around the present illness, the past history, the family history, and the review of systems. Data concerning the personal life of the patient are considered important if they have possible bearing on the present illness. For example, if a patient describes unsafe sex practices, the interviewer will ask if the patient has ever had a venereal disease or been tested for HIV. However, if the patient's concern for the privacy of the written record is in doubt, such information can remain unwritten. The psychiatrist is also interested in the patient's symptoms, their dates of onset, and significant factors in the patient's life that may be related. However, psychiatric diagnosis and treatment are based as much on the total life history of the patient as on the present illness. This includes the patient's lifestyle, self-appraisal, traditional coping patterns, and relationships with others.

The medical patient believes that his symptoms will help the doctor to understand his illness and to provide effective treatment. He is usually willing to tell the doctor anything that he thinks may be related to his illness. Many psychiatric symptoms, on the other hand, involve the defensive functions of the ego and represent unconscious psychological conflicts (see Chapter 2, "General Principles of Psychodynamics"). To the extent that the patient defends himself from awareness of these conflicts, he will also conceal them from the interviewer. Therefore, although the psychiatric patient is motivated to reveal himself in order to gain relief from his suffering, he is also motivated to conceal his innermost feelings and the fundamental causes of his psychological disturbance.

The patient's fear of looking beneath his defenses is not the only basis for concealment in the interview. Every person is concerned with the impression he makes on others. The clinician, as a figure of authority, often symbolically represents the patient's parents, and consequently his or her reactions are particularly important to the patient. Most often the patient wishes to obtain the clinician's love or respect, but other patterns occur. If the patient suspects that some of the less admirable aspects of his personality are involved in his illness, he may be unwilling to disclose such material until he is certain that he will not lose the interviewer's respect as he exposes himself.

Diagnostic and Therapeutic Interviews

An artificial distinction between diagnostic and therapeutic interviews is frequently made. The interview that is oriented only toward establishing a diagnosis gives the patient the feeling that he is a specimen of pathology being examined, and therefore actually inhibits him from revealing his problems. If there is any single mark of a successful interview, it is the degree to which the patient and clinician develop a shared feeling of understanding. The beginner frequently misinterprets this statement as advice to provide reassurance or approval. As an example, statements that begin "Don't worry" or "That's perfectly normal" are reassuring but not understanding. Remarks such as "I can see how badly you feel about…," or those that pinpoint the circumstances in which the patient became "upset," are understanding. An interview that is centered on understanding the patient provides more valuable diagnostic information than one that seeks to elicit psychopathology. Even though the interviewer may see a patient only once, a truly therapeutic interaction is possible.

Initial and Later Interviews

At first glance, the initial interview might logically be defined as the patient's first interview with a professional, but in one sense such a definition is inaccurate. Every adult has had prior contact with a clinician and has a characteristic mode of relating in this setting. The first contact with a mental health professional is only the most recent in a series of interviews with health professionals. The situation is further complicated by the patient who has had prior psychotherapy or has studied psychology, thereby arriving, before his initial psychiatric interview, at a point of self-understanding that would require several months of treatment for another person. There is also the question of time: How long is the initial interview? One hour, 2 hours, or 5 hours? Certainly there are issues that differentiate initial from later interviews; however, these often prevail for more than one session. Topics that may be discussed with one patient in the first or second interview might not be discussed with another patient until the second year of treatment. We provide advice from time to time regarding those issues that should be discussed in the first few sessions and those that are better left for later stages of treatment. Greater precision would require discussion of specific sessions with specific patients. Examples from our own consultation rooms are provided throughout the book.

This book discusses the consultation and initial phase of therapy, which may last a few hours, a few months, or even longer. The interviewer uses the same basic principles in the first few interviews as in more prolonged treatment.

Data of the Interview

Content and Process

The *content* of an interview refers both to the factual information provided by the patient and to the specific interventions of the interviewer. Much of the content can be transmitted verbally, although both parties also communicate through nonverbal behavior. Often the verbal content may be unrelated to the real message of the interview. Some common examples are the patient who tears a piece of paper into small pieces or sits with a rigid posture and clenched fists or the seductive woman who exposes her thighs and elicits a guilty nonverbal peek from the interviewer. Content involves more than the dictionary meanings of the patient's words. For example, it also concerns his language style—his use of the active or passive verb forms, technical jargon, colloquialisms, or frequent injunctives.

The *process* of the interview refers to the developing relationship between interviewer and patient. It is particularly concerned with the implicit meaning of the communications. The patient has varying degrees of awareness of the process, experienced chiefly in the form of his fantasies about the doctor and a sense of confidence and trust in him. Some patients analyze the clinician, speculating on why he says particular things at particular times. The interviewer strives for a continuing awareness of the process aspects of the interview. He asks himself questions that illuminate this process, such as "Why did I phrase my remark in those words?" or "Why did the patient interrupt me at this time?"

Process includes the manner in which the patient relates to the interviewer. Is he isolated, seductive, ingratiating, charming, arrogant, or evasive? His mode of relating may be fixed, or it may change frequently during the interview. The interviewer learns to become aware of his own emotional responses to the patient. If he examines these in the light of what the patient has just said or done, he may broaden his understanding of the interaction. For example, he may begin to have difficulty concentrating on the dissertation of an obsessive-compulsive patient, thereby recognizing that the patient is using words in order to avoid contact rather than to communicate. In another situation, the clinician's own emotional response may help him recognize a patient's underlying depression or that the patient is quite narcissistic or borderline.

Introspective and Inspective Data

The data communicated in the psychiatric interview are both introspective and inspective. *Introspective* data include the patient's report of his feelings and experiences. This material is usually expressed verbally. *Inspective* data involve the nonverbal behavior of the patient and the interviewer. The patient is largely unaware of the significance of his nonverbal communications and their timing in relation to verbal content. Common nonverbal communications involve the patient's emotional responses, such as crying, laughing, blushing, and being restless. A very important way in which the patient communicates feelings is through the physical qualities of his voice. The interviewer also observes the patient's motor behavior in order to infer more specific thought processes that have not been verbalized. For example, the patient who plays with his wedding ring or looks at his watch has communicated more than diffuse anxiety.

Affect and Thought

The patient's decision to consult a mental health expert is usually experienced with some ambivalence, even when the patient has had prior experience with that situation. It is scary to open oneself up to a stranger. This is particularly true if the stranger does little to put the patient at ease or feels ill at ease himself. The patient fears embarrassment, or premature or critical judgments on the part of the interviewer. Inexperienced interviewers are more apt to feel anxious when meeting a patient for the first time. The patient is anxious about his illness and about the practical problems of psychiatric treatment. Many people find the idea of consulting a mental health professional extremely upsetting, which further complicates the situation. The clinician's anxiety usually centers on his new patient's reaction to him as well as on his ability to provide help. If the interviewer is also a student, the opinions of his teachers will be of great importance.

The patient may express other affects, such as sadness, anger, guilt, shame, pride, or joy. The interviewer should ask the patient what he feels and what he thinks elicited that feeling. If the emotion is obvious, the interviewer need not ask what the patient is feeling but rather what has led to this emotion now. If the patient denies the emotion named by the interviewer but uses a synonym, the interviewer accepts the correction and asks what stimulated that feeling instead of arguing with the patient. Some patients are quite open about their emotional responses, whereas others conceal them even from themselves. Although the patient's thoughts are important, his emotional responses are the key to understanding the interview. For instance, one patient who was describing details of her current life situation fought back her tears when she mentioned her mother-in-law. The interviewer might remark, "This seems to be an upsetting topic" or "Are you fighting back tears?"

The patient's thought processes can be observed in terms of quantity, rate of production, content, and organization. Is his thinking constricted? If so, to what topics does he limit himself? Are his ideas organized and coherently expressed? Gross disturbances in the pattern of associations, rate of production, and total quantity of thought are easily recognized.

The Patient

Psychopathology. *Psychopathology* refers to the phenomenology of emotional disorders. It includes neurotic or psychotic symptoms as well as behavioral or characterological disturbances. In the latter categories are defects in the patient's capacities for functioning in the areas of love, sex, work, play, socialization, family life, and physiological regulation.

Psychopathology also deals with the effectiveness of defense mechanisms, the interrelationships between them, and their overall integration into the personality.

Psychodynamics. *Psychodynamics* is a science that attempts to explain the patient's total psychic development. Not only are his symptoms and character pathology explained but also his strengths and personality assets. The patient's reactions to internal and external stimuli over the entire course of his lifetime provide the data for psychodynamic explanations. These topics are discussed in detail in Chapter 2 as well as in specific applications in the various clinical chapters in Part II. In recent years, neuroscientific research has provided useful understanding of brain function. For example, in the case of posttraumatic stress disorder, brain imaging techniques identify areas of the brain that are damaged as a result of severe psychological stress. This does not negate the psychological meaning of the experience for the patient. The lone survivor of a company wiped out by the enemy in battle suffers more than just witnessing the death of his friends and companions. He wonders why he was spared and what he could have done differently to help his comrades. Guilt is an essential component of the human psychic apparatus, and the patient can usually find a conscious or unconscious reason to blame himself for his suffering.

Personality strengths. Frequently, a patient comes to the consultation with the expectation that the interviewer is only concerned with symptoms and deficiencies of character. It can be reassuring when the clinician expresses interest in assets, talents, and personality strengths. With some patients such information is volunteered, but with others the interviewer may have to inquire, "Can you tell me some things you like about yourself or of which you are the most proud?" Often the patient's most important assets can be discovered through his reactions during the interview. The interviewer can help the patient to reveal his healthier attributes. It is normal to be tense, anxious, embarrassed, or guilty when revealing shortcomings to a stranger. There is little likelihood that the patient will demonstrate his capacity for joy and pride if, just after he has tearfully revealed some painful material, he is asked, "What do you do for fun?" It is often necessary to lead the patient away from upsetting topics gently, allowing him the opportunity for a transition period, before exploring more pleasant areas.

In this area, more than any other, the nonreactive interviewer will miss important data. For example, if a patient asks, "Would you like to see a picture of my children?" and the interviewer appears neutral, the patient will experience this as indifference. If the clinician looks at the pictures and returns them without comment, it is unlikely that the patient will show his full capacity for warm feelings. Usually the pictures provide clues to appropriate remarks that will be responsive and will help to put the patient at ease. The interviewer could comment on the family resemblances or what feelings are apparent in the picture, indicating that he takes the patient's offering sincerely. He could also ask the patient to name the persons in the picture.

Transference.   *Transference* is a process whereby the patient unconsciously displaces onto individuals in his current life those patterns of behavior and emotional reactions that originated with significant figures from his childhood. The relative anonymity of the interviewer and his role of parent-surrogate facilitate this displacement to him. These transference themes are integrated with the patient's realistic and appropriate reactions to the interview and together form the total relationship.

Many psychoanalysts believe that all responses in human relations are transferentially based. Others make a distinction between transference and the *therapeutic alliance,* which is the real relationship between the interviewer's professional persona and the healthy, observing, rational component of the patient. The realistic cooperative therapeutic alliance also has its origin during infancy and is based on the bond of real trust between the child and his mother. *Positive transference* is often employed loosely to refer to all of the patient's positive emotional responses to the therapist, but strictly speaking the term should be limited to responses that are truly transference—that is, attitudes or feelings that are displaced from childhood relationships and are unrealistic in the therapeutic setting. An example is the delegated omnipotence with which the therapist is commonly endowed. A stronger therapeutic alliance is desirable for treatment so that the patient will place his trust and confidence in the clinician—a process that is mistakenly referred to as "maintaining a positive transference." The beginner may misconstrue such advice to mean that the patient should be encouraged to love him or to express only positive feelings. This leads to "courting" behavior on the part of the interviewer. Certain patients, such as one who is paranoid, are more comfortable, particularly early in treatment, if they maintain a moderately negative transference exemplified in suspiciousness. For other patients, such as many with psychosomatic or depressive disorders, negative transference must be recognized and resolved promptly or the patient will flee treatment.

Transference neurosis refers to the development of a new dynamic constellation during intensive psychotherapy. The therapist becomes the central character in a dramatization of the emotional conflicts that began in the patient's childhood. Whereas transference involves fragmentary reproductions of attitudes from the past, the transference neurosis is a constant and pervasive theme of the patient's life. His fantasies and dreams center on the clinician.

Realistic factors concerning the clinician can be starting points for the initial transference. Age, sex, personal manner, and social and ethnic background all influence the rapidity and direction of the patient's responses. The female clinician is likely to elicit competitive reactions from female patients and erotic responses from male patients. If the clinician's youth and appearance indicate that she is a trainee or a student, these factors also influence the initial transference. With male clinicians the reverse holds true. Transference is not simply positive or negative but rather a re-creation of the various stages of the patient's emotional development or a reflection of his complex attitudes toward key figures of importance in his life. In terms of clinical phenomenology, some common patterns of transference can be recognized.

Desire for affection, respect, and the gratification of dependent needs is the most widespread form of transference. The patient seeks evidence that the interviewer can, does, or will love him. Requesting special time or financial considerations, borrowing a magazine from the waiting room, and asking for a glass of water can be common examples of the symbolic expressions of transference wishes. The inexperienced interviewer tries to differentiate "legitimate," realistic requests from "irrational" transference demands and then to respond to the former while frustrating and interpreting the latter. As a result, many errors are made in the management of such episodes. The problem could be simplified if it is assumed that all requests include unconscious transference meaning. The question then becomes the appropriate mixture of gratification and interpretation. The decision depends on the timing of the request, its content, the type of patient, the nature of the treatment, and the reality of the situation. One is wise not to make most transference interpretations until a therapeutic alliance has been firmly established.

For example, at their first meeting a new patient might greet the interviewer saying, "Do you have a tissue?" This patient begins his relationship by making a request. The clinician should simply respond to this request, since refusals or interpretations would be premature and quickly alienate the patient. However, once an initial relationship has been established, the patient might ask for a tissue and add parenthetically, "I think I have one somewhere, but I'd have to look for it." If the interviewer chose to explore this behavior, he could simply raise his eyebrows and wait. Usually the patient will search for his own while commenting, "You probably attribute some significance to this!" "Such as?" the interviewer might reply. This provides an opportunity for further inquiry into the patient's motives.

The interviewer who has provided tissues on several occasions might comment, "I notice that you often ask me for tissues." The discussion will then explore whether this request reflects a general practice or occurs only in the therapist's office. In either event, the dialogue can progress to the patient's attitude toward self-reliance and dependency on others.

On occasion, early transference feelings may appear in the form of a question, such as "How can you stand to listen to people complain all day?" The patient is trying to dissociate himself from aspects of his personality that he holds in contempt and that he fears will not be accepted by the clinician. The interviewer might reply, "Perhaps you are concerned about my reaction to you?" or "Patients do other things besides complain," thereby opening the topic of how the treatment time can be utilized.

Omnipotent transference feelings are revealed by remarks such as "I know you can help me!"; "You must know the answer"; or "What does my dream mean?" Hollywood has worn out the standard gambit of "What do you think?" Instead, the interviewer can reply, "You feel that I know the answers?" or "Do you feel that I am withholding?" A more difficult manifestation of this problem is seen in the younger patient who consistently refers to the interviewer with an ingratiating manner as "Ma'am" or "Doctor." The interviewer meets great resistance if he attempts to interpret this behavior prematurely, particularly if the patient grew up in an environment where this was the polite tradition.

Questions about the interviewer's personal life may involve several different types of transference. However, they most often reveal concern about his experience or his ability to understand the patient. Such questions include "Are you married?"; "Do you have children?"; "How old are you?"; "Are you Jewish?"; or "Do you live in the city?" The experienced interviewer often knows the meaning of the question from prior experience and his knowledge of the patient and might intuitively recognize when it is preferable to answer the question directly. For the most part, the beginner is best advised to inquire, "What did you have in mind?" or "What leads to your question?" The patient's reply may reveal transference feelings. At that point, the interviewer could interpret the meaning of the patient's question by stating, "Perhaps you ask about my age because you're not sure if I am experienced enough to help you?" or "Your question about my having children sounds as if it means, am I able to understand what it is like to be a parent?" On other occasions these questions signify the patient's desire to become a social friend rather than a patient, since he dislikes the asymmetry of the patient role and believes that a symmetrical friendship will provide the contact that he craves. Here the interviewer can explore the subject of the patient's friendships and inquire whether he has attempted to discuss his problems with friends and whether they were helpful. If this had helped sufficiently, the patient would not be in the clinician's office.

Later in the process, the therapist often becomes an ego-ideal for the patient. This type of positive transference is often not interpreted. The patient may imitate the mannerisms, speech, or dress of the therapist, usually without conscious awareness. Some patients openly admire the clinician's clothing, furniture, or pictures. Questions such as "Where did you buy that chair?" can be answered with "What leads to your question?" The patient usually replies that he admires the item and wants to obtain one for himself. If the therapist wishes to foster this transference, he may provide the information; if he wants to interpret it, he will explore the patient's desire to emulate him. With increasing experience the interviewer is more comfortable occasionally answering such questions, first because he grows more at ease in his therapist role and second because he is more likely to find an opportunity to refer to the episode in an interpretation later in the session or in a subsequent session after he has accumulated additional similar material.

Competitive feelings stemming from earlier relations with parents or siblings can be expressed in the transference. An illustration occurred with a young man who regularly arrived for morning appointments earlier than the therapist. One day he uncharacteristically arrived a few minutes late and remarked, "Well, you beat me today." He experienced everything as a competitive struggle. The therapist replied, "I didn't realize that we were having a race," thereby calling attention to the patient's construction of the event and connecting it with a theme that had been discussed in the past.

Other common manifestations of competitive transferences include disparaging remarks about the therapist's office, manners, and dress; dogmatic, challenging pronouncements; or attempts to assess the clinician's memory, his vocabulary, or his fund of knowledge. Belittling attitudes may also appear in other forms, such as referring to a clinician as "Doc" or constantly interrupting him. Other examples include using the therapist's first name without invitation or talking down to the interviewer. The clinician can directly approach the underlying feeling by asking, "Do you feel there is something demeaning about talking to me?" In general, competitive behavior is usually best ignored in the initial interview because the patient is vulnerable to what will be experienced as a criticism.

Male patients show interest in the male clinician's power, status, or economic success; with a female clinician they are more concerned with her motherliness, her seduceability, and how she is able to have a career and a family. Female patients are concerned about a male therapist's attitude concerning the role of women, whether he can be seduced, what sort of father he is, and what his wife is like. The female patient is interested in a female therapist's career and in her adequacy as a woman and mother. She may ask, "How do you manage it all?" or "How do you make the difficult choices?"

Competitive themes may reflect sibling rivalry as well as oedipal conflicts. The patient's competitive feelings may become manifest when he responds to the therapist's other patients as though they were siblings. Spontaneous disparaging remarks such as "How could you treat someone like that?" or "I hate the smell of cheap perfume" are common examples. In initial interviews no response is preferable.

Older patients may treat a young interviewer as a child. Maternal female patients may bring a therapist food or caution him about his health, working too hard, and so on. Paternal male patients may offer fatherly advice about investments, insurance, automobiles, and so on. Early attention to either the ingratiating or the patronizing dimensions of these comments would be disruptive to the developing relationship. These transference attitudes can also occur with younger patients. Such advice is well intentioned at the conscious level and is indicative of positive conscious feelings. It is therefore often not interpreted, particularly in the first few interviews. Older interviewers with younger patients often elicit parental transferences. If the patient has a positive relationship with his parents, he may develop an early positive transference, deferring to the interviewer's wisdom and experience or seeking advice in a specific situation. Older patients usually prefer older clinicians, and high-status patients generally seek high-status professionals. Older men of importance are particularly prone to address the male interviewer early on by his first name, sometimes asking or stating, "I hope that you don't mind that I call you John!" This situation can be handled with a reply such as "Whatever you prefer." This is unlikely to happen with a female patient unless it is with a female interviewer.

Some therapists use first names with their patients. This is neither inherently good nor inherently bad, but it always means something, and that meaning should be understood. Symbols used in the relationship should reflect mutual respect and comfortable social forms. Generally, therapists call children or adolescents by first name, as do other adults. Patients who would expect to be on a first-name basis with the therapist outside the therapeutic situation may prefer to use first names in the professional setting, and there is no reason not to do so. However, this should always be symmetrical. The patient who wants to be called by his or her first name but calls the therapist "Dr. ——" is expressing a desire for an asymmetric relationship that has important transference meaning that should be explored but not enacted by the therapist. It usually suggests the patient's offer to submit to the therapist, with the submission entailing authority or social, racial, generational, sexual, or other power. The therapist who accepts such an invitation not only abuses the patient but also misses an important therapeutic opportunity. Conversely, the therapist who, uninvited, has the impulse to call an adult patient by his or her first name should explore that impulse for countertransference significance. This occurs most commonly with patients of perceived lower status—socially, economically, or because of pathology or great age. Understanding the temptation can help the patient; acting on it is destructive.

In general, transference is not discussed early in treatment except in the context of resistance. This does not mean that only negative transference is discussed; positive transference can also become a powerful resistance. For example, if the patient discusses only affection for the clinician, the interviewer can remark, "You spend much more time discussing your feelings about me than talking about yourself or your problems." Other patients avoid mentioning anything that is related to the interviewer. In this case, one waits until the patient seems to suppress or avoid a conscious thought and then inquires, "You seemed to hesitate for a moment. Did you avoid some thought?" When a patient who has spoken freely suddenly becomes silent, it is usually because of thoughts or feelings about the clinician. The patient may remark, "I have run out of things to talk about." If the silence persists, the interviewer could comment, "Perhaps there is something you are uncomfortable talking about?"

Resistance.   *Resistance* is any attitude on the part of the patient that opposes the objectives of the treatment. Insight-oriented psychotherapy necessitates the exploration of symptoms and behavior patterns, and this leads to anxiety. Therefore the patient is motivated to resist the therapy in order to maintain repression, ward off insight, and avoid anxiety. The concept of resistance is one of the cornerstones of all dynamic psychotherapy.

Resistance can develop from any of the transference attitudes previously described. Each of the major types of transference is at times used as a resistance. The patient attempts to elicit evidence of the clinician's love or expects a magical cure through his omnipotent power. Rather than resolving his basic conflicts, the patient may merely attempt an identification with the therapist, or he may adopt an attitude of competition with the therapist instead of working together with him. These processes may assume subtle forms—for example, the patient may present material that he thinks is of particular interest to the clinician simply to please him. Just as transference can be used as a resistance, so too can it serve as a motivating factor for the patient to work together with the clinician.

> For example, a resident came to one of us for analysis. Soon the patient was informing the therapist (who held an important administrative position in the program) of the misbehavior of other residents. Attempts to explore the meaning of the tattling were useful, but the behavior continued. Finally, the therapist suggested that the patient omit the names of the other residents. This was after exploring the obvious fantasy that the analyst received gratification from this private source of information. The patient replied angrily, "Aren't I supposed to say whatever comes to mind?" The therapist replied, "You can continue to discuss the incidents and their meanings to you, but I don't need to have the names." At that point the patient stopped tattling on colleagues.

Another example of resistance is reflected by the patient's unwillingness to relinquish the secondary benefits that accompany his illness. Thus the patient with a conversion symptom of back pain is legitimately unable to carry out her unwanted household tasks as long as she is sick, and at the same time she receives attention and sympathy.

A different resistance is manifested by the patient's unconscious need for punishment. The patient's symptoms inflict suffering on himself that he is reluctant to relinquish. This is particularly prominent in the treatment of depressed patients or patients who feel intensely guilty when they encounter critical feelings toward a loved one.

It is a valid clinical observation that patients maintain fixed maladaptive patterns of behavior despite insight and the undoing of repression. Neuroscientists explain this phenomenon in terms of the persistence of established patterns of neurocircuitry. This means that the therapist and patient must learn to accept that which cannot change despite multiple repetitions of alternate patterns.[1]

Clinical examples of resistance.   Clinical examples of resistance are overdetermined and represent mixtures of several mechanisms. They are classified in terms of their manifestations during the interview rather than according to hypothetical underlying psychodynamics.

---

[1]Sandor Rado was decades ahead of his time with his belief in a neurobiological basis for resistance to change and that the patient had to actively change his behavior before he could develop new responses to old situations.

First are the resistances that are expressed by patterns of communication during the session. The one that is most easily recognized and most uncomfortable for many interviewers is silence. The patient may explain, "Nothing comes to my mind" or "I don't have anything to talk about." Once the initial phase of therapy is past, the doctor may sit quietly and wait for the patient. Such an approach is rarely helpful in the first few interviews.

The interviewer indicates his interest in the patient's silence. He might comment, "You're silent. What does that mean?" or "Tell me about your silence" if that is not successful. Depending on the emotional tone of the silence, as revealed by nonverbal communication, the clinician may decide on a tentative meaning and then remark accordingly. For example, he could say, "Shame makes people hide" or "Perhaps there is something that is difficult for you to discuss." If the patient seems to feel helpless and is floundering for direction, the interviewer might interpret, "You seem to feel lost." The patient might respond, "Could you ask me some questions?" The interviewer's goal is to teach the patient how to participate without provoking the feeling that his performance thus far has been inadequate. One possible response is, "It is often helpful to find out just what was on your mind when it went blank. The last thing we were talking about was your children. What were you thinking then?"

If the silence is more a manifestation of the patient's defiance or retentive obstinacy, an appropriate remark would be, "You may resent having to expose your problems to me" or "You seem to feel like holding back."

Beginning interviewers often unwittingly provoke silences by assuming a disproportionate responsibility for keeping the interview going. Asking the patient questions that can be answered "yes" or "no" or providing the patient with multiple-choice answers for a question discourages his sense of responsibility for the interview. Such questions limit the patient's spontaneity and constrict the flow of ideas. The patient retreats to passivity while the interviewer struggles for the right question that will "open the patient up."

The patient who speaks garrulously may use words as a means of avoiding engagement with the interviewer as well as of warding off his own emotions. If the interviewer is unable to get a word in edgewise, he can interrupt the patient and comment, "I find it difficult to say anything without interrupting you." The literal-minded patient may reply, "Oh, did you want to say something?" A suitable response would be, "I was wondering what makes it so difficult for us to talk together?"

Censoring or editing thoughts is universal. Clues to this include interruptions in the free flow of speech and abrupt changes of subject, facial expressions, and other motor behavior. These are usually not interpreted directly, but the interviewer sometimes remarks, "You don't seem free to say everything that comes to your mind"; "What was it that interrupted your thought?"; or "It seems that you're screening your thoughts." These comments emphasize the process of editing rather than the content. Another form of editing occurs when the patient comes to the appointment with a prepared agenda, thereby making certain that spontaneous behavior during the interview will be at a minimum. This resistance is not to be interpreted in the first few interviews, since the patient will be unable to accept that it is a resistance until later. Further discussion of this issue appears in Chapter 2.

The patient who brings notes to the interview may utilize them as a way of controlling the interview or of avoiding interaction with the interviewer. However, bringing notes to the interview is not always a manifestation of resistance. For example, a disorganized patient may use the notes to help organize himself, or an older patient may use them to compensate for memory impairment.

Intellectualization is a form of resistance encouraged by the fact that psychotherapy is a "talking" therapy that utilizes intellectual constructs. Beginning interviewers have particular difficulty in recognizing the defensive use of the patient's intellect except when it occurs in obsessive or schizophrenic patients, in whom the absence of affect is an obvious clue. However, in the case of the histrionic patient who speaks in a lively manner, often with more "emotion" than the interviewer, the process may go undetected. If the patient offers some insight into his behavior and then asks the interviewer, "Is that right?" resistance is operating regardless of how much affect was present. Although the insight may be valid, the side comment reveals the patient's concern with the interviewer's concurrence or approval. It is the use of intellectualization to win the therapist's emotional support that demonstrates the patient's resistance. The patient is simultaneously opening issues related to the therapeutic alliance as he attempts to collaborate with the clinician in learning the therapist's "language" and concepts for the purpose of winning the therapist's approval. The interviewer can address the transference resistance while supporting the therapeutic alliance. He might say to the patient, "Finding answers that are meaningful to you not only helps you understand yourself, but it also builds your self-confidence." The patient might not accept this answer and might respond with "But I need you to tell me whether I'm right or not." This is one of the most common problems in psychotherapy, and one that will be analyzed repeatedly in a variety of different contexts. The therapist, by recognizing and accepting the patient's need for reassurance and guidance, offers some emotional support without infantilizing the patient.

There are several ways in which the interviewer can discourage intellectualization. First, he can avoid asking the patient questions that begin with "Why?" The patient usually does not know why he became sick at this time or in this particular way, or even why he feels as he does. The clinician wants to learn why, but in order to do so he must find ways to encourage the patient to reveal more about himself. When "Why?" comes to the clinician's mind, he could ask the patient to elaborate or provide more details. Asking "Exactly what happened?" or "How did this come about?" is more likely to elicit an answer to a "why" question than asking "Why?" "Why" questions also tend to place the patient in a defensive position.

Any question that suggests the "right" answer will invite intellectualization. Furthermore, it will give the patient the idea that the interviewer is not interested in his true feelings but is attempting to fit him into a textbook category. The use of professional jargon or technical terms such as "Oedipus complex," "resistance," or "masochistic" also encourages intellectualized discussions.

Patients who use rhetorical questions for the effect that they produce on the interviewer invite intellectualization. For example, a patient says, "Why do you suppose I get so angry whenever Jane brings up the subject of money?" Any attempt to deal with the manifest question ensures intellectualization. If the interviewer remains quiet, the patient usually continues to speak. The experienced interviewer may see this as an opportunity to find out the details and asks, "Would you give me a recent example?" The meaning of a pattern is hidden in the details of particular episodes. The interviewer, on the other hand, may strategically utilize rhetorical questions on occasion when he wishes to stimulate the patient's curiosity or leave him with something to ponder. For instance, "I wonder if there is any pattern to your anxiety attacks?"

Reading about psychotherapy and psychodynamics is at times used as an intellectual resistance or a desire to please the therapist. It also may be a manifestation of a competitive or dependent transference. The patient may be attempting to keep "one up" on the clinician or may be looking for the "additional help." Some therapists used to give the patient injunctions against reading. Usually this avoided the issue. The popular literature is now filled with information for patients, as are Web sites, and a generation of people are trained to look things up. If the patient finds it helpful, go with the flow. If it largely has a transferential message, let it emerge.

Generalization is a resistance in which the patient describes his life and reactions in general terms but avoids the specific details of each situation. When this occurs, the interviewer can ask the patient to give additional details or to be more specific. Occasionally, it may be necessary to pin the patient down to a "yes" or "no" answer to a particular question. If the patient continues to generalize despite repeated requests to be specific, the therapist interprets the resistant aspect of the patient's behavior. That does not mean telling the patient, "This is a resistance" or "You are being resistant." Such comments are experienced only as criticisms and will not be helpful. Instead, the clinician could say, "You speak in generalities when discussing your husband. Perhaps there are details concerning the relationship that you have trouble telling me." Such a comment, because it is specific, illustrates one of the most important principles in coping with generalization. The interviewer who makes vague interpretations such as "Perhaps you generalize in order to avoid upsetting details" will encourage the very resistance he seeks to remove.

The patient's preoccupation with one aspect of his life, such as symptoms, current events, or past history, is a common resistance. Focusing on symptoms is particularly common with psychosomatic and panic attack patients. The clinician can interpret, "You seem to find it difficult to discuss matters other than your symptoms" or "It is easier for you to talk about your symptoms than about other aspects of your life." The interviewer must find ways to demonstrate to the patient that constant reiteration of symptoms is not helpful and will not lead to the relief he seeks. The same principle applies to other preoccupations.

Concentrating on trivial details while avoiding the important topics is a frequent resistance with obsessive patients. If the interviewer comments on this behavior, the patient insists that the material is pertinent and that he must include such information for "background." One patient, for instance, reported, "I had a dream last night, but first I must tell you some background." Left to his own devices, the patient spoke most of the session before telling his dream. The interviewer can make the patient more aware of this resistance if he replies, "Tell me the dream first." In psychoanalysis, the patient might be permitted to discover for himself that he never allowed enough time to explore his dreams.

Affective display may serve as a resistance to meaningful communication. Hyperemotionality is common in histrionic patients; affects such as boredom are more likely in obsessive-compulsive patients. The histrionic patient uses one emotion to ward off deeper painful affects; for example, constant anger may be used to defend against injured pride. Frequent "happy sessions" indicate resistance in that the patient obtains sufficient emotional gratification during the session to ward off depression or anxiety. This can be dealt with by exploring the process with the patient and by no longer providing such gratification.

In addition to resistances that involve patterns of communication, there is a second major group of resistances called *acting out.* These involve behavior that has meaning in relation to the therapist and the treatment process. It does not necessarily occur during the session, but the clinician is directly involved in the phenomenon, although he may be unaware of its significance. An *enactment* is a little drama in which the patient's transference fantasy is played out rather than verbalized or even consciously recognized by the patient. Examples would be the patient who answers his cell phone during the session to dramatize his own importance compared with that of the therapist or the woman who has her secretary call to check the time of the next appointment, which she was too preoccupied to write in her appointment book.

Acting out is a form of resistance in which feelings or drives pertaining to treatment or to the clinician are unconsciously displaced to a person or situation outside the therapy. The patient's behavior is usually ego-syntonic, and it involves the acting out of emotions instead of experiencing them as part of the therapeutic process. Genetically, these feelings involve the reenactment of childhood experiences that are now re-created in the transference relationship and then displaced into the outside world. Two common examples involve patients who discuss their problems with persons other than the therapist and patients who displace negative transference feeling to other figures of authority and become angry with them rather than with the therapist. This resistance usually is not apparent during the first few hours of treatment, but when the opportunity presents itself, the interviewer may explore the patient's motives for the behavior. In most cases the patient will change, but at times the clinician may have to point out the patient's inability to give up the behavior despite his recognition that it is irrational.

Requests to change the time of the appointment may be a resistance. The patient may communicate his unconscious priorities by saying, "Can we change Thursday's appointment? My wife can't pick up the kids at school that day." To interpret this simply as resistance can miss an opportunity to help the patient recognize that he is saying that he is more afraid of his wife than of his therapist. One patient may look for an excuse to miss the appointment altogether, whereas another may become involved in a competitive power struggle with the clinician, saying, in effect, "We will meet when it is convenient for me." A third patient may view the clinician's willingness to change the time as proof that he really wants to see the patient and therefore will be a loving, indulgent parent. Before interpreting such requests, the clinician needs to understand the deeper motivation. The clinician may indicate that he is *unwilling* to grant such a request. The claim that he is *unable* to grant them often reveals a fear of displeasing the patient. Special problems exist for the patient whose job demands change abruptly so that absence on short notice occurs. Keeping one's job is more important than pleasing the therapist. The clinician's best response is empathy for the situation.

The use of minor physical symptoms as an excuse in missing sessions is a common resistance in narcissistic, phobic, histrionic, and somatization disorder patients. Frequently, the patient telephones the clinician prior to the interview to report a minor illness and to ask if he should come. This behavior is discussed in Chapter 15, "The Psychosomatic Patient." When the patient returns, the clinician explores how the patient felt about missing the meeting before he interprets the resistance.

Arriving late and forgetting appointments altogether are obvious manifestations of resistance. Early attempts at interpretation will be met with statements such as "I'm sorry I missed the appointment, but it had nothing to do with you"; "I'm late for everything; it has no bearing on how I feel about treatment"; "I've always been absentminded about appointments"; or "How can you expect me to be on time? Punctuality is one of my problems." If the interviewer does not extend the length of the appointment, the lateness will become a real problem that the patient must face. It will often become clear that the patient who arrives late expects to see the clinician the moment he arrives. It is not appropriate for the interviewer to retaliate, but it is not expected that he sit idly, waiting for the patient's arrival. If the clinician has engaged in some activity and the patient has to wait for a few minutes when arriving late, additional information concerning the meaning of the lateness will emerge. In general, the motive for lateness involves either fear or anger.

Failing or forgetting to pay the clinician's bill is another reflection of both resistance and transference. This topic is considered in greater detail later in this chapter (see "Fees").

Second-guessing or getting "one up" on the clinician is a manifestation of a *competitive* transference and resistance. The patient triumphantly announces, "I bet I know what you are going to say next" or "You said the same thing last week." The interviewer can simply remain silent, or he can ask, "What will I say?" If the patient has already verbalized his theory, the clinician might comment, "Why should I think that?" It is generally not a good idea to tell the patient if he was correct in second-guessing the interviewer, but as with every rule, there are exceptions.

Seductive behavior is designed either to please and gratify the interviewer, thereby winning his love and magical protection, or to disarm him and obtain power over him. Further illustrations are such questions as "Would you like to hear a dream?" or "Are you interested in a problem I have with sex?" The interviewer might reply, "I am interested in anything that is on your mind." If these questions occur repeatedly, he could add, "You seem concerned with what I want to hear." Various "bribes" offered to the interviewer, such as gifts or advice, are common examples of seductive resistance.

Beginning interviewers are often made anxious by overt or covert sexual propositions. Most frequently these propositions involve a male therapist and a female patient. The clinician knows that accepting such an invitation is a boundary violation, and he recognizes it as transference resistances. Nevertheless, discomfort is frequent. Most often, it stems from guilt that he is pleased by the invitation, and he fears that his feelings may interfere with proper management of the patient. Frequently, this is revealed by statements such as "That would not be appropriate in a doctor–patient relationship" or by a comment to the supervisor that "I don't want to hurt the patient's feelings by rejecting her." The clinician must explore in his own mind whether he subtly invited such behavior from the patient, as is often the case. If he did not elicit the invitation, he can ask the patient, "How would that help you?" If the patient indicates that she needs love and reassurance, the clinician can reply, "But we both know that accepting your invitation would mean the opposite. My job is to help you work out your problem, but your plan would make that impossible." When a therapist has an adequate amount of professional self-confidence, he or she will no longer respond to overt seduction by feeling flattered and anxious, provided he or she also has adequate self-confidence as a man or woman.

Asking the clinician for favors, such as borrowing small sums of money or requesting the name of his lawyer, dentist, accountant, or insurance broker, is a form of resistance. It attempts to shift the therapy from helping the patient to cope more effectively to becoming dependent on the therapist's coping skills. It often involves the erroneous assumption, on the part of both, that the therapist knows more than the patient about how to get along in the outside world. One makes exceptions, at times, in the treatment of patients who may have deficiencies in this area, such as adolescent, depressed, cognitively impaired, or psychotic patients (see the appropriate chapters).

Other examples of the patient's acting out (often erroneously called "acting in") include behavior during the interview that is unconsciously motivated to ward off threatening feelings while allowing partial discharge of tension. Common illustrations include leaving the interview to get a drink of water or go to the bathroom or walking around the office. For instance, the patient may be recounting a sad experience and be on the verge of tears when he interrupts himself to ask for a glass of water. In the process he gains control of his emotions and continues the story, but without the same affect. The interviewer could comment, "Taking the drink of water helped you to control your feelings." The patient often experiences these interpretations as criticisms or as being treated like a child. Rigidity of posture and other ritualized behavior during the session are other indications of resistance. For example, one patient always said "Thank you" at the end of each session. Another went to the bathroom before each appointment. When asked about the "routine," she indicated that she did not wish to experience any sensations in that part of her body during a session.

Another group of resistances clearly show the patient's reluctance to participate in the treatment but do not predominantly involve the transference. For example, the usual transferences do not seem to develop with many antisocial patients, with some who are forced into treatment by external pressures, or with some who have other motives for treatment, such as avoiding some responsibility. With certain combinations of therapist and patient, the true personality and background of the therapist are either too far removed or too similar to those of the patient. In such cases, a change in therapists is indicated.

Some patients do not change as a result of insight into their behavior. This is common in certain character disorders and is to be differentiated from the patient who is psychologically obtuse and cannot accept insight. This resistance is related to the clinical phenomenon that led Freud to formulate the "repetition compulsion." Neuroscientists understand this phenomenon as due to biological determinants of behavior, either genetically programmed or related to early neurocircuitry patterns that are fixed.

A common resistance in depressed patients is that the patient only accepts insights and interpretations in order to further flagellate himself. He then says, "What's the use?" or "I'm hopeless; nothing I do is right." This behavior, the "negative therapeutic reaction," is further discussed in Chapter 6, "The Masochistic Patient," and Chapter 7, "The Depressed Patient."

Despite the complexity of these concepts, it is important to understand the major psychodynamic issues that are useful in discussing the therapist–patient relationship.

The Interviewer

The inexperienced interviewer. Psychotherapy is a very intense experience not only for the patient but also for the interviewer. Each clinician brings a different personal and professional background to the interview. His character structure, values, and sensitivity to the feelings of others influence his attitudes toward fellow human beings—patients and nonpatients alike. The therapeutic use of the self is a complex concept that evolves in each clinician over the training years and early practice. It is frequently said that it takes about 10 years for an individual to reach maturity in the therapeutic role. No two trainees progress at exactly the same rate, and there will be as many somewhat different clinicians as there are trainees. The clinician's life experiences—past, present, and future—all affect this very personal work. Mistakes are part of the learning curve, and if the beginner is too fearful of making mistakes, he is doomed to remain a beginner indefinitely.

In the beginner's interview, the theoretical persuasion of his teacher will exert an influence on his approach to the patient. However, as the novice interviewer becomes more experienced, that factor fades into the background and his own personality has a much greater influence.

A skilled clinician is something one becomes. It cannot be mastered by reading about the principles. Nevertheless, there are particular problems that beginning interviewers have in common. The beginning interviewer is more anxious than his experienced colleague. The defense mechanisms that he employs to keep his anxiety under control diminish his sensitivity to subtle fluctuations in the emotional responses of the patient. Since the beginner is usually in a training institution, one major source of his anxiety is his fear that he will do something wrong and lose the approval of his teacher. There may also be resentment, which results from not winning a supervisor's praise. His fear of being inadequate is often displaced onto the patient, who he imagines will become aware of his "student" status and lose confidence in him as a competent clinician. The patient's references to such matters are best handled in an open and forthright manner, because patients are usually aware when they have gone to a teaching institution. The young clinician's calm acceptance of the patient's fears that he is inexperienced will strengthen the patient's trust and confidence.

The beginner commonly feels a desire to perform better than his peers in the eyes of the faculty. Not all of his competitive feelings are related to his sibling rivalry; he also wishes to perform more skillfully than his teacher. Defiant attitudes toward authority figures are another manifestation of competitiveness that prevent the novice interviewer from feeling at ease with his patient.

The inexperienced clinician in any specialty feels guilty about "practicing" on the patient. This guilt is exaggerated in the medical student who fails three or four times while performing his first venipuncture, knowing that the intern could have succeeded at his first attempt. In every area of medicine, the young doctor has conscious and unconscious guilt feelings when he thinks that someone else could have provided better care. In many medical specialties, a resident under supervision can provide approximately the same quality of treatment as a senior physician. However, the psychiatric interview cannot be supervised in the same way, and it takes years to acquire skill in interviewing. Although his teacher may reassure him that he exaggerates the importance of this factor, the beginner continues to imagine how much faster the patient would recover if he were treated by the supervisor. The young clinician projects the same feelings of omniscience onto his supervisor that the patient has projected onto the therapist.

The beginning clinician's attitude toward diagnosis has been discussed. He may become preoccupied with diagnosis and often focuses on ruling out organic factors in every case because he is more experienced and comfortable in the traditional medical role. He goes through the outline for psychiatric examination with obsessive completeness, lest he overlook something important.

In other situations, the interviewer becomes so intrigued with psychodynamics that he neglects to elicit an adequate description of the psychopathology. One resident questioned a patient at length about her compulsive hair pulling. He asked questions pertaining to its origins, precipitating events in her daily life, how she felt about it, where she was when she did it, and so on. He failed to notice that she was wearing a wig and was surprised when she later told his supervisor that she was bald. Since the patient seemed to be quite "intact" and the resident had not encountered this syndrome previously, he would not have thought to ask the supervisor's next question: "Do you ever put the hair in your mouth?" The patient replied that she did and went on to disclose her fantasy that the hair roots were lice that she was compelled to eat. A comprehensive knowledge of both psychopathology and psychodynamics facilitates exploration of the patient's symptoms.

In some respects the inexperienced interviewer is similar to the histology student who first peers into the microscope and sees only myriad pretty colors. As his experience increases, he becomes aware of structures and relationships that previously escaped his attention and recognizes an ever-increasing number of subtleties.

The tendency of the novice is to interrupt the patient in order to include all his questions. With more experience, he learns whether a patient has completed his answer to a question or merely requires slight encouragement to continue his story. As the novice interviewer's competence grows, it becomes possible for him to hear the content of what the patient is saying and at the same time to consider how he feels and what he is telling about himself through inference or omission. For example, if the patient spontaneously reports several experiences in the past in which he felt that he was mistreated by the medical profession, the interviewer could remark, "No wonder you're uneasy with doctors."

The interview is most effectively organized around the clues provided by the patient and not around the outline for psychiatric examination. The novice often feels more comfortable if he can follow a formal guide, but this gives the interview a jerky, disconnected quality and results in little feeling of rapport.

Although the neophyte may talk too much and not listen, he also tends toward passivity. His professional insecurity makes it difficult to know when to offer reassurance, advice, explanations, or interpretations. Wary of saying the wrong thing, the interviewer often finds it easier to overlook situations in which some active intervention is required.

A professional self-image is acquired through identification with teachers. The young clinician often emulates the gestures, mannerisms, and intonations of an admired supervisor. These identifications are multiple and shifting until after several years the interviewer integrates them into a style that is all his own. Then it is possible for him to relax while he is working and to be himself. In the meantime, he often resorts to gimmicks, which are sometimes used in a stereotyped manner—for example, repeating the patient's last word or phrase at frequent intervals or overusing clichés such as "I don't understand"; "What do you think?"; "Uh huh"; or "And then what happened?" As the interviewer becomes more relaxed, he will naturally employ a variety of different responses with which he is comfortable.

Countertransference. Interviewers have two classes of emotional responses to their patients. First are reactions to the patient as he actually is. The clinician may like the patient, feel sympathetic toward him, or even be antagonized by him, which are reactions that the patient would elicit in most people. Countertransference responses can be specific for the individual interviewer. They occur when the interviewer responds to the patient as if he were an important figure from the interviewer's past. The more intense the interviewer's neurotic patterns, and the more the patient actually resembles such figures, the greater the likelihood of such countertransference responses. In other words, the interviewer who had an intensely competitive relationship with her sister is more likely than other therapists to have irrational responses to female patients of her own age. If she reacts in this way to all patients, regardless of their age, sex, or personality type, the problem is more serious. Countertransference responses can also be a valuable vehicle for an understanding of the patient's unconscious (see Chapter 9, "The Borderline Patient"). These countertransference responses are less related to the interviewer's psychology and more a manifestation of the patient's psychodynamics.

Countertransference responses could be classified into the same categories as are used in the discussion of transference. The clinician may become dependent on his patient's affection and praise as sources of his own self-esteem or, conversely, may feel frustrated and angry when the patient is hostile or critical. Any therapist may use the patient in this way occasionally. The clinician may unconsciously seek the patient's affection and only come to recognize that he is doing so when the patient responds. Beginning male clinicians may find female patients writing love notes or poems or proposing marriage. One trainee commented that his prior model for male–female relationships was that of dating. There are more subtle manifestations of this problem, such as offering excessive reassurance, helping the patient obtain housing or a job, and so forth, when such assistance is not really necessary and serves as a bribe to earn the patient's love rather than an appropriate therapeutic intervention. Going out of one's way to rearrange time or fees, providing extra time, and being overly kind may all be ways of courting the patient's favor. Not allowing the patient to get angry is the other side of the same coin. On the other hand, clinicians are people, and some are warmer or friendlier or more helpful than others. There is nothing wrong with being nice.

The clinician can utilize exhibitionism as a way of soliciting affection or admiration from patients. Displaying one's knowledge or social or professional status to an inappropriate degree is an example, and it usually stems from the therapist's wish to be omniscient to compensate for some deep feeling of inadequacy.

Experienced therapists have commented that it is difficult to have only one case in long-term therapy, because that patient becomes too important to them. Other factors can cause a clinician to experience a particular patient as having special importance. The "VIP" creates so much difficulty for the clinician that a later subsection (see "The Special Patient") is devoted to the discussion of these patients.

All persons in the healing arts react to the patient's need to endow them with magical power. The nature of the clinician–patient relationship reawakens the clinician's desire to be all-knowing and all-powerful. This is a reciprocal aspect of the patient's wish for an omnipotent and omniscient therapist who can cure him by magical powers. If the interviewer assumes such a role, the patient will not be able to overcome his basic feelings of helplessness and inferiority. Nevertheless, the wish to become omnipotent is universal and can often be recognized in the clinician's behavior. For instance, the interviewer may be unable to see inconsistencies or inaccuracies in certain interpretations, or he may refuse to examine his own comments. An insistence on his own infallibility may lead to his implying that previous psychotherapists did not conduct therapy properly or did not accurately understand the patient.

A similar mechanism is demonstrated by the clinician who tells a spouse a clinical vignette that reveals how kind and understanding he was, tells how desirable and attractive his patients find him, or relates his brilliant interpretation. Discouraged with the slow progress of psychotherapy, he may subtly exaggerate and distort material from the sessions in order to impress his colleagues. He may exert pressure on the patient to improve for the purpose of enhancing his prestige and reputation. At times he may try to impress colleagues with the wealth, brilliance, or importance of his patients.

Countertransference is operating when the therapist is unable to recognize or refuses to acknowledge the real significance of his own attitudes and behavior. Such an admission might be phrased "Yes, I was preoccupied last time" or "My remark does sound belittling." The clinician is often concerned that the patient will try to turn the tables and analyze him further. In this situation the interviewer might reply, "Finding out why I said that is important, but it is really my problem. It would be unfair to burden our treatment with it, but to the extent that it is relevant, I will share it with you. Instead, let's understand as much as we can about your reactions to me." The patient is concerned about whether the therapist lives by a double standard, analyzing his patient's behavior but not his own. Occasionally a patient may exploit his therapist's openness concerning a mistake. The clinician who allows the patient to treat him sadistically also has a countertransference problem. Similar issues are raised when the patient has information regarding his therapist that comes from outside the treatment situation. Common examples are the patient who lives in the same neighborhood, has children in the same school as the therapist's children, or works in the same institution as the therapist. The most common example in the life of the psychiatric resident is the hospitalized patient who obtains information about his doctor from other patients, staff, bulletin boards, or his own direct observations.

In an attempt to maintain a professional role, the clinician is defensively tempted to hide behind analytical clichés such as "How do you feel about that?" or "What meaning did that have for you?" Often more subtle examples occur when the therapist's wording or the tone of his voice is crucial in revealing the implication of his remark. For example, "Your idea that I was flirting with the ward nurse upset you" implies that the flirtation existed only in the patient's mind. However, if the interviewer remarks, "The image of me flirting with the ward nurse upset you," the patient's perception is not challenged, and the interviewer can explore the impact of the experience on the patient.

A common manifestation of countertransference is overidentification with the patient. In this situation, the interviewer attempts to make the patient over in his own image. Perhaps the universal pitfall for psychotherapists is to indulge their Pygmalion fantasies. Difficulty in paying attention or remembering what the patient has said may be the interviewer's first clue to his countertransference. The clinician who overidentifies with his patient may have difficulty recognizing or understanding problems that are similar to his own, or he may have an immediate understanding of the problem but be unable to deal with it. For example, an obsessive interviewer who is preoccupied with time says after each hour, "I'll see you tomorrow at 3:30." It is unlikely that he will be able to help his patient work through a similar difficulty.

The beginning therapist may experience vicarious pleasure in the sexual or aggressive behavior of his patient. He may subtly encourage the patient to stand up to his parents in a manner that he himself admires. He may cater to the patient's dependent needs because he would like to be treated in a similar fashion. Psychotherapists who are undergoing analytic treatment themselves find that their patients are often working on the same problem that they are.

Power struggles, competition, and arguing with or badgering the patient are familiar examples of countertransference. The interviewer's task is to understand how the patient views the world and to help the patient better understand himself. It is not useful to force the interviewer's concepts on the patient. More subtle manifestations of this problem include the use of words or concepts that are slightly over the patient's head and thereby demonstrate the clinician's "one up" position. Other illustrations include the tendency to say "I told you so" when the patient discovers that the clinician has been correct or laughing at the patient's discomfort.

The countertransference response of wishing to be the patient's child or younger sibling most often occurs with patients who are older than the interviewer. Once again, the more the patient actually resembles the therapist's parent or sibling, the greater the likelihood of such responses. With female patients the therapist might accept gifts of food or clothing; with a male patient he might accept business advice or other such assistance. There is a fine line in this area with behavior that violates professional ethical boundaries.

There are a variety of nonspecific manifestations of countertransference. Sometimes an interviewer will experience anxiety, excitement, or depression, either while he is with a certain patient or after the patient leaves the office. His reaction might involve a countertransference problem, or it might reflect anxiety or neurotic triumph about the way in which he dealt with the patient.

Boredom or inability to concentrate on what the patient is saying most often reflects unconscious anger or anxiety on the part of the interviewer. If the interviewer regularly is late or forgets the session, this behavior usually indicates avoidance of hostile or sexual feelings toward the patient.

Another common countertransference problem stems from the therapist's failing to see occasions when the apparent "observing ego of the patient" together with an enthusiastic curiosity about the meaning of dreams, the recovery of early memories, and insight into unconscious dynamics is actually a transference enactment. The result is an overly intellectualized therapy that is relatively devoid of emotion.

The direct expression of emotion in the transference will frequently provide an opportunity for countertransference enactments. For example, one therapist told his patient, "It isn't really me you love (or hate); it's your father." Transference does not mean that the patient's feelings toward the therapist are not real. Telling the patient that his feelings are displaced is disrespectful and belittling. Similarly, beginning therapists sometimes respond to the patient's expression of anger by a comment such as "It is a real sign of progress that you are able to get angry at me." Remarks of this type are contemptuous of the patient's feelings. Although the transference neurosis involves the repetition of past attitudes, the emotional response is real; in fact, it is often stronger than it was in the original setting because less defense is necessary. The therapist's discomfort with the patient's intense emotional reactions may lead to a subtle defensiveness. An example is provided by the clinician who asks, "Isn't this the same way you felt toward your sister?" or says, "We know that you have had similar feelings in the past." These comments divert the discussion away from the transference rather than encouraging exploration of it. Both the clinician and the patient will understand the patient's feelings better if the interviewer asks, "How am I a son-of-a-bitch?" or "What is it that you love about me?" Such an approach takes the patient's feeling seriously. When the patient elaborates his feeling, he will usually discover the transference aspect of his response by himself. As he fully delineates the details of his reaction, he often volunteers, "You don't react the way my father did when I felt like this" or "This makes me think of something that happened years ago with my sister." Then the interviewer can demonstrate the transference component of the patient's feeling.

In the pursuit of the details of the patient's emotional reactions, distorted perceptions of the therapist frequently emerge. For instance, when describing why she felt that she loved her therapist, a patient said, "For some strange reason I pictured you with a mustache." Exploration of such clues identified the original object of the transference feeling from the patient's past.

Discussions of countertransference typically leave the beginner feeling that this reaction is bad and must be eliminated. It would be more accurate to say that the therapist tries to minimize the extent to which his neurotic responses interfere with the treatment. The clinician who is aware of his countertransference can use it as another source of information about the patient. In interviews with borderline patients, the mutual recognition of the clinician's countertransference can be particularly useful in the process of therapy (see Chapter 9, "The Borderline Patient").

The special patient.   The special patient is discussed at this point because the chief distinguishing features of this interview center on the interviewer's reactions to the status of his patient. The problem continues to occur throughout a clinician's career, although the criteria that define the patient as "special" may change. In the early years of a clinician's training, this patient may be a medical student, a fellow house staff officer, the relative of a staff member, or a patient who is known by a prestigious teacher.

As the clinician's experience and status increase, so does the status of his special patients. No matter how experienced the interviewer, or how secure, there always exists a person of such renown that the clinician will feel uneasy with him. There is as much variety in the attitude of special patients about their status as there is in any other group of people. Those whose special status depends on their personal significance to the interviewer usually expect to be treated like any other patient.

Some patients do expect and warrant special consideration. The interviewer may be uncertain where reality ends and neurotic expectations begin. Resolution of the quandary involves a consideration of the rights of the ordinary patient. The status of the special patient may deprive him of basic rights. The clinician's extraordinary arrangements that, in effect, place this patient on a par with other patients are not likely to harm the treatment. For example, consider the nationally prominent political figure whose position could be jeopardized if the public discovered that he had consulted a mental health professional. The clinician, by conducting a consultation in the patient's home, offers the same privacy that another patient can maintain while seeing the clinician in his office. In this case the application of the principle is clear, but in other instances the clinician must decide whether to side with the reality situation of the patient's life or with the principle that the interviewer should not go out of his way to gratify neurotic demands. If the consequences are high, it is preferable to risk erring by gratifying the patient's neurosis.

Problems arise in the treatment of this patient not only because his situation is special but also because he is special to the clinician. The success of his treatment assumes an urgent importance, and the clinician is overly concerned with maintaining the goodwill of the patient, his relatives, and his associates. One protection for both the patient and clinician is to make special arrangements in the selection of a therapist. The senior physician who is hospitalized for a major depression or the psychotic son of a prominent person should be assigned to someone who will not be intimidated by the patient's status. By choosing a clinician who is less likely to be made insecure, many problems are minimized.

The physician-patient presents particular problems. The treating clinician offers more detailed explanations on some occasions but no explanation at all on others, assuming that the patient already has sufficient knowledge. The physician-patient sometimes expects to be treated as a colleague and to have a "medical" discussion about his own case. He may fear asking questions that would make him appear ignorant or frightened. He may feel that he should not complain, express anger, or take too much of his clinician's time. The young clinician is prone to use jargon or to give intellectualized formulations to physician-patients. One physician-patient described a terrifying experience during which a urologist gave a continuous monologue of his maneuvers while passing a cystoscope and then described the clinical findings in the doctor's bladder, which, unbeknownst to the patient, had little pathological significance. The urologist apparently felt that a physician-patient might be reassured by this extra information.

The role of the interviewer.　The most important function of the interviewer is to listen and to understand the patient so that he may help. An occasional nod or "Uh-huh" is sufficient to let the patient know that the interviewer is paying attention. Furthermore, a sympathetic comment, when appropriate, aids in the establishment of rapport. The clinician can use remarks such as "Of course," "I see," or "Naturally" to support attitudes that have been communicated by the patient. When the patient's feeling is quite clear, the clinician can indicate his understanding with statements such as "You must have felt terribly alone" or "That must have been very upsetting." In general, the interviewer is nonjudgmental, interested, concerned, and kind.

The interviewer frequently asks questions. These may serve to obtain information or to clarify his own or the patient's understanding. Questions can be a subtle form of suggestion, or by the tone of voice in which they are asked, they may give the patient permission to do something. For example, the interviewer might ask, "Did you ever tell your boss that you felt you deserved a raise?" Regardless of the answer, the interviewer has indicated that such an act would be conceivable, permissible, and perhaps even expected.

The interviewer frequently makes suggestions to the patient either implicitly or explicitly. The recommendation of a specific form of treatment carries the clinician's implied suggestion that he expects it to be helpful. The questions that the clinician asks often give the patient the feeling that he is expected to discuss certain topics, such as dreams or sex. In psychotherapy, the clinician suggests that the patient discuss any major decisions before acting on them, and he may suggest that the patient should or should not discuss certain feelings with important persons in his life.

Clinicians may help patients with practical matters. For instance, a young married couple requested psychological counseling because of difficulty getting along with each other. At the end of the consultation, they asked whether it would be helpful if they tried to have a baby. A well-intentioned clergyman had suggested that a child might bring the couple closer together. The clinician advised that a baby could be a source of additional stress to have at that time and recommended that they wait until their relationship had improved.

The clinician provides the patient with certain gratifications and frustrations in the process of treatment. He helps the patient with his interest, understanding, encouragement, and support. He is the patient's ally and in that sense offers him opportunities to experience closeness. When the patient becomes unsure of himself, he may provide reassurance with a comment such as "Go ahead, you're doing fine." Generalized reassurance such as "Don't worry, it will all work out" is of limited value for most patients. This is because the interviewer does not know that whatever the patient fears *will* work out. Therefore he loses credibility both with the patient and with himself, as a result of offering false promises. It is preferable to offer support in the form of understanding that is founded on specific formulations of the patient's problem. At the same time, the clinician seeks to alleviate the patient's symptoms and the unconscious gratification that they provide. He makes the patient aware of conflicts—an awareness that can be painful and frustrating unless he is able to offer possible solutions for the patient's conflicts. Often the patient can imagine new solutions once the conflict has been thoroughly explored.

The most important activity in psychoanalytically oriented psychotherapy is interpretation. The aim of an interpretation is to undo the process of repression and allow unconscious thoughts and feelings to become conscious, thereby enabling the patient to develop new methods of coping with his conflicts without the formation of symptoms (see Chapter 2 discussion on the formation of symptoms). The preliminary steps of an interpretation are confrontation, which is pointing out that the patient is avoiding something, and clarification, which is formulating the area to be explored.

A "complete" interpretation delineates a pattern of behavior in the patient's current life showing the basic conflict between an unconscious wish and fear, the defenses that are involved, and any resulting symptom formation. This pattern is traced to its origin in his early life, its manifestation in the transference is pointed out, and the secondary gain is formulated. It is never possible to encompass all of these aspects at the same time. A similar interpretation using the object relations model would place less emphasis on the unconscious wish and defense component. Instead, the therapist traces the patient's conscious and unconscious introjections of one or both of the parents, accepting or defensively rejecting that parent. This formulation occurs repeatedly, to the point where the therapist remarks, "It sounds as though the mother in your head is still telling you what to do, and you seem unable to give up that angry attachment."

> A male patient reported having a rageful fit when his wife threw out a pair of his old shoes without his permission. He revealed that he did not completely understand his reaction because the shoes no longer fit, and he had planned to throw them out himself. Relevant family history included his description of his anger with his mother for her repeated violations of his space, privacy, and possessions. The interviewer, who already had elicited that information, said to the patient, "So your worst nightmare came true; your wife turned into your mother." "That's it," replied the patient, "she made me feel I was still a little boy. I may have had something to do with that," the patient added. "I may have set her up by dressing in a manner that is inappropriate to a man of my age in Manhattan." The patient fell silent, reflecting on his comment. The therapist remarked, "So you are devoting your life to changing your mother into the mother you wish you had." The patient was visibly moved and remarked, "I have to get over this or I'll ruin my marriage."

Interpretations can be directed at resistances and defenses or at content. In general, the interpretation is aimed at the material closest to consciousness, which means that defenses are interpreted earlier than the unconscious impulse that they help to ward off. In practice, any single interpretation involves both resistance and content and is usually repeated many times, although with varying emphasis; the therapist shifts back and forth as he works on a given problem. The earliest interpretations are aimed at the area in which the conscious anxiety is greatest, which usually is the patient's presenting symptoms, his resistance, or his transference. Unconscious material is not interpreted until it has become preconscious. To illustrate these issues, consider a young man with panic attacks:

> The therapist's first confrontation was aimed at the patient's resistance, with the remark, "You spend a good portion of our time talking about your symptoms." The patient answered, "What would you like me to talk about?" and the interviewer indicated that he would like to know more about what had been happening just before the last attack began. The patient's reply led to a clarification by the interviewer: "This is the third time this week that you had an attack after becoming angry with your wife." The patient accepted this remark, but it was not until a subsequent session that he added that he became angry whenever he felt that his wife was closer to her mother than to him. Still later it was learned that the patient felt intensely competitive with his sister and had always feared that their mother preferred her to him. At this time it was possible to interpret the patient's wish to attack his sister and his fear that he would be rejected by his mother as punishment. The same feelings were re-created in his current relationship with his wife. The clinician interpreted not only the patient's jealousy of his wife's attention to her mother but also his envy of the love that his mother-in-law bestowed on her daughter. At a different time, the secondary gain of the patient's symptom was interpreted as the fact that his panic attack invariably brought forth sympathetic indulgence from his wife. The entire process was repeated in the transference, in which the patient became enraged that the therapist did not demonstrate more sympathy for his symptoms and then described a dream in which he was the therapist's favorite patient.

Interpretations are more effective when they are more specific. In this example, a specific interpretation is "You became angry when you felt that your wife cared more about her mother than about you." A general statement would have been "Your anger seems to be directed at women." An initial interpretation is, of necessity, incomplete. As shown in the example, many steps are required before one can formulate a complete interpretation. When the interviewer is uncertain, interpretations are better offered as possibilities for the patient's consideration than as dogmatic pronouncements. One might introduce an interpretation with "Perhaps" or "It seems to me."

Timing is a critical aspect of interpretation. A premature interpretation is threatening; it increases the patient's anxiety and intensifies his resistance. A delayed interpretation slows treatment, and the clinician is of little help to the patient. The optimal time to interpret is when the patient is not yet aware of the material but is able to recognize and accept it—in other words, when the patient will not find it too threatening.

Whenever there is a strong resistance operating in the transference, it is essential that the interviewer direct his first interpretations to this area. One patient began each session with a discussion of her most recent dates. She felt that the therapist, like her father, was concerned about her sexual activity. A more obvious example is the patient who only wishes to discuss her erotic interest in the clinician. The interviewer might comment, "It seems that your feelings for me are disturbing you more than your symptoms."

The impact of an interpretation on a patient may be viewed in three main ways: first, the significance of the content of the interpretation on the patient's conflicts and defenses; second, the effect of the interpretation on the transference relationship; and third, the effect on the therapeutic alliance, which is the relationship between the clinician and the healthy, observing portion of the patient's ego. Each interpretation simultaneously operates in all three areas, although sometimes more in one than another.

The clinical manifestations of the patient's responses are quite varied. The patient may display emotional responses such as laughter, tears, blushing, or anger, indicating that the interpretation was effective. New material might emerge, such as additional historical data or a dream. The patient sometimes reports that his behavior in the outside world has changed. He may or may not have awareness of the confirmatory significance of such material. In fact, the patient may vigorously deny that the interpretation is correct only to change his mind later, or he may agree immediately but only as a gesture to please the therapist. If the patient negates or rejects an interpretation, the interviewer should not pursue the matter. Argument is ineffective, and therapeutic impact is not necessarily correlated with the patient's conscious acceptance.

Interpretations are deprivations insofar as they are aimed at removing a patient's defense or blocking a symbolic or substitute route for obtaining gratification of a forbidden wish. Certain patients are able to defend themselves against this aspect of an interpretation by accepting it as another form of gratification—that is, the interviewer is talking to them, wants to help them, and therefore will use his omnipotent power to cure them. This is easily recognized when the clinician makes an interpretation and the patient replies, "You're so smart; you really understand my problems." A change may take place in the quality of the therapeutic alliance after a correct interpretation because of an increased feeling of trust in the therapist. One patient was less preoccupied with fantasies about the clinician as the result of a transference interpretation.

The interviewer is expected to set limits on the patient's behavior in the office anytime the patient seems unable to control himself or uses inappropriate judgment. For example, if an enraged patient gets out of his seat and walks menacingly toward the interviewer, this is not the time to interpret, "You seem angry." Instead, the interviewer would say, "Sit down!" or "I am not going to be able to help if you are threatening me, so why don't you sit down." Likewise, the patient who refuses to leave at the end of the session, uses the shower in the doctor's bathroom, reads his mail, or listens at his office door should be told that such behavior is not permitted before the clinician attempts to analyze its meaning.

THE PSYCHIATRIC EXAMINATION[2]

The outline for organizing the data of the interview is referred to as the *psychiatric examination*. It is emphasized in a number of psychiatric textbooks and is therefore discussed here in terms of its influences on the interview. It is usually divided into the *history* (or anamnesis) and the *mental status*. Although this organization is modeled after the medical history and physical examination, it is actually much more arbitrary. The medical history includes subjective findings such as pain, shortness of breath, or digestive problems; the physical examination is limited to objective findings such as heart sounds, reflexes, skin discoloration, and so forth. Many of the findings pertaining to the mental status are subjectively revealed, and the interviewer may not be able to observe them directly. Hallucinations, phobias, obsessions, feelings of depersonalization, previous delusions, and affective states are examples. Furthermore, the general description of the patient is technically part of the mental status. However, it is more useful if it is placed at the start of the written record.

The Psychiatric History

Purpose

A careful history is the foundation for the diagnosis and treatment of every patient. Each branch of medicine has its own method for gathering and organizing an accurate, comprehensive story of the patient's illness and its impact on his life. In the general practice of medicine, the usual

---

[2]This section ("The Psychiatric Examination") is closely adapted from MacKinnon RA, Yudofsky SC: *Principles of the Psychiatric Evaluation*. Baltimore, MD, Lippincott Williams & Wilkins, 1986, pp. 40–57. Copyright 1986, Lippincott Williams & Wilkins. Used with permission.

technique is to secure, in the patient's own words, the onset, duration, and severity of his present complaints; to review his past medical problems; and to question the patient regarding the present function of his organs and anatomical systems. This focus is designed essentially to investigate the function of the tissues and organ systems as they maintain the internal economy of the body, and emphasis is placed on how malfunctions affect the patient's physical state or social patterns. In psychiatry, the history must also convey the more elusive picture of the patient's individual personality characteristics, including his strengths and his weaknesses. The psychiatric history includes the nature of the patient's relationships as well as information about important people in his past and present life. A complete story of the patient's life is impossible because it would require another lifetime to tell. Nevertheless, a useful portrayal of the patient's development from his earliest years through the present usually can be developed.

Like other professionals, the novice mental health clinician must progress through certain stages in the mastery of his profession. Whether it be school figures for the skater, finger exercises for the pianist, or the classic third-year medical student history for the future physician, these techniques are time-proven steps to be mastered in the pursuit of professionalism. The relevant historical data that the third-year medical student requires 3 hours to elicit usually can be obtained by the resident in 1 hour and by the professor in 20 minutes. Similarly, time and experience are required before the novice can respond quickly and directly to the initial cues provided by the patient that tell the senior clinician how and where to proceed with the history.

Techniques

The most important technique in obtaining the psychiatric history is to allow the patient to tell his story in his own words and in the order he chooses. Both the content of and the order in which the patient presents his history reveal valuable information. As the patient relates his story, the skillful interviewer recognizes points at which he can introduce relevant questions concerning the various areas described in the outline of the psychiatric history and the mental status examination.

Although the clinician's questions or comments are relevant, it is not uncommon for the patient to become confused or perplexed. The interviewer realizes this when the patient knits his eyebrows or says, "I don't understand why you need to know that." The interview will proceed more smoothly if the clinician takes the time to explain what he had in mind and show the patient the relevance of his question. On occasion, as the result of inexperience or an error in judgment, the clinician has pursued an issue that in fact was irrelevant. In that case he can say, "It just occurred to me, but perhaps you are right and it is unimportant." The patient will accept such occurrences without losing confidence in his clinician, provided irrelevant questioning does not occur to excess. Every clinician will, on occasion, ask the patient a question that elicits information the patient had provided earlier. Often the interviewer continues, hoping the patient will not notice or will not care. It is always preferable to remark, "Oh yes, I asked you that earlier" or "Oh yes, you already told me" and then repeat what the patient had said. Successful clinicians often keep a summary sheet of the patient's identifying life data, personal habits, and the names and ages of the spouse and children, if any. They review this material prior to the appointment for patients they follow irregularly. In this way they not only keep up with the patient's clinical condition but also avoid asking the same questions time and time again, such as "Is your child a boy or a girl?" or "Who is Susan?" Although this advice seems simple and obvious, many experienced and competent clinicians neglect to follow it.

Some clinicians obtain the history by providing the patient with a questionnaire to complete prior to the first meeting. Although that technique saves time and may be useful in clinics or other places where professional resources are severely limited, that efficiency is obtained at a significant price: it deprives the clinician and the patient of the opportunity to explore feelings that are elicited while answering the questions. Questionnaires may also inject an artificial quality to the interview. When the patient finally meets the clinician, he may experience him as yet another bureaucratic functionary, more interested in pieces of paper than in his patient. A good clinician can overcome this undesirable mental set, but it is an undesirable bit of pseudo-efficiency to create it in the first place.

Psychiatric histories are vital in delineating and diagnosing major neurotic or psychotic illnesses. Nevertheless, in the realm of personality diagnosis, many psychiatric histories are of minimal value. This is particularly true when they are limited to superficial reports such as historical questionnaires filled out by the patient.

Another frequent deficiency in the psychiatric history is when it is presented as a collection of facts and events that are organized according to date, with relatively little attention to the impact of those experiences on the patient or the role that the patient may have played in bringing them about. The history often reveals that the patient went to a certain school, held a certain number of jobs, married at a certain age, and had a certain number of children. Often, none of that material provides distinctive characteristics about the person that would help to distinguish him from another human being with similar vital statistics.

In most training programs, there is relatively little formal psychiatric training in the techniques involved in eliciting historical data. The novice clinician is given an outline and is expected somehow to learn to acquire the information requested. It is unusual for each of his written records to be corrected by his teachers and still more unusual for him to be required to rewrite the report and to incorporate any suggested corrections. In his supervised psychotherapy training, the trainee usually begins with a presentation of the history as it has been organized for the written record rather than as it flowed from the patient. The supervisor is often unaware of the trainee's skill in the process of eliciting historical information. Supervisors are usually more interested in the manifestations of early transference and resistance than in teaching the technique of eliciting a smooth, flowing history. As a result, this deficit in the supervisor's own training is unintentionally passed on to another generation of young clinicians.

The psychotic patient. Major modifications in techniques may be necessary for interviewing a disorganized patient. In the case of the patient with a psychotic process or severe personality disorder, the psychiatrist should provide more structure to elicit a coherent, chronological, organized story of the patient's present illness. The patient's lack of an organizing ego requires the interviewer to provide that support. The purpose is not merely to enable the interviewer to construct a more coherent story; the technique also has a therapeutic value: the patient is able to use the clinician's ego to compensate for his own deficit and experience relief from a frightening state of confusion. In this fashion the therapeutic alliance is formed at the same time that the requisite historical data are secured.

This advice should not be interpreted to suggest that the clinician ignore or become insensitive to leads provided by the psychotic patient at the time the patient offers them. When the clinician does not understand the meaning of something the patient volunteers, he should put his own agenda aside temporarily in order to establish better contact with the patient.

Organization of Data

The organization used in this chapter is solely for the purpose of preparing the written record. It is not to be used as an outline for conducting the interview, as stated earlier.

Preliminary Identification

The clinician should begin the written history by stating the patient's name, age, marital status, sex, occupation, language (if other than English), race, nationality, religion, and a brief statement about the patient's place of residence and circumstances of living. Comments such as "The patient lives alone in a furnished room" or "The patient lives with her husband and three children in a three-bedroom apartment" provide adequate detail for this part. If the patient is hospitalized, a statement can be included as to the number of previous admissions for similar conditions.

Although a detailed description of the patient appears at the beginning of the mental status portion of the record, it is useful to have a brief nontechnical description of the patient's appearance and behavior as it might be written by a novelist. What is required is not a stereotyped medical description of a "well-developed, well-nourished white male" but rather a description that brings the person to life in the eyes of the reader. The following description is a good illustration of what is desired:

> Mr. A is a 5-foot, 5-inch tall, powerfully built, heavyset man with coarse features and a swarthy complexion who appears quite unfriendly. His short, curly, dark brown hair is parted on the side, and one is immediately aware that his gaze follows the interviewer's every move. He creates an intimidating image as he nervously paces the floor and repeatedly looks at his watch. He spontaneously says, "I gotta get outta here, Doc. They're comin' to get me, Doc!" His perspiration-drenched T-shirt is dirty and is tucked into his paint-stained, faded jeans. He appears younger than his stated age of 30, and he obviously has not shaved for several days.

This information focuses the reader's attention and serves as the innermost of a series of concentric circles that, at each step, expand the story while maintaining the focus.

Chief Complaint

The chief complaint is the presenting problem for which the patient seeks professional help (or has been referred for it). The chief complaint should be stated in the patient's own words if possible. Certain patients, particularly those with psychoses or certain character disorders, have difficulty in formulating a chief complaint. In such situations the interviewer can work with the patient to help him uncover or formulate his reason for seeking treatment as well as understand the separate issue, "Why now?" If the chief complaint is not supplied by the patient, the record should contain a description of the person who supplied it and his relationship to the patient. At first glance, this part appears to be the briefest and simplest of the various subdivisions of the psychiatric history; however, in actuality it is often one of the most complex.

In many cases the patient begins his story with a vague chief complaint. One or more sessions may be required for the clinician to learn what it is that the patient finds most disturbing or why he seeks treatment at this particular time. In other situations, the chief complaint is provided by someone other than the patient. For example, an acutely confused and disoriented patient may be brought in by someone who provides the chief complaint concerning the patient's confusion. Occasionally, a patient with multiple symptoms of long duration has great difficulty explaining precisely why he seeks treatment at a particular time. Ideally, the chief complaint should provide the explanation of why the patient seeks help now. That concept must not be confused with the precipitating stress (often unconscious in nature) that resulted in the collapse of the patient's defenses at a particular time. The precipitating stress may be difficult to determine. Usually, the ease of determining the chief complaint correlates directly with the ease of determining the precipitating stress. At times the clinician uncovers the chief complaint in the course of looking for a precipitating stress or in considering what the patient unconsciously hoped to accomplish in pursuing the consultation. An example illustrating the usefulness of determining the patient's expectation of a consultation follows:

> A woman arrived at a clinician's office feeling distraught after her husband confronted her with the fact that he had been unhappy with their relationship for the past 10 years. She felt depressed and upset at his request for a separation and was convinced that her husband was going through a midlife crisis. She was certain that he did not know what he had "really" felt and that in actuality they had been happily married during all their years together. Although she had consulted the clinician voluntarily, she did not believe that she felt any emotional conflict. She believed that her reaction to the confrontation with her husband was quite normal. She wanted the clinician to interview her husband, convince him that he was going through a phase for which he might require treatment, and advise him that he should remain with her. Although she did not see herself as a patient, she had some striking personality pathology that, at the time, was ego-syntonic and not directly involved in her reason for seeking help. She was unaware of her inability to look critically at her own behavior and its effects on others or at her tendency to project her own tension state onto her husband. These traits were central aspects of her neurotic character and accounted for the fact that she was never able to accept treatment for herself.

History of Present Illness

Onset.   The clinician must provide an adequate amount of time during the initial interview to explore those details of the presenting symptoms that are most relevant to the patient's decision to consult a professional at this time. Inexperienced clinicians, particularly those with an interest in psychodynamics, often have difficulty determining precisely when an illness began. They frequently feel that the present illness must have begun sometime in the patient's early life, perhaps even during the first 2 years. Although such developmental concepts are useful in understanding the patient's psychodynamics, they are of relatively little value in determining when the patient's current failure in adaptation began. For that reason it is essential to evaluate the patient's highest level of functioning, even though this may not be considered healthy by normative standards. The patient's best level of adaptation must be considered the baseline for measuring his current loss of functioning and determining when maladaptive patterns first appeared. Most often, a relatively unstructured question such as "How did it all begin?" leads to an unfolding of the present illness. A well-organized patient is able to present a chronological account of his difficulties.

Precipitating factors.   As the patient recounts the development of the symptoms and behavioral changes that culminated in his seeking assistance, the interviewer should attempt to learn the details of the patient's life circumstances at the time these changes began. When asked to describe these relationships directly, the patient is often unable to give correlations between the beginning of his illness and the stresses that occurred in his life. A technique referred to as the *parallel history* is particularly useful with the patient who cannot accept the relationship between psychological determinants and psycho-physiological symptoms. In eliciting a parallel history, the interviewer returns to the same time period covered by the present illness, but later in the interview. He specifically avoids making his inquiry in phrases that suggest that he is searching for connections between what was happening in the patient's life and the development of the patient's symptoms. The clinician, without the patient's awareness, makes connections (i.e., the parallel history) between stresses that the patient experienced and the development of his disorder. The patient may notice some temporal connection between a particular stress and the appearance of his symptoms that impresses him and arouses his curiosity about the role of emotional factors in his illness. Nevertheless, premature psychological interpretations concerning the interrelationship of the stress and the symptom may undermine that process and intensify the patient's resistance. Unless the patient makes a spontaneous connection between his emotional reaction to a life event and the appearance of his symptoms, the clinician should proceed slowly.

Impact of the patient's illness.   The patient's psychiatric symptoms or behavioral changes have an impact on the patient and his family. The patient should describe how his problems have interfered with his life and how he and his family have adapted to these challenges. These are the *secondary losses* of the symptoms.

The *secondary gain* of a symptom may be defined as the indirect benefits of illness, such as obtaining extra affection from loved ones, being excused from unpleasant responsibilities, or obtaining extra gratification of one's dependency needs, as opposed to the primary gain that results from the unconscious meaning of the symptom.

The ways in which the patient's illness has affected his life activities and personal relationships highlight both the secondary loss and the secondary gain of the patient's illness. In attempting to understand the secondary gain, the interviewer must explore, in a sympathetic and empathic fashion, the impact of the patient's illness on his own life and the lives of his loved ones. The clinician must be careful to communicate to the patient an understanding of the pain of the patient's illness and the many losses that result from his symptoms. An implication that the patient may unconsciously benefit from being ill would immediately destroy the rapport the clinician has established.

> A married woman with three children complained of severe backaches with no apparent physical abnormalities. After listening to the description of her pain, the clinician asked, in a sympathetic voice, "How do you manage to take care of the housework?" "Oh," replied the patient, "my husband has been very kind; ever since I have been sick, he helps after he comes home from work." The clinician did not interpret the obvious secondary gain but mentally stored, for later use, the clue that the husband may not have been very kind before the onset of her backaches. In subsequent meetings, the clinician explored that area with the patient, who, after her resentment unfolded, became aware of the secondary gain of her backaches.

Psychiatric Review of Systems

After the clinician has completed his initial study of the patient's present illness, he can inquire about the patient's general medical health and carefully review the functioning of the patient's organ systems. Emotional disturbances are often accompanied by physical symptoms. A *systems review* is a traditional medical step in which the interviewer learns the medical problems that the patient has not volunteered or that are not part of the chief complaint or present illness. The systems review is the same as that performed by an internist, but through the particular perspective of a psychiatrist. No psychiatric evaluation is complete without statements concerning the patient's sleep patterns, weight regulation, appetite, bowel functioning, and sexual functioning. If the patient has experienced a sleep disturbance, it would be described here unless it is part of the present illness. The clinician should inquire about whether the insomnia is initial, middle, terminal, or a combination. Insomnia can be an extremely disturbing problem, and the interviewer is well advised to explore in detail the circumstances that aggravate it and the various remedies the patient has attempted and their results. Other organ systems commonly involved in psychiatric complaints are the gastrointestinal, cardiovascular, respiratory, urogenital, musculoskeletal, and neurological systems.

It is logical to inquire about dreams while asking the patient about sleep patterns. Freud stated that the dream is the royal road to the unconscious. Dreams provide valuable insight into the patient's unconscious fears, wishes, and conflicts. Repetitive dreams and nightmares are of particular value. Some of the most common themes are of food (either the patient is being gratified or the patient is being denied while others eat), aggression (the patient is involved in adventures, battles, or chases, most often in the defensive position), examinations (the patient feels unprepared, is late for the examination, or cannot find the proper room), helplessness or impotence (the patient is shooting at someone with a gun that is ineffective, the patient is fighting and his blows seem to have no effect on the opponent, or the patient is being chased and is unable to run or to cry for help), and sexual dreams of all varieties, both with and without orgasm. The clinician should also record the residual feelings of the patient regarding anxiety and revealing associations or feelings while recounting the dream.

It is useful to ask the patient for a recent dream. If the patient cannot recall one, the interviewer might say, "Perhaps you will have one between now and our next appointment." The patient frequently produces a dream in the second interview that reveals his unconscious fantasies about his illness, the clinician, the treatment, or all three.

Fantasies or daydreams are another valuable source of unconscious material. As with dreams, the clinician can explore and record all manifest details and attendant feelings.

Previous Psychiatric Illnesses

The section on previous psychiatric illnesses is a transition between the story of the present illness and the personal history. Here, prior episodes of emotional or mental disturbances are described. The extent of incapacity, the type of treatment received, the names of hospitals, the length of each illness, and the effects of prior treatments should all be explored and recorded chronologically.

Personal History

In addition to studying the patient's present illness and current life situation, the clinician needs an equally thorough understanding of the patient's past life and its relationship to his presenting emotional problem.

In the usual medical history, the present illness gives the physician important information that enables him to focus his questions in his "review of systems." Similarly, because it is impossible to obtain a complete history of a person's life, the clinician uses the patient's present illness to provide significant clues to guide him in further exploration of the personal history. When the interviewer has acquired a general impression of the most likely diagnosis, he can then direct his attention to the areas that are pertinent to the patient's major complaints and to defining the patient's underlying personality structure. Each interview is modified according to the patient's underlying character type as well as according to important situational factors relating to the setting and circumstances of the interview. To modify the form of the interview, the clinician must be familiar with the psychodynamic theory of psychological development and with the phases and conflicts that are most important for each condition. In that way, he may concentrate the questions in the areas that will be most significant in explaining the patient's psychological development and the evolution of the patient's problems.

A thorough psychodynamic explanation of the patient's illness and personality structure requires an understanding of the ways in which the patient reacts to the stresses of his environment along with the recognition that the patient has played a major role in selecting his current situation and choice of environment. Through an understanding of the interrelationship between external stress and the patient's tendency to seek out situations that frustrate him, the clinician develops a concept of the patient's core intrapsychic conflict.

The personal history is perhaps the most deficient section of the typical psychiatric record. A statement about whether the patient was breast- or bottle-fed, followed by statements of questionable accuracy concerning the patient's toilet training or early developmental landmarks such as sitting, walking, and talking, is of limited value. That entire area may be condensed in a statement such as "Developmental landmarks were normal." The clinician might replace these routine and often meaningless inquiries by an attempt to understand and utilize new areas of knowledge germane to child development, as explained in the next subsections.

Prenatal history. In the prenatal history, the clinician considers the nature of the home situation into which the patient was born and whether the patient was planned and wanted. Were there any problems with the mother's pregnancy and delivery? Was there any evidence of defect or injury at birth? What were the parents' reactions to the gender of the patient? How was the patient's name selected?

Early childhood. The early childhood period considers the first 3 years of the patient's life. The quality of the mother–child interaction during feeding is more important than whether the child was breast or bottle fed. Although an accurate account of this experience is difficult to obtain, it is frequently possible to learn whether, as an infant, the patient presented problems in feeding, was colicky, or required special formulas. Early disturbances in sleep patterns or signs of unmet needs, such as head banging or body rocking, provide clues about possible maternal deprivation. In addition, it is important to obtain a history of caretakers during the first 3 years. Were there auxiliary maternal objects? The clinician should discover who was living in the patient's home during early childhood and should try to determine the role that each person played in the patient's upbringing. Did the patient exhibit problems with stranger anxiety or separation anxiety?

It is helpful to know if the loving parent and the disciplining parent were one and the same person. In one case, a child received most of her love from a grandmother but was trained and disciplined by a maid. In her adult life she rejected housework, which was associated with the cold punitive authority of the maid, but pursued a career in music, which had served in her childhood as a connection to her loving grandmother. The fact that her actual mother had not enjoyed childrearing and had been emotionally distant caused further problems in maternal identification. It was not surprising that the patient did not have a cohesive sense of herself as a woman and had great difficulty integrating her career with being a wife and mother.

Toilet training is another traditional area that is of limited value in the initial history. Although an age may be quoted, useful and accurate information concerning the more important interaction between parent and child usually is not remembered. Toilet training is one of the areas in which the will of the parent and the will of the child are pitted against each other. Whether the child experienced toilet training chiefly as a defeat in the power struggle or as enhancing his own mastery is of critical importance for characterological development. However, this information usually is not possible to obtain during the evaluation.

The patient's siblings and the details of his relationships with them are other important areas that often are underemphasized in the psychiatric history. The same deficiency is often reflected in psychodynamic formulations as well. Psychodynamics is too often conceptualized only in terms of oedipal or preoedipal conflicts. Other psychological factors, such as sibling rivalries and positive sibling relationships, may significantly influence the patient's social adaptation. The death of a sibling before the patient's birth or during his formative years has profound impact on developmental experience. The parents, particularly the mother, may have responded to the sibling's death with depression, fear, or anger, which may have resulted in diminished emotional nourishment to their other children. Siblings may also play a critical role in supporting one another emotionally and may provide an opportunity to develop alliances and to have support at times when the patient experiences feelings of rejection or isolation from the parents.

The child's evolving personality is a topic of crucial importance. Was the child shy, restless, overactive, withdrawn, studious, outgoing, timid, athletic, friendly, a risk taker, or risk avoidant? Play is a useful area to explore in studying the development of the child's personality. The story begins with the earliest activities of the infant who plays with parts of his body and gradually evolves into the complex sports and games of adolescents. This portion of the history not only reveals the child's growing capacity for social relationships but also provides information concerning his developing ego structures. The clinician should seek data concerning the child's increasing ability to concentrate, to tolerate frustration, and to postpone gratification, and as he became older, to cooperate with peers, to be fair, to understand and comply with rules, and to develop mature conscience mechanisms. The child's preference for active or passive roles in physical play also should be noted. The development of intellectual play becomes crucial as the child becomes older. His capacity to entertain himself—playing alone in contrast to his need for companionship—reveals important information concerning his developing personality. It is useful to learn which fairy tales and stories were the patient's favorites. Such childhood stories contain all of the conflicts, wishes, and fears of the various developmental phases, and their themes provide clues concerning the patient's most significant problem areas during those particular years.

The clinician can ask the patient for his earliest memory and for any recurrent dreams or fantasies that occurred during childhood. The patient's earliest memory is significant, often revealing an affective tone. Memories that involve being held, loved, fed, or playing carry a positive connotation for the overall quality of the patient's earliest years. On the other hand, memories that contain themes of abandonment, fear, loneliness, injury, criticism, punishment, and so forth have the negative implication of a traumatic childhood.

Middle childhood (ages 3–11 years). The clinician can address such important middle childhood subjects as gender identification, punishments used in the home, who provided the discipline, and who influenced early conscience formation. He can inquire about early school experiences, especially about how the patient first tolerated being separated from his mother. Data about the patient's earliest friendships and peer relations are valuable. The interviewer can ask about the number and the closeness of the patient's friends, whether the patient took the role of leader or follower, his social popularity, and his participation in group or gang activities. Early patterns of assertion, impulsiveness, aggression, passivity, anxiety, or antisocial behavior often emerge in the context of school relationships. A history of the patient's learning to read and the development of other intellectual and motor skills is important. A history of hyperactivity or of learning disabilities, their management, and their impact on the child is of particular significance. A history of nightmares, phobias, bed wetting, fire setting, cruelty to animals, or compulsive masturbation is also important in recognizing early signs of psychological disturbance.

Later childhood (prepuberty through adolescence). The unfolding and consolidation of the adult personality occur during later childhood, an important period of development. The clinician should continue to trace the evolution of social relationships as they achieve increasing importance. During this time, through relationships with peers and in group activities, a person begins to develop independence from his parents. The clinician should attempt to define the values of the patient's social groups and determine whom the patient idealized. That information provides useful clues concerning the patient's emerging idealized self-image.

He should explore the patient's academic history, his relationships with teachers, and his favorite curricular and extracurricular interests. He asks about hobbies and participation in sports and inquires about emotional or physical problems that may make their first appearance during this phase. Common examples include feelings of inferiority, weight problems, running away from home, smoking, and drug or alcohol use. Questions about childhood illnesses, accidents, or injuries are always included in thorough history taking.

Psychosexual history. The sexual history is a personal and embarrassing area for most patients. It will be easier for the patient to answer the physician's questions if they are asked in a matter-of-fact, professional manner. Such a concentration of attention on the patient's sexual history provides a therapeutic structure that is supportive of the patient and that makes sure the therapist will not fail, as a result of countertransference, to obtain relevant sexual data. Much of the history of infantile sexuality is not recoverable, although many patients are able to recollect sexual curiosities and sexual games played during the ages of 3–6 years. The interviewer should ask how the patient learned about sex and what attitudes he felt his parents had about his sexual development and sex in general. The interviewer can inquire about sexual transgressions against the patient during childhood. Those important incidents are conflict laden and are seldom voluntarily reported by the patient. The patient often experiences relief when a sensitively phrased question allows him to reveal some particularly difficult material that he otherwise might not have recounted to the clinician for months or even years. An example is "Were you ever touched by an adult in an inappropriate manner?"

No history is complete without a discussion of the onset of puberty and the patient's feelings about this important milestone. Female patients should be questioned about preparation for their menarche as well as about their feelings concerning the development of the secondary sexual changes. The story of a woman's first brassiere is often enlightening. Who decided it was the proper time, who accompanied her to the store, and what was the experience like? A man may discuss beginning to shave, reacting to changes in his voice, or how he learned about masturbation and his reaction to his first ejaculation.

Children who develop unusually early or unusually late typically suffer embarrassment and often take elaborate measures to conceal their differences from their peer group. Any exception to that general principle is well worth understanding. Adolescent masturbatory history, including the content of fantasies and the patient's feelings about them, is significant. The interviewer should routinely inquire about dating, petting, crushes, parties, and sexual games. Attitudes toward the sexes should be examined in detail. Was the patient shy and timid, or was he aggressive and boastful, with the need to impress others by his sexual conquests? Did the patient experience anxiety in sexual settings? Was there promiscuity? Did he participate in homosexual, group masturbatory, incestuous, aggressive, or perverse sexual behavior?

Religious, cultural, and moral background. The interviewer should describe the religious and cultural background of both parents as well as the patient's religious instruction. Was the family attitude toward religion strict or permissive, and were there conflicts between the two parents over the religious education of the child? The clinician should trace the evolution of the patient's adolescent religious practices to his present beliefs and activities. Even though the patient may have been raised without formal religious affiliation, most families have some sense of identification with a religious tradition. Furthermore, each family has a sense of social and moral values. These typically involve attitudes toward work, play, community, country, the role of parents, children, friends, and cultural concerns or interests.

Adulthood

Occupational and educational history. The interviewer should explore the patient's school experiences. Where did he go, why, how far, and what were his areas of enjoyment, success, failure? His choice of occupation, the requisite training and preparation, his ambitions, and long-range goals are important. What is the patient's current job, and what are his feelings about it? The interviewer should also review the patient's relationships at work with authorities, peers, and, if applicable, subordinates. He should describe the number of jobs the patient has had, their duration, and the reasons for changes in jobs or job status.

Social relationships. The clinician should describe the patient's relationships, with emphasis on their depth, duration, and quality. What is the nature of his social life and his friendships? What types of social, intellectual, and physical interests does he share with his friends? By *depth of relationships* we refer to the degree of mutual openness and sharing of one's inner mental life as measured by norms of the patient's cultural background. By *quality of relationships* we refer to the patient's capacity to give to others and his capacity to receive from them. How much are his relationships colored by idealization or devaluation? Are people used narcissistically to enhance the patient's sense of status and power, or does he truly care about the inner well-being of others?

Questions often arise concerning the patient who has few, if any, friends. First, the clinician explores the nature of the few relationships that the patient has maintained, even if they are limited to one or two family members. Next, he attempts to understand why the patient has so few friendships. Does a fear of rejection cause him to remain aloof from others? Does he passively wait for others to take the initiative in friendships? Does he feel unlikable and reject overtures from others? Does he lack the requisite social skills to negotiate a friendship? Does he overwhelm people with excessive needs for intimacy and thereby alienate himself from potential friends? The major character disorders all show some disturbance in this crucial area of functioning. For example, the obsessive-compulsive personality typically is excessively controlling in his relationships with others, whereas the histrionic is seductive and manipulative.

Adult sexuality. Although the written record organizes adult sexuality and marriage in separate categories, in the conduct of the clinical interview it is often easier to elicit that material together. The premarital sexual history should include sexual symptoms such as frigidity, vaginismus, impotence, and premature or retarded ejaculation as well as preferred fantasies and patterns of foreplay. Both premarital and marital sexual experiences should be described. Responses to menopause are described here when appropriate.

Marital history. In the marital history the clinician describes each marriage or other sustained sexual relationship that the patient has had. The story of the marriage should include a description of the courtship and the role played by each partner. The evolution of the relationship, including areas of agreement and disagreement, the management of money, the roles of the in-laws, attitudes toward raising children, and a description of the couple's sexual adjustment, should be described. The last description should include who usually initiates sexual activity and in what manner, the frequency of sexual relations, sexual preferences, variations, techniques, and areas of satisfaction and dissatisfaction for each partner. It usually is appropriate to inquire whether either party has engaged in extramarital relationships and, if so, under what circumstances and whether the spouse learned of the affair. If the spouse did learn of the affair, describe what happened. The reasons underlying an extramarital affair are as important as its subsequent effect on the marriage. Of course, these questions should be applied to the spouse's behavior as well as the patient's. In the written record care should be taken not to include material that could be harmful to the patient if it were revealed to an insurance company or a court.

In the event that a marriage has terminated in divorce, it is indicated to inquire about the problems that led to this. Has there been a continuing relationship with the former spouse, and what are the details? Have similar problems arisen with subsequent relationships? Has the patient been monogamous in his or her relationships? Does he maintain triangular relationships or simultaneous multiple relationships? The latter implies little commitment, whereas the pattern of triangular relationships involves betrayal, mistrust, split commitments, secret liaisons, or competition for someone else's partner.

Homosexual marriages, or sustained sexual relationships in which one's life is shared with a person of the same sex, are now an accepted and legal part of the contemporary cultural landscape. In such cases, it is appropriate to explore most of the same areas suggested for heterosexual marriages.

No marital history is complete without describing the patient's children or stepchildren. Include the sex and ages of all children, living or dead; a brief description of each; and a discussion of his or her relationship to the patient. Make an assessment of the patient's functioning in the parental role. Attitudes toward contraception and family planning are also important.

Current social situations. The clinician should inquire about where the patient lives and include details about the neighborhood and the patient's particular residence. Include the number and types of rooms, the other persons living in the home, the sleeping arrangements, and how issues of privacy are handled. Particular emphasis should be placed on nudity of family members and bathroom arrangements. Ask about family income, its sources, and any financial hardships. If there has been outside support, inquire about its source and the patient's feelings about it. If the patient is hospitalized, have provisions been made so that he will not lose his job or home? Will financial problems emerge because of the illness and associated medical bills? The interviewer should inquire about who is caring for the home, children, pets, and even plants as well as who visits the patient in the hospital and how frequently visits occur.

Military history. For those patients who have been in the military, it has usually been a significant experience. The interviewer should inquire about the patient's general adjustment to the military, his rank, and whether he saw combat or sustained an injury. Was he ever referred for psychiatric consultation, did he suffer any disciplinary action during his period of service, and what was the nature of his discharge?

Family history. Hereditary factors are important in a variety of psychiatric disorders. A statement about any psychiatric illness, hospitalizations, and treatments of family members, particularly the patient's parents, siblings, and children or any other important family members, should be placed in this part of the report. In addition, the family history should describe the personalities of the various people living in the patient's home from childhood to the present. The clinician should also define the role each has played in the patient's upbringing, and their current relationship with the patient. Informants other than the patient may be available to contribute to the family history, and the sources should be cited in the written record. Frequently, data concerning the background and upbringing of the patient's parents suggest behaviors that they may have exhibited toward the patient, despite their wishes to the contrary. Finally, the clinician should determine the family's attitude toward and insight into the patient's illness. Does the patient feel that they are customarily supportive, indifferent, or destructive?

Summary

In summary, we want to emphasize the following points: 1) There is no single method to obtain a history that is appropriate for all patients or all clinical situations. 2) It is necessary to establish rapport and to obtain the patient's trust and confidence before the patient will cooperate with a treatment plan. 3) The history is never complete or fully accurate. 4) The description of the patient, the psychopathology, and the developmental history should all fit together, creating a cohesive picture. 5) The clinician should link the patient's mental life with his symptoms and behaviors. 6) Psychodynamics and developmental psychology help us to understand the important connections between past and present. Without this as a foundation, dynamic psychotherapy is based only on concepts about communication and the therapeutic relationship. Therefore the clinician is unable to exploit the potential of reconstructive or psychogenetic approaches. 7) This discussion is far more comprehensive than any real clinical history. No clinician can respond to every issue raised in this chapter for any patient he interviews.

The Mental Status

The lack of standardization for mental status evaluations has gradually led to their virtual replacement by formal rating scales. These scales are valuable for research in that they are reliable, valid, objective, and quantifiable. Nevertheless, the clinician needs a format to guide his clinical evaluation.

The mental status is the systematic organization and evaluation of a description of the patient's current psychological functioning. The developmental picture of the person revealed by the history is thus supplemented by a description of the patient's current behavior, including aspects of his intrapsychic life. Although the mental status is separated in the written record, such a separation is artificial in the interview and will be resented by the patient. The experienced interviewer develops skill in evaluating the patient's mental status while simultaneously eliciting the history.

At some point in the interview, the neophyte may say, "Now I'm going to ask you some questions that may sound silly." This apology usually precedes mental status questions that the clinician consciously or unconsciously realizes are most likely inappropriate. There is no excuse for asking a patient "silly questions." Instead, the interviewer might pursue a more detailed discussion of problems in the patient's daily living that reflect potential difficulties in his mental processes. A cognitively impaired woman became distressed during an interview by a noise from a steam pipe. She asked, "Do you hear that?" The clinician replied, "Yes, I do. Do noises bother you?" She nodded, and the interviewer inquired further, "Do you sometimes hear things when other people don't?" In this way the inquiry followed a natural course in the interview. Another patient seemed unaware that she was in a hospital and thought that she was in a hotel. In that case the interviewer's questions about orientation seemed quite appropriate. An elderly man revealed some memory difficulties, and the clinician asked if he had any problem counting change when shopping. The patient answered, "Well, most people are honest, you know." At this point, a question about change from $10 after a $3 purchase would not seem silly.

One would no more ask an obviously nonpsychotic patient if he hears voices than ask an obviously comfortable medical patient if he is in great pain. The interviewer will inhibit the development of rapport by asking a patient who has no suggestion of impaired orientation or cognition to subtract serial 7's or to identify today's date. However, any discussion of the patient's history offers innumerable opportunities to assess orientation and simple cognitive skills. (See Chapter 16, "The Cognitively Impaired Patient," for use of specific mental status assessment instruments.)

Detailed instruction on this subject can only be provided by the demonstration and supervision of interviews. For further consideration of specific examples, the reader is referred to the appropriate chapters.

Therapeutic Formulation

Although the techniques of case formulation exceed the scope of this book, it has been demonstrated that those clinicians who have carefully formulated their understanding of the patient make more successful therapists. Statements about the patient's clinical condition (psychopathology) should be kept separate from speculative hypotheses that attempt to explain the intrapsychic forces at work (psychodynamics) and from constructs that suggest how the patient became the person he is (psychogenetics).

As the interviewer attempts a psychodynamic formulation, he will quickly become aware of the areas of the patient's life about which he has obtained the least knowledge. He can then decide whether these omissions are caused by his lack of experience or by countertransference, or are manifestations of the patient's defenses. In any case, he will be well rewarded for his efforts.

Practical Issues

Time Factors

Duration of the session.   Psychiatric interviews last for varying lengths of time. The average therapeutic interview is about 45–50 minutes. Often, interviews with psychotic or medically ill patients are more brief, whereas in the emergency department longer interviews may be required. This is discussed in the appropriate chapters.

Frequently, new patients will ask about the length of the appointment. Such questions usually represent more than simple curiosity, and the clinician might follow his answer with "What makes you ask?" For example, the patient may be making a comparison between the interviewer and previous clinicians or checking to see if his insurance will cover the cost. Another common experience is for patients to wait until near the end of an interview and then ask, "How much time is left?" When the interviewer inquires, "What did you have in mind?' the patient usually explains that there is something he does not wish to talk about if there are only a few minutes remaining. Delaying an important subject until the last few minutes has significance—a resistance the interviewer might want to discuss now or at some time in the future. He might suggest that the patient bring the topic up at the beginning of the next appointment or, if there is enough time, that he begin now and then continue in the following interview.

The patient.   The patient's management of time reveals an important facet of his personality. Most patients arrive a few minutes early for their appointments. Very anxious patients may arrive as much as half an hour early. This behavior usually causes little problem for the interviewer, and it is often not noted unless the patient mentions it. Likewise, the patient who comes precisely on time or even a few minutes late does not often provide an opportunity to explore the meaning of his behavior in the early weeks of treatment.

A difficult problem is created by the patient who arrives very late. The first time this occurs, the interviewer might listen to the patient's explanation, if one is volunteered, but avoid making comments such as "Oh, it's quite all right"; "That's OK"; or "No problem." Instead he may call the patient's attention to the limitations this creates with a remark such as "Well, we'll cover as much as we can in the time remaining." It is important that this is said in a pleasant tone of voice! On occasion, the patient's reason for being late is a blatant resistance. For instance, he might explain, "I forgot all about the appointment until it was time to leave." In this situation the interviewer can ask, "Did you feel some reluctance about coming?" If the answer is "Yes," the clinician might continue his exploration of the patient's feeling. If the answer is "No," he should allow the matter to rest for the time being. It is important that the interview be terminated promptly in order to avoid collaborating with the patient in an attempt to avoid the limitations of reality.

An even more difficult situation exists when the patient arrives quite late for several interviews, each time showing no awareness that his actions might be caused by factors within himself. After the second or third time, the clinician might remark, "Your explanations for being late emphasize factors outside yourself. Do you think that the lateness may have something to do with your feelings about coming here?" Another method is to explore the patient's reaction to the lateness. The clinician could ask, "How did you feel when you realized you would be late today?"; "Did it bother you that you were late?"; or "How did you imagine I would react to your lateness?" Such questions may uncover the meaning of the lateness. The main concern is that the clinician respond with interest in the meaning of the behavior rather than with criticism or even anger.

The clinician. The interviewer's handling of time is also an important factor in the interview. Chronic carelessness regarding time indicates a characterological or a countertransference problem, a specific one if it involves only a particular patient or a general one if the interviewer is regularly late for most patients. However, on occasion the interviewer is detained. If it is the first interview, it is appropriate for the clinician to express his regret that the patient was kept waiting. After the first few interviews, other factors must be considered before the interviewer offers an apology for lateness. For certain patients, any apologetic comment from the clinician only creates more difficulty in expressing their annoyance. With such patients, the clinician could call attention to his lateness by glancing at his watch and remarking on the number of minutes remaining. Unless the patient appears annoyed or has nothing to say, the interviewer can allow the matter to drop. Depending on the effectiveness of his repression and reaction formation, the patient may either acknowledge some mild irritation or say that he did not mind waiting. The interviewer can listen for indications that the patient had some unconscious response that should be explored. When the clinician is late, he should extend the length of the interview to make up the time. He will show respect for the patient's other time commitments if he inquires, "Will you be able to remain 10 minutes longer today?"

The transition between interviews.   It is a good idea for the interviewer to have a few minutes to himself between interviews. This provides an opportunity to "shift gears" and to be ready to start fresh with the next interview rather than continue to think about the patient who has just left. A telephone call or glancing at the mail or at a magazine will facilitate this transition. One can also provide a brief extension of the interview when that is clinically indicated. An example is the patient who is crying uncontrollably at the end of the session. Telling the patient "We will have to stop shortly" allows the patient time to re-compose himself.

Space Considerations

Privacy.   Most patients will not speak freely if they feel that their conversation might be overheard. Quiet surroundings also offer fewer distractions that might interfere with the interview, and clinicians try to avoid interruptions. Privacy and some degree of physical comfort are minimal requirements.

Seating arrangements.   Many clinicians prefer to conduct interviews while seated at a desk, but even then it is preferable not to place the chairs so that there is furniture between the interviewer and patient. Both chairs should be of approximately equal height so that neither party is looking down on the other. If the room contains several chairs, the interviewer can indicate which chair is for himself and then allow the patient to select the location in which he will feel most comfortable. The main factors that influence the patient's choice involve the physical distance and location in relation to the clinician's chair. Patients who seek more intimacy, for example, prefer to sit as close to the interviewer as possible. Oppositional or competitive patients will sit farther away and often directly across from the clinician.

Fees

Money is the common unit of value for goods and services in our culture, and the fee that the patient pays symbolizes the value of treatment to both patient and clinician. The fee signifies that the relationship is mutually advantageous, and the payment of a fee can reflect the patient's desire to be helped, but it is not true that a patient must undergo some financial hardship or sacrifice in order to benefit from psychotherapy.

The average clinician has little opportunity to determine and collect fees before he has completed his training. For example, it is easy for a trainee to remain aloof from the fee-setting arrangements of the clinic registrar, with the unfortunate result that the entire subject is ignored in the therapy.

Therapists ignore financial arrangements with patients who do not pay them directly, something that would never be permitted with those who do. The clinician may not care that the patient pays little or nothing. A beginner may feel that because he is so inexperienced, his services are not worth money; that he owes the patient something because he is learning at the patient's expense; or even that he is underpaid by the institution, in which case he retaliates by allowing the patient to cheat the "establishment." In one case, a patient had concealed financial assets from the registrar only to confess to the staff therapist, who then passively became a collaborator in "stealing from the institution." It was some months before he realized that, in the patient's unconscious, he was the "institution." Supervisors also often pay insufficient attention to the handling of fees, thereby losing valuable opportunities to explore transference and countertransference.

The fee has various meanings in the therapeutic relationship. The patient may view the fee as a bribe, offering to pay a larger fee than the clinician would customarily charge. In the era when psychiatric evaluation was a prerequisite for an abortion, one woman stated, "I hope you realize that I would be willing to pay you any fee you ask." The clinician replied, "I will do whatever is appropriate to help you. I understand that you feel desperate, but a bribe isn't necessary and won't have any impact anyway." Another patient utilized the fee as a means of control. He had already determined the clinician's fee per session; he multiplied it by the number of visits and presented the doctor with a check before receiving his bill. He was symbolically in control; the clinician was not charging him; he was giving the clinician money.

Masochism or submissiveness may be expressed by payment of inordinately high fees without protest. The patient may express anger or defiance to the therapist by not paying or by paying late. He may test the therapist's honesty by asking if there is a discount by paying cash, with the inference that the clinician will be able to conceal it on his income tax. These maneuvers are discussed in greater detail in Chapter 12, "The Antisocial Patient."

With private patients, the subject of fees usually does not arise until the end of the interview. The clinician can wait until the patient raises the issue, which may not happen for two or three visits. If the interviewer suspects that his usual fee will be difficult for the patient, he should mention the subject at the time when the patient is on the topic of his finances. If the patient describes difficult financial problems but plans to continue therapy, the clinician might ask, "How do you feel about the cost of treatment?" If the patient has no realistic plan, the interviewer could explore the meaning of this behavior.

Occasionally, a patient will ask about the clinician's fee at the beginning of the interview or on the telephone. The easiest response is to give the cost of a consultation, adding that any further fees can be discussed at that time. During the consultation the interviewer might inquire if the patient is worried about the cost of treatment. If such is the case, the clinician could suggest that the subject of cost be deferred until the treatment plan is discussed, because the major factors of frequency of visits and possible duration of treatment must also be taken into account, and those questions must wait until the clinician has learned about the problems. Affluent patients may never ask about the fee, but if the patient should be concerned about the cost of therapy and does not inquire after several sessions, the clinician might say, "We have not discussed the fee." In this way the interviewer may learn something about the patient's attitude toward money.

Chance Meeting of the Patient Outside the Interview

Occasionally the clinician may accidentally meet his new patient outside the consultation room either before or after the interview, in a lobby, hospital dining room, elevator, or subway. This situation may be uncomfortable for the young therapist, who is not sure whether to speak or what to say. The simplest procedure is to take one's cue from the patient. The clinician is not obligated to make small talk, and he is well advised to wait until he is inside the office before entering into any discussion of the patient's problems. In most situations the patient will feel uncomfortable in the presence of his therapist outside the office. If the patient makes small talk, the interviewer can reply in a brief but friendly manner without extending the conversation. When the patient does ask a question that the therapist feels should not be answered, he can suggest that they wait to discuss that until they have more time or are in more private surroundings. When the therapist meets the patient outside the office and the patient becomes intrusive, the clinician can use small talk to control the situation and keep the conversation on neutral ground. Occasionally the therapist's admission of his own uneasiness after meeting a patient outside the office can be useful for the therapy.

Our perspectives on this subject reflect life in the big city, where anonymity is the rule rather than the exception. Nevertheless, mental health professionals live and work in a variety of settings, including large or small cities or small towns where they may regularly encounter their patients in local stores, restaurants, sporting events, or back to school nights. In these settings both the patient and the interviewer have a natural inclination to protect the privacy of the treatment and comfortably establish the appropriate social boundaries. If the patient becomes intrusive in a social setting, the clinician may suggest, "This is a topic best left for our next session."

MANAGEMENT OF THE INTERVIEW

Pre-Interview Considerations

The Patient's Expectations

The patient's prior knowledge and expectations of the clinician play a role in the unfolding of the transference. During the clinician's early years of training, these factors are less often significant, because the patient did not select the clinician personally. On the other hand, the "institutional transference" is of considerable importance, and the clinician can explore the reasons for the patient's selection of a particular outpatient facility. In addition, the patient usually has a mental image of a mental health professional. This pre-interview transference may be disclosed if the patient seems surprised by the clinician's appearance or remarks, "You don't look like a psychiatrist." The clinician could ask, "What did you expect a psychiatrist to be like?" If the patient replies, "Well, someone much older," the clinician might answer, "Would it be easier to speak to an older person?" The patient may indicate that he is actually relieved and that he had imagined the psychiatrist to be a more frightening figure. At times a patient enters the clinician's office and jokes, "Well, where are the guys with the white coats?" thereby revealing his fear of being considered crazy. He sees the clinician as a dangerous and authoritarian person.

In private practice, patients are usually referred to a specific clinician. The interviewer is interested to learn what the patient was told at the time of the referral. Was he given one name or a list of names? In the latter case, how did he decide which one to call first, and was the interviewer the first one he contacted? One patient may indicate that he was influenced by the location of the office, whereas in another situation the clinician's name may have suggested an ethnic background similar to his own.

The Interviewer's Expectations

The interviewer usually has some knowledge of the patient prior to their first meeting. This may have been provided by the person who referred the patient. Some clues about the patient have often been obtained directly by the clinician during the initial telephone call that led to the appointment.

Experienced clinicians have personal preferences concerning the amount of information they want from the referring source. Some prefer to learn as much as possible; others desire only the bare minimum, on the grounds that it allows them to interview with a fully open mind. Anytime the interviewer experiences a feeling of surprise when he meets his new patient, he must question himself. Was he misled about the patient by the person who referred him, or was his surprise due to some unrealistic anticipation of his own?

The Opening Phase

Meeting the Patient

The clinician obtains much information when he first meets a new patient. He can observe who, if anyone, has accompanied the patient and how the patient was passing the time while waiting for the interview to begin.

One interviewer begins by introducing himself; another prefers to address the patient by his name and then introduce himself. The latter technique will indicate that the clinician is expecting the patient, and most people like to be greeted by name. As a rule, social pleasantries such as "It is nice to meet you" are not warranted in the professional situation. However, if the patient is unduly anxious, the clinician might introduce a brief social comment. It is inappropriate to use most patients' first names except in the case of children or young teenagers. Such familiarity would put the patient in the "one down" position, unless the patient were also expected to use the clinician's first name.

Important clues to the conduct of the interview can often be obtained during these few moments of introduction. The patient's spontaneity and warmth may be revealed in his handshake or greeting. Patients who like direction and are eager to please ask where to sit and what to do with their coats. Hostile, competitive patients may sit in the chair that quite obviously is reserved for the interviewer. Suspicious patients might carefully glance around the office searching for "clues" about the clinician. The specific behavior of different patients is elaborated in the chapters in Part II.

Developing Rapport

The experienced interviewer learns enough about the patient during the initial greeting that he may appropriately vary the opening minutes of the interview according to the needs of the patient. The beginner usually develops a routine way of starting the interview and then attempts variations later in his training.

A suitable beginning is to ask the patient to be seated and then inquire, "What problem brings you here?" or "Could you tell me about your difficulty?" If the patient is likely to be a candidate for dynamic psychotherapy, it can be helpful to bring the therapeutic relationship in from the start: "How can I help you?" A less directive approach would be to ask the patient, "Where shall we start?" or "Where would you prefer to begin?" Sometimes a very anxious patient will speak first, inquiring, "Where shall I begin?" As indicated, the beginner will do better to reply, "Let's start with a discussion of your problem." After some years of experience, the clinician knows when the patient will continue easily without a reply and when to say, "Begin anywhere you like." Many interviewers begin by asking the patient's home address, telephone numbers, and billing address if that is different from the home address. Some interviewers continue further, obtaining other basic identifying data such as age, occupation, marital status and number of children, and names and ages of spouse and children and any other members of the household. This can be accomplished in 5 minutes and provides the interviewer with the cast of characters prior to moving on with the story. Next the interviewer asks about what problem has led to the patient's seeking a consultation. The interviewer may choose to postpone these questions, but sooner or later this information is needed. This can also be done at the end of the first transition period when the clinician leaves the topic of the chief complaint and present illness to learn more about the details of the patient's life. Both systems have their advantages and drawbacks. The most important factor is that the patient feel as comfortable as possible, and a comfortable interviewer is the single most important factor in facilitating that process.

Sullivan discussed the value of a summary statement about the referring person's communications concerning the patient or a restatement of what the clinician learned during the initial telephone conversation. It is comforting for the patient who is not self-referred to feel that the clinician already knows something about his problem. A presentation of all the details is likely to be harmful, because it will rarely seem completely accurate to the patient, and the interview gets under way with the patient defending himself from misunderstanding. General statements are preferable. For example, the clinician might say, "Dr. Jones has told me that you and your husband have had some difficulties" or "I understand that you have been depressed." Most patients will continue the story at this point. Occasionally, the patient may ask, "Didn't he tell you the whole story?" The interviewer could reply, "He went into some of the details, but I would like to hear more about it directly from you." If the patient has difficulty continuing, the clinician might remark sympathetically, "I know it is difficult to talk about some things." This gives the patient a feeling that the clinician understands him, but depending on how he chooses to interpret the remark, he might take it as permission to begin by discussing some less painful material.

In the event that the patient brings something with him to the interview, it will help the development of rapport to examine what the patient has brought. For example, one patient was referred for treatment by a psychologist who had tested him for career aptitude. The clinician refused to read the psychologist's report, and the patient was offended. Another clinician never asked about some artwork that a young woman had brought to show him. She failed to return for a second visit.

To establish rapport, the interviewer must communicate a feeling of understanding the patient. This is accomplished both by the clinician's attitude and by the expertise of his remarks. He does not wish to create the impression that he can read the patient's mind, but he does want the patient to realize that he has treated other people with emotional difficulties and that he understands them. This includes not only neurotic and psychotic symptoms but also ordinary problems in living. For example, if a harried housewife reveals that she has six children under the age of 10 and no household help, the interviewer might remark, "How do you manage?" The young clinician who has had little experience in life and has no imagination might ask, "Do you ever find your children a strain?" The successful interviewer will broaden his knowledge of life and human existence through the empathic experience associated with gaining an intimate understanding of the lives of so many others.

The clinician's interest helps the patient to talk. However, the more the interviewer speaks, the more the patient is concerned with what the interviewer wants to hear instead of what is on his own mind. On the other hand, if the clinician is unresponsive, the patient will be inhibited from revealing his feelings.

Some patients are reluctant to speak freely because they fear that the clinician might betray their confidence. The patient might say, "I don't want you to tell this to my wife" or "I hope you won't mention my homosexuality to my internist." The interviewer might reply, "Everything you tell me is in confidence, but it seems that you are particularly concerned about certain things." When this behavior occurs in later sessions, the patient's mistrust and fear of betrayal can be explored.

Sometimes a patient will ask, "Are you Freudian?" Usually this means, "Do I have to do all the talking and get little feedback?" In any event, the patient is not really interested in the clinician's theoretical orientation, and such questions require exploration of their meaning to the patient instead of a literal reply.

The Middle Phase

An abrupt transition is sometimes required after the patient has discussed the present illness. For example, the clinician can say, "Now I would like to learn more about you as a person," or "Can you tell me something about yourself other than the problems that brought you here?" The interviewer now devotes his attention to the history, filling in relevant information that has not yet been discussed. Just where to start depends on what aspects of the patient's life have already been revealed. Most patients talk about their current life before revealing their past. If the patient has not already mentioned his age; marital status; length of marriage; ages and names of spouse, children, and parents; occupational history; description of current living circumstances; and so on, the interviewer can ask for these details. It is preferable to obtain as much of this information during the description of the present illness as possible. Rather than following the outline used for the organization of the written record, it is much easier for the clinician to draw conclusions about the significance and interrelationship of these data if the patient offers them in his own way. For instance, if the interviewer asks, "How do your symptoms interfere with your life?" the patient may provide information pertaining to any or all of the topics just mentioned.

It is a mistake to permit the first interview to end without knowing the patient's marital status, occupation, and so forth. These basic identifying data are the skeleton of the patient's life on which all the other information is placed. When this material does not emerge spontaneously during the discussion of the present illness, it is often possible to obtain much of it with one or two questions. The interviewer could inquire, "Tell me about your present life." The patient may then interpret the question as he sees fit, or he may ask, "Do you mean, am I married and what sort of work do I do, things like that?" The interviewer merely has to nod and then see if the patient omits anything, at which time he can point out that the patient has not mentioned thus and such. Most patients will provide more useful information if they are given a topic to discuss rather than a list of questions that can be answered briefly. Specific exceptions are discussed in Chapter 14, "The Psychotic Patient," and Chapter 16, "The Cognitively Impaired Patient."

The number of possibilities in the middle portion of the interview are infinite, and thus it is impossible to provide precise instructions about which choices to make. For example, the patient might indicate that she is married and has three children, that her father is dead, and that her mother lives with her. Experience, skill, and personal style all influence what the interviewer will do now. He could be quiet and permit the patient to continue, or he could ask about the marriage, the children, the mother, or the father's death or ask the patient, "Could you elaborate?" without indicating a specific choice. The feeling tone of the patient's description is another important aspect that could be focused on. If she seems anxious and pressured, the interviewer might remark, "It sounds as if you have your hands full." In such a case, some clinicians would argue in favor of one approach over the others. However, we feel that there is no single right answer, and we would probably make different choices with different patients and even with the same patient on different occasions.

Most leads provided by the patient should be followed up at the time of presentation. This gives smooth continuity to the interview even though there may be numerous topical digressions. To continue with the last vignette, let us suppose that the patient goes on to reveal that her mother has only been living with her family for a year. It would be logical to assume that the patient's father had died at that time, and therefore the interviewer might ask, "Is that when your father died?" If the patient replies, "Yes," the clinician might assume that the patient's parents had lived together until that time, but rather than jump to false conclusions, it is better to ask, "How did it happen that your mother came to live with you after your father's death?" The patient might surprise the interviewer by saying, "You see, Mother and Dad were divorced 10 years ago, and she moved in with my brother's family, but now that Dad is gone, my brother moved to Chicago to take over his business. Mother's friends are all in this area and she didn't want to move to Chicago, so she moved in with us." The interviewer might ask, "What was the effect on your family?" or "How did your husband feel about this arrangement?" At the same time, the interviewer notices that the patient did not provide any information about the circumstances of the father's death. When the patient "runs down" on the present topic, the clinician could reopen that area.

Now that the interviewer has some ideas concerning the present illness and the patient's current life situation, he might turn his attention to what sort of person the patient is. A question such as "What sort of person are you?" will come as a surprise to most people, since they are not accustomed to thinking of themselves in that fashion. Some patients will respond easily, and others may become uncomfortable or offer concrete details that reiterate facts of their current life situation such as, "Well, I'm an accountant" or "I'm just a housewife." Nevertheless, such replies provide both phenomenological and dynamic information. The first reply was made by an obsessive-compulsive man who was preoccupied with numbers and facts, not merely in his job but also in his human relationships. What he was telling the interviewer was "I am first and always an accountant, and in fact, I can never cease being an accountant." The second reply was offered by a phobic woman who had secret ambitions for a career. She was letting the clinician know that she had a deprecatory view of women and, in particular, of women who are housewives. Like the first patient, she was never able to forget herself.

Often the patient's self-perception will vary depending on the situation. Consider the businessman who is a forceful leader in his job but is timid and passive at home or the laboratory scientist who is active and creative in his work but feels shy and reserved in social situations. Then there is the man who is a sexual athlete with numerous affairs who perceives himself as inadequate and ineffectual at work. The interviewer does not elicit all of the material pertinent to the patient's self-perception in one interview. However, a more complete picture gradually emerges. Another patient revealed in the third interview, "There is something I haven't told you that really bothers me. I have a terrible temper, often with a member of the family." The interviewer replied, "Could you give me the details of some recent examples?"

Other questions that pertain to the patient's view of himself include "Tell me the things you like about yourself"; "What would you consider your greatest assets?"; or "What things bring you the most pleasure?" The interviewer might ask the patient to describe himself as he appears to others, and to himself, in the major areas of his life, including family, work, social situations, sex, and situations of stress. It is often revealing to ask the patient to describe a typical 24-hour day. The patient may even experience some increase in his self-awareness while reflecting on this question. Topics and questions that have a direct bearing on the present illness and current life situation are most meaningful to the patient.

Depending on the amount of time available and whether there will be more than one interview, the clinician will plan his inquiry into the patient's past. The question of which past issues are most significant varies with the problems of the patient and the nature of the consultation.

At various times during the interview, the patient may become uncomfortable with the material he is discussing. This is due not only to his wish to be accepted by the interviewer but also, and often more importantly, to his fear concerning partial insights into himself. For example, the patient may pause and remark, "I know lots of people who do the same thing"; "Isn't that normal?"; or "Do you think I'm a bad father?" Certain patients may require reassurance in order to become engaged in the interview, whereas others will profit by the clinician's asking, "What did you have in mind?" or "Just what are you concerned about?"

Stimulating the patient's curiosity is a fundamental technique in all interviews aimed at uncovering deeper feelings. Basically, the clinician uses his own genuine curiosity to awaken the patient's interest in himself. The question of where the clinician can best direct his curiosity is related to the principles of interpretation discussed earlier in the chapter. In summary, the curiosity is not directed at the most deeply repressed or most highly defended issues but rather at the most superficial layer of the patient's conflict. For instance, a young man describes how he first experienced his panic attack after he saw a man collapse in a railroad station. Later he reveals that he often experiences attacks in situations in which he feels that he is winning an argument with someone he considers an inferior. The interviewer would not express curiosity about an unconscious wish on the part of the patient to destroy his father, whom he considered passive and helpless, but would instead direct his curiosity to situations that seem to be exceptions for the patient. Thus he might ask, "You mentioned that on some occasions, winning an argument doesn't seem to bother you; I wonder what could be different about those situations?"

The clinician's expressed curiosity about concealed motives of both the patient and his loved ones is seldom therapeutic in the first few interviews because it is too threatening to the patient's defenses. For example, the clinician might say, "I wonder why your husband spends more time at his office than is necessary?" Although the interviewer has the right to be curious about this phenomenon, a direct question could be construed by the patient as an accusation or innuendo.

The Closing Phase

The closing phase of the initial interview varies in length, but 10 minutes is generally sufficient. The interviewer might indicate that time is drawing to a close by saying, "We have to stop soon; are there some questions that you would like to ask?" If the patient has no questions, the interviewer could comment, "Would you suggest something you think we should discuss further?" Most often the patient will raise questions pertaining to his illness and treatment.

Each person who consults an expert expects and is entitled to an expert opinion about his situation as well as recommendations for therapy or some other helpful advice. It was once customary to tell the patient as little as possible about his diagnosis and the therapeutic rationale of the treatment plan. In recent years, the publication of information through the Internet and lay press as well as changes in the training of clinicians has led to a better-informed and more questioning public. Psychiatry particularly has been the recipient of such attention, and many patients have questions about psychotherapy, various drug therapies, cognitive-behavioral therapy, and psychoanalysis. Although the patient has a right to receive direct answers about such issues at the completion of the consultation, the interviewer can assume that these questions will reveal important transference attitudes as well.

Although it is artificial to distinguish between diagnostic and therapeutic interviews, it is expected that clinicians will present the patient with a clinical formulation and available treatments or other plans when the consultation is completed. Usually this presentation occurs at the end of the second or third interview, but in some cases it may require weeks of exploratory meetings. Beginning therapists often neglect this phase, and much to their surprise, a patient they have been seeing for 6 months will suddenly ask, "Why am I still coming?" or say, "I don't think I need to see you anymore!" Such neglect is disrespectful of the patient's right to question the clinician's prescription and to participate in formulating a treatment plan and selecting a therapist. The patient is entitled to state his own goals for treatment. He may only desire symptomatic improvement, and this may be good judgment; there are patients whose basic character structure is best left alone. An example is the elderly patient who has had a successful life but recently developed panic attacks who asks for medication to control the attacks and does not want exploratory psychotherapy.

This phase of the interview provides a useful opportunity for the clinician to uncover resistances and to alter his treatment plan accordingly. Although the clinician is the expert, his recommendations cannot be handed down like royal decrees. Often the clinician must modify his treatment plan as he learns more about the patient. By presenting a treatment plan in a stepwise fashion, the interviewer can discover in what areas the patient has questions, confusion, or disagreement. This cannot happen if the clinician makes a speech.

If the consultation is limited to one interview, more of that interview must be devoted to such matters than if a second or third meeting can be arranged. The clinician often tries to avoid giving the patient a formal diagnostic label. Such terms have little use for the patient and may be quite harmful, because the interviewer may be unaware of the meaning that the patient or his family attaches to them. The patient often provides clues to the proper terms to use in giving the formulation. One patient acknowledges a "psychological problem"; another says, "I realize it's something emotional" or "I know I haven't completely grown up" or "I realize it isn't right for me to have these fears." Although the patient's statement may have been made earlier in the session, the clinician can utilize it as a springboard for his own formulation, provided the patient truly believes what he is saying. This is not the case with the psychosomatic patient who says, "I know it is all in my mind, doctor."

The clinician might begin, "As you have already said, you do have a psychological problem." He might refer to what he considers the chief symptoms and indicate that they are all related and part of the same condition. He might separate acute problems from those that are chronic and concentrate first on treatment for the acute ones. Because it is not a good idea to overwhelm the patient with a comprehensive statement of all his pathology, the formulation should be confined to the major disturbance. For example, in the case of a young man who has difficulty getting along with authority figures, including his father, the interviewer would state, "It appears that you do have a problem getting along with your father, which has influenced your attitude toward all figures of authority."

In the current era, the patient is often caught in a dilemma. He may have insurance that will provide support for treatment, but in order to receive such benefits he must provide consent for the clinician to communicate with the insurer. Current law requires the medical profession to provide the patient with a written statement regarding his right to privacy. Any information the clinician provides to a third party, whether verbally or in writing, should be discussed with the patient before it is given to others. For a discussion of diagnostic codes and procedures, the reader is referred to DSM-5.

Now that the clinician and patient are both clear on what they believe constitutes the problem, it is time to consider the subject of treatment. The clinician may be confident of his opinion without making a dogmatic pronouncement. For example, he might state, "In my experience, the most effective approach is..." or "A variety of therapies are used for this condition, but I would suggest..." This response pays proper respect to the fact that whatever the interviewer's therapeutic orientation, the patient should be told that there are other treatments available. Often the patient will bring up a question he has kept back pertaining to the effectiveness of one of the other therapies.

It is rarely useful in analytically oriented psychotherapy to give the patient lengthy prepared speeches about the method of treatment, how psychotherapy works, or free association. However, the less sophisticated patient does require some preparation. This may involve an explanation that the interviewer is interested in all of his thoughts and feelings, whether or not they seem important. It takes a long time and a great deal of trust before a patient can associate freely. Some patients may ask, "Shall I just talk?" or "Shall I just say anything that comes to mind?" The interviewer can answer such questions affirmatively.

Frequently the patient will inquire, "How long will treatment take?" or "It isn't serious, is it?" Once again, the best indication is found in the patient's own productions. It is usually helpful, when acute symptoms can be differentiated from chronic ones, to point out that more recent symptoms are usually the first to improve and that problems of long duration often require long treatment. Sometimes the patient will ask about a more specific period of time. It is unfair to make misleading statements concerning the duration of therapy in order to reassure the patient. Few patients respond favorably to learning in the first interview that they require years of treatment. The patient's concern with the duration of treatment is not entirely a manifestation of resistance or the desire for a magical cure. Therapy is costly in terms of both expense and time involved that interferes with other activities in the patient's life. If there is a time limit on the duration of therapy, as is often the case in clinics, or if the clinician is not going to be available as long as the patient expects treatment to last, the patient should be told so at once. Also, the patient deserves to know from the outset if the consultant will not be the treating clinician. This is the time in the interview to consider the financial aspects of treatment, which were discussed earlier in the chapter.

If the patient was upset during the interview, the closing phase also serves as an opportunity for him to pull himself together again prior to leaving the clinician's office and returning to the outside world.

Some patients ask about prognosis, either seriously or in a pseudo-jest. Common examples are "Well, is there any hope?"; "Have you ever treated anyone like me?"; or "Is there anything I can do to speed things up?" The clinician is advised to be careful in dealing with these questions. The patient may not have revealed all of his problems. In cases in which statements about prognosis are indicated, such as with the depressed patient, the clinician's encouraging reassurance is of great importance.

Before the interview is terminated, the interviewer can set the time and date of the next appointment. The end of the session is indicated by the clinician's saying, "Let's stop now"; "We can go on from here next time"; or "Our time is up for now." It is common courtesy to arise and escort the patient to the door.

Occasionally an interview must be terminated prematurely because the clinician receives an emergency call. This is a more common experience for resident psychiatrists who are on call. The clinician can explain the situation to the patient and arrange to make up the time on another occasion. A related but more infrequent occurrence is that the patient gets angry and leaves before the session is over. The clinician can attempt to stop the patient verbally by saying firmly, "Just a minute!" If the patient waits, he can continue, "If you are angry with me, it is better that we discuss it now." The clinician neither rises from his chair nor indicates that he condones the patient's action.

Later Interviews

Often the consultation is completed within two interviews, but it may take longer. The second interview is best scheduled from 2 days to a week later. A single meeting with the patient permits only a cross-sectional study. If several days are allowed to intervene before the next session, the clinician will be able to learn about the patient's reactions to the first visit. In this way he can determine how the patient will handle treatment. There is also an opportunity for the patient to correct any misinformation that he provided in the first meeting. One way to begin the second interview is for the clinician to comment, "I suspect that you have thought about some of the things we discussed last time" or "What thoughts have you had about our meeting?" When the patient answers "Yes" to the former, the clinician might say, "I would like to hear about that" or "Let's start there today." If the patient says "No," the clinician might raise his eyebrows questioningly and wait for the patient to continue. There are several common patterns of response. The patient might have pursued the self-inquiry that began in the previous meeting, often providing additional pertinent history related to a previously raised point. He might have reflected further on a question or on suggestions of the clinician and come to some greater understanding. Such activity is subtly rewarded by interviewers who in one way or another let the patient know that he is on the right track. This response has more important prognostic significance for analytically oriented psychotherapy than whether the patient felt better or worse after the session.

Another group of responses have more negative implications. The patient might have thought about what he reported the first time and decided that it was wrong, that he did not understand why the interviewer had asked about a certain topic, or that the clinician did not understand him. He might state that he had ruminated about something the interviewer had said and felt depressed. Frequently these responses occur when the patient feels guilty after talking "too freely" in the first interview. He then either withdraws or becomes angry with the interviewer. In this patient's mind, criticizing his loved ones or expressing strong emotions in the clinician's presence is personally humiliating.

While on the topic of the patient's reactions to the first interview, the clinician might inquire whether the patient discussed the session with anyone else. If he did, the interviewer will be enlightened by learning with whom the patient spoke and the content of the conversation. After this topic has been explored, the clinician will continue the interview. There are no set rules concerning the questions that are better put off until the second meeting. Whatever inquiries the clinician senses to be most embarrassing for this patient may be postponed unless the patient has already approached this material himself or is consciously preoccupied with it. If the interviewer asks about dreams in the first interview, the patient will frequently report dreams in the second meeting. It is useful to inquire directly about such dreams, because they reveal the patient's unconscious reactions to the clinician as well as showing key emotional problems and dominant transference attitudes.

CONCLUSION

This chapter considers the broader aspects and general techniques of the psychiatric interview. Subsequent chapters discuss specific variations that are determined either by the type of patient or by the clinical setting of the interview. It must be emphasized that real people do not fit into the discrete diagnostic categories outlined in this book. Every person is unique, integrating a variety of pathological and healthy mechanisms in a characteristic way. In discussing different clinical syndromes, we are not merely considering patients who fall into the associated diagnostic categories. For example, obsessive defenses will be encountered in anxious, histrionic, depressive, paranoid, cognitively impaired, psychotic, and antisocial patients and may be integrated into neurotic or psychotic patterns. The techniques of working with a patient who has a given cluster of defenses will be similar regardless of his diagnosis. The reader is left with the task of resynthesizing the material that has been separated for pedagogic purposes. In any given interview the patient will utilize defensive patterns that are described in several different chapters, and he may shift his defenses during the course of treatment or even within a single interview.

The interviewer may function effectively without having a conceptualized understanding of resistance, transference, countertransference, and so forth. Furthermore, intellectual mastery of these concepts does not itself produce clinical proficiency. However, an organized framework is necessary for the systematic study and conceptualization of the factors that contribute to the success or failure of an interview. A theoretical understanding of psychodynamics is vital if the student plans to study his own intuitive functioning and thereby improve his clinical skill. It will allow each interview to contribute to the professional growth of the clinician.

CHAPTER 2

GENERAL PRINCIPLES OF PSYCHODYNAMICS

Psychiatry is the medical specialty that studies disorders of behavior and experience, both affective and cognitive. Like other branches of medicine, it considers 1) the phenomenology of the normal and abnormal, 2) systems of classification and epidemiological information, 3) etiology, 4) diagnosis, and 5) prevention and treatment. Because human behavior is complex, psychiatry draws on many fields of knowledge, ranging from biochemistry, genetics, and neuroscience to psychology, anthropology, and sociology, in order to understand its subject matter.

The interview is a basic technique of psychiatry and most other clinical specialties. Other methods may also be employed, such as biological or psychological tests, symptom rating scales, or pharmacological or physical treatments, but even these usually occur within the context of a clinical interview. The psychiatric interview is by far the most important diagnostic tool of today's psychiatrist. With our current knowledge, physiological and biochemical studies of behavior offer little assistance in understanding interviews, whereas psychodynamic concepts have proved valuable.

In the psychodynamic frame of reference, behavior is viewed as the product of hypothetical mental processes, wishes, fears, emotions, internal representations, and fantasies and the psychological processes that regulate, control, and channel them. Subjective experience, thoughts, and feelings are of central importance, and overt behavior is understood as the product of inner psychological processes that can be inferred from the patient's words and acts.

A psychodynamic formulation offers a description of mental experience, underlying psychological processes, their hypothetical origins, and their clinical significance. It provides a rational basis for the patient. As long as the interview is the central tool of psychiatry, psychodynamics will remain an essential basic science. At present it also provides the most comprehensive and clinically useful understanding of human motivation, pathology, pathogenesis, and treatment of many disorders.

This chapter presents the basic assumptions of psychodynamics and psychoanalysis, the school of psychodynamics started by Sigmund Freud that has been the source of most of our knowledge and has almost become synonymous with psychodynamics. In recent years alternative psychodynamic models have been found clinically useful and also are described briefly. It discusses basic psychodynamic models of psychopathology, various types of pathological formations, and those psychoanalytic concepts that are most crucial in understanding the interview. Space does not permit a complete consideration of psychoanalysis, which includes a theory of personality development, a technique of treatment, specific methods for obtaining information about the psychodynamic determinants of behavior, and a metapsychology or series of abstract hypotheses about the basis of mental functioning and the source of human motives. These aspects of psychoanalysis go beyond the scope of a book on interviewing and are discussed in the books on psychoanalytic theory listed in the bibliography at the end of the book.

BASIC ASSUMPTIONS OF PSYCHODYNAMICS AND PSYCHOANALYSIS

Motivation

Behavior is seen as purposeful or goal-directed and as a product of hypothetical forces—drives, urges, impulses, or motives. *Motives* are represented subjectively by thoughts and feelings and objectively by a tendency toward certain patterns of action. Hunger, sex, aggression, and the desire to be cared for are examples of important motives.

The early years of psychoanalysis were extensively concerned with the origins of basic human motives and, specifically, with developing a model that would relate them to their biological roots. Freud used the German term *trieb*, which has usually been translated as "instinct," to refer to these basic drives, which were assumed to involve a form of "psychic energy." This drive theory was helpful in focusing on the complex shifts or "vicissitudes" in motivations that occur in the course of development, and it was a useful framework for understanding the psychodynamic basis of neurotic behavior. For example, the idea of a sexual drive with many and varied manifestations makes it possible to conceptualize the links among hysterical seizures, sexual inhibitions, and infantile sexual behavior. However, in recent years, some aspects of psychoanalytic drive theory have been criticized as tautological and unscientific hypotheses that cannot be tested or refuted. At the same time the attention of psychoanalysts has shifted from the origins of basic human motives to their psychological manifestations and the various means by which they are expressed. To many, the biological basis of motivations is a physiological problem that cannot be explored by psychoanalysis, a psychological method. In any event, it is an issue that has little direct bearing on the interview. By the time a child is able to talk, he has strong psychological motives that will be present for the rest of his life, motives represented by the wishes that form the basis of our psychodynamic understanding. The extent to which their origin is constitutional or acquired is of great theoretical, but little immediate clinical, importance.

Dynamic Unconscious

Many of the important inner determinants of behavior occur outside the individual's subjective awareness and are normally not recognized by him. The existence of unconscious mental activity was apparent long before Freud—events that are forgotten but later remembered are obviously stored in some form during the interim. However, this would be of little clinical importance were it not for the dynamic significance of these unconscious mental processes—that is, the great influence they exert on behavior and particularly the important role they play in determining both pathological and normal behavior.

The early history of psychoanalysis is a record of the progressive discovery of the role of unconscious mental processes in determining almost every area of human behavior—neurotic symptoms, dreams, jokes, parapraxes, artistic creations, myths, religion, character structure, and so forth.

Psychic Determinism

Science in general—and late-nineteenth-century positivist science in particular—views all phenomena as determined in accordance with "laws" of nature. If one knows these laws, and the initial conditions, one can predict subsequent conditions. However, commonsense psychology and the romantic tradition largely exempted subjective experience from such determinism. One of Freud's central contributions was to apply strict determinism to the realm of subjective experience. Mental events were determined and were set in motion by prior mental events (not simply by neural events, as in currently popular neurobiological reductionist models). The challenge for psychoanalysis as a science was to discover the psychological laws that governed these processes and to develop the methods necessary to apply them to our understanding of human mental life.

Regulatory Principles

Behavior is regulated in accordance with certain basic principles. These organize the expression of specific motives and determine priority when they come into conflict with each other or with external reality. For example, someone may feel angry or violent, but his awareness of the painful consequences of a direct expression of these feelings leads to a modification of his behavior. This illustrates the *pleasure–pain principle* (or simply, "pleasure principle"), which states that behavior is designed to pursue pleasure and to avoid pain. Although this seems obvious, much of the behavior that psychiatry studies appears to violate this principle. Pathological or maladaptive behavior frequently seems destined to lead to pain, and often even a casual observer will tell the patient that he is acting "foolishly" and that he would be much happier if he simply changed his ways. Every paranoid person has been told that his suspiciousness is self-defeating, every obsessive that his rituals are a waste of time, and every phobic that there is no reason to be frightened. Perhaps one of the major contributions of dynamic psychiatry has been to demonstrate that these apparent paradoxes are really confirmations of the pleasure principle once the underlying unconscious emotional logic is revealed, and that even the individual with an apparently inexplicable desire to be beaten or tortured can be seen to be following the basic pleasure principle when his unconscious wishes and fears are understood.

Each individual has his own personal hierarchy of pleasure and pain. For example, people who have been raised in painful circumstances develop a view of life as a series of inevitable choices among painful alternatives. Their pursuit of the lesser of two evils conforms to the pleasure principle. The self-defeating personality provides an illustration. The little girl who was scolded more than she was praised received love and affection when she was sick or in danger from the same parent who scolded her. Scolding thus became the symbol of love. Years later, her predilection for abusive relationships seems incomprehensible until one recognizes their unconscious meaning of love, affection, and security.

With maturity, the capacity for abstract symbolic thought provides the basis for mental representations of the distant future. The elementary pleasure–pain principle, rooted in the immediate present, is modified as reason dictates that one tolerate current discomfort in order to achieve future greater pleasure. This is called the *reality principle*, which is basically a modification of the pleasure principle. However, at an unconscious level, much behavior continues to be regulated by the more primitive pleasure principle.

Fixation and Regression

Childhood experiences are critical in determining later adult behavior. Neurotic psychopathology can often be understood as the persistence or reemergence of fragments or patterns of behavior that were prevalent and often adaptive during childhood but that are maladaptive in the adult. *Fixation* describes the failure to mature beyond a given developmental stage, whereas *regression* refers to the return to an earlier adaptive mode after one has progressed beyond it. Both are selective processes and affect only certain aspects of mental functioning. The result is that the neurotic individual has a mixture of age-appropriate and more childish behavior patterns. For example, his cognitive functioning might be unimpaired, but his sexual fantasy life may be immature. Of course, psychological development is complex, and even the most disturbed adult patient has many aspects of mature functioning, whereas healthy people have many aspects of behavior that are characteristic of earlier developmental stages. For example, all adults have a proclivity for wishful or magical thinking. Rituals related to good luck, such as "knocking on wood" or avoiding the number 13, are everyday examples.

Fixation and regression can affect motives, ego functions, conscience mechanisms, or any combination of these. Often the most important marker of pathology, especially in children, is not the extent of the regression but the unevenness with which it has affected some psychological processes while sparing others. Regression is universal during illness, stress, sleep, intense pleasure, love, strong religious feeling, artistic creativity, and many other unusual states, and it is not always pathological. Creativity, sexual pleasure, and spiritual experiences all involve regressive aspects, as suggested by the concept of "adaptive regression in the service of the ego." In fact, the capacity to regress and to make adaptive use of regressive experiences is an essential prerequisite for creative thinking and empathic understanding and thus also for conducting a psychiatric interview. To be able to feel what the patient feels while at the same time observing and studying that feeling is the essence of the psychiatrist's skills and is an example of regression in the service of the most mature aspects of the personality.

Emotions

Emotions are states of the organism that involve both the mind and the body. They include characteristic physiological responses; subjective affects, thoughts, and fantasies; modes of interpersonal relations; and styles of overt action. Anxiety, a key emotion in the development of psychopathology, serves as an example. The anxious individual is aware of inner feelings of diffuse, unpleasant anticipatory fear or dread. His cognitive functioning is impaired, and he is likely to be preoccupied with fantasies of magical protection, retaliation, or escape. His overt behavior is dominated by his own characteristic response to threat—fight, flight, or helpless surrender. There are alterations in pulse, blood pressure, respiratory rate, gastrointestinal functioning, bladder control, endocrine function, muscle tone, the electrical activity of the brain, and other physiological functions. No one of these phenomena is itself the emotion, but the syndrome as a whole constitutes the organismic state that we call *anxiety*. Emotions proliferate and differentiate with development, so that the adult has a much larger and more subtle array of emotions than the young child. These play a critical role in the development of the personality as a whole, and especially of symptoms, which will be explored in greater detail later.

Fantasies of Danger

The newborn infant has no internal psychological conflict about seeking pleasure from drive gratification; it is only that he needs the understanding and assistance of a caretaker in order to do so. When this is available, he is "as happy as a baby." However, frustration is inevitable regardless of the caretaker's skill. Overstimulation can interfere with pleasure seeking, the child may be separated from the caretaker, or the caretaker may be experienced as disinterested or hostile, and as development proceeds, the child may come to fear loss of pleasure-seeking capacity or experiences of inner psychological anguish in the form of shame or guilt. In time virtually every wish is accompanied by one of the fears that develop in the context of the child–caretaker relationship. The result is that, in the adult, we rarely see pure wishes or pure fears but rather conflicts between wishes and the fears that accompany them, with the former sometimes and the latter usually unconscious.

Representations

Subjective experience involves patterns, images, or representations as well as drives or wishes and emotions or feelings. Foremost among these are representations of one's self and of important others such as parents or primary caretakers. Current developmental theory suggests that these self and other representations differentiate out of an original amorphous subjectivity—that, in Winnicott's words, there is no such thing as a baby but rather from the beginning a mother–baby constellation. The representation of the self evolves throughout development and is a core feature of the personality, whereas the representations of others in relation to the self also evolve, are shaped and refined, and become the templates of the various transference phenomena that are central to psychodynamic thinking and that are discussed throughout this book. Whereas Freud's original hypothesis placed drives in a central position and viewed representation born of self and of others as secondary, several post-Freudian thinkers have reversed this model, with self and object representations seen as central and drives as secondary.

Objects

The term *object* seems like the wrong word to refer to other people, or even the inner mental representations of other people, as is its meaning in psychodynamics. However, it makes sense in terms of the history of psychodynamic thinking. After an initial interest in neurosis as the result of childhood trauma, Freud's attention shifted to the centrality of drives and to psychological development as largely based on the maturation of innate drive predispositions, with the environment serving as the context for this maturation. Drives generally required some aspect of the external world for their gratification—hence their "object"—and this was often (but not always) another person—for example, a mother or a lover. The emphasis, however, was not on the human characteristics of the object but rather on its drive-gratifying potential. However, in time a number of psychoanalysts, especially those who worked with children, recognized that significant others in the child's life were more than targets: they made a difference. The term *object* stuck, but it was increasingly recognized that the object had an active role in shaping the child's growth and experience and that the maturational unfolding of innate predisposition was part of an interactive developmental process to which objects made important contributions.

Today some schools of psychodynamics continue to see drives as central, whereas others focus on relations between the child (or later adult) and important objects. Each group recognizes that both are aspects of any full account of personality. Conceptual models based on object relations have been particularly influential in the study of infants and children, of more serious psychopathology such as psychotic and borderline conditions, and of psychotherapy and interviewing, with their inescapable attention to the relationship between individuals.

Freud's original notion was that patients suffered from *reminiscences*—memories of earlier pathogenic experiences. He quickly decided, on the basis of his clinical experience, that these memories stemmed from childhood and were primarily sexual. Many of his patients had reported memories, often hazy, partial, or fragmented, of what seemed to be childhood sexual experiences—traumas—that Freud believed to be at the core of their neurotic symptoms. However, the nature of the memories, their omnipresence, and his discovery that at least some of them had to be "false" led to a basic revision of his theory beginning in 1897. He still believed that his patients suffered from memories, but no longer from memories of "real" events. Rather, they suffered from memories of childhood fantasies, fantasies that had the dynamic power of psychic reality and were rooted in the hitherto unrecognized psychosexual life of children. From that point on, psychodynamics was no longer primarily about the representation of external events; it was increasingly about the internal predisposition to formulate one's experience of the external world in terms of wishes, fears, and fantasies. The therapeutic process continued to emphasize the recovery of repressed memories, but these were now memories of fantasies, of subjective experience, rather than memories of the external events of childhood. As a corollary, psychoanalytic interest in developmental psychology continued, but the focus shifted to include not only how the growing child interacts with the world but also how the child's fantasies unfold and how they influence the processing and recording of interactions with the world.

Contemporary psychodynamic thinking, like Freud's, is interested in childhood. However, in working with adult patients it recognizes that it has no direct access to the "facts" of childhood, and indeed that even if it did, they might not be very useful. Rather, it is interested in the adult patient's memories, beliefs, and fantasies about childhood, both unconscious and conscious. It recognizes that, like all memories, these are contemporary constructions, or perhaps reconstructions—the adult reworking of the adolescent reworking of the childhood reworking of the infantile interpretation of the experience. These memories are dynamically powerful, and one way of understanding the mechanism of action of psychodynamic treatment is that it uncovers them; explores them; understands the extent to which they are creations influenced by the patient's developmental stage, major conflicts, and character structure rather than veridical copies of reality; and therefore recognizes that although they are memories they can be changed. In effect, the treatment succeeds to the extent that the patient can change his history, or at least loosen the grip that the particular version of his history that has controlled him continues to exert on his life.

The psychodynamic psychotherapist's interest is not simply in the events of childhood but much more in the memories that adults have of childhood, the memories that serve as the templates for their neurotic patterns and transference responses. For the most part, in all but the most disturbed patients, these memories are compatible with what "really" happened, but they are only one of the many possible versions of what "really" happened. The well-educated therapist knows something about what developmental psychologists have learned about childhood and even more about the impact of development on the recording of childhood memories and the kinds of transformations that occur with each subsequent developmental step. He knows the familiar narratives of childhood, the memories that are frequently associated with specific syndromes or character types, and also knows that when these are transformed into hypotheses about developmental dynamics, although in theory they may be testable, for the most part they have not yet been tested. However, he further knows that their clinical value and their therapeutic leverage depend not on their historical validity but rather on their fit with the subjective mental lives of patients and their ability to facilitate the patients' reformulation of their personal histories.

PSYCHODYNAMICS OF PSYCHOPATHOLOGICAL CONDITIONS

Normality and Pathology: The Nature of Neurotic Behavior

There are no generally accepted definitions of the terms *normal* and *pathological* or *health* and *disease*, and yet the daily practice of medicine requires frequent decisions based on these concepts. *Psychopathology* refers to behavior that is less than optimally adaptive for a given individual at a given stage of his life and in a given setting. Psychodynamics studies the mental processes that underlie all behavior, adaptive and maladaptive, healthy and pathological. There is, of course, psychopathology that cannot be understood in psychodynamic terms alone—the automatic behavior of a psychomotor seizure and the hallucinations that result from taking a psychedelic drug are examples. Psychodynamics may help to understand the content but has little to do with the form of such behavior. The description of a given behavior as resulting from the resolution of an inner conflict or as the product of mental mechanisms of defense does not distinguish whether it is normal or pathological. The critical question is whether the individual, in resolving his conflict, has unnecessarily impaired his capacity to adapt to his environment or interfered with his capacity for pleasure. Everyone has inner psychological conflicts, and everyone responds to the anxiety that they evoke by the use of mental mechanisms. A discussion of the psychodynamics of a piece of behavior is independent of whether it is normal or pathological. This is somewhat more complex in practice because some psychodynamic constellations and some mental mechanisms are more often associated with psychopathology. In general, any defense that threatens the individual's contact with reality, the maintenance of interpersonal relationships, or the possibility of pleasurable affects is likely to be pathological. However, there is no defense mechanism that is never found in healthy individuals.

In clinical practice, the physician is not primarily concerned with assessing whether the patient's interview behavior is healthy or sick. He is more interested in what it means and what it tells him about the patient. Psychiatrists are frequently called upon to interview, and even to treat, healthy individuals who may be coping with major crises or facing extraordinary circumstances. Knowledge of psychodynamics is vital for the skillful conduct and thorough understanding of interviews with these psychiatrically normal individuals. However, it is important for every clinical interviewer to study psychopathology as well as psychodynamics, not only to understand interviews with patients who are not psychiatrically normal but also to understand psychodynamic principles, which are learned most easily from individuals with emotional difficulties.

The Structure of Neurotic Pathology

Basic motives, such as sex, aggression, the quest for power, or dependency, impel the individual toward behavior that would lead to their gratification. However, because of internal psychological conflict, the expression of this behavior may be partially or completely blocked, with a resulting increase of intrapsychic tension. The opposing forces in this conflict result from the anticipation of both the pleasant and the unpleasant or dangerous consequences of acting on the motive involved. In the simplest situation, common in childhood, external danger is real and its perception leads to an emotional state, fear. For example, a boy may feel angry and want to attack the adult whom he feels is treating him unfairly; however, his fear of retaliation will lead him to control and suppress his rage. In this example, the outcome is highly adaptive, and it makes little difference whether the perception of danger and the resulting inhibition of the impulse occurred consciously or unconsciously.

The situation becomes more complex when the dangerous consequences that are feared are neither real nor immediate but rather fantasies, imaginary fears that have resulted from formative experiences in childhood—when the shadow of the past falls on the present. Such fears are almost always unconscious, and since they result from dynamically significant unconscious memories rather than conscious current perception, they are not easily corrected even by repeated exposure to a contradictory reality. It is difficult to unlearn attitudes that are rooted in unconscious mental processes. The fear of an unconsciously imagined danger, called *anxiety*, leads to an inhibition of the relevant motive. In this case, the inhibition is not a response to the real world in which the individual is currently living and therefore is more likely to be maladaptive or pathological. However, there are exceptions. Inhibitions of basic motives that stem from unconscious fantasies of imagined dangers may be highly adaptive if the original unconscious fantasies themselves developed in a situation that is closely analogous to the individual's current reality. In simple terms, if one's current situation is similar to the world of one's childhood, seemingly neurotic patterns may actually be adaptive.

An example will illustrate this. A man who has warm and loving feelings toward his wife has unconscious fears of being castrated should he participate in adult sexual activity. A potency disturbance and inhibition of sexual impulses result, an obviously maladaptive solution in his current life, however understandable it might have been in the childhood setting in which it originally developed. Another man who is momentarily sexually attracted to a woman at a party loses interest when he learns that she is his boss's wife. This may also be the result of an inhibition of sexual impulses based on the unconscious fear of castration, but the result is now adaptive, because the setting closely parallels that of his fantasy, which stems from early childhood, when the expression of such impulses was clearly limited.

The anxiety that results from a conflict between a wish and an unconscious fear is one of the most common symptoms of psychological distress. It is the dominant feature of the classic anxiety disorder and is also found in many of the symptomatic neuroses. Patients may become anxious about the possibility of future anxiety—that is, "anticipatory anxiety," particularly characteristic of phobic disorders. They also may experience brief, circumscribed episodes of severe anxiety, "panic," with no conscious precipitant or mental content. Many investigators believe that this suggests an altered neurobiological threshold to anxiety, and both pharmacological and psychological interventions have been effective in its treatment. Some people with symptomatic neurotic psychopathology, and many individuals with personality or character disorders, experience little or no conscious anxiety. Their problems are manifested by neurotic symptoms such as phobias, obsessions, compulsions, or conversion phenomena or by various character traits, and anxiety may be a less important part of the clinical picture or may even be absent altogether.

The psychoanalyst understands these more complex conditions as the result of defense mechanisms. These are automatic unconscious psychological patterns elicited by conflicts that threaten the individual's emotional equilibrium. The resulting threat or anticipation of anxiety, called *signal anxiety*, never becomes conscious because of the mental mechanisms that defend the individual from it. In other words, the individual responds to the unconscious threat of anxiety resulting from a psychological conflict by utilizing mechanisms that lead to a symptom or behavior pattern in order to ward off that anxiety. A clinical example illustrates this theory:

> A young woman who had had a somewhat restrictive and puritanical upbringing developed a phobia, a fear of going outdoors alone. She recalled a brief period of anxiety at the time that her phobia began. However, she experienced no anxiety at present as long as she remained indoors. When asked why she was afraid of going outdoors, she described episodes of palpitations and dizziness and her concern about what would happen if these occurred while she was on the street. Later, she told of women in her neighborhood who had been accosted by strange men and of her fear of being attacked. She had repressed sexual impulses toward attractive men whom she saw on the street, and she feared disapproval and punishment for these impulses, although both her wish and her fear were unconscious.

Here we see a number of defenses: repression of sexual wishes, the displacement of a fear of sex to a fear of the outdoors, avoidance of the outdoors, and the projection of sexual impulses onto strange men. These mechanisms were effective in controlling the patient's anxiety, but at the price of sexual inhibitions, frigidity, and the restriction of her freedom to travel. This inhibition of healthy behavior is a constant feature of symptom formation. It is often the "secondary loss" from the symptom that elicits the patient's feeling of inadequacy, helplessness, or even depression.

Symptoms not only defend against forbidden wishes; they also serve, symbolically and partially, to gratify them. This is necessary if symptoms are to be effective in protecting the individual from discomfort, because the ungratified wish would continue to press for satisfaction until the psychological equilibrium was disturbed and the fear and anxiety returned. An example of the gratification provided by symptoms is seen in the case of the woman just described. She was only able to venture outdoors in the company of her older brother, who had always been a romantic partner in her unconscious fantasies. Symptoms may also provide symbolic punishment related to the original unconscious fear. As a small child, the same young lady had been punished for naughtiness by being locked in her room, and her phobic symptom re-created that experience.

Symptom and Character

Neurotic psychopathology represents a compromise between a repressed unacceptable wish and an unconscious fear. Although all behavior represents an attempt to compromise between the demands of inner drives and external reality, neurotic behavior is a second-best solution, reflecting the individual's effort to accommodate not only to the external world but also to the restrictions imposed by inner unconscious fears. The two basic ways in which these neurotic patterns can be integrated into the personality are described by the terms *symptom* and *character*.

Neurotic *symptoms* are relatively sharply delineated behavior patterns that are experienced by the individual as undesirable "ego-alien" phenomena, not truly part of his self or personality. He consciously desires to be free from them, and they not infrequently lead him to seek help. Anxiety, depression, phobias, obsessions, compulsions, and conversion phenomena are typical examples. In time the patient may adjust to his symptoms and learn to live with them and even to exploit them ("secondary gain"), but they always remain foreign to the self—fundamentally experienced as "not me."

Character traits are more generalized behavior patterns that merge imperceptibly into the individual's total personality. They are ego-syntonic because he sees them as part of himself and either fails to recognize them as pathological or, realizing that they are undesirable, simply feels that they reflect his "nature." These traits rarely lead the individual to seek assistance, although their indirect secondary social consequences are frequent precipitants of psychiatric consultations. Mistrust, stinginess, irresponsibility, impulsiveness, aggressiveness, compulsiveness, and timidity are illustrations of troublesome character traits, whereas perseverance, generosity, prudence, and courage are more desirable ones.

Although the underlying psychodynamic structures of symptoms and character traits are closely related, they present quite different technical problems in psychiatric interviews and in treatment. In general, when treating patients who seek relief from symptoms, the clinician considers the underlying character structure along with such factors as motivation and life setting in planning the therapy, since it is only by viewing the symptoms in terms of the individual's overall functioning that a rational program for treatment can be developed. For instance, two men may experience depressive symptoms of the same severity. One is single, young, articulate, and intelligent; has an obsessive personality structure; and has considerable motivation for treatment, some flexibility, and few irreversible life commitments. Intensive exploratory, analytically oriented psychotherapy may be recommended for this person, with the goal of modifying predisposing character traits as well as relieving symptoms. The other person is older and has married a woman whose personality problems complement his, and they have several children. She responded quite negatively to an earlier attempt at treatment on his part. He is now suspicious and mistrustful of psychiatry and has little interest in his inner life, focusing on concrete externals. For this person, a more symptom-focused treatment is preferable. Symptom relief is an important goal with both patients, and pharmacological interventions may be useful with either, but psychodynamic considerations are important in evaluating the potential benefits and risks of employing a character-focused psychotherapy.

Conversely, with individuals who present with predominantly characterological pathology, the interviewer searches for symptoms that the patient may have not recognized or acknowledged. Improvement of such symptoms may enhance the patient's motivation for treatment. As therapy progresses, in a sense, the clinician tries to shift the patient's attitude toward his character problems to that seen with symptoms, attempting to help the patient experience his pathological character traits as separate from his "self." This has led to the often misunderstood maxim that treatment is not really working until the patient becomes symptomatic. It would be more accurate to say that as a patient with a character disorder begins to gain some insight into his pathology, he experiences it as more ego-alien. The tragedy of certain character traits is not in what the patient suffers but rather in what he misses.

An extremely obsessive man prided himself on his punctuality and his general perfectionism. One day he arrived at his session exactly on the hour, proudly explaining to the therapist that he had timed it perfectly, just glancing at his watch in time to make the train. Later he revealed that he had been lunching with his daughter, an unusual event, and that she had been somewhat surprised and hurt when he had left so abruptly. He had offered her neither an explanation nor an apology. The therapist agreed that he had made the appointment on time but suggested that he had traded a potential experience of intimacy and warmth for a "perfect record." The patient became quite gloomy at the suggestion that his treasured virtue could be seen as the surface manifestation of an underlying pervasive psychological problem—in effect, that his traits were symptomatic. As the treatment proceeded, they explored the many possibilities for combining his punctuality and precision, obsessional traits that he valued, with warmth and intimacy, newly acquired values that he was no longer willing to sacrifice, thus preserving the adaptive aspects of his traits while diminishing the pathological effects that he now experienced as symptomatic.

In the interview, symptoms are most clearly reflected in what the patient talks about; character traits are revealed in the way he talks and the way he relates to significant other people, particularly to the interviewer. From another point of view, the patient describes his symptoms, whereas his character traits are observed by the clinician. The beginning interviewer tends to focus on symptoms, since they are emphasized by the patient, are similar to the focus of interviews in other areas of medicine, and are easiest to recognize and to understand. The more experienced interviewer will also listen to the patient's description of symptoms, but more of his attention is directed to the patient's character structure as it emerges during this discussion. One of the major contributions of psychoanalysis is the recognition of the importance of dealing with the patient's characterological structure if the interview is to be maximally productive.

Neurosis and Psychosis

There is no single criterion that differentiates psychotic from neurotic patients. In general, psychotic patients are sicker—that is, they have more pervasive and widespread difficulties in adaptation. More specifically, areas of functioning that are considered to be essential for a minimal level of adaptation and that are usually intact in neurotic patients may be impaired in psychotic patients. These would include the perception and testing of reality, the capacity for sustained interpersonal relations, and the maintenance of autonomous ego functions such as memory, communication, and motor control. The distinction between psychotic and nonpsychotic organic brain syndromes is based on related criteria and is discussed in Chapter 16, "The Cognitively Impaired Patient."

Studies of the psychological processes involved in neuroses and psychoses have repeatedly raised the question of whether these are qualitatively different or merely quantitative variations of the same basic mechanisms. Those who hold the former view may suggest that one or another basic defect is primary in the psychotic process (usually viewed as genetic or neurobiological in origin) and that the other phenomena of the illness can then be explained as the result of defensive and reparative psychological responses similar to those seen in neuroses. For example, in schizophrenia this central defect has variously been described as a diminished capacity for affectivity, a disturbance in the perception or testing of reality, abnormal cognitive processes, poor interpersonal relations, or a primary deficit in the synthetic function of the ego, which integrates other mental functions into a harmonious whole.

Specific mechanisms of defense are neither psychotic nor neurotic, or for that matter, neither pathological nor healthy. However, some mental mechanisms, such as projection and denial, interfere with autonomous ego functions and the relationship with reality and are therefore commonly associated with psychotic processes. Hallucinations and illusions are gross disorders in the perception of reality, and delusions represent severe disturbances in reality testing; all three of these symptoms are usually associated with psychosis. However, subtler disturbances in the subjective sense of the "real" world, such as derealization or depersonalization, are common in neuroses as well as in psychoses. Furthermore, all neurotic symptoms, insofar as they are maladaptive, are in some sense "unrealistic." However, the defective contact with reality found in neurosis is more sharply circumscribed, usually unconscious, and most areas of the patient's life are unaffected.

The disturbance in interpersonal relations found in psychotic disorders may stem from earlier stages of the patient's development, because the beginnings of the child's capacity for perception and testing of reality, thought, language, and affectivity all grow out of the early relationship with the mother. The neurotic patient tends to force current relationships into the mold created by later childhood experiences, and the result can be a serious disturbance in friendships and love lives. However, the neurotic patient does have the capacity to develop and maintain relationships with others, and if the neurotic problems are overcome, these are major sources of gratification. Many psychotic individuals (particularly those with schizophrenia) have more basic defects in their capacity for relating to others. This is seen clinically in their tendency toward isolation and withdrawal, having few lasting friendships and a shallowness and superficiality in those that do develop. Friends and acquaintances will often find them less stable and less reliable parts of their lives.

The clinician may experience this defect in the nature of the patient's relationships during the interview. The psychotic patient may "feel" different; it is harder to make contact with him and to empathize with his emotional responses. For example, if the clinician is unable to remember the patient several hours after the first visit, it may reveal in retrospect that little real contact was established. The patient's shifting sense of personal identity may leave the clinician feeling that there is not a specific other person there with him. Experienced psychiatrists detect psychosis by this kind of feeling as well as by the psychopathological criteria that are used to justify the diagnosis. However, every relationship that the psychotic patient establishes need not be shallow or superficial. There are striking exceptions, and often there is one person with whom the patient has an intense symbiotic relationship that is far more all-encompassing than any that the neurotic develops. This person may be the psychotherapist, and therefore this has special relevance to the interview.

When sufficient information about the patient's life is available, most neurotic psychopathology can be understood in great detail within the psychodynamic frame of reference. Even with this information, however, much psychotic psychopathology is difficult to understand. This has led to the view that psychoses have major nonpsychodynamic determinants, whereas neuroses do not. In any case, the psychodynamic explanation of any type of pathology is more helpful in understanding its meaning than in clarifying its etiology. Indeed, it should be recalled that Freud felt that there was a biological basis to neuroses as well as to psychoses.

Psychotic patients can, and usually do, have neurotic problems in the form of both symptoms and character traits in addition to their more basic psychopathology. Thus the interviewer must take into account both the psychotic and the neurotic pathology of the psychotic patient. This may be quite difficult, since the psychotic disturbance can interfere with the capacity of the patient to participate in the interview itself. The patient's tendency to be mistrustful of others may make it difficult for him to feel comfortable with the interviewer, and his diminished capacity for interpersonal relations, together with his disturbed thought processes, leads to major problems in communication.

Psychosis is not a constant phenomenon, and many psychotic patients move in and out of psychotic states over a span of days, weeks, or even within a single interview. Often the dilemma in treatment is to work on the patient's conflicts and problems while providing enough emotional support that the stress of the therapy does not push him further into psychosis. Two clinical examples may help to illustrate these issues:

A young man arrived at a hospital emergency room in a state of extreme anxiety. He believed that he had had a heart attack and was dying and complained of chest pains and a choking sensation. Although cooperative, he was sweating and trembling with fear. He denied any psychological or emotional difficulties. There had been several similar episodes in the past, each ending quickly and without incident. The remainder of the brief initial history was unremarkable, and as the interviewer proceeded, the patient's symptoms subsided and he began to feel better. A normal electrocardiogram offered further reassurance, and after the intern told him that he seemed to be in good physical health, the patient began to relax and to speak more comfortably. He spoke of his family and early life experiences and revealed that he had led a sheltered and protected childhood. He was still closely tied to his family, and particularly to his mother, who strongly disapproved of the girl he had been seeing recently. It was while on his way to visit the girl that the attack occurred.

A second young man also arrived at the hospital in a panicky state. He complained of strange feelings in his back and "electric shocks" in his legs, which he thought might be related to physical exhaustion. He had not slept for several days, staying up in order to protect his apartment and possessions from attack. He was vague about who might want to hurt him but felt certain that he had been followed on the street in recent days. As he discussed these thoughts, he lowered his voice and leaned forward to tell the interviewer that several men had made homosexual advances toward him earlier that day. The doctor, inexperienced in psychiatry, asked if the patient had ever had homosexual experiences. The patient became agitated, screaming that the doctor was trying to frame him, and tried to run from the examining room. Later, after he had received some tranquilizing medication, he readily agreed to hospitalization in order to protect himself from his enemies.

The first patient had a classic panic attack with hyperventilation, and the second had an early psychotic paranoid schizophrenic break, although they both had virtually the same initial complaints.

PSYCHOANALYTIC MODELS OF MENTAL FUNCTIONING

Structural Model and Ego Psychology

As psychoanalytic theory has been applied to the study of psychopathology, personality development, dreams, art, culture, and other areas of human activity, a number of theoretical models have been developed. The earliest of these, the so-called topographic model, described mental activity as conscious, preconscious, or unconscious. Although this scheme was easy to apply, it soon became apparent that it was not helpful in discussing a central psychodynamic issue, that of intrapsychic conflict. Many conflicts in clinical practice are entirely unconscious, with the patient unaware of the basic drive or motive, the fantasized danger, and the psychological strategy employed to resolve them.

As a result, Freud developed a later "structural" theory that has largely supplanted his earlier topographic one and that remains one of the most commonly used models in contemporary psychoanalytic thought. In it the mind is viewed as consisting of more or less autonomous structures that are most sharply defined at times of conflict. Each structure consists of a complex array of psychological functions that act in concert during conflict. Therefore most (but not all) conflict is seen as occurring between these structures. Three structures are generally recognized: the *id*, which consists of the basic drives, impulses, and needs; the *ego*, which includes the psychological functions that control and regulate these drives, the defenses, as well as all other psychological adaptive and coping strategies and all relationships with the external world; and the *superego*, which is a specialized aspect of the ego that develops in the early relationship with the parents and embodies the conscience and the conscious and unconscious ethical, moral, and cultural standards acquired during socialization. The *ego ideal*, usually considered a component of the superego, refers to the goals and aspirations that the individual develops through identification with parents and that are elaborated and modified through his later contact with peers and the larger culture. Most conflicts of clinical significance occur between one of these structures and the other two, with each of the three combinations possible. Thus anxiety and guilt over sexual impulses that were forbidden in childhood would be an example of ego and superego against id; sadistic revenge against a friend who has been guilty of a minor infraction would be superego and id against ego; and an ascetic self-denying lifestyle would be the characterological manifestation of superego against ego and id.

Ego

The term *ego* describes those psychological functions that help the individual to adapt to the environment, respond to stimuli, and regulate basic biological functions while ensuring survival and the satisfaction of needs. Historically, the concept originated from studies of psychological conflict in which the ego represented those forces that opposed and controlled basic biological drives. Later it was extended to include functions that were not involved with conflict and that could even operate in concert with basic drives to serve the organism's adaptive needs. The ego is the executive organ of the mind, mediating between the internal demands of the biologically determined motives (the id), the socially determined goals and values (the superego), and the external demands of reality. It is the final common pathway that integrates all of these determinants and then controls the organism's response. The ego develops through interaction of the maturing infantile psyche with external reality, particularly that portion of external reality that consists of significant other humans. There is on the one hand an unfolding biological potential that leads to the maturation of memory, learning, perception, cognition, communication, and other vital adaptive functions and on the other hand a highly specialized environment composed of a need-gratifying and stimulus-controlling object, a good-enough, attentive, and responsive mother or caretaker.

The ego includes both conscious and automatic unconscious psychological processes. Before Freud the conscious portion was considered to be the subject matter of psychology. The ego also includes the unconscious defense mechanisms and the forces of repression that Freud discovered in his early work. Although they operate outside the patient's awareness, they are directed against the expression of basic needs and drives and are therefore considered part of the ego.

Id

The term *id* describes the biologically based drives and motives that are at the source of much behavior. Sex, aggression, and the craving for security are examples of such motives. Other needs develop as the result of exposure to society and are determined by the demands of that society. Status, prestige, and power are examples of the goals related to such needs. Classic psychoanalytic theory believed that these needs could directly be traced to biologically determined origins. As these motives press for satisfaction, they become one of the major factors impinging on the ego and therefore determining the individual's behavior. Freud's early explorations of the unconscious determinants of neurotic symptoms uncovered the phenomena encompassed by the term *id*. Evolutionary biologists postulate that earliest primates lived in groups that were organized for the purpose of survival. The acquisition of food was more efficient when it was hunted by an organized group, as was protection from natural enemies and from rival bands of primates. These groups were run by the strongest members so that a hierarchy evolved. The hierarchical order determined who ate first and who had preferred mating rights. Despite the enormous complexity of human beings, these same basic instincts in both real and symbolic forms still drive much of our behavior.

In more recent years, psychoanalytic investigation has been directed toward the psychology of unconscious mechanisms of adaptation and patterns of behavioral integration in addition to the influence of unconscious drives. In other words, there has been a shift from a primarily id psychology to a more balanced view that includes ego psychology. This shift became possible as the unconscious determinants of behavior were better understood, and it was paralleled by a growing clinical interest in psychiatric problems that involve ego pathology, such as character disorders and psychoses.

Freud described the primitive mental activity of the id and the unconscious ego with the phrase "primary process," in contrast to the "secondary process" thinking of the conscious adult ego. Primary process thinking is childlike, prelogical, and self-centered. It is controlled by the pleasure principle, tolerates contradictions and inconsistencies, and employs such mental mechanisms as symbolization, condensation, and displacement. Secondary process thinking, in contrast, is logical, rational, reality-centered, goal-directed, and relatively free of emotional control. Most thought processes combine elements of both. One of the clinically important discoveries of psychoanalysis is the astonishing extent to which even the most rational-seeming behavior may involve unconscious primary process.

Superego

Superego refers to psychological functions that involve standards of right and wrong together with the evaluation and judgment of the self in terms of these standards. In general usage, it also includes the ego ideal, the psychological representation of what a person wishes to be like, his ideal self. The superego was originally considered to be a portion of the ego, but it operates independently of, and often at odds with, other ego functions, particularly in conflict situations and pathological conditions. It develops out of the young child's relationship with his parents, who initially provide him with external judgments, criticism, and praise for his behavior. As he grows away from his parents, he nevertheless maintains a relationship with his internalized psychological representation of them, establishing an internal mental structure, a dynamically significant psychic agency—the superego—that carries on those functions that formerly belonged to the parents.

The superego is further influenced by parental surrogates such as teachers, by peers, and by society at large. This is even more true of the ego ideal, which at the age of latency is often concretely symbolized by popular cultural heroes.

Reality

At first it might seem superfluous to include a section on reality in a discussion of psychological functioning, but a distinction must be made between psychic reality and the more familiar concept of physical reality. The real world influences psychological functions only as it is registered and perceived by the individual. This can be illustrated by considering the most important aspect of external reality: the social reality of important other people. An individual reacts not to his real mother or father but rather to his internal representations of them, which inevitably involve selections, distortions, and constructions. There has been repeated misunderstanding of this critical distinction, even by Freud himself. During their childhoods, neurotic patients frequently experienced adults as either highly seductive or callously indifferent. It took Freud some time to recognize that this was not necessarily an accurate portrayal of their "real" experiences. However, it is even more misleading to disregard this internal psychic reality because it may not be historically valid, for without it, both the child's fears and the adult's neuroses are meaningless. The conclusion is that reality must be considered as a psychic structure that is responsive to the external environment but that involves a creative personal interpretation of that environment. When we tell someone "Don't be silly" (i.e., "You're crazy"), it usually means that we do not perceive that person's psychological reality but only our own. One of the central tenets of psychoanalysis is that behavior that seems irrational from the perspective of the observer makes sense in the context of the other person's own (usually unconscious) psychic reality.

Behavior results from the interaction of innate and socially determined motives, the goals and standards acquired during early socialization, the subjective experience of external reality, and the individual's own unique temperament, personality, talents, defensive style, and integrative capacity. In terms of the structural theory, it is the product of id, ego, superego, and psychic reality.

This framework provides a means of thinking about clinical data in general and about psychiatric interviews in particular. One can consider the patient's predominant wishes or motives, his unconscious fears, and his characteristic defenses. How are these integrated, and what symptoms or character traits are present? How do these interfere with adaptation, and what secondary adjustments have been necessary? Each individual is unique, but there are certain typical patterns of drive, fear, and defense; symptoms; and character style that have led to the description of well-known clinical syndromes in psychiatry. Our discussion of more specific problems in the psychiatric interview includes the most common patterns seen in clinical practice.

Some contemporary psychoanalysts collaborating with neurobiologists are developing alternative models of "mind" that attempt to bridge psychology and neuroscience.

Object Relations Models

Freud's earliest model emphasized motivational forces and particularly their biological roots—the instincts or drives. The organism matured, and the environment was little more than the setting or context for this maturation. The term *object* originally stemmed from the view that various external "objects" were targets of the drives and essential for their discharge. The fact that among the most important early objects were the people critical for the child's development, particularly the mother, and that these "objects" had major influence on the child's developing personality, was largely ignored. However, several factors led to an interest in the child's relationship with "objects" and with the development of internal representations of objects; this eventually led to a major reformulation of psychoanalytic theory with a central focus on object relations and representations rather than drives and their discharge.

These factors included 1) studies of children and of child development, and the recognition of the immense importance of the caretaker; 2) studies of more severe psychopathology—psychotic and borderline conditions—that was understood as involving disturbance in the capacity to construct internal objects as much as conflicts regarding the discharge of drives; and 3) new views of the treatment process that emphasized the relationship of patient to therapist (reflecting the new models of development) as well as the patient's insight into intrapsychic conflict.

Object relations models conceive of psychic structures as developing through the child's construction of internal representations of self and others. These representations are originally primitive and fantastic, often combining several individuals into a single representation or splitting a single individual into several representations. With time, they gradually become more realistic. They are associated with widely varying affects (e.g., anger, sadness, feelings of safety, fear, pleasure) as well as with various wishes and fantasies (e.g., of sex, of control, or of devouring and being devoured). The growing child struggles with contradictory representations and feelings of self and others, tending to separate good and bad experiences, constructing all-good and all-bad internal objects. At this early level of development, one may feel that one has two different mothers, for example—a good, gratifying one and a bad, frustrating one. In the more mature individual, these images are integrated into coherent representations with multiple complex qualities, selected and formed in part to help self-esteem, make affects tolerable, and satisfy wishes. Traditional fairy tales and ancient myths clearly depict figures such as the fairy godmother, the wicked witch, the all-good god, and the all-evil devil.

Psychodynamic formulations that employ this model focus on the nature of the self and object representations and the prominent conflicts and contradictions among them. A special emphasis is given to developmental failures in integrating the various partial and contradictory representations of self and others and to the displacement and defensive misattribution of aspects of self or others. Object relations models are especially useful for formulating the fragmented inner world of psychotic and borderline patients who experience themselves and others as unintegrated parts; however, the models may be less useful for relatively healthier patients in whom conflict may more easily be described in terms of traditional ego psychology. These models have also been influential in studies of patterns of attachment and in studies of the role of early relationships in the development of mentalization and a theory of the mind, the awareness that others have an independent existence and that both oneself and others have minds (wishes, fears, thoughts, and feelings) and that individuals make constant inferences about the minds of others.

Self Psychological Model

The self psychological model postulates a psychological structure, the self, that develops toward the realization of goals that are both innate and learned. Two broad classes of these goals can be identified: one consists of the individual's ambitions, the other of his or her ideals. Normal development involves the child's grandiose idealization of self and others, the exhibitionistic expression of strivings and ambitions, and the empathic responsiveness of parents and others to these needs. Under these conditions, the child's unfolding skills, talents, and internalization of empathic objects will lead to the development of a sturdy self with capacities for creativity, joy, and continuing empathic relationships. In this model, genetic formulations trace character problems to specific empathic failures in the child's environment that distorted and inhibited the development of the self and the capacity to maintain object ties. These formulations also describe how the individual has defensively compensated for these failures of self-development and suggest therapeutic strategies needed to support the resumption of self-development that had been arrested in the past, emphasizing the special transference needs of the patient. The self psychological model is especially useful for formulating the narcissistic difficulties present in many types of patients (not only those with narcissistic personality disorder); however, the model lacks a clear conception of intrapsychic structure, and it is less useful for formulating fixed repetitive symptoms that arise from conflicts between one's conscience and sexual or aggressive wishes.

In many ways these three models can be seen as logically contradictory. However, the clinician is not disturbed by such contradictions. He draws on insights garnered from each of them—from his own life and from clinical experience; from teachers, supervisors, and colleagues; from the professional literature; from myths; and from works of art and literature—in order to understand his patients and the meaning of his interaction with them. Different models may be useful for different clinicians, for different patients, or for different phases of contact with a single patient. Many believe that the conviction that behavior is meaningful, the process of collaboration with the patient in the attempt to discover or construct that meaning, and the understanding of unconscious processes such as transference and resistance are far more important than the specific model of psychological processes that the clinician employs. Our discussions draw most heavily on structural models and often employ notions from object relations or self psychological models, but, most importantly, view all of these models as tools to be employed when useful and to be discarded when they interfere with the clinician's relationship with the patient.

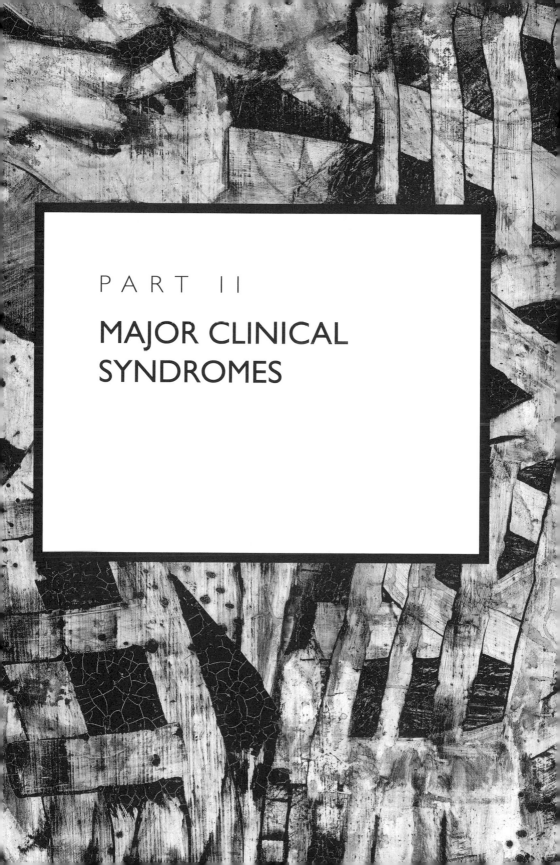

PART II

MAJOR CLINICAL SYNDROMES

CHAPTER 3

THE OBSESSIVE-COMPULSIVE PATIENT

The obsessive-compulsive personality is encountered frequently in clinical practice. The patient with this personality possesses one of the most consistent, rigid, and consequently predictable personality types. The obsessive-compulsive patient's controlling nature, procrastination, ambivalence, indecisiveness, perfectionism, and absence of emotional warmth makes him easily recognizable. The presenting clinical picture is well described in DSM-5.

The DSM-5 diagnostic criteria for obsessive-compulsive personality disorder are presented in Box 3–1.

BOX 3–1. DSM-5 Diagnostic Criteria for Obsessive-Compulsive Personality Disorder

---

A pervasive pattern of preoccupation with orderliness, perfectionism, and mental and interpersonal control, at the expense of flexibility, openness, and efficiency, beginning by early adulthood and present in a variety of contexts, as indicated by four (or more) of the following:

1. Is preoccupied with details, rules, lists, order, organization, or schedules to the extent that the major point of the activity is lost.
2. Shows perfectionism that interferes with task completion (e.g., is unable to complete a project because his or her own overly strict standards are not met).
3. Is excessively devoted to work and productivity to the exclusion of leisure activities and friendships (not accounted for by obvious economic necessity).
4. Is overconscientious, scrupulous, and inflexible about matters of morality, ethics, or values (not accounted for by cultural or religious identification).

5. Is unable to discard worn-out or worthless objects even when they have no sentimental value.
6. Is reluctant to delegate tasks or to work with others unless they submit to exactly his or her way of doing things.
7. Adopts a miserly spending style toward both self and others; money is viewed as something to be hoarded for future catastrophes.
8. Shows rigidity and stubbornness.

Source. Reprinted from American Psychiatric Association: *Diagnostic and Statistical Manual of Mental Disorders,* 5th Edition. Arlington, VA, American Psychiatric Association, 2013. Copyright 2013, American Psychiatric Association. Used with permission.

Obsessive-compulsive disorder (OCD) was historically seen as being the anlage of obsessive-compulsive personality disorder but is now believed to be a separate entity with a significant neurobiological substrate. In DSM-IV-TR, OCD was classified with the anxiety disorders. In DSM-5, obsessive-compulsive and related disorders became an independent diagnostic category, and OCD was included there (Box 3–2).

BOX 3–2. DSM-5 Diagnostic Criteria for Obsessive-Compulsive Disorder

---

A. Presence of obsessions, compulsions, or both:

Obsessions are defined by (1) and (2):

1. Recurrent and persistent thoughts, urges, or images that are experienced, at some time during the disturbance, as intrusive and unwanted, and that in most individuals cause marked anxiety or distress.
2. The individual attempts to ignore or suppress such thoughts, urges, or images, or to neutralize them with some other thought or action (i.e., by performing a compulsion).

Compulsions are defined by (1) and (2):

1. Repetitive behaviors (e.g., hand washing, ordering, checking) or mental acts (e.g., praying, counting, repeating words silently) that the individual feels driven to perform in response to an obsession or according to rules that must be applied rigidly.
2. The behaviors or mental acts are aimed at preventing or reducing anxiety or distress, or preventing some dreaded event or situation; however, these behaviors or mental acts are not connected in a realistic way with what they are designed to neutralize or prevent, or are clearly excessive.
   Note: Young children may not be able to articulate the aims of these behaviors or mental acts.
B. The obsessions or compulsions are time-consuming (e.g., take more than 1 hour per day) or cause clinically significant distress or impairment in social, occupational, or other important areas of functioning.

C. The obsessive-compulsive symptoms are not attributable to the physiological effects of a substance (e.g., a drug of abuse, a medication) or another medical condition.

D. The disturbance is not better explained by the symptoms of another mental disorder (e.g., excessive worries, as in generalized anxiety disorder; preoccupation with appearance, as in body dysmorphic disorder; difficulty discarding or parting with possessions, as in hoarding disorder; hair pulling, as in trichotillomania [hair-pulling disorder]; skin picking, as in excoriation [skin-picking] disorder; stereotypies, as in stereotypic movement disorder; ritualized eating behavior, as in eating disorders; preoccupation with substances or gambling, as in substance-related and addictive disorders; preoccupation with having an illness, as in illness anxiety disorder; sexual urges or fantasies, as in paraphilic disorders; impulses, as in disruptive, impulse-control, and conduct disorders; guilty ruminations, as in major depressive disorder; thought insertion or delusional preoccupations, as in schizophrenia spectrum and other psychotic disorders; or repetitive patterns of behavior, as in autism spectrum disorder).

Specify if:

With good or fair insight: The individual recognizes that obsessive-compulsive disorder beliefs are definitely or probably not true or that they may or may not be true.

With poor insight: The individual thinks obsessive-compulsive disorder beliefs are probably true.

With absent insight/delusional beliefs: The individual is completely convinced that obsessive-compulsive disorder beliefs are true.

Specify if:

Tic-related: The individual has a current or past history of a tic disorder.

Source. Reprinted from American Psychiatric Association: *Diagnostic and Statistical Manual of Mental Disorders,* 5th Edition. Arlington, VA, American Psychiatric Association, 2013. Copyright 2013, American Psychiatric Association. Used with permission.

OCD may begin in early childhood but usually appears in adolescence or early adulthood. OCD is viewed by some as the behavioral sequelae of a brain disorder involving basal ganglia and thus related to tic disorders and Tourette's syndrome. Obsessive-compulsive personality disorder can be seen as a psychological adaptation to growing up with OCD, both exploiting its adaptive potential and adapting to its challenges. Obsessive-compulsive personality disorder can develop in other ways, however, and preexisting OCD is only one of multiple pathways that may lead to the personality disorder. Although OCD undoubtedly possesses a neurobiological basis, a psychodynamic understanding of the OCD patient's psychopathology is useful. This includes pervasive ambivalence, a need for control, magical thinking, rituals of doing and undoing, and a confusion between thought and action. Hoarding in the extreme degree is pathognomonic for OCD as are other behavioral rituals that are not required as regular aspects of a particular religion. Examples include showering three or more times a day, having to check that the stove is turned off immediately after one has just done so, and incessant compulsive hand washing. Effective treatment of OCD will usually include the use of appropriate medication and cognitive-behavioral therapy. The psychodynamic elements found in OCD, and hence aspects of the interview, are in common with those of the obsessive-compulsive personality. However, individuals with OCD, in contrast to those with obsessive-compulsive personality disorder, are seldom responsive to psychodynamic psychotherapy.

Freud wrote extensively about obsessive-compulsive syndromes, most notably in the Rat Man case (1909). He described obsessional dynamics such as ambivalence, the regression to preoedipal anal-sadistic conflicts over control, and the emergence in the obsessional patient of ego defenses such as reaction formation, intellectualization, isolation, undoing, and the pervasive presence of magical thinking. He conflated "obsessional neurosis" (i.e., OCD) with obsessional personality disorder, but, as noted earlier, this is no longer done. Nonetheless, his insights have relevance to a psychodynamic understanding of both disorders and to the interview.

PSYCHOPATHOLOGY AND PSYCHODYNAMICS

The concept of *personality* traditionally refers to aspects of an individual as viewed by others, whereas *character* refers to a person's internal psychological organization. This is in contrast to the term *self* that is used to refer to the inner representation of one's personality and character. In the psychotherapy of character disorders it is essential that the therapist understand and work empathically with the discordance between the patient's view of his self and that held by others. This is of particular importance in the treatment of the person with obsessive-compulsive personality who sees himself as intelligent, rational, organized, goal-directed, thorough, persevering, self-sufficient, emotionally well controlled, respected, loyal, devoted, conscientious, ethical, reliable, consistent, punctual, thrifty, orderly, and a witty tease.

As perceived by others, a more negative picture appears. He is experienced as emotionally isolated, cold, excessively controlling, indecisive, procrastinating, demanding, perfectionistic, stubborn, insensitive to the feelings of others, arrogant, pedantic, moralistic, rigid, and stingy—

a covertly sadistic person who is preoccupied with trivia and always planning for future pleasure that never arrives.

The obsessive-compulsive patient is quite aware of his emotions of fear, rage, and guilt. However, he has difficulty experiencing feelings of warmth, love, and tenderness. He feels strong when angry and defiant and weak when fearful and guilty. Perhaps his greatest impairment is in accepting his warm, tender, loving emotions. They cause him to feel exposed, embarrassed, vulnerable, and weak. His fantasy life is preoccupied with themes of aggression, power, or controlling others. He holds many imaginary conversations in preparation for real-life interactions that never turn out quite according to his plan. He lives out roles in his imagination of a folk hero such as the Lone Ranger, or rescuer, or leader. Similar themes of dominance and submission are prominent in his sexual fantasies, although obsessive-compulsive females are more interested in being loved.

The obsessive-compulsive patient is often unable to commit himself to a relationship, and therefore he is usually doing at least two things at once. An example occurs at a party where he pretends to be listening to the person with whom he is conversing while simultaneously listening to another conversation beside or in back of him. He gives himself away with a blank stare or a blank smile that is a bit out of sync with what the other person is saying. This occurs during the interview, and after the first few interviews, the clinician can ask, "Do I have your undivided attention?" The patient will say, "Of course," and can repeat the interviewer's last words. The interviewer says, in friendly tone of voice, "I know that you were listening but what else were you thinking about at the same time?"

This confrontation of such a defense must be done gently because it will cause the patient to feel exposed, guilty, and fearful of the clinician's disapproval. It is these fears and guilt that contribute to the patient's basic low self-esteem.

It may simplify the process of understanding the obsessive-compulsive personality to consider the multitude of traits as stemming from several basic patterns. First is the emotional isolation that accounts for the rigidity, coldness, and disturbance in human relations. Next is the obsessive-compulsive patient's fear of making a mistake. This leads to indecisiveness and obsessing excessively and the accompanying manifestation of procrastination or making lists as a substitute for action. The "list" is treated as though something has been accomplished, and it assumes a magical power in the patient's mind. Misplacing the list produces anxiety and guilt so that more time may be devoted to finding the list than to re-creating it. Obsessive-compulsive patients love to save things (anal retentiveness), a function of indecision and fear of making a mistake: "Who knows, someday I might need this." The patient treats his possessions as though they were important people and his important people as though they were possessions.

Next is his excessive morality and preoccupation with rules, ethics, and procedures, including rituals. His rigidity and fear of making a mistake are expressed in this area as well. His way is the "right way," and he stubbornly resists change. He does not delegate well unless he is certain that the other person will do it the way that he believes to be the best way. This perfectionist approach to life breaks down when creativity, imagination, and spontaneity are part of the task. Also related to this area are the traits of overconscientiousness, overcommitment to work, and postponing pleasure.

Obsessive-Compulsive Traits and Their Miscarriage

It is crucial that the clinician understand and respect the virtues of the obsessive-compulsive patient. It is through a precise understanding of how each of these traits gets the patient into trouble that one is able to establish a therapeutic alliance in which the patient does not feel he is being judged and criticized. It will be around these points that the patient's transference projections onto his therapist will occur, and it is through the analysis of these transference projections that the treatment will proceed. Examining each of the traits individually develops understanding of how they get the patient into difficulty with himself and his environment.

First, the patient's preoccupation with intellectual mastery is accompanied by emotional isolation and the loss of human experience. His rational thinking and concern with logic lead to rationalization and indecisiveness, since rational processes fail to solve problems that are basically emotional in nature. His excellent organizational capacity leads to his being excessively controlling of others, which causes much of his interpersonal difficulty. His goal-directed planning for the future is usually done to an extreme, leading to the postponement of pleasure. The patient's preoccupation with work adds to the barrenness of his emotional life. The obsessive patient's thoroughness, carried to extremes, leads to perfectionism. This occurs at the point at which there is a lack of reasonable return for the effort expended. The patient is particularly sensitive to the clinician's understanding that he cannot decide at what point there is no reasonable return for his continuing effort. The patient's tenacity, a fine trait, is confused with his stubbornness, which reflects the influence of emotions that he cannot understand logically because there is nothing rational about being stubborn, which is anger driven.

As stated earlier, the patient's perfectionism is accompanied by a preoccupation with self-sufficiency. In the patient's belief that he can do everything better himself, he is unaware that he hurts the feelings of others. His desire for self-sufficiency leads to condescension to others, and he feels important while ignoring the self-esteem others gain by feeling needed. He also feels contemptuous of those who appear helpless and lack confidence.

In his pursuit of continual emotional control, the obsessive-compulsive patient easily becomes emotionally isolated. The patient feels proud of his ability to control his angry or hurt feelings. However, the process of emotional isolation requires that he control his warm and tender feelings as well. The result is that he emotionally starves those who are dependent on him for warmth. The clinician must develop the patient's awareness of this problem early in the treatment in a supportive manner that will not humiliate the patient. It is important that the clinician word his comments in such a way as to recognize the patient's warm and caring feelings, which he fears expressing in an openly emotional manner. Otherwise, the patient will feel that he is considered defective. It is necessary to do so even when the patient believes he is defective. The interviewer can search quite diligently to show the patient behavioral evidence of his deeper feelings of love and devotion even though he does not consciously allow himself to experience such emotions. Often feelings of devotion and loyalty are carried to extremes, so that the patient becomes fanatical and unwilling to see that in his excessive devotion he becomes too controlling of the other person.

The obsessive-compulsive patient's conscientiousness and high ethical values are easily miscarried to become moral rigidity and scrupulosity. These attitudes introduce barriers in his interpersonal relations. His reliability and consistency—again, virtues—can easily be carried to the extreme and then become indistinguishable from inflexibility. Punctuality, also a virtue, can be pursued as an end in itself with the resulting loss of human experiences and inconsideration of the feelings of others. The patient realizes he is missing something, but he is not certain how it happened.

Every obsessive-compulsive patient is proud of his thriftiness. However, he is not proud when he suspects that he has been selfish and stingy. The patient is also proud of his sense of humor, which typically involves teasing. Unfortunately, he lacks the warmth to carry it off well, and he often comes across as mean or sadistic. The clinician's sensitive handling of the patient's social ataxia eventually strengthens the patient's capacity to analyze this trait. This becomes accessible in treatment when the patient worries that his teasing was misunderstood and he feels guilty. His usual defense is to blame the other person for taking it the wrong way or lacking a sense of humor.

Finally, the orderliness of the obsessive-compulsive patient, when pursued to excess, becomes a preoccupation with order and trivia, and the purpose of the organization becomes lost. The result is an overall loss of efficiency and a feeling of failure.

The Central Conflict

The obsessive-compulsive patient is involved in a conflict between obedience and defiance. It is as though he constantly asks himself, "Shall I be good, or may I be naughty?" This leads to a continuing alternation between the emotions of fear and rage—fear that he will be caught at his naughtiness and punished for it, and rage at relinquishing his desires and submitting to authority. The fear, stemming from defiance, leads to obedience, whereas the rage, derived from enforced submission, leads back again to defiance.

This conflict has its origins in childhood experience and therefore is couched in childish terms. Obedience and defiance are equated with humiliating subjugation and murder. Issues lose their proportion, and the problem of whether one finishes a sentence or permits an interruption is a problem of whether one annihilates the other or is annihilated by him. Vital issues require extreme defenses, and the rigidity and totality of obsessive defenses are extreme.

Most of the character traits that classically define the obsessive-compulsive personality can be traced to this central conflict. Thus his punctuality, conscientiousness, tidiness, orderliness, and reliability are derived from his fear of authority. These can be highly adaptive traits of great social value when they are derived through healthy identification with a parent who has them. It is important to realize that, for the obsessive-compulsive individual, such behavior is not always motivated by mature, healthy, constructive forces but stems from unrealistic fear. This understanding will bring much behavior that appears at first to be uninvolved in psychopathology into dynamic significance, as will appreciating the source of this patient's constant anxiety. If the patient is early for the appointment, it is not simply an accident or a sign of enthusiasm but a symbolic placation to avoid punishment for transgressions of which he is quite aware, even if the clinician is not. If the interviewer asks the patient his preference in arranging the time of the next appointment, the patient does not respond to the consideration or interest but inwardly feels he has obtained a special privilege.

Another set of obsessive-compulsive traits is derived from the rage portion of the conflict. Untidiness, negligence, obstinacy, parsimony, and sadism can be traced to defiant anger. It is apparent by now that this list of traits includes many opposites—conscientiousness and negligence, orderliness and untidiness, and so on. These contradictory traits not only are essential features of the obsessive-compulsive individual but also may appear in the same person at the same time! He may meticulously clean his shoes before entering the office but later create a mess with the residue of his coffee and doughnut. Contradictory motives can be seen within a single act. The patient, in his eagerness to pay the bill as soon as he receives it, will delay the therapist for several minutes while he carefully fills out his check and the stub. The apparent contradictions vanish when one remembers that the origin of these traits is embedded in the conflicts of defiance and obedience and rage and fear. The essence of the obsessive patient is not either side of this conflict, but rather the conflict itself.

Issues Involved in the Conflict

Three key issues are inevitably involved and frequently appear in the interview situation. They are dirt, time, and money. Although the earliest power struggles between parent and child center around feeding and sleeping, the battle soon includes toilet training. Parental concern with the child's bowel habits extends into other areas that involve dirt, cleanliness, and orderliness. These include the struggles that develop over the child's washing behind his ears, cleaning his room, watching television, and going to bed. Dirt and time provide the most common issues for the content of the child's struggles that develop with parental authority. The child develops magical concepts that associate dirt with aggression and defiance. The defiance then leads to guilty fear and expectation of punishment through illness or even death. These concepts are based on parental and cultural edicts concerning the dangers of dirt, germs, and the defiance of authority. The obsessive patient will be fearful to reveal his secret dirty habits, whether picking his nose or wearing yesterday's socks. He will be particularly concerned about the dirt he brings into the interview—the mud on his shoes and his dirty hands. Both sides of the conflict may be seen as he states, "I just want to wash my hands before we start," and then leaves the sink a mess and wipes his wet, dirty hands on the towel. Exposure of this behavior leads to intense shame and humiliation. It can only be discussed after many sessions, and even then the therapist must use tact. The clinician could inquire, "What behaviors did your mother repeatedly criticize?" If the patient draws a blank, the interviewer could ask about issues such as cleanliness, lateness, disorderliness, tracking in dirt, or not hanging up his things. When the patient initially draws a blank to the general question but has recollections when asked the specifics, this is a matter worthy of further exploration. The clinician's attitude is one of curiosity rather than criticism.

Time is another key area in the child's battle with his parents. Dawdling and procrastination are prominent in the battles at bedtime, mealtime, playtime, and homework time. It is also prominent in current power struggles, because it deals so directly with control and mastery. The amount of time that is spent in the interview has a special significance to the obsessive-compulsive patient. He will want to know how long the interviews last, as though there is a direct correlation between quantity and quality. At the close of the session, the obsessive-compulsive patient will consult his watch to be sure he "got his money's worth," as though his watch would measure the value of the experience. An additional 2 minutes could cause him to leave feeling expanded and important, as though he were the recipient of a gift. It could also lead to a sense of having gotten away with something and to fear that the interviewer is unable to maintain proper control over his time. The obsessive-compulsive patient looks to his watch rather than his feelings to see what he will do next. In this way, the motivation of behavior is externalized. He may look at his watch shortly before the end of a session to see if there is enough time to bring up a matter he has been avoiding. The clinician can empathically recognize this by asking, "Are you checking to see if there is sufficient time left to open up another topic?" The patient may proceed or reply, "I'd rather wait until next time." The clinician could respond, "Let's start it now, because it is probably connected to something going on now. Let's not lose the moment of relevance."

The obsessive-compulsive patient tends to use money and status rather than love as his foundation for emotional security. Finances are one of the most threatening topics for discussion, and the clinician's motivation for prying into such matters is immediately suspect. Money comes to represent the innermost source of self-esteem and is treated with the secrecy and privilege that others reserve for the intimate details of love relationships. This is all the more striking when love relationships can be discussed with an apparent lack of anxiety or emotion. Social prohibitions against the discussion of money may lead the interviewer to collaborate with the obsessive-compulsive patient in avoiding this important area.

Indeed, in many ways the obsessive-compulsive patient is a caricature of social tact. Customs of etiquette are designed to avoid hurting or offending others. The exaggerated etiquette of the obsessive-compulsive patient is designed to control his hostile impulses. The skillful interviewer is working for emotional rapport and honesty rather than a sham of social form. This requires maneuvers that may seem tactless or rude to the beginner. This directness strives for an understanding relationship that is sympathetic with the patient's difficulty with fear, anger, and guilt as well as his feelings of warmth and tenderness.

In his preoccupation with time, money, status, and power struggles, the obsessive-compulsive patient is an intensely competitive individual. Although he fears the consequences of open competition with anyone of equal or greater status, he imagines himself to be in competition with everyone. All behavior is viewed in terms of its competitive implications. This is related to a developmentally later phase of his conflict with parental authority. He struggles with his mothering person over sleeping, feeding, toilet training, and the other issues of the first 2 years of life. In homes in which the father's authority is dominant, the boy's fear of authority then comes to represent a fear of competition with a more powerful male figure. The emerging dynamics of the oedipal stage are superimposed on this struggle. The boy symbolically experiences fear of retaliation for his oedipal desires as a fear of castration. It is therefore easy to understand how the anxiety manifested in the clinical interview often relates to fears of castration rather than to fears of loss of dependency. The initial power struggle often is similar with the female obsessive-compulsive patient in homes in which the mother's authority predominates, and the battle with the father may not occur until a later age or may never occur if the girl perceives her father as a protector from the mother's anger and control.

Defenses Derived From the Conflict

The obsessive-compulsive patient must keep his conflicting emotions, and indeed all emotion, as secret as possible—secret not only from the therapist but also from himself. This leads to one of his most characteristic defense mechanisms: *emotional isolation*. He prefers to operate as though emotion did not exist and tries to "feel with his mind."

The obsessive-compulsive patient uses his intellect to avoid his emotions—his feelings are converted to thoughts, so he thinks rather than feels. Conflicts involving emotion are reflected by his rational doubting. He struggles to engage other people on the level of theories and concepts, leading to an endless discussion of details and situations in order to avoid true engagement on the level of feelings and emotions. Thoughts should be related to motives, emotions, and actions in the real world. For the obsessive-compulsive patient, thought serves to avoid awareness of motives and emotions and to delay adaptive action.

Rationalization—a common defense of the obsessive-compulsive patient—is defined as the intellectual substitution of words, language, and concepts to control and express affects selectively, chiefly in derivative form. Emotional isolation logically accompanies this defense because the patient feels threatened by any expression of emotion. This process takes one of four basic forms: 1) emotion after the fact; 2) emotions that are hidden behind token representations of their opposites (as in the process of doing and undoing); 3) the defensive use of anger, which increases the sense of strength and power, thereby avoiding dangerous feelings of warmth and love but with the result that the patient believes that he is bad; and 4) the displacement of emotions to other persons or situations from those that stimulated the feeling.

Words and language, the tools of thought, are utilized in a special way by the obsessive-compulsive patient. They are used in order not to communicate. The obsessive-compulsive patient will provide a flood of speech, but the interviewer is left with useless residue. Details are used to obscure rather than enlighten, producing a great deal of data but not useful, real information. Boredom is a common response to the patient's preoccupation with minutiae, his struggle to find just the right word, and his emphasis on irrelevant detail. The clinician's boredom is a signal that the patient is successfully avoiding emotion and that the interviewer has not been able to challenge this defensive behavior effectively.

The avoidance of such painful affects as fear and rage is easily understood, but the obsessive patient is even more anxious to avoid affection, warmth, and love. His sense of strength and pride are tied to his ever-present, defiant rage, causing him to mistrust any feelings of warmth or tenderness. In his earlier life, the emotions that normally accompany closeness occurred in the context of dependency relations. Therefore, he reacts to his warm emotions with dependent and passive helpless feelings that stimulate fears of possible ridicule and rejection. Pleasurable experiences are postponed, because pleasure is also dangerous. The obsessive-compulsive patient is intensely efficient in planning for future happiness but cannot relax enough to enjoy it when that time arrives. His avoidance of pleasure is based on unconscious guilt. He atones for his transgressions, appeases his conscience, and rigidly controls his forbidden impulses.

In the initial interviews, the obsessive-compulsive patient usually denies problems in his sexual relations. His inhibition will become conscious only as he perceives his general constriction of pleasurable functioning. The partner of the obsessive-compulsive patient knows that sexual relations are always the same. There is either little variety or compulsive variety, because true spontaneity is viewed as dangerous. The obsessive-compulsive patient has a particular fixation and conflict in the area of masturbation, which has become projected onto heterosexual experience. The partner becomes a new and more exciting instrument for accomplishing masturbation. The partner is expected to be under the control of the obsessive-compulsive patient during the sexual relationship, and neither is allowed to do anything different. This kind of control is a direct extension of the masturbatory fantasy, where the fantasy partner is exclusively controlled by the individual creating the fantasy. It comes as a startling revelation to the obsessive-compulsive patient that no two people make love exactly the same way. The concept of the sexual relation as an opportunity for two persons to discover and explore one another while expressing feelings of love and tenderness is quite foreign. Instead, the obsessive-compulsive patient experiences the bed as a proving ground where he must demonstrate his prowess and work to conceal his inadequacy. The obsessive-compulsive man is preoccupied with his performance; the obsessive-compulsive woman is more likely planning the next day's grocery list. Either may be preoccupied with getting into just the right position, and if both are obsessive-compulsive, a power struggle will ensue over that issue. Performance, for the obsessive-compulsive person, can be measured: it is measured by the duration, frequency, or number of orgasms. Often the number of orgasms given to the partner is more important than the pleasurable aspects of the experience.

The need to avoid feelings leads to evasiveness and suspiciousness. Emotions are frequently hidden behind token representatives of their opposite. Angry at the therapist's lateness, the patient will thank the clinician for managing to find time for him in a busy schedule. Moved by the therapist's warm spontaneity in response to a tragedy in his life, the obsessive-compulsive patient may complain that the interviewer is only pretending to be concerned as a paid listener. These token emotions are coupled with a kind of deviousness. An apparent gift usually contains a hidden dagger. The patient who compliments a drab piece of furniture may be indirectly telling the interviewer that he has no taste. The patient is even more likely to disguise warm feelings and consequently suffers from loneliness, social isolation, and diminished capacity for pleasure. He pays a heavy price for avoiding his fear and rage by minimizing emotional contact with others.

Analogous to the use of token emotions is the experience of emotions after the fact. Unresponsive during the interview, the patient will experience feelings of rage after leaving the office. Once he has left the interview, the need for repression is no longer so great. Depending on the severity of the isolation, only the ideas may come to consciousness.

An illustration is the patient who says, "After the last session, the thought of punching you in the nose came to mind." If the interviewer inquires whether this was accompanied by anger, the patient might reply, "No, the thought just passed through my head." The less severe obsessive-compulsive patient might work himself into a rage and declare, "If only he were here, I would really tell him." It will be ancient history by the next appointment, back in the box with the lid nailed down. The obsessive-compulsive patient lives a secret inner life that he fears sharing with anyone. The interviewer must convince the patient that he can accept and understand these feelings without disapproval. The patient's shame and mistrust make this difficult, and he often provokes the angry or disapproving behavior that he fears. Every obsessive-compulsive patient is somewhat paranoid.

Unable to experience love and affection, the obsessive-compulsive patient substitutes respect and security. This leads to a desire for dependent attachments to others, but such dependency is experienced as a form of inadequacy and submission. The obsessive-compulsive patient usually responds by avoiding the dependency gratification that he craves; therefore, he is frequently depressed. This is aggravated by the diminished self-confidence and self-esteem that follow his inhibition of assertion and aggression. The depression may not be apparent to the patient, because he handles depression, along with other emotions, by isolation. The interviewer should anticipate its appearance as soon as the isolation is broken through. From this renunciation of dependency gratification, together with his need for respect from others, the obsessive-compulsive patient forges a subjective sense of moral superiority. This compensates for his refusal to accept dependency gratification from others by providing a fantasy of constant approval from internalized objects. Moral superiority colors the obsessive-compulsive patient's every act. This can be a particularly difficult resistance to interpret, because it converts many symptoms and character traits, however painful or maladaptive, into ethical virtues

It has already been mentioned that the obsessive-compulsive patient has exaggerated feelings of dependence and helplessness. Dynamically, such feelings occur whenever his omnipotent status is threatened. Obsessional omnipotence is a function of two people who are joined together in symbiotic partnership. The original omnipotent partnership was that of the infant and his mother, who seemed to be all-knowing, all-powerful, and all-providing. He continually seeks to reestablish such a partnership, in which he can again substitute grandiose omnipotence for effective coping mechanisms. This alliance does not have to be with an individual but can be with a system of thought, a religion, a scientific doctrine, and so forth. When you separate the obsessive-compulsive patient from his omnipotent partner, he becomes clinically anxious, overwhelmed with feelings of helplessness, inadequacy, and dependence. The scientist who feels insecure when away from his laboratory is a clear example. Not infrequently, the obsessive-compulsive patient will attempt to reestablish his grandiosity by appearing to be an expert in matters about which he actually knows very little. In each new situation, he will quickly rush about amassing facts, on which he then proceeds to exhibit expertise. Typical of the obsessive-compulsive patient in his compensatory grandiosity is his refusal to delegate. He feels he can do everything better for himself than anyone else can do it for him, and he hates to admit to himself that he needs another person. Both the possessiveness and the need to save everything relate to his fear of separation from any loved object as well as to the defiant aspects of his power struggles.

Obsessive *indecisiveness* is a major defense involving both the problem of commitment and the fear of making a mistake. Frequently, these mechanisms are intertwined. Any situation in which the patient encounters the pronouncement "All sales final, no exchange or refunds" will cause hesitation even when the patient has found exactly what he wants at exactly the price he wants to pay. This example is used both in a literal sense and as a metaphor. Although the interviewer can interpret the patient's fear of making a mistake, the patient requires active encouragement on the part of the clinician in order to make decisions. The clinician can support whichever decision the patient seems to want at the particular moment, especially when either side of the decision can work out for the patient's success. The clinician can emphasize, "Your problem is more in making a decision rather than in finding the right or wrong answer." It is also useful to point out that the hidden affective or emotional implication of the decision cannot be resolved through intellectual processes. It is important that the therapist refrain from making decisions for the patient.

An important therapeutic opportunity develops when the patient begins to complain about not having much fun or always working while other people seem to be having a good time. The patient defensively utilizes his high moral standards as an excuse to avoid pleasure. He fears corruption, with the resultant loss of his virtues. Moral masochism typically occurs as part of the obsessive-compulsive personality disorder, sometimes mixed with mildly paranoid or narcissistic traits as well. The clinician frequently is viewed in early dreams in the role of a seducer or corrupter. This pattern may be interpreted in the transference early in the treatment.

Although the patient's compulsive talking, not listening, interrupting the clinician, finishing his sentence for him, or asking him to repeat what he just said is apparent in the initial interview, it is not a behavior pattern to interpret until well after the initial engagement, because doing so makes the patient feel put down and criticized. This is an area in which the interviewer's countertransference frequently causes him to intervene prematurely in a nonsupportive fashion. Eventually, such confrontations will become necessary and may provide constructive emotional experiences for the patient.

It is useful to consider the patient's defensive use of teasing and sadism. Although one is countertransferentially tempted to focus on those behaviors early in the treatment, this is rarely productive and invariably leads to the patient feeling hurt and misunderstood. Using the term *sadism* rather than anger or aggression can be useful for several reasons that become clear if we examine the origins of sadism. First, the young child may sense the parents' sadistic pleasure when they tease the child, causing embarrassment or humiliation. The child, through the process of identification, then gains the notion that he, too, can gain pleasure from teasing others in some way. This sadistic play involves hiding the child's favorite toy, making a scary noise, and pushing a game to the point that the child cries rather than laughs. The child learns that he, too, can play this way. For example, throwing the toy out of the crib so that the parent will bring it back. After several rounds, the parent pretends to suffer ("Oh no, not again!"), and the child laughs gleefully. The same child, like his parents, lacks the subtle social skill of knowing when he has gone "too far" in these supposedly fun games and feels ashamed, humiliated, and guilty when he is scolded for the behavior.

Sadism thus develops from the child identifying with the sadistic powerful controlling behavior of the parent. Sadism is also a derivative of inhibited anger and aggression. The repressed affect of chronic anger returns in the form of deliberate meanness. In the midphase of treatment, the therapist begins to show the patient that some of his behavior is mean and that he was mean because of some earlier anger that he could not express. Next, one interprets the patient's expectation that others will feel loved when he is teasing them, and last, the patient develops awareness of his identification with a powerful and sadistic parent. Intense feelings of guilt, with or without depression, often develop during this phase of the treatment. In fact, obsessive-compulsive patients often become depressed during the course of treatment as they begin to relinquish some of their defenses.

Differential Diagnosis

Obsessive-compulsive symptoms are found in a wide variety of patients, including the phobic patient, the depressed patient, the cognitively impaired patient, and the narcissistic patient. In Chapter 5, "The Narcissistic Patient," there is a detailed discussion concerning the similarities and differences between the narcissistic and the obsessive-compulsive patient. Narcissistic and obsessive-compulsive features frequently occur in the same patient. The patient with an eating disorder has obsessive-compulsive ideas concerning food that result in ritualized behavior with regard to his food and exercise. Purging and vomiting are often prominent features. The phobic patient is obsessed with the situations he finds frightening, and he has developed elaborate rituals designed to symbolically provide safety and protection against frightening situations. The paranoid patient also has many obsessive-compulsive defense mechanisms. He, too, is filled with mistrust of others and assigns meanings to other people's behavior as it pertains to himself. However, he lacks friends, and he has much more trouble in the workplace getting along with people, whom he correctly feels do not like him but incorrectly believes are conspiring against him. He is litigious and has little insight into his situation, unlike the obsessive-compulsive person who has some friends and performs well in tasks that require attention to detail. The passive-aggressive personality can be confused with the obsessive-compulsive patient because of the resistance expressed by procrastination, stubbornness, forgetfulness, and related self-defeating behavior in work-related and social areas. Like the paranoid person, the passive-aggressive person is unappreciated at work and is a chronic complainer. He blames others and can be openly argumentative, irritable, and oppositional. The passive-aggressive personality often expresses his anger through a sullen, sulking, unpleasant attitude. He seeks out others like himself, and together they complain about the unfairness of life, the job, marriage, and so on. His presentation differs from the masochistic patient in that his aggression and anger are focused on authority figures, whereas the masochistic patient's negativity is focused on himself.

Masochistic features are found in the obsessive-compulsive patient who suffers more from what he misses in life. He has trouble having fun, relaxing, and enjoying the pleasures of love and companionship. He never feels there is time for fun when there is so much work to do. When he takes a vacation, he pays off his guilty conscience by bringing work along. Although his partner may experience that behavior as sadistic, it is more driven by the patient's guilt than his repressed anger. This is an important distinction to draw for the patient in the interview situation, and the clinician can help the obsessive-compulsive patient to understand how his partner could suffer by not sharing his value system regarding work and his fear of losing his virtue.

MANAGEMENT OF THE INTERVIEW

The obsessive-compulsive patient may approach the interviewer by attempting to reverse roles. He may begin by asking, "How are you today?" and then continue with other questions, seizing the controlling role. Another pattern is to wait for the clinician to initiate the interview and then turn the tables by saying, "Could you explain what you mean by that?" It is not unusual for the beginning clinician to respond with annoyance to the patient's maneuvers. It is more useful to respond sympathetically with a casual comment such as, "Your interest in interviewing me suggests that it must be difficult for you to be the patient." Later in the interview, the clinician responds to these maneuvers by telling the patient that there are no right or wrong answers and that he should respond with whatever comes into his mind rather than trying to get the question exactly right so that he can answer it correctly.

The chief problem in the interview is to establish genuine emotional contact. The subjective emotional responses of the interviewer are an excellent guide to success. If the interviewer is interested, involved, and "tuned in," contact has been established. If he is anxious or angry, contact has been established, but the secondary defenses of the patient are at work. If the interviewer is bored or indifferent, there is little contact.

The obsessive-compulsive patient will misuse every mode of communication in the service of emotional isolation. To reach someone, it is necessary to look at the person, talk to him, listen to him, and attend to what he says; it is also necessary to be spontaneous and expressive and to avoid silence. The obsessive-compulsive patient may avoid direct eye contact with the interviewer. Eyes are important mediators of emotional contact with people. To avoid looking helps to avoid emotional contact. On occasion the patient may appear to be looking at the interviewer but is only pretending and is really looking beyond the interviewer. It is the same avoidance, but with token appeasement added. He can also avoid engagement with his voice. He can whisper, mumble, or speak in such a way that the interviewer will have difficulty hearing what is said. The patient will not listen. He will not hear the interviewer's comment and will ask to have them repeated. When the interviewer repeats, the patient will interrupt to complete the sentence and then ask for verification. The patient may hear the words but not comprehend their meaning. The obsessive-compulsive patient is a master at concealing his inattentiveness. While appearing to pay complete attention, in reality he is thinking about something totally different. Some individuals are highly skilled at this and are able to repeat the interviewer's exact words on request. However, although the words were registered in the patient's mind, the significance of their content was not registered until the patient repeated the statement.

Repeating the interviewer's phrases and questions allows the obsessive-compulsive patient to avoid contact; he is really talking to himself, not to the other person. He is not answering questions or following rules, but in his unconscious fantasy he is controlling the entire interchange by minimizing the interviewer's participation. Another common way of accomplishing this is by lecturing to the interviewer. It is important that one not hurt the patient unnecessarily when interrupting this behavior. Rather than utilize the patient's device of phony tact, it is more to the point to comment in an accepting tone, "I feel like I'm being scolded. Did I do something that offended you?"

The patient will utilize a variety of defenses for the same purpose. The interviewer should avoid interpreting every defense, or the patient will feel attacked and the interview will have the quality of constantly putting the patient down, increasing his self-consciousness. Instead, the interviewer observes what is happening and directs his comments to a key or central defense. It is far better to err by choosing a less important defense than to bombard the patient with the table of contents of a psychodynamics textbook. This error is more likely to occur when one has had enough training to recognize the many defensive maneuvers but has not yet had the experience to use this knowledge at the proper time.

Another technique for concealing feelings is the use of denial. The obsessive-compulsive patient will frequently tell more about himself in the negative than in the positive: "It isn't that I feel thus and such" or "It isn't that this happened to be troubling me at such and such a time." In the unconscious there are no negatives; he is revealing the underlying problem in his own way. The interviewer should not directly challenge this denial but encourage him to elaborate. The more this is done, the more he begins to reverse himself. When the reversal is complete, the interviewer is in a position to return to the original statement and expose the conflict. He may say to the patient, "You are describing the feelings that you denied only a few minutes before, and I find this puzzling."

Another common means of avoiding involvement is the use of notes or lists consisting of topics to be discussed or questions to be asked. These may appear at any time during the interview, and they represent a key defense against the patient's anxiety. In an initial interview an understanding interviewer allows the patient his defenses, particularly a patient who needs to feel in control of the interview. The interviewer can suggest to the patient, "It is best if you tell your story in whatever order it comes to you and then consult your notes to see what you forgot. This approach could be more helpful." It is not appropriate to engage the patient in a power struggle before he has even had a chance to tell his story. The older patient may need the assistance of a list or notes because he no longer trusts his memory, and he is unclear about how long the interview will last.

When it is apparent that the patient is following an outline, the interviewer can ask, "Did you plan the interview in advance?" If the reply is affirmative, the clinician can ask, "Were you anxious about the interview? How did planning the interview reduce that anxiety?"

One of the obsessive-compulsive patient's favorite techniques involves his particular use of intellect and language. He is preoccupied with finding just the right word to describe the quantitative aspect of emotion. Words have become more than symbols and have an importance of their own. He was not "angry"; he was "annoyed." Or he was not "angry" or "annoyed"; he was "perturbed." A related way of avoiding emotion is through the use of scientific terms and technical jargon. The clinician must avoid such terms in his own comments and should translate the patient's technical terms into everyday language. The obsessive-compulsive patient will often use euphemisms to describe a basically unpleasant or embarrassing situation. These misleading terms should also be rephrased by the clinician in basic, direct words. For example, if the patient states that he and his wife had a "slight tiff," the interviewer might reply, "How did the fight begin?" In another instance, a patient might refer to a recent sexual experience by saying, "We were close last night." The interviewer can reply, "Do you mean you had sex?"

The patient's tendency toward intellectualization can also be minimized if the clinician avoids asking questions that contain the word "think." "What did you think about this?" is a typical obsessive question and leads to intellectualization. Instead, the interviewer asks, "How did you feel?" When the obsessive-compulsive patient is asked how he feels, he will relate what he thinks. The interviewer can interpret this, saying, "I didn't mean, 'What did you think?' I meant, 'How did you feel?'" It requires persistence to reach feelings if the person has no awareness of them himself. The clinician should also avoid asking questions that require the patient to make a decision, thereby triggering the doubting mechanism in the intellectual defenses. If the patient is asked, "Who are you closer to, your mother or your father?" his answer may offend someone, and therefore his doubting serves as a defense. It is better to say, "Tell me about your parents," and notice which parent is mentioned first and what information is volunteered.

A patient described her eagerness to visit her sister as motivated by fondness for her and not by any feeling of competition between them. Inquiry about the relationship led to a discussion of the sister's dependence on their parents and finally to the patient's irritation that the sister received more than her share of presents from the parents. The visit emerged as an attempt to ascertain what recent gifts her sister might have received. At this point the interviewer said, "I'm not sure I understand. You said that there is not competition, but it seems that you are envious of the things she receives from your parents." The patient struggled to explain that there was no contradiction, but finally admitted that the visit would help to suppress her competitive feelings, since the sister's gifts were always more attractive in the patient's fantasies than in reality.

A specific type of denial commonly found is the introductory or parenthetical statement, such as "To tell the truth"; "My real feelings are…"; or "Let me be frank with you." These apparently innocuous assurances are purposeful. The patient has something to hide and is denying it. Again, direct confrontation will only lead to more indignant denial, but these are invaluable clues to distortions and hidden feelings that the patient feels are reprehensible.

Even the most carefully guarded obsessive-compulsive patient has two episodes of spontaneous behavior in each interview: the beginning and the end. Most patients exclude these episodes from their mental picture of an interview, and as a result they provide a wealth of information to the attentive interviewer who excludes nothing. The patient reveals feelings in the corridor or the waiting room that he carefully conceals in the office. Rather than start a new conversation after the patient and interviewer are seated, the clinician might continue the original conversation. The patient's activity in the waiting room should be observed, for example, the magazine he reads, the chair he selects, and the objects in which he becomes interested. He will compliment or criticize the office furniture as a means of communicating his feelings about the interviewer. When the session is finished, he will relax, and with this relaxation his feelings will emerge. He may allude to the secret he has been guarding ("I wonder why you didn't ask me about such-and-such") or reveal his disappointment in the interviewer by saying, "I thought you were going to tell me what to do."

The obsessive-compulsive patient will waste time on irrelevant detail. He is so convinced that the interviewer will not understand him that he must provide volumes of background information before he can come to the point of his story. This becomes so complex that when the patient finally arrives at what he wanted to say, either the interviewer has lost interest or the interview is over. Eventually, this defense must be interpreted; it is an error to let the patient finish, although he will plead that it will only take another minute. He is inordinately sensitive to criticism, which makes interruptions or admonitions to get to the point particularly difficult. The interviewer can say, "I don't understand how this is related to the question that I asked you," to which the patient may respond, "Oh, it's related. You've got to know about this and this and this." The clinician's reply might be, "Do you feel that I won't be able to understand you if I don't have all this detailed background?" "Indeed," the patient will answer, to which the interviewer comments, "Well, let's try going directly to the heart of the matter, and if I don't understand, I'll ask you for more background information." The patient may hesitate while deciding whether to appease the interviewer or to proceed as before. If he persists with irrelevant details, the interviewer should not pursue the matter further at that time. Patience on the interviewer's part is crucial with the obsessive-compulsive patient.

Silence is another technique for avoiding emotional rapport. The obsessive-compulsive patient can endure prolonged silence to a greater extent than most other patients, with the exception of those who are grossly psychotic or deeply depressed. The interviewer must learn to tolerate these silences. When the patient breaks the silence, a piece of spontaneous behavior emerges from an individual who avoids spontaneity. If the patient remains silent, the interviewer may comment, "You feel quiet now?" or "You're silent." The patient may reply, "I was just waiting for your next question." If this is indeed what the patient was doing, and it is very unlikely, the reply might be, "Yes, I can see that you were waiting for me to do something next. Perhaps you are concerned about something that might be upsetting?" If the therapist interrupts the silence, it is not to introduce a topic but rather to focus on the possible meaning of the silence itself, for example, "Have you run out of things you want to talk about?" "I guess so," the patient replies. The interviewer continues with, "Only you can decide whether it is worse pain to face your embarrassment or to feel bad about yourself that you weren't able to share your pain."

The obsessive-compulsive patient's attempts to do the interviewing do not all occur at the beginning of the session. He may refer to a comment the interviewer made earlier, with a request that some confusing aspect be explained. When the interviewer complies, more questions ensue, and soon the patient has the interview well in hand—his hand. This both assures him that he will not be caught off guard saying the wrong things and allows him to control and direct the interview.

Toward the middle or later portion of the interview, one could explore the patient's financial status. This is useful in exposing the patient's fear and mistrust of the clinician. It is equally productive with private patients and those with whom the clinician may not have direct responsibility for setting the fee. Fees and the hours of the appointments are two issues that the interviewer should not allow to become simply commodities to be managed through bargaining. The obsessive-compulsive patient is a "wheedler." If the fee is reduced, the patient feels either that the clinician was overcharging him in the first place or that he, the patient, has succeeded in gaining an advantage, which may increase his guilt feelings.

DEVELOPMENT OF THE THERAPEUTIC ALLIANCE

The interviewer should help the patient to develop an awareness of emotions other than fear, rage, and guilt. When the patient describes an emotion, the clinician can name it. This particularly includes love, shame, tenderness, sadness, or hurt feelings. Reinforcing the experience of such feelings provides evidence to the patient that he is emotionally alive. Contrary to standard advice given to beginning therapists, it is useful for the interviewer to name the feeling for the patient when the patient cannot do so himself. The patient can correct the clinician if he is wrong. The obsessive-compulsive patient's lack of awareness of these other emotions in himself contributes to his social disconnection and feeds his devalued sense of self-worth. He has a secret admiration for people who seem strong and at the same time experience warmth and tenderness. The interviewer makes it clear to the patient that the goal is not merely to behave as though he has the feelings but actually to experience them, although for many obsessive-compulsive patients the behavior facilitates the awareness of the emotion. The interviewer can look for displaced emotions or their somatic equivalents, such as vasomotor responses. It is important to notice and to remark on them, with a comment such as "You are blushing." The patient should be asked to report emotional incidents that occur outside of the therapy as well, because they represent opportunities to understand the patient's feelings and at the same time enable the patient to bring a different body of data to the session. This is preferable to criticizing the patient with interpretations of his absence of emotional response. It may not always be possible to learn immediately what produced the emotional reaction, but it has at least been established that the patient had an emotional response.

The therapist's spontaneity and emotional reactivity have an important impact on the obsessive-compulsive patient. Beginning clinicians often misunderstand the principle of technical neutrality, adopting an attitude with their patients that is bland, noncommittal, and emotionally unresponsive. The clinician's use of his own emotional responses sets an example for the patient, who not infrequently remarks, "You seem to have more feelings about this subject than I do."

The clinician should avoid stereotyped ways of starting and finishing a session. Clinicians tend to develop routines, ending their sessions each time with the same phrase, which sets a model for the patient that fits in neatly with the obsessive-compulsive patient's character structure.

> A patient with many obsessive-compulsive personality traits had been discussing during the session his need to control the important people in his life. He presented convincing data supporting the idea that he was somewhat grudgingly acknowledging that he was not the omnipotent person to which he aspired. At the end of the session, as he walked toward the door, he performed a quick "pat down" on his jacket. "Did you lose something?" asked the clinician. "No," the patient replied in a questioning tone. The interviewer responded, "Do you *feel* as though you have lost something?" "That's it. You got it." The patient demonstrated, through a nonverbal communication, the subjective sense of something being physically removed from him as he began to relinquish his all-consuming need to see himself as omnipotent.

When the patient seems to be confusing the clinician with elaborate or unnecessary detail, it is important to avoid making critical comments. The patient is trying to be more precise and to avoid errors and control his own wish to distort his presentation. One explores the patient's fear of distortion. After all, everyone does it, and the patient must understand that he, too, is "entitled" to distort when it is based on authentic emotional perceptions. This is part of encouraging the patient to take emotional viewpoints. There may be times when the patient is unconsciously attempting to obfuscate and confuse the clinician. On those occasions it is appropriate to remark, "We have 10 minutes left, and I sense you have something you very much want to discuss and we may not be able to get to it today." On other occasions, when this mechanism is operating, it is appropriate to ask the patient at the beginning of the story, "Tell me the bottom line." It may be necessary to persuade the patient that it is in his own best interest to attempt this exercise. This is not something to do in the initial meetings. The patient has a need to be long-winded. However, eventually blocking the behavior can enable the patient to become conscious of the emotional need that is reflected in his long-windedness. The patient desires a monologue rather than a dialogue or interaction in order to hold the attention and maintain control of the clinician, a mechanism of which the patient is quite unconscious. An empathic interpretation is made after the patient experiences a feeling in response to being brought more directly to his point. Without such an interpretation a power struggle will ensue. Rather than point out the patient's aggressive and controlling character, it is possible to allow the patient to become aware of this in response to his own feeling of wanting not to listen to the therapist and only wanting the therapist to listen to him. The clinician can then try to understand, together with the patient, what it is that the patient fears. As indicated earlier, it is important to interact with this patient whenever possible rather than appearing detached, aloof, and objective.

TRANSFERENCE AND COUNTERTRANSFERENCE

The obsessive-compulsive patient often feels that he has come to an omniscient clinician who has all the answers to his problems. When the clinician comments, "You feel I know the answers to your problems and are annoyed that I am arbitrarily making you work them out for yourself," the patient comments, "That is correct, so why don't you speed things up and be more helpful?" The beginning therapist then falls silent, and the patient feels frustrated and discouraged or angry. This type of interaction only slows the development of a working alliance. Furthermore, it tends to be taken by the patient as a criticism of his emotional needs, with an implication that he makes insatiable demands. By the therapist's providing answers to the patient's questions when possible, a therapeutic alliance is fostered. In due time the patient will become aware that his needs are, at times, insatiable, and then the therapist can help the patient understand himself better, from the vantage point of an ally rather than an adversary.

Secrets and withholding for this patient represent problems with power, control, submission, and defiance rather than the separation-individuation issues seen in sicker patients. They also reflect his incomplete commitment to the treatment. Often the patient maintains a secret list of the clinician's mistakes and deficiencies for use at the proper time. It is necessary to uncover this process while being sensitive to the patient's criticisms and disappointments that have not yet been verbalized. It is important to explain to the patient that these feelings should be discussed as they occur, because that is when the patient's feelings are most available. Nevertheless, it is precisely at that time that the patient feels most vulnerable and therefore is inclined to withhold. For example, the clinician might say, "I just noticed that I mixed up the names of your brothers." The patient will typically respond, "I noticed it too." The interviewer can reply, "But you didn't mention it. Perhaps you didn't want me to know that you were disappointed in me." Later, the clinician can show the patient that his collection of these negative feelings ultimately has a destructive impact on his relationships. The defensive use of criticism of others to ward off intimacy can be interpreted relatively early in treatment, but it is often more useful to do this outside of the transference, because the patient will deny feelings of intimacy with the therapist early in the treatment. As the patient becomes a more sophisticated participant in the treatment and the therapist comments on his own error, the patient may remark, "You said that I shouldn't be such a perfectionist; I'm just trying to be tolerant and overlook your mistakes as you suggested." At this point, it is better to keep quiet than to engage in a debate. If the patient was joking, the interviewer can smile and say, "Touché."

In the inevitable battle that develops between clinician and patient over issues of money and time, try to get the battle where it belongs—that is, inside the patient. The clinician can ask the patient, "What would you consider fair for both of us?" or "How do you suggest we resolve this?" This is to expose a conflict within the patient rather than in the dyadic relationship.

As treatment progresses, the clinician should be alert for regressive wishes on the part of the patient to make a mess, to be nurtured, to control the world, and so on. The clinician's empathy with these regressive wishes causes the patient to fear he will lose control of himself. He becomes uncomfortable. The patient will be reassured to learn that a little gratification will not lead to a total collapse of all of his virtues and that when he feels more gratified, he will be less angry and better able to share himself with others.

Avoid spending much time on the discovery of the meanings of the rituals and their origins. This is only rarely helpful. Why the patient continues to engage in them is always more important. Instead, concentrate on recent events, present frustrations, and resentment. This avoids the dry, historical account of the patient's past. This patient will frequently attempt to leave the present to discuss the past in a defensive way. The therapist may interpret that defense with a comment such as, "You seem to feel more comfortable discussing the past because the feelings that were attached to those experiences have now subsided."

The clinician can be supportive when the patient's grandiose self-expectations make him dissatisfied with small gains and slow progress. The patient wants magical gains and an instant cure. His criticism of his progress can be interpreted as an unwillingness to relinquish his excessive demands on himself and those persons who are most important to him, including the clinician.

It is necessary to convince the patient of the need to change the behavior to which he clings rigidly and that he rationalizes. At times, when all else fails, the clinician can say to the patient, "Try to experiment; you have nothing to lose. If it doesn't work, you can always go back and do it your way." If the patient is unable to follow such a suggestion, the clinician must further explore the patient's fear. It is particularly helpful to do this in the case of major life events such as births, funerals, weddings, birthdays, graduations, and other significant experiences for which the patient will have no second chance.

> A female patient began a session expressing anger with her mother, who had just advised her of the mother's pending remarriage 3 days hence in a distant city. For years the patient had had an angry, dependent relationship with her mother. The clinician commented, "Your feelings are hurt because your mother didn't invite you. She probably believed you would say no and was sparing herself hurt feelings." "I never thought of that," the patient answered. The patient's anger subsided, but it was clear that nothing further was about to happen, so the clinician suggested, "You could call her back, congratulate her, and tell her that you felt hurt not to be invited." The patient said, "I'll think about it." The following week the patient thanked the clinician and reported, "When I told my mother how I felt, she said she wanted me to come but was afraid I'd say no. I cried, she cried, and she offered to pay for my ticket, then I said I'd pay for it, and we agreed to each pay half. If I hadn't done that, it would be a wound that would never have healed."

> A married female attorney in her mid-30s with two children presented with mild depression and feelings of anxiety at work that began in response to a job situation in which she felt she was losing control. Shortly into the treatment, she reported that her child was sick, which had made it necessary for her to remain away from work for a day to care for her. The clinician began the next session by asking about the child's condition. The patient replied that her daughter had a streptococcal infection, and after giving a detailed commentary on the daughter's medical condition, the patient remarked, "I found it difficult being home with her all day long. She likes to play imaginative games and fritters away time on mindless activities. I try to teach her to play with the computer so that she will learn something more useful and practical for her later life. She doesn't want to do that, and we get into a power struggle." She went on to describe her 4-year-old daughter as clinging and demanding, which meant that she liked to climb into her lap while watching television. The patient felt that affection must be rationed, and only the appropriate amount should be given, much like the medication for her daughter's infection.
>
> This commentary evoked a countertransference response in the clinician, who inwardly and critically thought to himself, "Is all life to be understood in terms of dominance and submission, power and control?" Instead of giving voice to some version of this inner thought, which the patient would have experienced as both critical and contemptuous, the clinician asked, "Don't you like to cuddle and feel close?" In response, the patient said, "I wonder what my children will remember

about me as a mother when they grow up?" At this juncture the patient was emotionally accessible; her rationalizations for control over her daughter were being inwardly questioned. The clinician asked, "How would you like them to remember you?" "Perhaps I should allow myself to enjoy their imagination and affection more." The patient's emotional isolation and rationalized need for control and perfectionism had been brought into question. This paralleled the transference, in which emotion, imagination, and creativity made the patient feel uncomfortable. She could not allow herself to be a playful child with the clinician. Her own mother had neglected her and allowed her to play in the street and do things that were dangerous. She had felt uncared for and abandoned. She developed a reaction-formation against identifying with that aspect of her mother, thereby becoming excessively controlling. She did not realize that her children did not experience her controlling attitude as her means of giving love in a manner she once imagined would have made her feel more secure.

In a following session, the patient talked about her lack of connectedness with her peers and elaborated on her stubborn pursuit of her "rights" in her law firm, but now with some awareness that she was being insensitive and aggressive with her colleagues and how she might be undermining herself. "You seem both tolerant and caring," she said to the clinician. "You've put up with me and my demands about changing times, even the argument over the fee." The clinician had carefully monitored his countertransference responses to this patient. Right at the beginning she had engaged in a power struggle over time and money in an attempt to control him. His response had been to say, "We have to work this out collaboratively. Let's see what times we can both agree on. The same is true for the fee. What can we agree on?" In this manner the patient's paranoid fear that she would be controlled and abused was initially addressed by empathically responding to her anxieties. Ultimately, this was a productive treatment; the patient became curious about her controlling behavior and finally allowed herself the pleasure of feeling love and enjoying her husband and children.

CONCLUSION

Because of their emotional isolation, rigidity, psychological inflexibility, and tendency to engage in overt or covert power struggles with the clinician and the world at large, the obsessive-compulsive patient presents a considerable therapeutic challenge. An empathic awareness of the patient's inner central conflicts and the misery that they engender in the patient's everyday life makes it possible for the clinician to engage in a productive treatment that offers the patient the possibility of freeing himself from an internal mental tyranny that cripples enjoyment of the ordinary pleasures of life.

CHAPTER 4

THE HISTRIONIC PATIENT

Many patients have histrionic features in their makeup, and in general, histrionic patients are attractive people who add much to their surrounding environment through their imagination and sensitivity. Consciously, the histrionic patient wants to be seen as an attractive, charming, lively, warm, intuitive, sensitive, generous, imaginative person who enhances the lives of others and who does not waste time on the trivial details and mechanics of life. However, to those around them, the histrionic patient can appear exhibitionistic, attention seeking, manipulative, superficial, overly dramatic, given to exaggeration, easily hurt, impulsive, inconsiderate of the feelings of others, demanding, and readily given to scenes of tears or anger. Histrionic patients possess a capacity to experience one emotional state after another in very rapid order. In this sense, their affective experience resembles that of the small child who can quickly turn from laughter to tears.

Histrionic personality disorder occurs equally in both sexes. The common transgender features are those of wishing to be seen as glamorous and sexually exciting. The histrionic patient is frequently charismatic and charming. The histrionic patient elicits different responses in other people dependent on their gender. The female histrionic patient is frequently found appealing by male clinicians but is often disliked by female clinicians. Conversely, the male histrionic patient often appeals to female clinicians but not to male clinicians. When a histrionic patient is hospitalized, this gender split is reflected in professional staff discussions. The staff gender polarization that occurs is highly suggestive evidence that the patient's diagnosis is that of histrionic personality disorder.

The histrionic patient presents himself to the world in three domains. One is the *dramatic*—the exhibitionistic, extravagant, emotionally labile, intense, and overly generous constellation. A second is the *manipulative,* in which the interpersonal world is controlled and gratification is extracted from it. This is the attention-seeking, demanding, easily hurt, inconsiderate of others, socially promiscuous, and dependent constellation. The third has to do with aspects of *ego functions*. The histrionic patient is often impulsive, scattered, disorganized, easily bored by detail, rarely punctual, and difficult to rely on. The DSM-5 criteria for histrionic personality disorder focus on a more primitive variant than that described in the older literature (Box 4–1).

BOX 4–1. DSM-5 Diagnostic Criteria for Histrionic Personality Disorder

---

A pervasive pattern of excessive emotionality and attention seeking, beginning by early adulthood and present in a variety of contexts, as indicated by five (or more) of the following:

1. Is uncomfortable in situations in which he or she is not the center of attention.
2. Interaction with others is often characterized by inappropriate sexually seductive or provocative behavior.
3. Displays rapidly shifting and shallow expression of emotions.
4. Consistently uses physical appearance to draw attention to self.
5. Has a style of speech that is excessively impressionistic and lacking in detail.
6. Shows self-dramatization, theatricality, and exaggerated expression of emotion.
7. Is suggestible (i.e., easily influenced by others or circumstances).
8. Considers relationships to be more intimate than they actually are.

Source. Reprinted from American Psychiatric Association: *Diagnostic and Statistical Manual of Mental Disorders,* 5th Edition. Arlington, VA, American Psychiatric Association, 2013. Copyright 2013, American Psychiatric Association. Used with permission.

Although this describes one end of a continuum that overlaps with the borderline patient, it excludes the well-integrated and better-functioning histrionic patient, who represents a personality type rather than a disorder and tends to be more stable, with better impulse control. The seductiveness is less overt in better-functioning histrionic patients, and they may possess a strict superego, healthier object relations, and higher-level ego defenses in contrast to the more primitive, and hence more disturbed, histrionic patient. In this disorder, clinical attention to underlying dynamics rather than the manifest behavior is crucial in establishing the diagnosis and differentiating the healthier from the sicker histrionic patient. The unifying features of the continuum of histrionic patients are emotionality and theatricality, which can be charming in those on the healthier end of the spectrum but unappealing in those pa-

TABLE 4–1. Gabbard's differentiation of hysterical personality disorder from histrionic personality disorder

Hysterical personality disorder	Histrionic personality disorder
Restrained and circumscribed emotionality	Florid and generalized emotionality
Sexualized exhibitionism and need to be loved	Greedy exhibitionism with a demanding, oral quality that is "cold" and less engaging
Good impulse control	Generalized impulsivity
Subtly appealing seductiveness	Crude, inappropriate, and distancing seductiveness
Ambition and competitiveness	Aimlessness and helplessness
Mature, triangular object relations	Primitive, dyadic object relations characterized by clinging, masochism, and paranoia
Separations from love objects can be tolerated	Overwhelming separation anxiety occurs when abandoned by love objects
Strict superego and some obsessional defenses	Lax superego and a predominance of primitive defenses, such as splitting and idealization
Sexualized transference wishes develop gradually and are viewed as unrealistic	Intense sexualized transference wishes develop rapidly and are viewed as realistic

Source. Adapted from Gabbard GO: *Psychodynamic Psychiatry in Clinical Practice*, 5th Edition. Washington, DC, American Psychiatric Publishing, 2014, p. 550. Copyright 2014, American Psychiatric Publishing. Used with permission.

tients found at the more disturbed end, who often seem crude in their seductiveness and more dependent, demanding, and helpless.

We agree with Gabbard (2014) that the elimination of the DSM-II diagnosis of hysterical personality disorder and its replacement by histrionic personality disorder in DSM-III essentially removed a clearly identified diagnostic entity and replaced it with the more primitive variant. Gabbard has tabulated the clinical differences between the better-functioning histrionic patient, which he continues to refer to as having "hysterical personality disorder," and the patient with DSM-IV-TR (and DSM-5) histrionic personality disorder (Table 4–1). Gabbard's chart summarizes the distinction between the primitive, oral, "hysteroid" histrionic patient and the mature, oedipal, "hysterical" histrionic patient, a clinical distinction first made by Zetzel (1968) and by Easser and Lesser (1965).

In this chapter we use the DSM-IV-TR (and DSM-5) term *histrionic personality disorder* but apply it in a wider sense to the continuum of histrionic patients, which includes that subsumed under Gabbard's definition of hysterical personality disorder.

PSYCHOPATHOLOGY AND PSYCHODYNAMICS

Histrionic Characteristics

Self-Dramatization

The speech, physical appearance, and general manner of the histrionic patient are dramatic and exhibitionistic. Communication is expressive, and descriptors emphasize feelings and inner experience rather than facts or details. Language patterns reflect a heavy use of superlatives; emphatic phrases may be used so repetitively that they acquire a stereotyped quality. The listener finds himself drawn in by the patient's view of the world. The patient exaggerates in order to dramatize a viewpoint and is unconcerned about rigid adherence to truth if a distortion will better accomplish the drama. These patients are often attractive and may appear younger than their age. In both sexes there is a strong interest in style and fashion, which immediately calls attention to their physical appearance. In the woman there is an overdramatization of femininity; in the man there may be a quality of foppishness or excessive masculinity.

Emotionality

Although the histrionic patient has difficulty experiencing deep feelings of love and intimacy, his superficial presentation is quite to the contrary. This patient is charming and relates to others with apparent warmth, although his emotional responses are labile, easily changeable, and at times excessive. His seeming ease at establishing close relationships quickly causes others to feel like old friends, even though the patient may actually feel uncomfortable. This becomes clearer when further intimacy fails to develop after the first few meetings. Whereas the obsessive-compulsive patient attempts to avoid emotional contact, the histrionic patient constantly strives for personal rapport. In any relationship in which the histrionic patient feels no emotional contact, he experiences feelings of rejection and failure and often blames the other individual, considering him to be boring, cold, and unresponsive. He reacts strongly to disappointment, showing a low tolerance for frustration. A failure to elicit sympathetic responses from others can often lead either to depression or to anger, which may be expressed as a temper tantrum. His charm and verbal expressiveness create an outward impression of poise and self-confidence, but usually the patient's self-image is one of apprehension and insecurity.

Since it is impossible to objectively measure the depth of another person's emotions, it is a quality that one infers from the stability, continuity, and maturity of emotional commitments. A perfectly normal 8-year-old child may change "best friends" with some regularity. Such fickleness in an adult suggests a histrionic character. Relationships with the histrionic patient can be transient and reactive to an immediate event, from loving someone to dismissing them much as a child can move from crying to smiling in a short span of time. There is an underlying instability to the histrionic patient's emotional attachments.

Seductiveness

The histrionic patient creates the impression of using the body as an instrument for the expression of love and tenderness, but this stems from a desire to obtain approval, admiration, and protection rather than a feeling of intimacy or genital sexual desire. Physical closeness is substituted for emotional closeness. The attractive and seductive behavior serves to obtain the love or approval of others rather than to give sexual pleasure to the patient. Histrionic patients respond to others of the same sex with competitive antagonism, particularly if the other person is attractive and utilizes the same devices to obtain affection and attention.

Dependency and Helplessness

Since Western society has different attitudes toward manifest patterns of dependency in men and women, there are striking differences between the superficial behavior of male and female histrionic patients, but these disappear at a deeper level. The male histrionic patient is more likely to exhibit pseudo-independent behavior, which can be recognized as defensive because of the accompanying emotional responses of excessive fear or anger.

In the interview situation, the histrionic woman presents herself as helpless and dependent, relying on the constant responses of the clinician in order to guide her every action. She is possessive in her relationship to him and resents any competitive threat to this parent–child relationship. The interviewer is viewed as magically omnipotent and capable of solving all of her problems in some mysterious fashion. The practitioner, as a parent surrogate, is expected to take care of the patient, to do all of the worrying, and to assume all responsibility; the patient's obligation then is to entertain and charm in response. In working out solutions to her problems, she acts helpless, as though her own efforts do not count. This leads to major countertransference problems in the clinician who enjoys the opportunity to enter an omnipotent alliance. Histrionic patients also adopt a particularly helpless posture when in the presence of their mothers. They are frequently regarded by their families as lovable, cute, ineffective, and "still a child." The seductiveness and pseudo-helplessness are used to manipulate others.

These patients require a great deal of attention from others and are unable to entertain themselves. Boredom is, therefore, a constant problem for histrionic patients, because they consider their inner selves to be dull and unstimulating. External stimulation is constantly pursued, and the theatrical, seductive, overly emotional, helpless, and dependent behavior of the histrionic patient is designed to subtly involve others so that their continued interest and affection are assured. "I just don't know what to do about my boyfriend," exclaimed a histrionic patient. "He's fickle and unreliable, but I'm confused because he's so attractive. Tell me what to do; shouldn't I break up with him? You're experienced, knowledgeable. You must have the answer."

The histrionic patient denies responsibility for the plight in which he finds himself, complaining, "I don't know why it always has to happen to me." He feels that all of his problems stem from some impossible life situation. If this were to be magically changed, he would have no complaint. When dependent needs are not met, these patients typically become angry, demanding, and coercive. However, as soon as it becomes apparent that one technique for obtaining dependent care is not likely to succeed, the patient will abandon it and abruptly switch to another approach.

Noncompliance

In this important group of character traits, the histrionic patient again appears to be the antithesis of the rigid obsessive character, showing disorderliness, a lack of concern with punctuality, and difficulty in planning the mechanical details of life. This group of dynamically organized traits are frequently flaunted by the histrionic patient in an arrogant or passive-aggressive manner.

Whereas the obsessive-compulsive patient feels anxious without his watch, the histrionic patient prefers not wearing a watch. He trusts that there will be a clock in the window of a jewelry store or on top of a billboard or that he can ask a passing pedestrian the time. Management of the time during the session is delegated to the interviewer.

Record keeping and other mundane tasks are viewed by the histrionic patient as burdensome and unnecessary. The obsessive-compulsive patient must always keep his checkbook in order, but the histrionic patient does not bother to do so because the bank keeps a record of the money and will notify him if he is overdrawn. For an obsessive-compulsive person, such an occurrence would be a shameful humiliation.

Histrionic thinking has been described as impulsive, with the patient relying on quick hunches and impressions rather than critical judgments that arise from firm convictions. The patient is often not well informed on politics or world affairs. His main intellectual pursuits are in cultural and artistic areas. He does not usually persevere at routine work, considering it unimportant drudgery. When confronted with a task that is exciting or inspiring and in which the patient can attract attention to himself as a result of his achievement, he reveals a capacity for organization and perseverance. The task can be done particularly well if it requires imagination, a quality that rarely is found in the obsessive character.

Self-Indulgence

The histrionic patient's intense need for love and admiration creates an aura of egocentricity. The narcissistic and vain aspects of his personality are manifested in a concern with external appearance and with the amount of attention received from others. His needs must be immediately gratified, a trait that makes it difficult for the histrionic patient to be a good financial planner, because he buys impulsively. Whereas the histrionic patient is extravagant, the obsessive-compulsive patient is parsimonious.

Suggestibility

Although it has traditionally been said that histrionic patients are overly suggestible, we agree with Easser and Lesser that the histrionic patient is suggestible only as long as the interviewer supplies the right suggestions, those that the patient has subtly indicated that he desires but for which he wants someone else to assume the responsibility.

Sexual and Marital Problems

The histrionic patient usually has disturbed sexual functioning, although there is considerable variation in the form this takes. In the woman, partial frigidity is a reaction to the patient's fear of her own sexual feelings. Also, sexual excitement interferes with her use of sex to control others. This fear is reflected in her hostile, competitive relationships with women and her desire to achieve power over men through seductive conquest. She has great conflict over these goals, with resulting sexual inhibition. Other patients are sexually responsive, but their sexual behavior is accompanied by masochistic fantasies. Promiscuity is not unusual, because the patient uses sex as a means of attracting and controlling men.

The man whom the histrionic woman loves is quickly endowed with the traits of an ideal, all-powerful father who will not make demands on her. However, she always fears losing him as she lost her father, and consequently, she selects a man whom she can hold because of his dependent needs. She may marry "down" socially or marry a man of a different cultural, racial, or religious background, both as an expression of hostility to her father and as a defense against her oedipal strivings. In this way she substitutes a social taboo for the incest taboo. The group who marry older men are also acting out oedipal fantasies but have a greater need to avoid sex. Another dynamic mechanism that often influences the choice of a mate is the defense against castration fear, expressed by selecting a man who is symbolically weaker than the patient.

The male histrionic patient also has disturbances of sexual functioning. These include potency disturbances and Don Juanism. In each of these, there is often an intense neurotic relationship with the mother. Like the female patients, they have been unable to resolve their oedipal conflicts.

It is often observed that the histrionic patient and obsessive-compulsive patient marry each other, seeking in the partner what they are lacking in themselves. The histrionic patient provides emotional expressiveness; the obsessive-compulsive patient offers control and regulations. Typically, the partner of the female histrionic patient is obsessive, with strong passive-dependent trends. These latter traits are not recognized by either party, and particularly not by the histrionic patient, who sees him as a selfish, controlling tyrant who wants to keep her a prisoner. There is usually some degree of validity in this perception, because the partner views her as a status symbol because of her attractiveness, seductive behavior, and appeal to other men. Unconsciously, he views her more as an ideal mother who will gratify both his sexual and dependent needs while he remains passive. The relationship may be stormy and often soon leads to mutual disappointment. Interpersonal conflicts have a characteristic pattern: The woman is angered by her partner's cold detachment, parsimony, and controlling attitudes. He becomes irritated with her demanding behavior, extravagance, and refusal to submit to his domination. In their arguments, he attempts to engage her through intellectualization and appeals to rational logic. She may initially engage in his debate but soon becomes emotional, displaying her anger or her hurt feelings of rejection. The partner either withdraws, feeling bewildered and frustrated, or erupts in a rage reaction of his own. Both parties compete for the role of the "much-loved child." Because she has selected a man who will not desire her as a woman and an equal partner, she has no choice but to shift alternately between being his mother and his child.

The female patient usually reports that her sexual life deteriorated after marriage, with loss of desire for her husband, frigidity, or an extramarital affair. The relationship with her husband leads to disillusionment as she discovers that he is not the ideal man of whom she had dreamed. In her frustration and depression, she retreats to romantic fantasies. This often leads to the fear of impulsive infidelity, which, if it occurs, further complicates her life with added guilt and depression. Flirtatiousness and seductive charm are reparative attempts that fail to enhance her self-esteem, leading to additional disappointment. Similar patterns occur with the male histrionic patient who becomes disillusioned with his partner and either develops potency disturbances or pursues new and more exciting partners.

Somatic Symptoms

Somatic complaints involving multiple organ systems usually begin in the patient's adolescence and continue throughout life. The symptoms are dramatically described and include headaches, backaches, conversion symptoms, and in the female, pelvic pain and menstrual disorders. In patients with more serious ego pathology, there may be frequent hospitalizations and surgery; gynecological procedures are common in women. It is unusual for these patients to feel physically well for a sustained period of time. Pain is by far the most common symptom and often involves an appeal for help.

Male histrionic patients may also complain of headaches, back pain, gastrointestinal disturbances, and other somatic symptoms. Frequently, histrionic patients possess the fantasy that they have a disorder that is beyond the ken of ordinary physicians. They will often resort to herbal remedies and alternative medical practices in the belief that their physical distress will only respond to an unconventional or exotic treatment.

Mechanisms of Defense

The mechanisms of defense utilized by the histrionic patient are less fixed or stable than those employed by the obsessive-compulsive patient. They shift in response to social cues, which partially explains the difference in diagnostic impression among different mental health practitioners seeing the same patient. Histrionic character traits and symptoms provide more secondary gains than most other defensive patterns. The derisive attitude that typically characterizes both medical and social reaction to this group of people is related to the fact that the secondary gains and special attention received are not only great but also transparent to everyone but the patient. Successful histrionic defenses, unlike most other neurotic symptoms, are not in themselves directly painful, and therefore they potentially offer great relief of mental pain. However, lack of mature gratification, loneliness, and depression develop as a result of the patient's inhibition. In the case of conversion symptoms, the secondary loss is reflected in the painful and self-punishing aspect of the symptom.

Repression

Histrionic symptoms defend the ego from the reawakening of repressed sexuality. Although repression is a basic defense in all patients, it is most often encountered in pure form in the histrionic patient. Memory lacunae, histrionic amnesia, and lack of sexual feeling are clinical manifestations of repression. Developmentally, the erotic feelings and the competitive rage of both the positive and the negative oedipal situations are dealt with by this mechanism. When repression fails to control the anxiety, other defense mechanisms are utilized. Any therapeutic resolution of the other histrionic defenses is incomplete until the initial repression has been accepted by the patient.

Daydreaming and Fantasy

Daydreaming and fantasy are normal mental activities that play an important role in the emotional life of every person. Rational thinking is predominantly organized and logical and prepares the organism for action based on the reality principle. Daydreaming, on the other hand, is a continuation of childhood thinking and is based on primitive, magical wish fulfillment processes that follow the pleasure principle.

Daydreaming is particularly prominent in the emotional life of the histrionic patient. The content centers around receiving love or attention, whereas in the obsessive-compulsive patient, fantasies usually involve respect, power, and aggression. Daydreaming and its derivative character traits serve a defensive function. The histrionic patient prefers the symbolic gratification provided by fantasy to the gratification available in his real life, because the latter stimulates oedipal anxiety. The central role of the oedipal conflict in the genesis of the higher-functioning histrionic personality is discussed later in this chapter under the heading "Developmental Psychodynamics."

Most patients consider this aspect of their mental lives particularly private, and it is seldom revealed during initial interviews. The histrionic patient is no exception as far as the conscious disclosure of his fantasies is concerned. However, the content of the histrionic patient's daydreams is revealed indirectly. His infantile fantasies are projected onto the outside world through the use of dramatic behavior. Emotionally significant persons in the patient's life are involved as participants.

(These phenomena are ubiquitous, however, and can be observed in obsessive-compulsive, narcissistic, paranoid, and masochistic patients as well.) When the histrionic patient is successful, these persons interact with the patient so that his real world conforms to the daydream, with the patient as the central character in the drama. The self-dramatization and the overt daydreaming defend the patient against the imagined dangers associated with mature involvement in the adult world. At the same time, the patient is assured that his narcissistic and oral needs will be supplied. By acting out daydreams, the patient reduces the loneliness of the fantasy world and yet avoids the oedipal anxiety and guilt associated with mature adult behavior. The dissociative reaction is an extreme example of this process.

Misrepresentation or lying also defends against real involvement in the world by attempting to substitute the fantasy world. Elaborate falsehoods often contain factual elements that have psychological significance in terms of the past and reveal both the oedipal wish and the defense.

> A young woman frequently exaggerated or confabulated experiences concerning her cultural and artistic activities. She reported a feeling of elation while recounting such stories. She would begin to believe the story herself if it were told often enough. In the attempt to turn her daydreams into reality, fact and fantasy had become intertwined. In analyzing these stories, it was learned that the patient's father was a patron of the arts and that her most frequent and intense contact with him in childhood involved discussions of music and art. In acting out the mother's role, she feigned knowledge and understanding in order to better please her father. The present-day confabulations symbolized past experiences of closeness to her father, while repression and denial blocked her awareness of the erotic feelings. This elation was the affectual residue that escaped into consciousness and represented the feeling of magical rapport that she had achieved with her father. In daydreams, the patient symbolically defeated her mother by sharing her father's interests to a greater degree than her mother did. At the same time, she avoided real competition with her mother.

When the interviewer attempts to challenge such confabulations, the patient will often indignantly cling to the distortion and even confabulate further to escape detection. Intense emotional reactions of guilt, fear, or anger may occur when the falsehood is finally acknowledged. The nature of the emotional response will tell the interviewer how the patient has experienced the confrontation. In this example, responses of guilt or fear would reveal the patient's expectation of punishment, whereas a response of anger would indicate that she was enraged at the thought of having to relinquish her fantasized relationship with her father or possibly narcissistically humiliated by being caught.

Daydreaming assumes its greatest psychic importance during the oedipal phase of development and may be associated with masturbatory activity. Because histrionic patients often come from families in which sexual activity is associated with great anxiety, it is no surprise that they often recall either real or imagined maternal prohibitions against masturbation during childhood. The child, striving to control his masturbatory temptations, utilizes daydreaming as a substitute means for obtaining pleasurable self-stimulation. In the oedipal phase, the child's sexuality is focused on his erotic desire toward his parents. This desire cannot be directly gratified and is displaced to the masturbatory activity. Therefore, the fantasies that accompany or substitute for masturbation offer a symbolic gratification of the child's oedipal wishes. In other situations, the parents are exhibitionistic and seductive themselves, overstimulating their child. Depending on the culture, this behavior may lead to sexual precocity, thus incurring negative reactions from peers or other authority figures.

Emotionality as a Defense

The histrionic patient utilizes intense emotionality as a defense against unconscious, frightening feelings. Seductiveness and superficial warmth with the opposite sex permit the avoidance of deeper feelings of closeness, with consequent vulnerability to rejection. Affective outbursts may serve as a protection from sexual feelings or from the fear of rejection. These dramatic emotional displays also relate to identification with an aggressive parent. Playacting and role-playing ward off the dangers inherent in a real participation in life. This explains the quick development of transference as well as the pseudo-intensity and transience of the relationships that these patients develop. This mechanism also leads to the self-dramatization and labile emotionality that are so readily observed. Similar mechanisms are involved between homosexual partners when one or both has prominent histrionic traits.

Identification

Identification plays a prominent role in the development of histrionic symptoms and character traits. First, the histrionic patient may identify with the parent of the same sex or a symbolic representative in a wishful attempt to defeat that parent in the competitive struggle for the love of the parent of the opposite sex. At the same time, this identification also maintains the child's relationship to the parent of the same sex. An example of identification with a symbolic representative is the man who developed cardiac conversion symptoms after seeing a man his own age collapse with a heart attack. Although this person was a complete stranger, the patient imagined that the heart attack had occurred because the man was driving himself too much in his work. The patient's father also had succumbed to a heart attack at a young age, and he identified with his father and feared punishment by death for his competitive oedipal desires. The patient had unconsciously made this equation when his mother explained to him, "Your father died because he aggressively drove himself. He was too competitive."

Second, the histrionic patient can identify with the much-desired parent of the opposite sex or his symbolic representative. This occurs when the patient feels less chance of success in the oedipal competition. Although on the surface the patient relinquishes the parent of the opposite sex, he unconsciously maintains the attachment through identification. In either of these two cases, the symbolic representative of the parent could be an older sibling.

A third type of identification is based on competitive rivalry and envy. Here the other person's significance to the patient lies in the fact that some experience in this person's life stimulates envious feelings in the patient. A common example occurs at any rock concert. One young woman will scream ecstatically, and immediately several others will emulate her as they unconsciously seek the sexual gratification symbolized by her behavior, in addition to attracting attention.

Identification is as important a mechanism as conversion in the production of histrionic pain. The identification through pain includes both preoedipal and oedipal components. The pain provides the symbolic gratification of the oedipal wish as well as the compromise of healthy functioning and punishment for the associated feelings of guilt.

Identification is a complex mechanism that is utilized by everyone. Although many persons may identify predominantly with one parent, there are always partial identifications with the other parent as well as with other significant figures. In the mature adult, these partial identifications have fused, but in the histrionic patient this does not occur. This lack of fusion is particularly important in understanding the histrionic patient. Through successful treatment, the patient's partial identifications become fused into a new self-image.

Somatization and Conversion

Histrionic patients often express repressed impulses and affects through somatic symptoms. Conversion is not merely a somatic expression of affect but also a specific representation of fantasies that can be retranslated from their somatic language into their symbolic language. Conversion symptoms are not confined to histrionic patients, however, as was once thought, but can occur in a whole range of patients, including borderline and narcissistic individuals.

The process of conversion, although it is not thoroughly understood, has its origin in early life and is influenced by constitutional factors as well as by the environment. The fundamental step in this mechanism can be briefly explained as follows: Thinking represents trial action and, later, abortive action. For the young child, acting, feeling, thinking, and speaking are all intertwined. Gradually, with development, these become distinct, and thinking and speaking—communicating in symbols—become separate from feeling and acting. However, the potential for expressing thoughts and fantasies through action persists and is reawakened in conversion. In the beginning, thinking is mental talking accompanied by communicative behavior. Gradually there is a less fixed relationship between mental talking and the related motor activity. The child thereby learns that both his behavior and his thoughts have symbolic as well as concrete meanings. When the child's actions are prohibited or rewarded by his parents, he equates this with prohibition or reward for the related thoughts and affects. Therefore, the inhibitions of action that result from parental restriction usually are associated with repression of the accompanying thought and affect. In the infant, affect expression is directly accompanied by motor, sensory, and autonomic discharge. Since the parental prohibitions involve both the sexual and aggressive feelings of the child, it is the conflicts over the expression of these impulses that are dealt with through the conversion process.

Later, partial repression leads to a separation, so that the affect may remain repressed but the motor, sensory, or autonomic discharge may break through. The term *conversion symptom* refers to the selective malfunction of the motor or sensory nervous system, whereas the persisting abnormal autonomic discharge has been called *somatization*. The impairment has features of inhibition as well as pathological discharge, the relative proportion varying with different symptoms. For example, conversion paralysis reflects a greater degree of inhibition, and a "hysterical seizure" manifests a greater discharge of the unacceptable impulse. Blushing demonstrates both inhibition and release through the autonomic nervous system.

The affected organ is often an unconscious substitute for the genital. For example, a woman developed hysterical blindness when exposed to the temptation of an extramarital affair. During the course of treatment, she revealed that as a child she had been caught watching her parents' sexual activities. A traumatic confrontation ensued, with the result that the patient repressed both her visual memory and the accompanying sexual arousal. For her, visual perception and genital excitement were equated, with the result that the conversion symptom had served as a symbolic compromise for sexual gratification and punishment for that forbidden pleasure.

In another instance, the sexual excitement is repressed but the accompanying cardiorespiratory discharge breaks into consciousness, or perhaps an itching sensation affects the genital area. The protracted nature of these symptoms is explained by the fact that a vicarious means of discharge has a limited value in contrast with more direct expression.

The patient's particular choice of symptoms is influenced by many factors, including both physical and psychological determinants. The physical factors include organic predispositions or the direct effect of illness or injury on a particular organ system. Psychological factors influencing organ choice include historical events, the general symbolic significance of the affected organ, and the particular meaning it has to the patient because of some traumatic episode or because of identification with persons who have had a related physical symptom. Conversion symptoms tend to reflect the patient's concept of disease. Gross symptoms are, therefore, more common in individuals with less medical sophistication. Patients who are in a health profession may simulate complex syndromes, such as lupus erythematosus, on a conversion basis. Conversion operates with varying degrees of effectiveness in binding the patient's anxiety, which accounts for the controversial opinions concerning the classic *la belle indifférence* or apparent lack of concern. In our experience, this attitude is relatively uncommon, because depression and anxiety usually break through the defense. The exception would be patients with a gross conversion reaction, and even then, depression soon becomes apparent. *La belle indifférence* may be seen with those minor somatic complaints that form part of the character structure of the histrionic patient, or in persons with primitive character structure, for whom the secondary gain of dependent care is of great importance.

Regression

In the histrionic patient there is a selective regression by which the patient abandons adult adaptation in favor of the period of childhood during which his inhibitions were established. The conflicts over his emotional experiences caused him to treat certain aspects of his body and its sensations as ego-alien. The selective regression from conflicts over genital sexuality may lead to an oral or anal level of adaptation, although the same conflict will be expressed in the regressed symptom. Features of primitive incorporation are common, as has been shown by the prominent role of identification in the histrionic patient. This can be seen directly in one patient who had globus hystericus, in which there is an unconscious wish to perform fellatio. As treatment progressed, the pregenital incorporative aspect became clear in the patient's associations of a penis with her fantasy of oral impregnation by her father—and, ultimately, with her mother's breast. Regressive behavior is particularly common when the patient is confronted by powerful authority figures of the same sex.

In another example, the patient began the third session stating, "I had a dream last night but I can't tell you about it." This was followed by an extended silence. The patient remained quiet, and the clinician, responding to the patient's coyness and curled-up "little-girl" posture, commented, "It feels like you are teasing me." "My father always teased me. I guess I want to do it to you," replied the patient, changing her posture and attitude and reverting to adulthood. This patient had illustrated through her childlike posture and behavior a dramatic and regressive linkage between body and mind.

Denial and Isolation

Histrionic patients deny awareness of the significance of their own behavior as well as the behavior of others. This unawareness is greatest in the areas of seductive and manipulative behavior and the secondary gain associated with their symptoms. They also deny their strengths and skills, further contributing to the façade of helplessness. These patients also deny painful emotions, with the result that isolation develops as a defense against depression, and if it is unsuccessful, they will resort to distortion and misrepresentation to escape facing their unhappiness.

Externalization

Externalization, the avoidance of responsibility for one's own behavior, is closely related to denial. The patient feels that his own actions do not count and views both success and suffering as being caused by other people in his life.

Developmental Psychodynamics

The developmental patterns of histrionic patients are less consistent than those of obsessive-compulsive patients. One common feature is that the patient occupied a special position in the family, perhaps with the prolonged role of "baby," as sometimes happens with the youngest child. Physical illnesses that led to special indulgence are often described, and frequently another family member suffered from ill health, which offered the patient an opportunity to observe and envy the privilege accorded to the sickly.

When the future female histrionic patient enters the infantile struggles with her parents over sleeping, feeding, and being held, she discovers that crying and dramatic scenes lead to getting her own way. Her mother gives in, albeit with some annoyance. Her father is more likely to withdraw, often criticizing the mother's behavior and occasionally intervening with even more indulgence "because the poor child is so upset." The child is soon aware of the conflict between her parents, and she learns to play each against the other. This pattern interacts with the normal development of conscience, as she learns to escape punishment by indicating that she is sorry or "feels bad." The mother responds either by making no attempt to punish the child or by not enforcing the punishment. The child escapes the consequences of misbehavior and is left with unresolved feelings of guilt as a result of avoiding punishment.

The typical mother of the female histrionic patient is competitive, cold, and either overtly argumentative or subtly resentful. She unconsciously resents being a woman and envies the masculine role. Overprotection and overindulgence of her daughter compensate for her inability to give real love. Her most tender warmth is expressed when the child is depressed, sick, or upset, which helps to establish depression, physical illness, and tantrums as means of obtaining dependent care. The patient's need to maintain a dependent relationship with her mother makes it difficult for her to mature. She fails to develop an internalized ego ideal, as is clinically evidenced by the histrionic patient's continued reliance on the approval of others in order to maintain her own self-esteem.

In families in which special privileges and status are still accorded to men, the little girl becomes sensitive to this sexist prejudice. The female histrionic patient reacts with competitive envy that may be expressed through symbolically castrating behavior, through imitation as expressed by being a tomboy, or through competing directly with men while retaining her feminine identity. The tomboy pattern is more likely if older brothers provide a readily available model. The histrionic patient may emulate her mother during childhood, but in early adolescence their relationship is marked by open strife. At that time she does not like or admire her mother as much as she does her father, and this also furthers her identification with men.

Since the histrionic patient is unable to obtain adequate nurturant warmth from her mother, she turns to her father as a substitute. He is most often charming, sensitive, seductive, and controlling. Mild alcoholism and other sociopathic trends are common. During the first 3 or 4 years of her life, she and her father are usually close to each other. If he feels rejected by his cold and competitive wife, he turns to his daughter as a safe and convenient source of gratification for his failing masculine self-esteem. He thereby rewards and emphasizes his daughter's flirtatiousness and emotionality. During her latency period, he becomes increasingly uncomfortable with her femininity and may therefore encourage her tomboyish behavior. As she becomes older, she finds her father a difficult man to please because he is easily manipulated on one occasion but may capriciously dominate her on another. At puberty, the romantic and erotic aspects of their relationship are denied by both father and daughter, because both are threatened by their incestuous feelings.

Her transient rejections by her father leave the patient feeling that she has no one, since she already feels alienated from her mother. She may express her rage with emotional outbursts and demanding behavior or she may intensify her seductive and manipulative efforts. Self-dramatization, hyperemotionality, simulated compliance, seductiveness, and physical illness serve to reestablish control in her relationship with her father. She is unwilling to relinquish her attachment to him, and consequently all sexuality must be inhibited. Her oedipal fantasies make her unable to experience sexual desires for any other man.

At puberty, as her sexuality unfolds, trouble begins. The father moves away from his daughter, sometimes finding a mistress but at the same time jealously guarding his daughter from young suitors. The girl feels that she must inhibit her sexuality and remain a little girl in order to retain Daddy's love and at the same time to ward off threatening, exciting impulses. In the healthier patient, the defense against the oedipal conflict is the most significant factor. Fear of maternal retaliation for her success with her father and the fear of incestuous involvement lead to regression to a more infantile level of functioning. The less healthy patient, with more prominent conflicts at an oral level, already views her father more as a maternal substitute.

Variant patterns of histrionic development exist in which the daughter has a greater degree of overt dependence on the mother as well as a father who is more aloof and less seductive. At puberty, the mother makes a strong bid to keep her daughter dependent on her and thereby defeats the child in the struggle for her father's love. These girls inhibit their basically histrionic character traits, and this personality organization may only emerge later in life or during the course of psychotherapy.

In some patients, the real mother is absent, and maternal deprivation may stem from a foster mother who fails to provide closeness. The child learns to simulate emotionality. The father, although erratic, often provides the genuine experience that offers the child a chance at further development.

Beginning in the teenage period, the less well-integrated female histrionic patient has poor relationships with other girls, particularly attractive girls. She is too jealous and competitive with them to be accepted. She is not comfortable with her budding femininity and fears sexual involvement. Therefore she may have only platonic relationships with boys. Everyone in the high school knows who she is, but she is not usually popular. She is often pretty herself and is preoccupied with her appearance. Unattractive girls are less likely to develop histrionic patterns, because they are less successful in using them. The histrionic woman prefers girlfriends who are less attractive and masochistic—an arrangement that offers mutual neurotic gratification. As she progresses through the teen years, she shifts her attention to men but classically overvalues them and selects men who are in some way unattainable. Disappointment, frustration, and disillusionment are inevitable, and she reacts with depression and anxiety.

In the case of the male histrionic patient, the situation is somewhat different. In these cases there is a strong identification with the mother, who was obviously the more powerful figure in the family. She typically had many histrionic traits herself, whereas the father tended to be more withdrawn and passive, avoiding arguments and attempting to maintain peace at any price. The father often expressed his own inhibited aggression through being hypercritical and overly controlling with his son. At times the father was relatively absent in the home or was disinterested in his son, or perhaps he was excessively competitive with his son. In either case, the boy fears castration as a retaliation for his oedipal striving. In adolescence he has less masculine self-confidence than the other boys and is fearful of physical competition. His feeling of masculine strength has been acquired through an identification with the personal strength of his mother, and consequently it is more likely to be manifested in intellectual than physical pursuits. The lack of a strong father figure with whom he can identify leads to faulty superego development and an inadequate ego ideal. When this restriction of oedipal sexuality continues into adolescence, there evolves a predisposition toward homosexuality. Homosexual object choice probably represents a continuum with biological and constitutional factors as determinants at one end. At the other end of this continuum, however, environmental factors, such as those described earlier, are likely to be crucial in determining same-sex preferences. Thus the boy, in his quest for paternal love and affection, adopts techniques utilized by his mother for gaining the admiration, attention, and affection of men. The greater the weakness, disinterest, or absence of the father, the more overtly effeminate the boy will become.

Differential Diagnosis

A distinguishing feature of histrionic patients lies in the emphasis they place in their personality, interactional manner, and dress for the transmission of sexual signals. This amounts to a type of self-dramatization through sexuality. Histrionic patients will often seem to exaggerate culture-bound gender symbols. In men and women this can take two disparate forms but with an underlying common theme: the dramatic highlighting of sexual stereotypes. In histrionic men one such form is the hypermasculine "cowboy." This contrasts with the effeminate "interior decorator" type. In histrionic women, one form is the hyperfeminine "charming hostess," which contrasts with the masculine "boardroom director" type.

The phallic narcissist can easily be confused with the histrionic:

> In his first interview, a patient exclaimed, "I just flew up here at 80 miles an hour on my brand-new bike, a Harley-Davidson of course, leaving all those nerds in their pathetic little cars in the dust." This middle-aged man entered the office armored in black leather. He proceeded to deposit his formidable, dark-tinted motorcycle helmet on the floor and proclaimed: "This felt like the right Wagnerian overture to my psychiatric treatment, the power of the bike, my obvious superiority to everyone else."
>
> At first sight this patient's clinical presentation seemed to be histrionic—dramatic, exhibitionistic, hypermasculine. However, the true diagnosis—phallic narcissism—became apparent in the patient's wish to dominate and feel superior to everyone else combined with a sadistic desire to pound his "inferiors" into the dust. He wanted to be feared rather than loved, and the exhibitionism was directed toward that end. Furthermore, this behavior was not personally focused on a particular person or group. His targets were randomly chosen, and his behavior was anonymous.

Differential diagnosis with the histrionic patient can be difficult, as this example demonstrates. Not only is there disagreement among professionals about whether a given patient is histrionic initially, but the clinician also may change his own diagnosis on different occasions in response to changes in the transference/countertransference paradigm. An example would be the young female histrionic patient who is hospitalized for suicidal threats. Such a patient, dramatically using gender signals of seductiveness, dependency, and infantile "little girl" behavior, can split the ward staff along countertransference gender lines. The male professionals may find her sympathetic and "histrionic," whereas the female professionals may dislike her and regard her as "borderline."

The major differential with the histrionic patient is thus with the higher-level borderline patient. Both types can be manipulative and demanding. The histrionic patient is more likely to begin the clinical encounter with charm and flattery, whereas the borderline patient more quickly resorts to threats. If charm is unsuccessful, the histrionic patient may also have temper outbursts and use threats to try to manipulate the person they seek to control. Both types of patients may find a real or imagined abandonment a threat, and both patients crave to be the center of attention.

Histrionic interaction with others is often characterized by inappropriate sexual or other provocative behavior. This can be confused with borderline impulsivity, which involves at least two behaviors that are potentially self-damaging (e.g., excessive spending, promiscuous sexual encounters, reckless driving, binge eating). Histrionic patients can be impulsive buyers to an extent that may approach spending binges. Differentiating this from a hypomanic spending binge requires an understanding of the patient's thoughts and affective experiences. The hypomanic patient is in an elated mood state and believes he can afford anything he desires. He has lost touch with reality. In contrast, the histrionic patient is most likely depressed or is angry with a spouse, and the spending is accompanied by a desire to feel better immediately. The interviewer inquires, "What were you feeling when you went on this shopping spree, and what was going on before you decided to shop?"

Although both histrionic and borderline patients are subject to affective instability or emotional lability, the borderline patient is more negative and vacillates more between fear and rage than between love and anger. The histrionic patient remains connected to significant others and does not have the feelings of emptiness that characterize borderline patients.

In all likelihood, lower-functioning histrionic patients and higher-functioning borderline patients represent much the same group. The differential is best made when the patient is functioning at his highest level rather than his lowest level. The level of psychological organization is the crucial variable. In all personality disorders there exists a dimension of relative health versus relative sickness, a quantitative measure. In the borderline patient there is a qualitative boundary that, when breached, is of greater clinical gravity and indicates the diagnosis through relentlessly self-destructive and "out-of-control" behavior that is not typical of the average less-disturbed histrionic patient.

The second most difficult differential diagnosis is with the narcissistic patient. Like the narcissistic patient, the histrionic patient desires excessive admiration and believes that he or she is special and unique and can only be understood by other special or glamorous people. The histrionic patient also possesses a sense of entitlement, may be envious of others, and in moments of stress, may display haughty behaviors and attitudes. Both types of patients may have romantic fantasies, but the narcissist is more concerned with power and admiration than with love. The narcissistic patient cannot fall in love, which is a key diagnostic element. The narcissistic patient possesses a more grandiose sense of himself that can be confused with the histrionic patient's fantasies of royal birth. Many histrionic patients have prominent narcissistic features, but the histrionic patient is more attached to significant others than the narcissist, is able to fall in love, and cares about the feelings of other people. The histrionic patient likes people who like him. The narcissist has no compunction in dismissing those who like him if they do not acknowledge his special status.

Finally, there is a type of "hypomanic" personality that can be confused with the histrionic patient. Such individuals can be charismatic, constantly "on," and live in a world of intense affect. They are more vivid than life, never bland, and can be quite charming and charismatic, although they are exhausting with their relentless enthusiasm, energy, and need for constant stimulation. This ill-defined personality type is probably constitutional, a type of low-level, contained hypomania, and its expression is not dynamically determined as it is in the histrionic patient.

MANAGEMENT OF THE INTERVIEW

The female histrionic patient usually arrives at the clinician's office after being disappointed or disillusioned by her husband or lover, resulting in an intensification of fantasy and the fear that an impulsive loss of control of sexual urges will occur. The clinician is unconsciously used as a safe substitute and an inhibiting force. Chief complaints involving depression or generalized anxiety occur in patients of either sex. On some occasions, particularly with male histrionic patients, somatic symptoms may be in the foreground, and the patient is referred for psychiatric help when no adequate organic basis can be found to explain his suffering. The somatic symptoms often screen depressed feelings, particularly if pain is prominent. Suicidal gestures may lead to the initial psychiatric contact in other cases.

Concern over sexual symptoms is expressed early in treatment. The patient may quickly acknowledge some degree of frigidity or impotence, although this did not lead to seeking treatment until it threatened a love relationship. In healthier patients there are also complaints of social anxiety and inhibition. These are discordant with the patient's actual performance in social situations. This same phenomenon occurs during the interview, in which the patient may conduct himself with apparent poise and composure but feels subjective discomfort.

> An attractive, stylishly dressed, professional woman, a veteran of a number of previous unsuccessful therapies, began her initial consultation by saying, "I have to tell you this dream I had last night. It will reveal much more about me than just relating my boring life history." Without waiting for the clinician's response, she launched into a description of a colorful dream that involved her presence at the opera, first as a disgruntled, overlooked member of the audience accompanied by her despised boyfriend and then magically transformed into the star of the performance, the beautiful courtesan Violetta in Verdi's *La Traviata*. "This was a happy dream. I hate being just an uninteresting member of the audience, passively watching." The clinician responded by saying, "What does the dream tell you beyond your life history?" The clinician recognized the patient's transference craving for center stage and her underlying fear that she was really of no interest to others. From the beginning, her exhibitionism and need to seduce by being a famous prostitute, yet unconscious fear of sexuality (Violetta is doomed to die, prematurely), all characteristic of the histrionic patient, were dramatically produced in the first 10 minutes of the session.

The beginning mental health practitioner finds the histrionic patient one of the easiest to interview; the experienced clinician finds him one of the most difficult. This is because it is so necessary for the patient to elicit a favorable response from the clinician. The beginner is reassured by the patient's eager compliance; the more experienced interviewer recognizes the inauthenticity of the affect and role-playing. The interviewer is usually pleased with his new patient, especially if the patient is young, attractive, and of the opposite sex. He may experience the vague aura that accompanies a new romance. Attempts on the part of the interviewer to explore the patient's role in his problems will threaten the patient's feeling of acceptance because of his strong need to feel that the clinician likes him. Focusing on this issue prematurely will drive the patient away, and yet he cannot be helped unless his role in his difficulties is explored. The interviewer must develop a relationship that will permit the patient to continue in treatment as well as encourage the unfolding of his problems.

The Opening Phase

Initial Rapport

The histrionic patient establishes "instant contact" at the beginning of the interview. He quickly develops apparent emotional rapport, creating an impression of a strong commitment to the interviewer, although feeling little involvement. The patient's first comments are frequently designed to please and flatter the interviewer, complimenting the clinician's office or remarking, "I'm so glad you were able to see me" or "What a relief finally to have someone I can talk to." A reply to such comments is unproductive, and instead the interviewer can shift the focus by asking, "What seems to be the problem?"

Dramatic or Seductive Behavior

The histrionic patient is obviously relieved by the opportunity to describe his suffering and does so with a dramatic quality. Before the interviewer can inquire about the chief complaint, the patient may begin by asking, "Shall I tell my story?" The drama unfolds as he describes his difficulties in vivid, colorful language, using many superlatives. The patient's behavior is designed to create an impression, and the interviewer begins to feel that the scene has been rehearsed and any questions will be an intrusion.

The histrionic patient usually prefers a clinician of the opposite sex. The female histrionic patient often is disappointed if she finds that her new interviewer is a woman. The disappointment is concealed, although the patient may remark, "Oh, I didn't expect a woman therapist!" There is no point in exploring the patient's disappointment in the first part of the interview, because it will only be denied. If the patient has already had a failed treatment with a therapist of the opposite sex, the patient may seek a same-sex therapist the second time around.

Even the inexperienced interviewer quickly recognizes the most common stereotype of the female histrionic patient. The patient is stylishly and often colorfully dressed and has a seductive manner, ranging from social charm to overt sexual propositions. Body language provides clues in understanding the patient. The patient who dresses up when coming to see the clinician employs a form of body language that lends itself to exploration early in treatment. The most frequent example of the use of the body is the female patient who sits in a provocative posture, exposing a portion of her anatomy in a suggestive way. This behavior is designed to engage and distract the interviewer sexually. It is an unconscious mechanism to equalize the power balance with the interviewer.

Self-dramatization can be interpreted relatively early in treatment, although not in the first few sessions. Premature interpretations cause the patient to feel rejected and are usually made because the clinician is anxious. When the male interviewer comments on the female patient's seductiveness and her tendency to sexualize every relationship, she will protest that her behavior is not sexual. She might say, "I just want to be friendly, but they always have other ideas." The interviewer should maintain his opinion without getting into an argument with the patient, who has difficulty accepting the idea that a pretty woman cannot initiate a casual conversation with strange men.

Early interpretations are often useful when the patient directs the interviewer's attention to her behavior in the initial interview. For example, an attractive young woman pulled up her dress and asked the clinician to admire her suntan. He replied, "Are you more confident about your appearance than about what you are telling me in regard to yourself?" This general, but supportive, interpretation is preferable to silence early in treatment because it is less of a rejection for the patient.

The dramatization of roles that are less obviously sexualized is more difficult to recognize.

> A young woman arrived for an interview in tattered jeans and a dirty sweatshirt. The interviewer asked about her problem, and she replied, "Well, I've been depressed for months, and a week ago I had a big fight with my husband, and got furious, and that's when I took the pills." The patient did not appear to be depressed, and she related her story with dramatic flourish. When the interviewer inquired about the pill episode, the patient answered, "First I started popping the Advil, and then I went for the Valium pills, and that's when he hit me and I got this lump on my head." The interviewer requested further details about the fight, and the patient said, "Actually he did not hit me, he shoved me against the wall and I bumped my head." Rather than the result of a depressive spell, the episode was the culmination of a dramatic free-for-all involving the patient, her husband, and her children.
>
> On several occasions this patient casually, but abruptly, introduced highly charged material, which is typical histrionic behavior. Early in the interview, she gave the ages of her five children as 12, 10, 6, 5, and 1. No explanation was given when, in the next sentence, she indicated that she had been married only 7 years. Later in the interview, she was asked about her relationship to her in-laws, and she replied, "Well, it is not too bad now, but at first they were not happy about Bill marrying a divorcée with two children."

Dramatic remarks are made frequently during the interview. For instance, the same patient, when volunteering that she was a housewife, added, "That's a glorified term." In the case example above, we can easily identify the patient as histrionic because the features of diagnostic significance have been abstracted from the interview. However, many interviewers do not recognize this behavior when it is mixed with non-histrionic material and the patient is not the stereotypic pretty, seductive young woman.

Another patient may dramatize indifference upon arriving 10 minutes late, showing no awareness of the time. This patient, unconcerned about small amounts of time, will feel that the clinician is being picayune in terminating the session on time even though the patient is in the middle of his story. The patient remarks with annoyance, "Can't I finish what I'm saying?" or "I had so much to tell you today." The interviewer can reply, "We had a late start" and let the matter drop. The interviewer wants the patient to become responsibly interested in the lateness and the motivation behind it.

Some histrionic patients will dramatize obsessiveness in the initial interviews, leading to errors in the clinician's understanding of the patient. An example would be the patient who brings a pad to the session and jots down notes about the clinician's remarks, but then loses the notes or never reads them. Beginning interviewers often mistake the patient's remarks that involve performance or competitiveness as evidence of an obsessive character. Although the histrionic patient can be just as competitive as the obsessive-compulsive patient, the goal of the histrionic patient's struggle is love or acceptance, whereas the obsessive-compulsive patient is more concerned with power, control, and respect. The histrionic patient may express anger over the doctor's fee or some other issue, but the subject is dropped when the emotional tone changes; the obsessive-compulsive patient remains inwardly angry for a much longer time, using intellectualization or displacement in order to keep his anger out of consciousness. The histrionic patient will often pay late, offering the excuse that he lost the bill.

Distortions and Exaggerations

When the first interview is almost over, the interviewer may realize that he has little historical data and almost no chronological sense of the patient's development. Instead, he has become immersed in the interesting and lively details of the present illness and dramatic episodes from the past and senses that he has already lost his neutrality. At some point in the first or second interview, the clinician must intervene in order to obtain more factual information. As he succeeds in getting behind the rehearsed facade, the patient will reveal feelings of depression and anxiety that can then be explored empathically.

Initially, the histrionic patient ascribes his suffering to the actions of others, denying any responsibility for his own plight. He tells what was said and done by the other person but leaves his own behavior a mystery. Rather than interpret these defenses in the initial interview, the clinician can simply ask the patient what he himself said or did in each situation. The patient's response to these confrontations will usually be vague and expressive of his lack of interest in his own role. The interviewer must be persistent if he is to obtain the information he seeks. In addition to gathering information, he subtly communicates that he considers the patient's role important and that the patient has the power to influence his human environment rather than merely being influenced by it. After the first few interviews, the clinician can comment, each time the patient leaves his own behavior a mystery, "You don't tell me what you contributed to this situation—it is as though you consider your own behavior unimportant" or "In describing each situation, you emphasize what the other person does, but you leave yourself out!"

Frequently the patient will contradict details of his own story or add further exaggeration when telling the story for the second time. The therapist should be alert to these occurrences because they provide excellent opportunities to interpret the patient's defensive misrepresentation. Usually it is the patient's desire for extra sympathy that underlies such distortions. The interviewer can then comment, "It appears that you feel you must dramatize your problems or I won't appreciate your suffering." It is through these openings that the therapist encourages the patient to share feelings of sadness and loneliness.

Early Confrontations

Exploration of the Problems

It is common for a histrionic patient to complete the initial interview without revealing the major symptoms that caused him to seek help. The patient frequently uses generalizations in describing his problems. These are accompanied by expressive emotionality, but specific difficulties are not defined. Intense affect conceals the vagueness of what is said. The interviewer finds that his questions are answered superficially and that the patient seems mildly annoyed when asked for further details. For example, a patient described her husband as a "wonderful person." The interviewer replied, "Tell me some of the ways in which he is wonderful." The patient hesitated briefly and then said, "Well, he is very considerate." The interviewer, realizing that he had actually learned nothing, asked for some examples. What emerged was that her husband never tried to force his attentions on her when she was not in the mood for sex. The interviewer could now ask the patient if she had difficulty with her enjoyment of sex. Without this step, it would have been easier for the patient to deny that she had a sexual problem.

Often the histrionic patient will discuss feelings of depression or anxiety without any outward manifestation of these emotions. The interviewer can indicate to the patient that he does not appear to be depressed or anxious. This must be said tactfully and in an empathic tone, or the patient will feel criticized. An example is, "You prefer not to allow your pain to show while describing it?" This confrontation invites the patient to share his true feelings rather than merely enlist the interviewer's sympathy with a sad story. The patient's fear of rejection leads to his attempt to gain sympathy without really sharing himself.

The relative prominence of physical symptoms in the interview to some extent reflects the patient's belief concerning the interests of the interviewer. It is a rare histrionic patient who does not have some mild physical complaints such as fatigue, headaches, backaches, and menstrual or gastrointestinal symptoms. The patient does not consider such symptoms to have important psychological determinants, and the interviewer should avoid challenging this view early in treatment. He can best inquire about the patient's physical health as part of his interest in the patient's life, without implying that he is seeking to find a psychological basis for such symptoms.

With the patient who has an extensive history of physical complaints, the interviewer must not interpret the secondary gain in the first few interviews, even though it may be quite transparent and is seemingly acknowledged by the patient. For example, a patient says, "My family certainly suffers because of my frequent hospitalizations." The interviewer can reply, "Yes, I'm sure that it is very hard on all of you," thereby emphasizing the patient's secondary loss rather than his secondary gain. The histrionic patient will occasionally state early in treatment that his physical symptoms are psychosomatic or are "all in my mind." The experienced interviewer recognizes this as a resistance, since the patient is making a glib statement that really has little meaning, trying to appeal to what he assumes the interviewer must believe.

Denial of Responsibility

Responsibility for the patient's feelings.   The histrionic patient attempts to avoid responsibility for his emotional responses and to elicit the interviewer's support and validation for doing so. The female histrionic patient finishes describing a fight with her husband and then asks, "Wasn't I right?" or "Wasn't that a terrible thing for him to say?" The patient will not be helped to better understand herself if the interviewer merely agrees with her. These questions are direct attempts to manipulate the clinician into taking sides with the patient against some other important figure in the patient's life. The therapist who participates in these enactments is assuming the parent role, which defeats the aim of treatment. The clinician who ignores these attempts at manipulation seems insensitive and uncaring in the patient's mind. It is for these reasons that exploratory questions are indicated. Examples include, "I'm not sure I understand what underlies your question"; "I feel I'm being put in the middle. If I say yes you are right, I am supporting a part of you but then I am critical of your husband. If I say no, then I don't appear to be sympathetic to your feelings"; or "Is there some element of self-doubt in this situation that we should explore?" The patient's desire for an ally is understandable, although underneath the patient has the feeling that she is not entitled to what she seeks. In the transference, the patient has reconstructed the triangular relationship that once existed with her parents, except that the therapist and the spouse now represent these parental objects in the patient's unconscious.

Frequently the patient will create a very negative picture of someone close to him. If the interviewer attempts to be supportive and comments that the patient's relative seems to be unfair or selfish, the patient will often repeat the interviewer's remark to the other person, stating, "My therapist says that you are unfair!" This can be minimized by remarking, "From your description, your mother sounds like quite a selfish person," or if the patient's remarks are sufficiently critical, "That is quite an indictment."

Responsibility for decisions. The histrionic patient will, whenever possible, attempt to have the clinician assume responsibility for his decisions. The wise clinician will not accede to these helpless appeals. Instead, he suggests that the patient explore the conflict that prevents him from making the decision for himself. The patient responds by seeming not to understand what factors are involved in making a decision. Even if the histrionic patient explores the psychological meaning of the decision, when all the discussion is over, he is likely to confront the practitioner with, "Now, what should I do?" If he is pressed to decide for himself, after doing so he will ask, "Is that right?" It is as though the discussion were something quite separate from the actual decision. In other situations, the patient has already made the decision in his own mind, but he wants the practitioner to share the responsibility for the consequences.

An example of one patient's helplessness occurred when the clinician changed the hour of an appointment. The patient made no record of the change and came at the wrong time. Then he said with annoyance, "How do you expect me to remember these things?" The clinician replied, "You are right, it is difficult, and I could never manage either if I hadn't written it in my appointment book!" The clinician should refrain from writing the time down for the patient, because this will only indulge his helplessness and reinforce the pattern. One patient telephoned to inquire if she had missed an appointment on the previous day. When the interviewer replied that she had, the patient sounded distraught and said, "I had so much to talk about; isn't there anything you can do?" The patient hoped that the therapist would take pity on her and find some way to squeeze her into his schedule. When he replied, "We can talk about it next time," she insisted, "There must be something you can do!" The interviewer answered, "No, there isn't." At this point it was clear that the manipulative effort had failed, and the patient said with a tone of resignation, "All right, I'll see you at the regular time tomorrow."

Another way in which the histrionic patient manifests attitudes of helplessness is the use of rhetorical questions. He exclaims, "What should I do about this problem?"; "Can't you help me?"; or "What do you think my dream means?" Stereotyped replies such as "What do you think?" are of little help to the patient. Often no reply is necessary, but early in treatment the interviewer could remark on the patient's feeling of helplessness. A different approach is for the clinician to demonstrate his honesty and humility with a statement such as "I don't know."

Interpretation of the Patient's Role

As the therapy progresses, the unconscious role that the histrionic patient lives out in life will emerge. The role that is most common and closest to consciousness is that of the injured party or the victim. Although the origins of this role lie in the distant past, the patient perceives it as a reflection of his current life situation. Other roles, such as that of Cinderella or a princess, are typically related to the patient's narcissism and grandiosity. The patient may elevate her self-esteem through exaggeration of her social status. The achievements of her more successful relatives or friends are inflated to create an overall impression of greater culture, romance, or aristocracy than is accurate. This attitude may manifest itself as a feeling of superiority to the clinician or a veiled reference to the lesser intellectual backgrounds of other people with whom she is involved.

This defense is not interpreted during early interviews. As the interviewer pursues the origin of these grandiose fantasies, he will find that they are oedipal. The female patient's father led her to believe that she was his little princess, and she dared not grow up. She compensates for her apparent helplessness in the adult female role through her pride in being a more feeling and sensitive person than those on whom she is dependent and who symbolically represent her mother. The histrionic patient feels that she has subtler tastes and finer sensibilities and appreciates the better things in life. She feels that it is herself, rather than her husband, whom their friends see as the interesting and attractive person. This attitude toward her husband also defends against sexual involvement with him. He is considered a crude and insensitive person who merely responds to basic animalistic drives. The male patient, on the other hand, is inclined to portray himself in the roles of hero, clown, or "macho," using some distortion of fact.

During therapy, there are shifts in the role that the patient dramatizes. These shifts reflect changes in the patient's current self-image as well as her style of re-creating part-object identifications from the past. Often, the changes in role are in response to the patient's attempts to elicit the interest of the interviewer.

The Patient Responds

Hyperemotionality as a Defense

Hyperemotionality, one of the histrionic patient's most important defenses, occupies a prominent position in the treatment. The emotionality influences the interviewer to empathize with the patient's feeling; however, the clinician is unable to gratify all of the patient's demands and instead offers interpretations, which serve to block some of the gratifications that the patient receives through his symptoms. As a result, the patient inevitably experiences frustration and may respond with anger to conceal his hurt feelings.

> A male histrionic patient elicited a feeling of sympathetic understanding while describing the "impossible situation" of a family business in which he was constantly put in the position of the baby. He went into considerable detail describing his father's tyrannical and excitable behavior. As the interviewer persisted in his questions, it became apparent that the patient had temper outbursts at work. At such times, his family would cater to him because he was upset. The patient's need to play the role of injured child because of his fear of the adult male role was interpreted. As would be expected, the patient reacted with an outburst of anger and depression. At the next session, the patient stated, "I was so upset after our last session, I felt much worse. I couldn't stop churning inside, but I finally felt better when I ate something on the way back to work." The interviewer then inquired, "What was it that you felt so badly about?" After the patient described his feeling of unhappiness, the clinician interpreted, "The food seems to provide a form of comfort and security." The patient revealed that he had been given food and extra privileges during his childhood when he felt badly or had been punished by his parents. The indulgence was associated with feelings of being loved by his parents and having been forgiven for his transgressions. In his adult life, the same experience was unconsciously repre-

sented by buying himself food. Rather than gratifying the patient's bid for love, the therapist offered only an interpretation, which blocked this area of gratification and required the patient to seek a new solution to his injured pride.

In working with this defense, however, the clinician must convince the patient that his traditional solutions offer no permanent resolution of the underlying problem, which is the patient's feeling of helplessness and damaged self-esteem. The clinician must then show the patient that the hyperemotional response that led to, in this case, the purchase of food also warded off a deeper and more disturbing emotion. At this point, the patient frequently becomes angry and asks, "Why should I have to change?" or "Why can't anyone accept me the way I am?" No comment is required on the part of the interviewer. Once again the histrionic patient utilizes his hyperemotional anger as a defense against his fear of the adult role.

In due time the patient will recognize that other people have less intense emotional reactions. It is then that the interviewer can point out the pride with which the patient regards his hyperemotional responses. This pride reflects a compensatory sense of superiority to the parent. The hyperemotionality is also a reaction to the emotional response expected by the parents. The reactions of feeling sorry, appreciative, or frightened were expected by the parent and produced by the child in order to gain parental approval. Later, these same processes operated intrapsychically as the ego attempted to obtain approval from internalized objects.

The interpretation of the histrionic patient's defensive patterns frequently leads to depression. If kept within reasonable limits, this emotion provides the motivation for therapeutic change. A premature urge to prescribe antidepressant medication may convey a message to the patient that the emotion of sadness must be controlled.

Regressive Behavior

Those histrionic patients who have more serious ego defects are particularly prone to regressive behavior as the clinician begins to interpret their defensive patterns. The patient may become even more helpless, depressed, and preoccupied with physical illness or may threaten suicide. These symptoms are associated with considerable secondary gain. When such infantile behavior emerges, it should occupy the central focus of the interviewer's interpretations. Thus it is not appropriate to interpret the female histrionic patient's fear of oedipal competition while she is depressed and threatening suicide. Instead, the clinician interprets her feeling of deprivation and need for dependent care. After the patient has improved and is experiencing the desire to compete in the adult feminine role, the therapist can explore her oedipal fears as a source of her inhibition.

Involvement and Pseudo-Involvement

The female histrionic patient is usually pleased with her therapist during the early phase of treatment. She eagerly anticipates her sessions and is prone to feel romantically involved with the clinician. She sees him as a strong and omnipotent figure who could provide the protection and support that she feels she needs. Similarly, she idealizes the female therapist for having the best of both worlds, a gratifying career as well as a husband and children.

The histrionic patient's enjoyment of treatment is accompanied by enthusiasm for psychological thinking. The patient is likely to acquire intellectual knowledge about emotional problems from books, friends, or from the clinician himself. Even the most experienced clinician may find himself pleased with the patient's early interest in treatment and the effort he applies to the work. Because of his emotionality, insights are related with feeling, in contrast to the intellectualization of the obsessive-compulsive patient. The inexperienced interviewer is convinced that this is true emotional insight, as contrasted with intellectual insight. However, after a year or two he discovers that the daily successes do not add up to long-term progress.

It requires experience to recognize when the histrionic patient is not really involved in changing his life and is only playing the role of psychotherapy patient. There are certain clues that are helpful in recognizing this process. For example, in his enthusiasm for analysis, the patient may bring in material about a spouse, mistress, lover, or friend. He may ask the clinician for advice concerning the other person's problem, or he might offer his own insights, hoping to win the interviewer's approval. If the patient receives any encouragement, he might bring in a friend's dream and request the practitioner's aid in interpreting it. The interviewer, rather than responding directly, can say to the patient, "What are your thoughts about bringing your friend's dream to me?"

Another instance is the patient who enlists the aid of auxiliary therapists. This process may take the form of reading books on psychology and psychiatry or it may involve the discussion of his problems with friends. On some occasions, the interviewer can point out that the patient has obtained a contradictory opinion from a friend by not describing the situation in the same way as he had presented it to the therapist. On other occasions, the clinician can interpret the patient's feeling that the therapist is not providing enough help, and that outside assistance from books and friends is necessary because he feels unable to work out his own answers.

Another example of the histrionic patient's style of involvement in treatment is his pleasure in watching the clinician "at work" while maintaining an emotional distance from the process. For instance, the patient asks, "Could you explain what you meant last time when you were talking about my mother?" His tone makes it clear that he is not asking for clarification of something he did not understand but that he wishes the clinician to provide sustenance in the form of explanations. When the clinician supplies this gratification, the patient may seem to become interested and involved, but he does not extend the perimeters of the clinician's explanation. He might even remark, "You seem so wise and understanding," indicating that he is responding to the clinician's strength rather than to the content of the interpretation. At these times, the clinician can say, "I get the feeling that you enjoy listening to me analyze you."

A more subtle clue to the incomplete involvement is provided by the patient's tendency to omit crucial data from his current life situation, such as the fact that he has started a new romance or that he is in danger of losing his job. When such omissions occur, the interviewer can interpret them as indications of the patient's partial involvement in treatment.

Recognition of the Patient's Distress

The histrionic patient's emotional display is not always a drama. When the interpretations of the defensive pattern are successful, the patient will experience genuine feelings of loneliness, depression, and anxiety. At such times, it is essential that the interviewer allow the patient to feel that the clinician cares, that he is able to help and will permit some measure of dependent gratification. The mature interviewer is able to accomplish this without abandoning his professional stance. The interviewer who fears being manipulated when the patient genuinely feels badly will miss appropriate opportunities for sympathy, kindness, and understanding. This failure will prevent the development of trust and insight. The interviewer may on occasion have an opportunity to share the patient's real pain before the end of the initial interview, but with many patients this does not occur for weeks or even months.

TRANSFERENCE AND COUNTERTRANSFERENCE

Transference is prominent in the behavior of the histrionic patient from the first interview. The transference is usually positive in the first few interviews and often assumes an erotic quality when interviewer and patient are of opposite sexes. Overtly sexual fantasies about the clinician at the very beginning of treatment often suggest borderline psychopathology.

The following paragraphs refer to the transference and countertransference phenomena seen between a female patient and male interviewer, but a similar relationship also develops between the female interviewer and the male histrionic patient. The patient soon refers to the interviewer as "my doctor," "my psychiatrist," or "my therapist." She may make flattering references to the clinician's clothing or the furnishings of his office. She is solicitous if he has a cold and takes pains to learn about his interests from clues provided by his office furnishings, books, magazines in the waiting room, and so forth. She is likely to bring newspaper or magazine articles or books that she feels might interest him. She will be particularly interested in the other women patients in the waiting room, with whom she feels intensely competitive. Her traits of possessiveness and jealousy are easily uncovered by exploring remarks that she makes concerning these competitors for the clinician's love.

Body language often reveals early indications of transference. For example, the female histrionic patient may ask for a glass of water or soda, rummage through her pocketbook in search of a tissue, or put the interviewer in the position of having to help her with her coat. Such behavior is difficult to interpret in an initial interview, although it provides important clues about the patient. On one occasion when the interviewer indicated that he had no soda, the patient responded by bringing a large bottle to the next interview as a deposit. The interviewer did not accept this offering, because it would have assured the patient that the clinician would provide gratification of her dependent needs on demand. In refusing, the interviewer remarked, "If you are able to bring your own soda today, I think you should be able to manage other times." Each interviewer must rely on his own personal background and personality style with regard to social formalities such as opening doors, shaking hands, and so on. Behavior that would be natural for a European-born practitioner might be forced for an American.

The histrionic patient makes demands on the clinician's time. As the treatment progresses, intrusions on the clinician increase. There are requests for extra time or telephone calls to his home. The patient quickly develops an interest in his professional and personal life. Questions such as "Are you married?"; "Do you have children?"; or "Do you live in the city?" are common in the first few interviews. If responded to they will lead to more questions: "What does your wife do?" or "Where do you go on vacation?" If the interviewer gives no reply, the patient will feel rejected or angry at the clinician's rudeness.

This therapeutic dilemma can best be addressed directly. The clinician might reply, "I appreciate your interest in me as a person, but I can be more helpful to you if we limit our focus to your life and what transpires between us here rather than on my outside life" or "Your questions about my outside life are only useful if we explore why you are asking them." A typical response by the histrionic patient to this rejoinder is, "In other words, I'm not allowed to ask anything about you." The patient is annoyed by the therapist's limit setting. This can now be directly addressed: "Are you unhappy with my answer?" or "Do you feel that this will not be a relationship between equals?"

> After several months of treatment, a patient related a dream of visiting the therapist and his family at home. She was particularly interested in the therapist's wife, and in the dream the patient was disappointed that the clinician did not seem as strong in his home as he did in the office. The dream was told late in the session, and the clinician's comments were limited to the patient's disappointment in him. A weekend intervened before another session, and the patient became upset and telephoned the clinician at home. In the following session, the telephone call was interpreted as an acting out of the wish in the dream—that is, to compete with the clinician's wife for his attention. With much embarrassment, the patient revealed that shortly before she had become upset, she had met a woman friend in the park who knew the clinician's wife and that the patient had made inquiries about her competitor. The patient was soon able to relate this behavior to the situation in her childhood home.

A borderline histrionic patient, having learned from the doorman that the clinician lived in the same building as his office, waited outside all day in order to discover the identity of his wife. If such behavior persists or becomes troublesome to the clinician, it may suggest a countertransference problem, with the patient receiving subtle encouragement from either the clinician's anxiety or his enjoyment of the patient's interest.

The histrionic patient evokes guilt in the interviewer by continually placing him in the position of having to choose between being an indulgent parent and a depriving, punitive one. Even the most skillful interviewer cannot always avoid this dilemma. The clinician can use a combination of sympathy and interpretation. The histrionic patient soon asks, either directly or indirectly, for special privileges. He may request a glass of water or ask to use the clinician's telephone. The female patient might ask to change her clothes in his bathroom or to have her friends meet her in his waiting room. One histrionic patient, who noted that a plant in the clinician's office was dying, brought a new one. Another patient began the session saying, "I didn't have time enough for lunch today. Would you mind if I ate my sandwich?" The interviewer is put in the position of choosing between denying the patient lunch or permitting her to eat during the session. The clinician could remark, "You are asking me to decide whether to accept your interfering with the treatment or to deprive you of your lunch." In general, the interviewer should explore the underlying motivation rather than grant these requests. Histrionic patients with more serious ego defects might be treated more indulgently early in the treatment. The clinician will be more successful if he avoids an unreasonable, rigid approach.

Sometimes the patient will mention that he has discussed his treatment with a friend. On other occasions, the patient may indicate that a friend made some particular comment about the patient's treatment or the patient's therapist, usually reflecting a response of the patient himself that he is disavowing. For example, the patient might say, "My friend does not agree with what you told me last time." The therapist inquires, "What did you tell your friend I said?" In this way, the therapist will learn the nature of the patient's distortions of his remarks. The interviewer can interrupt the patient to ask, "Is that what you thought I said?" Often the patient will be able to recall the clinician's actual statement but then add, "But I thought you meant…" or "What I repeated is almost what you said." It is important to demonstrate the distortion before attempting to analyze its meaning. A series of such experiences with the patient will quickly reveal the nature of the transference. An alternate method is to explore why the patient wants to discuss his treatment with someone else.

When the histrionic patient and the clinician are of the same sex, competitive behavior is more prominent in the transference. The female histrionic patient expresses feelings of envy about the woman clinician's "stimulating professional life." At the same time she looks for opportunities to imply that the clinician is not a good mother, dresses in poor taste, or is not very feminine. The patient often experiences disappointment that her therapist is a woman, and this can be interpreted quite early in treatment.

Countertransference problems with the histrionic patient vary according to the gender, personality, and degree of experience of the clinician. The less experienced interviewer is afraid of being manipulated by the patient and tends to assume a defensive posture that hampers the development of trust and a therapeutic alliance. Kindness, empathy, and at times, sympathy for the histrionic patient are essential for the treatment to progress. Empathizing with the histrionic patient's unconscious wish for dependent care, rather than reacting with self-righteous indignation, is crucial in this endeavor.

The therapist may allow himself to be set up against the patient's spouse, parents, boss, and so on, thereby assuming the role of key persons from the patient's past who were played off, one against the other. In the extension of this countertransference, the therapist plays the role of parent, protector, or lover in the patient's unconscious, enjoying the patient's quick insights, warmth, emotionality, or even helplessness. Erotic responses in the clinician are very common and may be quite frightening to the therapist. The warmth and seductive behavior of the patient may lead the clinician to be defensively aloof, cold, and business-like, allowing no emotional engagement in the interview. The clinician can look for opportunities to initiate engagement instead of merely responding to the patient's attempts at control.

Awkwardness in dealing with the patient's spontaneity leads the therapist to feel as though he has two left feet. The young clinician's spontaneity is often learned or rehearsed. An example occurred with a histrionic patient's second visit to a female resident. The patient began the session with, "Oh that is the same dress you were wearing last time." This savvy resident smiled and replied, "Well, how about that?" The balance of power was quickly reestablished. The competitive transference was not ready to be interpreted. If the interviewer allows a number of examples to unfold, the interpretation is more effective. A response by the interviewer of "touché" acknowledges, "You caught me off balance." One can then explore the patient's response, and the patient's covert reasons for the aggression will emerge.

Failure to see through the patient's intellectualizations that are designed to impress the therapist misses the fact that the patient is trying to please the clinician. Another common countertransference problem is to miss subtle inhibitions of self-expression. For example, not speaking up at a meeting or fear of asking questions in a class are examples of blind spots that allow the patient to remain a child.

Gratifying the patient excessively to avoid the patient's emotional storms or to keep the patient in treatment is obvious countertransference. Feeling guilty at being either too depriving or too indulgent is the rule, and errors on both sides should be analyzed in the transference. The errors on both sides tend to balance each other out.

There is the histrionic patient who brings gifts to the therapist. It might be a plant to replace one that is dying, or it may be something to eat. Then there is the patient who has a friend meet her in the clinician's waiting room or redoes her makeup in the bathroom or leaves a suitcase in the clinician's closet. Such behaviors by the histrionic patient have the capacity to make the interviewer feel gauche or petty about his response of annoyance. These obvious transference enactments provide countertransference traps. The easiest way of addressing this is when the patient brings it up, even if it is not until the following session, with a comment such as, "I hope you didn't mind that...?" It requires tact and comfort with one's own feelings to ask, "Did you have any reservations about it?" or "How did you think I felt about it?"

As the interviewer acquires experience and professional maturity, he finds it easier to be firm with the histrionic patient and at the same time to be kind and understanding. The histrionic patient always responds to the clinician's understanding by feeling loved. This feeling is followed by unreasonable demands. The clinician cannot gratify these demands, and the patient then feels rejected. The treatment of the patient typically alternates between these two extremes.

One of the easiest ways to avoid being manipulated in the matter of decisions is to admit to the patient that the interviewer does not know what would be best for the patient. At the same time, this challenges the patient's image of the clinician as an omniscient figure of authority. If the patient does succeed in manipulating the clinician, it is possible to use the experience constructively instead of becoming angry with the patient. The interviewer could ask, "Do you feel that this is the way that I can best help you?" or "Why is it so important to manipulate me in this way?" The patient will often misinterpret the firmness or control on the clinician's part as a rejection and as an attempt to inhibit the patient's spontaneous feelings. This misperception stems from the patient's inability to experience a subjective sense of emotional freedom and at the same time successfully regulate and control his life.

CONCLUSION

The histrionic patient is one of the most rewarding patients to treat. Although there are many stressful periods for the patient and the clinician, the experience is rarely boring. As treatment progresses, the patient will eventually develop his capacity for genuine emotional responses and also to manage his own life. His emotional swings will become less marked as he gradually is able to understand and accept his deeper feelings and repressed sexual wishes. The clinician will usually feel some personal enrichment from this therapeutic experience in addition to the satisfaction customarily derived from helping a patient.

CHAPTER 5

THE NARCISSISTIC PATIENT

Narcissism is a confusing psychiatric term. Originally it was used by Freud in a manner consonant with the ancient Greek myth of Narcissus. This was no accident, because the myth is profoundly insightful concerning the pathology of narcissism.

Narcissus was a beautiful youth, the product of the rape of the nymph Leiriope by the river god Cephisus. Leiriope was informed by a prophet that her son would live a long life provided he never knew himself. By the time he was 16 years old, as Robert Graves recounts, "his path was strewn with heartlessly rejected lovers of both sexes; for he had a stubborn pride in his own beauty." One of these repudiated lovers was the nymph Echo, who could no longer use her voice except to repeat the last sounds she heard. This was a punishment inflicted on her by Juno, whom she had deceived and distracted with beguiling stories while Juno's husband, Zeus, was unfaithful with the nymphs. Echo, who was lovelorn, approached Narcissus in the woods but could only repeat his words. "I will die before you ever lie with me," Narcissus cried. "Lie with me," she pleaded, repeating his words, but he abandoned her. Echo was heartbroken and pined away until only her voice remained. Later, a male suitor of Narcissus was spurned by him, and before killing himself he prayed to the gods, "Oh, may he love himself alone and yet fail in that great love." The goddess Artemis heard the plea and caused Narcissus to fall in love with his own image, which he saw in a reflecting pool and shattered every time he tried to embrace it. As Graves relates, "At first he tried to embrace and kiss the beautiful boy who confronted him, but presently recognized himself, and lay gazing enraptured into the pool, hour after hour. How could he endure both to possess and yet not to possess? Grief was destroying him, yet he rejoiced in his torments; knowing at least that his other self would remain true to him, whatever happened." Echo shared his grief and mourned as Narcissus plunged a dagger into his breast and died. From his blood sprang the flower that bears his name.

Many of the elements of pathological narcissism are cleverly incorporated into the myth: early psychological trauma and the consequent development of a sense of entitlement (Narcissus is the product of a rape); the absence of self-knowledge (most narcissists are oblivious to their pervasive and disabling disorder); egocentricity, arrogance, and insensitivity to the feelings of others (his treatment of Echo and the spurned youth); the desire and need of narcissists to have other people "echo" their thoughts and ideas; the absence of empathy for anyone but the self; disturbed object constancy (the fragmenting image in the reflecting pool); a mirroring transference (again the reflecting pool and the total love of only the self); and, finally, frustration and rage at the unattainable, leading to his suicide.

Freud initially viewed narcissism as a sexual perversion wherein the person's own body, as in the tale of Narcissus, was the object of desire. He subsequently used the term to delineate a normal developmental stage characteristic of infants and small children whose mental life is fundamentally egocentric. Gradually the concept evolved further to include a type of adult psychopathology characterized by grandiose self-importance, a failure to be concerned with the feelings of others, an inability to love someone else, and the exploitation of other people without any accompanying feelings of guilt.

Narcissism can be thought of as a universal dynamic theme of human psychology that is an essential and pervasive part of psychic structure. The concept possesses a spectrum of meanings. Narcissism organizes personality structure from the healthy to the pathological. Healthy narcissism is critical in maintaining basic self-esteem—the conviction that one is worthwhile—and the capacity to take pleasure in achievement, feel joy in being appreciated by others, and accept praise or rewards for one's accomplishments while sharing and acknowledging the role of others who were part of this success.

Narcissistic personality disorder is a relatively recent diagnostic category. Unlike most other personality disorders, it is not based on an extrapolation from the hypothetical psychodynamics of a symptomatic neurosis, on a description of nonpsychotic features of a psychotic disorder, or even on a cluster of maladaptive behavior traits. It began with psychoanalysts and psychoanalytic psychotherapists struggling to understand a group of particularly difficult patients who were not psychotic, not classically neurotic, and in general not responsive to traditional psychotherapeutic interventions and characterized not so much by observable psychopathological phenomenology as by inferred psychodynamic patterns. The other personality disorder with a similar history is borderline personality disorder, but whereas borderline patients were soon recognized to exhibit a characteristic cluster of affective instability, chaotic relationships, life course, and at times deficits in autonomous ego functions, narcissistic patients were often viewed by the world as high functioning and without obvious psychopathology. Their problems were internal and related to the way in which they experienced themselves and others. They suffered, although they often denied it, the rest of the world often failed to recognize it, and only their therapists realized its depth. It seemed from the beginning that narcissism was more of a theme in mental life than a distinct nosological category. It was essentially universal, although more prominent in some than in others, and it could be associated with a wide range of pathology, from relatively healthy to seriously disturbed.

Narcissistic pathology is thus on a continuum from a mild form to more serious forms. In more serious cases, grandiosity and self-centeredness preclude sensitivity to the feelings of others, who exist in the patient's mind only as a source of gratification and constant admiration. Such exploitation of others prevents any deep, caring relationship and reflects a vain and selfish individual who must constantly be the center of attention. When someone else is the celebrated person, the narcissist suffers inwardly, regardless of how unrealistic the competitive situation may actually be. For example, the severe narcissist may experience envy at the attention shown to a new baby, to a bride at her wedding, or to the eulogies given the deceased at a funeral. Pathological narcissism exhibits an oscillation between two feeling states: grandiosity and its opposite, a sense of nothingness.

The healthier, better-adapted, yet pathological narcissist is able to conform to social expectations. He seems comfortable with his accomplishments and has developed an outward appearance of modesty. Upon closer study, however, it is seen that he overestimates his importance and demands special treatment. These stronger wishes persist even though the person is considered to be successful. Secretly, he never feels satisfied with his achievements, and he experiences painful envy of the success of others.

The more subtle narcissist is a manipulator and can cause the other person to feel guilty for not offering whatever it was that he had wanted. The narcissist is easily hurt and responds with spiteful vindictiveness, which is often expressed with deliberate meanness. An example would be the mother who feels humiliated by some mild misbehavior by her child in front of others. She may smile and appear to offer gentle control of the situation while covertly pinching the child in a fashion not visible to others.

Superego pathology is characteristic of the narcissist. The person with a milder form of this disorder possesses a superego that enables him to do "the right thing," but he does not feel particularly good about it. In essence, this aspect of psychic structure—an amalgam of parental values, moral and ethical precepts, decency, kindness, and so on—is not idealized in the way it is by other people. Doing the right thing does not enhance the narcissistic person's sense of self-worth. He does not feel proud of himself, because he is far more preoccupied with power and acclaim. He has idealized the grandiose ego ideal, not the superego.

It is the narcissistic deep-seated, inner greediness that has been the downfall of many highly successful and powerful people who never feel that they have "enough" despite enormous wealth and power. Success seems to intensify feelings of entitlement rather than to allow a feeling of peace and fulfillment with accomplishments. The narcissistic person will lie or cheat effortlessly in order to escape exposure and humiliation.

The DSM-5 criteria for narcissistic personality disorder (Box 5–1) aptly capture the elements of the disorder in its more florid form. Milder variations, however, are common in clinical practice and can coexist with many other psychiatric disorders. A narcissistic individual can be quite charming, charismatic, self-confident, and superficially warm and entertaining. He has the ability to make another person, including the clinical interviewer, feel that he is also special. This reflects the narcissistic person's ability to psychologically incorporate another into his mental orbit of superiority and specialness as long as that person does not frustrate or contradict him. Over the course of time, this charming person reveals his lack of interest in the lives of others while expecting them to be interested in everything about him.

BOX 5–1. DSM-5 Diagnostic Criteria for Narcissistic Personality Disorder

---

A pervasive pattern of grandiosity (in fantasy or behavior), need for admiration, and lack of empathy, beginning by early adulthood and present in a variety of contexts, as indicated by five (or more) of the following:

1. Has a grandiose sense of self-importance (e.g., exaggerates achievements and talents, expects to be recognized as superior without commensurate achievements).
2. Is preoccupied with fantasies of unlimited success, power, brilliance, beauty, or ideal love.

3. Believes that he or she is "special" and unique and can only be understood by, or should associate with, other special or high-status people (or institutions).
4. Requires excessive admiration.
5. Has a sense of entitlement (i.e., unreasonable expectations of especially favorable treatment or automatic compliance with his or her expectations).
6. Is interpersonally exploitative (i.e., takes advantage of others to achieve his or her own ends).
7. Lacks empathy: is unwilling to recognize or identify with the feelings and needs of others.
8. Is often envious of others or believes that others are envious of him or her.
9. Shows arrogant, haughty behaviors or attitudes.

Source.   Reprinted from American Psychiatric Association: *Diagnostic and Statistical Manual of Mental Disorders*, 5th Edition. Arlington, VA, American Psychiatric Association, 2013. Copyright 2013, American Psychiatric Association. Used with permission.

Although not included in the DSM-5 nomenclature, a common subtype of narcissistic personality disorder, *shy or covert inner narcissism*, has been identified (Table 5–1). The shy narcissist is highly sensitive to slights or criticism. Where the criticisms are perceived as accurate, he responds with intense feelings of shame and humiliation. These same feelings of humiliation can be experienced when someone whom he views as a narcissistic extension—most likely a spouse, a child, or even a parent—performs poorly or embarrasses him. When the criticism or slight seems unjustified, he reacts inwardly with indignant rage and fantasies of exaggerated retaliation (e.g., .50-caliber machine guns mounted in the front fenders of his car to blast an aggressive driver who cut him off on the highway). The shy narcissist's arrogant counterpart is more apt to drive a couple of feet behind the other driver and make hand gestures or to swerve around him or even try to run him off the road. The shy narcissist tends toward periodic feelings of depression. He often feels best when doing things by himself. In this way, he avoids competitive feelings of inferiority, envy, or shame in the presence of others.

The shy narcissist may have many acquaintances and a capacity to appear friendly but rarely warm. He has very few, if any, friends (particularly men) from various periods of his life. This is due to his caring more about what others think of him than caring about them. He is unlikely to know the names of his children's friends or to have an interest in his "friends'" children. It is this incapacity to sustain long-term relations that contributes to his feelings of isolation and being disconnected from people. His incapacity for genuine empathy is masked by his awareness of social expectations and a set of learned appropriate

TABLE 5–1. Criteria for the shy or covert subtype of narcissistic personality disorder

The shy or covert inner narcissist
(1) is inhibited, shy, or even self-effacing.
(2) directs attention more toward others than toward self and is uncomfortable when he becomes the center of attention.
(3) is highly sensitive and listens to others carefully for evidence of slights or criticism or for praise and flattery.
(4) responds to slights or criticism with inner anger and/or intense shame, humiliation, and self-criticism; responds to flattery with an exaggerated feeling of pleasure mixed with a sense of superiority and a feeling of having fooled people, mistrusting their motives.
(5) is highly envious of the success and recognition achieved by others.
(6) is unable to commit to others with unconditional love; lacks appropriate responsiveness to others; may not return letters or telephone calls because of a desire to be pursued; needs a constant source of gratification, as in the old song, "When I'm not near the girl I love, I love the girl I'm near."
(7) lacks the capacity for empathy with others, or at best offers a calculated intellectualized empathy derived from figuring out the appropriate outward response; however, this response does not allow him to *feel* connected to the other person.
(8) has compensatory grandiose fantasies that substitute for real accomplishments.
(9) has a tendency toward hypochondria based on a response to feeling defective and inadequate; self-preoccupation easily focuses on health.

Source. Modified from Gabbard 1989.

responses that initially fool others into believing he cares more deeply than is the case. His feelings of entitlement and need to get his own way are concealed beneath his shy aloofness. On other occasions, he seems quite unaware of that to which he is actually entitled. A budding friendship will be abandoned because of a narcissistic injury that threatens the patient's deep feelings of grandiosity. He is too hurt, ashamed, and/or angry to even acknowledge his injured feeling, which quickly leads to his alienation from the other person.

Unlike the arrogant narcissist, the shy narcissist is able to feel, but rarely express, feelings of regret over his empathic failure. His "guilt" about his lack of concern for others is experienced as intense shame that compels him to hide. This contrasts with mature guilt that is accompanied by sorrow for the mistreatment of the other person and a desire to apologize and make amends. Nor can the shy narcissist accept the apology from someone who has hurt him. He collects these hurts on a score card and inwardly feels, "Now you owe me." Like his first cousin, the masochist, he revels in the role of the injured party and strategically utilizes this position to extract favors from people or to otherwise manipulate them. Akhtar noted that in contrast to the arrogant narcissist, the shy narcissist has a stricter conscience and higher moral standards, with less inclination toward inconsistency regarding rules or ethical and moral values.

PSYCHOPATHOLOGY AND PSYCHODYNAMICS

Narcissistic Characteristics

Grandiosity

An exaggerated sense of oneself as uniquely special, unusually talented, and superior to others is a regular characteristic of the narcissistic patient. This inflated view of one's importance, even genius, is usually at odds with reality. Sometimes, however, especially in the artistic, political, scientific, or business world, the narcissist may be quite professionally talented and will receive reinforcement for his grandiosity by the critical acclaim of others. However, the narcissist's sense of superiority functions as a fragile defense against inner feelings of weakness, and it commonly has little objective correlation. "I am more important than Virginia Woolf was to English literature," declared a 30-year-old writer in a first interview. It quickly emerged not only that she had never been published but also that her literary output was limited and fragmentary and had never been shown to fellow writers, editors, or critics, because "they would not understand or comprehend its brilliance. Worse, if they did get it, they would be incredibly envious."

The extreme case of the arrogant or flamboyant narcissist is easily recognized. Shy narcissists do not display themselves in an obvious fashion, but they are secretly ready to feel slighted if they do not obtain the recognition that they feel is their due. In essence, they believe that their special presence and aura should be automatically perceived and responded to by those around them. If treated like everyone else, they will inwardly seethe. The shy narcissist has the same desire as the flamboyant narcissist to be applauded for special virtues but has a deeper fear of potential humiliation and shame if his grandiose fantasies are exposed.

Unlike the arrogant narcissist, who may be highly successful in a way that reinforces his grandiosity, the shy narcissist has a grandiosity that usually exists largely in fantasy. His deepest ambition is to be the very best, but inhibitions based on a fear of failing protect him from intense feelings of shame and humiliation. Hence he does not really exert himself to achieve because to do so would carry the risk of failure or non-recognition. The grandiosity implicitly exists underneath his dissatisfaction with his every achievement. He can briefly feel happy or even elated over a small recognition, but it is never enough. He soon compares himself with someone who has done more. He both over- and undervalues the importance of his accomplishments. This leads to a spotty work record because he becomes less confident in himself as he rises in an organization. More success is experienced as a bigger opportunity to fail and to face a more public humiliation. The more arrogant narcissist experiences success as his entitlement and tacit permission to play fast and loose with ethics and rules.

Although the narcissist can sometimes be witty at other people's expense, the absence of a true sense of humor and an inability to laugh at oneself is characteristic of this disorder. The presence of fantasies of possessing transcendent charm, beauty, and intelligence are common. "My extraordinary radiance illuminates any room that I am in," one narcissistic patient smugly described it. A graduate student in molecular biology who had an erratic career and was on the brink of being dropped from his program confidently exclaimed, "It's inevitable that I will win the Nobel Prize. The fact that I have had problems with my advisors means nothing. Look at Einstein. He never got along with his professors." This example speaks to the organizing aspects of narcissism. All aspiring or accomplished scientists may desire to win the Nobel Prize. It may be considered a universal fantasy for scientists. The scientist with healthy narcissism may possess this desire but will realize that award of the prize is based on how others estimate the value of his works and will have an understanding of the complexity of the politics involved in giving awards. The pathological narcissist, in contrast, has the conviction that he deserves the prize and has a desperate need for this accolade to support his grandiosity, unrealistic as the possibility may be in reality.

Grandiosity and its opposite—a deep sense of inadequacy—coexist in the narcissistic person. The clinical presentation will begin with one or the other. The patient may present complaining of professional failure or ineptitude in love experiences, but shortly thereafter his grandiose, overbearing, and imperious side will emerge. Alternatively, the grandiose and inflated side may present initially, but later in treatment profound feelings of inadequacy and inner emptiness will come to the forefront.

Lack of Empathy

An inability to be empathic with others is characteristic of the narcissistic individual. *Empathy* is a complex psychological phenomenon that includes the capacity to identify with another person and to transiently experience the other's emotional state. Empathy should be distinguished from *sympathy*, which is the genuine feeling of compassion for another person's pain or suffering, for example, the loss of a loved one. Empathy enables the listener to experience being in the other person's shoes while at the same time maintaining separateness. This capacity requires one to focus attention away from oneself, and it is absent in most narcissistic persons.

> A narcissistic patient who was in the midst of a divorce, precipitated by his disclosure of an affair, bitterly complained, "I don't understand why my wife does not feel sorry for me. My life has been turned upside down, my kids are angry at me, my life is a mess. She just seems to want to persecute me, and that killer lawyer she is using is too much! How can she not care about how much pain I am in? I am suffering so much." He was incapable of feeling empathy for his wife's sense of loss, betrayal, and anger. He was the one for whom she should feel sorry, because he was suffering so much from the consequences of his actions.

More subtle failures of empathy are common. The narcissist is annoyed when his enjoyment of an evening is interfered with by some painful event in his partner's day. He may explode in a furious outburst if his partner, distracted by a family crisis, fails to praise his success. The accusation that the partner is "uncaring" will feel justified to the patient, who believes that he is the victim.

The ability to recognize what someone else is feeling does not, in itself, rule out the diagnosis of narcissism. The less extreme narcissistic person can identify another person's emotional state on some occasions. However, this is often based on inferences from external cues and not on inner feeling. On other occasions he has little or no emotional concern for the pain, distress, or feelings of the other person. While seeming to listen empathically, the narcissistic person is unconsciously storing information regarding the other person's vulnerable points to be used against that person on some future occasion when feeling criticized. These counterattacks are deliberate and show conscious meanness. Although the obsessive person may also engage in counterattacks when criticized, he does this from unconscious anger and a lack of tact, not the conscious sadism that is typical of the narcissist.

Entitlement

A profound sense of personal entitlement usually accompanies the narcissistic patient. "Of course I should not have to wait my turn," exclaimed a narcissistic patient. Trying to set up a mutually convenient time for the initial clinical interview may reveal the diagnosis in advance of the first meeting. "That time isn't good for me because of my workout schedule," stated a narcissistic patient. "I can only come before lunch. Can't you see me at 11:00?" The sense of entitlement is reflected in the conviction that the world should accommodate to him. Later in the interview the patient revealed, "My parents were cold and unfeeling. They gave me nothing emotionally. Of course I have to look out for number one; no one else will." The emotional deprivation that the narcissist believes he has experienced leads directly to a type of aloofness and contemptuous arrogance in dealing with people who are regarded as having no significance, thus reversing the narcissist's own experience of unimportance as a child.

> A highly intelligent graduate student was confronted with compelling evidence of his having plagiarized published material and came for psychiatric consultation. He did not arrive in the clinician's office of his own volition, but candidly admitted that seeing a mental health professional would bolster his defense against these charges and mitigate the consequences. Gradually, during the course of the interview, he conceded that "perhaps the files in my computer became confused so that I thought someone else's writing was really mine." He felt that the charges against him should be dismissed because it was simply an error of electronic transposition that whole pieces of a textbook had appeared in his papers as though they were his. "In any case, I'm the most brilliant student in the class. The authorities should make allowances for that fact." When asked by the interviewer what he thought the difference was between lying and a mistake, he became confused. It took some time for him to concede that it was a matter of intentionality.

This example speaks to the automatic sense of entitlement that the narcissistic patient possesses. "What belongs to someone else can be mine if I wish. Honesty is no virtue since it may prevent me from getting what I want."

Shame

Shame, as differentiated from guilt, is a common and painful affect for the narcissist. Morrison suggested that shame is an affect of equal importance to guilt in psychic life. Shame revolves around the experience of exposure of some failure or inadequacy and the consequent feeling of mortification. Morrison included within the designation of shame feelings of humiliation, embarrassment, and lowered self-esteem. The narcissist responds to criticism or failure in some attempted achievement with a feeling that the *self* is inadequate and defective. An intellectually accomplished narcissistic patient who had a number of important publications to her credit became mortified and depressed upon receiving a rejection of her latest paper from a prominent journal. "I am nothing. My work is trivial and worthless. There is no point to my life. I just want to hide from everyone," she exclaimed with bitterness and despair. The desire to hide is a classic response to the experience of shame. In some cultures in which shame is an excruciating and overwhelming affect, shamed and exposed individuals may feel that they have no recourse but to kill themselves, the ultimate form of "hiding."

Envy

Envy plagues the narcissist who constantly compares himself with others in the hope of reinforcing his sense of superiority. Frequent feelings of inferiority stimulate a desire to devalue the other. "I'm so angry that she got the promotion and I didn't," complained a junior book editor. "I'm prettier, sexier, and far more charming than she is. Just because she's smart and the writers she works with like her, she's so empty. Doesn't my company realize that image is everything? Looking good is what counts, not being likeable. I think I'm going to quit over this insult." A mental health professional revealed his envy of the interviewer by commenting in the first interview, "Well, I know you are prominent and admired. I can tell from talking with you that your success is a consequence of the fact that you are just more effective than I am at controlling and manipulating the psychiatric world."

Narcissistic Devaluation

Devaluation dominates the object relationships of the narcissistic patient. The distinctions are discussed in Chapter 9, "The Borderline Patient," in a comparison of the type of devaluation that is characteristic of the narcissistic and the borderline patients.

Severe Narcissism

The severely narcissistic patient represents the extreme end of the narcissistic spectrum. Such patients, because of the absence of even a modicum of conscience or guilt concerning their exploitative and often intensely aggressive (even violent) behavior, can seem repellent to the interviewer. Infamous tyrants such as Hitler and Stalin, whose indifference to their murder of millions is emblematic of their inhumanity, have been labeled malignant narcissists. Whether or not this is diagnostically accurate, it is consistent with the popular image of these dictators. Severe narcissism does overlap with the antisocial personality, and in some cases, severely narcissistic persons are capable of chilling acts of cruelty, violence, and even murder.

Two themes dominate the psychopathology of severely narcissistic patients. One reflects serious ego deficits that manifest themselves in impulsivity, low frustration tolerance, and an inability to delay gratification. The other is the absence of normal superego functioning. This combination of deficits is at the core of the violent outbursts that can occur with these patients. The superego exerts no control over unbridled impulsivity. Narcissistic rage of an explosive nature may thus color the life of the severe narcissist. Narcissistic rage can be global and unlimited. Such rage is precipitated by imagined or real slights that these individuals experience when they are thwarted or contradicted in everyday life. Opposition to their wishes evokes the fantasy of obliterating the individual who does not succumb to their demands and who thus challenges their underlying, but tenuous, feeling of omnipotence. In extreme cases, this may actually lead to the murder of a partner or spouse, for which act the severe narcissist feels no remorse because, within his extremely pathological inner world, it is completely warranted. Massive superego pathology, combined with impulsivity, is at the core of the severe narcissist's pathology and explains the absence of any feelings of guilt for his destructive actions.

Differential Diagnosis

The major differential diagnoses include borderline personality disorder, antisocial personality disorder, and bipolar spectrum disorders. Although there are relatively pure forms, it is not uncommon to see mixtures of narcissistic and borderline personality disorders.

Although in DSM-5 the distinctions between the obsessive-compulsive patient and the narcissistic patient seem clear, in actual clinical work they are frequently blurred. This is particularly true in those patients with mixed character disorders who have both obsessive and narcissistic aspects. These distinctions are particularly important in the treatment of a patient who has both features, so that the clinician does not make the interpretation of an obsessive dynamic when, at that particular moment, a narcissistic dynamic is driving the patient's behavior.

The first area of confusion is emotional isolation, which in the obsessive patient may be confused with the cool detachment of the narcissist. The obsessive person utilizes the mechanisms of minimization, intellectualization, and rationalization to deal with his own unwanted emotional responses. "I was not angry at my boss," the obsessive patient stated after his work had been criticized. "I was not pleased; I may have been a trifle piqued; but I certainly was not angry." The narcissistic person is quite aware of the rageful response he felt in a similar situation and has already begun to devalue the other person as stupid. The obsessive individual lacks tact and sensitivity to the feelings of others and is often unaware that he has said something that bothered someone. If it is brought to his attention, he feels guilty or defensive and attempts through logic and reason to persuade the offended party that he or she should not feel hurt. On other occasions, the obsessive person notices that he said or did something that might have upset another person, but he does not fully allow this to register in his mind, or if it does, he chooses to ignore it. The incident may later return to consciousness for further reflection or rumination. This does not happen with the narcissistic person, whose callous lack of concern for the feelings of others is genuine and is rationalized with an attitude of "that's how all people are; some are just better pretenders than others."

The obsessive person's pursuit of perfection differs from that of the narcissistic person, although this is perhaps one of the most difficult differential diagnostic features in understanding character pathology. The solution to the therapist's confusion lies in uncovering the latent object connection that is part of the perfectionistic pursuit or, in other words, understanding what unconscious motivation drives the behavior. What is it the patient expects to gain or lose—what conflict is involved in the perfectionistic drive? The obsessive person, when doing something perfectly, feels a sense of mastery, power, and control and anticipates praise or some positive reinforcement from his own internalized objects as well as from his parental figures. However, he feels the praise as an evidence of being respected—loved as a separate person even if he resents the feeling that he has to perform perfectly in order to win this respect. It is the firm sense of a separate identity that allows the obsessive individual to feel a genuine sense of accomplishment. This is due to his having internalized a good object image. He feels that he has been good and has lived up to his parents' perfectionistic standards. He deserves respect. At an unconscious level the obsessive person equates respect with love, and he believes that love must be earned. The narcissistic pursuit of perfection is a more exploitative event wherein the person is fulfilling a grandiose wish of his parent that will make the parent look good. The child is exploited as a device to enhance the brilliance, beauty, and success of the parent. When the narcissistic child is admired or praised, he does not feel this recognition as a separate person but feels that he merely enhanced the perfection that his parent pursues relentlessly. His mission on earth is to make the parent look good or, if he chooses, look bad. Therefore, when a narcissistic person fails to achieve perfection, he feels humiliated, ashamed, degraded, and worthless. The obsessive person, on the other hand, is more inclined to wonder if he did it wrong, did not follow instructions or try hard enough, or in some other covert way was disobedient. This is because the obsessive individual always has contradictory impulses to be defiant and oppositional. This is where the doing and undoing rituals arise and why obsessive people are always plagued by self-doubt.

At times the narcissistic person will unconsciously fail deliberately in order to embarrass and humiliate the parent who humiliated them. It is a masochistic way of getting even, and the act is motivated by spite. The sweetness of spiteful revenge offsets the personal pain and embarrassment from the failure. This is a common mechanism in narcissistic, masochistic adolescents who fail in school to get back at the parent for only caring that the child attends a prestigious college.

Another aspect of narcissistic perfectionism is related to the amount of work the patient is willing to do in order to win praise. The obsessive person is aware that success requires both skill and effort, and he is willing to put forth the effort. The narcissistic person wants maximum recognition in exchange for minimal effort.

Both obsessive and narcissistic individuals have inordinate drives to obtain power and control over others. However, the former is always plagued by self-doubt and feels conflicted about the consequences for those he may have hurt or damaged in his own pursuit of success. The latter seems conflict-free about the intensity of his drives. Both types of patient may have inhibitions of work performance that can only be distinguished on the basis of differing concepts of the unconsciously imaged danger accompanying success. The obsessive person unconsciously views work in terms of the conflict between being obedient and accepted but with a consequence of feeling simultaneously submissive and weak and being naughty and defiant but with a consequence of feeling strong and independent. This dynamic is most apparent in the procrastination component of the obsessive person's work problem. At the same time, oedipal dynamics express themselves in the obsessive patient in his ambivalent attitude toward same-sex competitors whom he views as more powerful than himself. This takes the form of losing his assertiveness and not being able to finish off an opponent despite being close to victory. He wants to be boss so that he will not be controlled by others. He wants his status, power, and control to be recognized by others. Typically, he assumes the responsibility that is appropriate to the power and sometimes even more than is appropriate. He will often complain about the responsibility but will feel great pride about it and be conscientious in discharging it. The narcissistic person desires the power in order to obtain the admiration of others and to be served by them, but he does not want the responsibility and looks for ways to push it off on some underling or otherwise to shirk it, sometimes under the guise of delegation of authority. This process becomes apparent when the narcissist delegates only the responsibility but never any of the glory that goes with successful achievement.

Consider the example of an obsessively indecisive graduate student. His ruminations involve "Which topic will please my thesis advisor the most and get me the best grade? Is there something I would really prefer to write about? Must I submit to his authority?" The narcissistic graduate student wonders which thesis advisor has the most power and glamour and wants a topic that will be flashy and bring him easy glory. A seeming exception to this principle occurred in the case of a narcissistic graduate student who chose to do her thesis in the Russian Department in preference to the German Department, where she had received higher grades and more encouragement as an undergraduate. However, the motive behind the choice was to spitefully demonstrate to the Russian Department that they had made a mistake about her brilliance, thereby vindicating herself and humiliating them. This can be contrasted with the obsessive person who argues over the meaning of a word and then goes to the dictionary. He wants recognition for his precision and implicit superiority, but his motive is not to humiliate his opponent. Paranoid personalities also wish to sadistically humiliate an adversary whom they feel has wronged them. The paranoid person wants recognition that he has been wronged, and he demands an apology—not just today, but again tomorrow, the next day, and on and on. However, if the offending party atones long enough, he eventually will be forgiven. The narcissistic character, on the other hand, merely writes off his adversary once and for all. The obsessive character, basically, wants to make up and will accept a sincere apology.

The histrionic character presents another difficult differential diagnostic dilemma. This type of patient is also attention seeking and may become quite flamboyant in order to remain the central focus of others. Narcissistic features are often mixed with histrionic character traits. The histrionic patient is quite capable of angry outbursts when these needs for recognition are frustrated. Nevertheless, this person is capable of genuine love and deep attachment to others. The histrionic patient has more charm, warmth, and capacity to not always put her own needs first. Manipulation of others usually involves charm, flattery, and a presentation of pseudo-helplessness. In contrast, the narcissistic patient uses entitlement and aggressive assertions that are quite inconsiderate of the feelings of another person. An illustrative example of this distinction occurred when two patients became concerned about the clinician's recent weight gain and what it might portend. The histrionic patient was genuinely concerned about the clinician's health, and being an expert on diet programs, she plied the clinician with effective regimens. She was worried on his behalf. The narcissistic patient was affronted that the therapist had become fat. "How can I have a therapist who looks like you? This reflects so badly on me. Please see my personal trainer and lose some weight. I'll pay for it." Another example of this differential diagnostic distinction occurs at the party where the histrionic patient is looking for her friends, whereas the narcissistic patient is looking for the "stars" who might be present while simultaneously thinking "Do I measure up to these people?"

The distinctions between narcissistic personality disorder and borderline personality disorder are discussed in Chapter 9. The differential diagnoses between antisocial personality and severe narcissistic personality disorder are imprecise, and there is significant comorbidity. Crime families, for example, represent a deviant antisocial subculture. A member of such a group can have lasting friendships and alliances with other members, pursuing codes of ethics that are well defined although at variance with the mainstream of society. They are capable of great loyalty, particularly to their biological family members. The television and motion picture industries exploit a public fascination for these groups. They are often ruthless and kill easily, but this behavior does not make them narcissists, although it is clearly antisocial. The "family business" does not tolerate the excessively narcissistic members of the group who do not fit in with the group cohesiveness and goals.

Bipolar spectrum disorder is one of the emerging diagnostic groups in which considerable controversy exists. The former (DSM-II) hypomanic personality was described as grandiose, boastful, exuberant, overoptimistic, overconfident, ambitious, high-achieving, and self-assertive. A person with hypomanic personality may have brief episodes of depression. Despite these qualities, he is warm and "people friendly" and can participate actively in give-and-take relationships. He is not the inwardly envious, devaluing, and vindictive person who is characteristic of the narcissist.

When a narcissistic person voluntarily seeks treatment, it is often because of depression. Narcissistic injuries in the form of occupational failure or a significant loss of face in a failed relationship are the usual precipitants. There is considerable overlap between dysthymia, narcissistic personality disorder (shy type), and masochistic personality disorder.

Developmental Psychodynamics

Healthy narcissism allows for a realistic appraisal of one's attributes and ambitions, the ability to have emotional attachments to other people while recognizing their separateness, and the capacity to love and to be loved. The awareness of the separate existence and the feelings of other people is a crucial aspect of healthy narcissism. When normal development fails, one finds the psychological disturbances characteristic of the narcissistic personality, ranging from the self-involved and mildly entitled individual to the flagrant egocentricity of the severe narcissist, who will tolerate no external challenge to his conviction of superiority and omnipotence. It is thought that this variation in degrees of narcissistic pathology reflects the amount of parental emotional neglect and absence of empathy as well as parental exploitation that the child experiences during early development, leading to varying deficits in the sense of self.

The evolution of healthy narcissism and the capacity to differentiate self from other are thought to be contingent upon empathic parenting coupled with limit setting presented in a kindly manner. The small infant experiences the external world as an extension of the self, a state of being that persists in pathological narcissism. Self–object differentiation occurs as an incremental process that evolves through interactions, both gratifying and frustrating, with the caretakers and the outside world. Over time, under normal conditions, a psychological inner awareness of the separateness of the self from other develops. Simultaneously, the psychological internalization of an image of the empathic, nurturing caretakers occurs and becomes part of the child's psychic structure. In a sense, this aspect of the external world becomes part of the child. This incorporation of representational aspects of the loving caretakers forms the underpinning for the child's gradual acquisition of empathy for others, healthy self-regard, and solid sense of self.

A failure of empathic caretaking, in particular the absence of parental mirroring, throws the small child back upon the self, which is tenuous and, in the young infant, always in danger of fragmenting, a type of emotional "falling apart" that one sees regularly in babies and young children when they are distressed. Mirroring is a complex parent–child interactive phenomenon that involves the parents receiving communications from the infant or small child, registering them, transforming them, imitating them, and reflecting them to the child. The parent echoes and elaborates the child's sounds or actions such as babbling, cooing, or banging her high chair with her hand. This is an emotional experience for both parent and child. The playful mood is the best example in which parental imitation elicits gales of laughter from the child and further laughter from the parent. This interplay bears a resemblance to what occurs among musicians when the initial simple melody is picked up and elaborated by the full orchestra. It is a natural emotional music-making between the child and parent. The child's experience interacts with the more psychologically highly organized parent, who integrates the child's communication from his or her perspective, reflects it back to the child, and thus helps the child's sense of self to evolve.

The message sent back to the child by the narcissistic or otherwise disturbed parent is not in empathic tune with the child's communication. It becomes a confusing message because it has nothing to do with the child's experience. Healthy mirroring implies a valid reflection of the child's more primitive experience; it is the parent responding to the as-yet unrealized potential of the child. For example, the normal mother hears the child's words in his babbling before he has language and will babble back in kind, thus reaching out to the infant who is struggling to communicate with the parent. The child's sense of self-wholeness is endangered by the absence of what has been termed "the gleam in the mother's eye," a poetic expression of the caretaker's delight in the infant's assertiveness and self-display. A heightened terror of fragmentation of the self is thought to arise from the caretaker's inability to respond approvingly to the demonstrative behavior of the infant. One theory claims that this failure also leads to the child's self-development becoming arrested, which continues into the adult life of the narcissist. The sense of self remains deficient, and an unconscious terror of potential self-fragmentation dominates the psyche, leading to compensatory defensive fantasies of grandiosity and omnipotence: "I am all-powerful. I cannot be destroyed." A state of inner emptiness and warded-off feelings of inadequacy and inferiority is also thought to be a consequence of these parental deprivations. "I have not been loved; therefore I am not lovable." The overvaluation by the narcissist of physical beauty, wealth, and power is a manifestation of the often desperate compensatory need to find external props that will reassure him that "I am the best, the most beautiful, the richest" and keep at bay the dread of confronting inner emotional poverty. This may begin when the child says, "Me do it, me do it," and the parent replies, "You can't do that; I'll do it." Except when the action is potentially dangerous, the more empathic parent says, "You can do it; let me help you."

Narcissists are commonly envious. From a developmental viewpoint, envy should be distinguished from jealousy. *Jealousy* is the desire to possess another person and triumph over a rival. It has a three-person quality and is typical of the oedipal period of development—the child's unconscious wish to have the opposite-sex parent to himself and remove the same-sex parent as a competitor. *Envy* occurs earlier in development and has a two-person nature. The child envies the parent for some quality he or she possesses—strength, size, power—that the child would like to have. In its more primitive manifestations, found in the narcissistic patient, envy can carry with it the active wish to destroy the person who arouses envious feelings in order to remove the source of feeling inferior.

The narcissistic patient usually can recall incidents in which one or both parents shamed the child in lieu of punishment. One patient recalled at the age of 4 or 5 hearing his mother say, "Young man, you should be ashamed of yourself." Such events occurred with regularity and instilled a deep sense of shame. This mother was narcissistic and viewed the child as an extension of herself. The child's imperfections were an exposure of her imperfections, about which she felt terribly ashamed. She frequently told her son, "You did that deliberately to humiliate me!" leaving the child feeling hurt, inadequate, and unable to understand the mother's response. Developmentally, the child experiences shame prior to acquiring a capacity to experience guilt. The child is ashamed when he is caught not living up to parental expectations. The more the parent humiliates the child or withdraws love, the more difficult it becomes for the child to internalize the parental values. The child needs to experience love-based criticism from the parents—that is, parents who are more concerned with the child's feeling than what other people will think of them as parents. When the child feels loved, he will internalize the parents' values and will feel guilty when he fails to live up to these values. This maturational step is not accomplished by the narcissistic person, who feels ashamed and humiliated when his mistakes or inadequacies are exposed by others. If he is not caught, he does not feel guilty. It is this same superego deficit that causes his low self-esteem, because he is unable to win the approval of his unloving internalized parents. The capacity to experience guilt has built-in mechanisms for the person to forgive himself. This is accomplished by confession and atonement, with the motive of obtaining forgiveness. The mature adult has learned how to manage guilt feelings and feels secure enough to apologize, to make amends, and to learn from the experience. In the small child, feelings of shame may occur concerning normal bodily functions if the child is scolded for accidents. The response to shame is to hide. This persists in the narcissistic adult, who will go to great lengths to disguise and thus not acknowledge misbehavior in order to escape exposure. Shame carries with it the related subjective experiences of humiliation and embarrassment, again all part of the child's experience of being small, losing control of his bladder or bowels, feeling weak and inferior, and being exposed and criticized. Shame is predicated on the expectation of exposure. It is wetting one's pants in public and being observed in the act. If the accident can be hidden, there is no shame. Shame results from being observed and thus humiliated by the observation of the other. If the narcissistic person can disguise or hide his sense of inadequacy, he will avoid the painful affect of shame. This propensity to hide perceived inadequacies with their potential for humiliation will inevitably distort the clinical interview with the narcissistic patient. The narcissist will go to great lengths to avoid revealing aspects of his history and present life that could recapitulate the experience of shame with the clinical interviewer.

One or both parents of the future narcissist tend to have prominent narcissistic features in their own character structure. One woman vividly recalled being criticized in a humiliating fashion by her mother, an arrogant woman who believed that she was always right. The patient described concluding, at a rather young age, that she was smarter than her mother. By identifying with her mother, she neutralized her mother's power to hurt her. In the process, she became contemptuous not only of her mother but also of all people whom she deemed less intelligent than herself.

Another psychodynamic contribution to the development of the *shy* narcissist is from the parents who consider their child to be perfect and overlook his mistakes or deficiencies. He becomes the parents' narcissistic projection of their own grandiosity. One patient said, "When I make a mistake, I try to cover it up. If I can't cover it up, I blame someone else. And if all else fails, I might admit that I did it, but I make up an excuse. I didn't feel I could live up to my parents' expectation of greatness. I always felt I had to fake it, that I was a fraud." The therapist's question that elicited this material was, "How do you feel when you discover that you have made a mistake?" In this case, the parents were never critical, settling for whatever the child did as "great." This person's inner shame developed without the parents ever telling him he should be ashamed of himself.

Failures of parental empathy occur throughout the entire developmental period. Consider the case of an 8-year-old girl who was using the family bathroom. A visiting aunt wanted to use the bathroom. Instead of knocking on the closed door, she asked the child's mother if there was anyone in the bathroom. The mother replied, "It's only Jane. Go right in; she won't mind." The child felt deeply humiliated, as though she were a nonperson.

Narcissism changes throughout the life cycle. As the narcissistic and emotionally deprived child grows and enters the world of school and peer relations, the already-present compensatory sense of superiority and entitlement may be perniciously fostered by parents. "This is my due; I am special and should be treated as such" can be pathologically reinforced by the parents' projected belief in the child's specialness. "My child should not have to conform to conventional strictures on behavior but should be given special attention." This parental sanction of entitlement in the school-age child can be a major contributing factor to the hypertrophied self-importance and smugness seen in the narcissistic adult. The child mirrors the parents' narcissism.

All adolescents, faced with the startling physiological changes and body alteration of puberty, respond with narcissistic patterns of adaptation. Conflicted about the upsurge of sexual desire and the all-too-obvious physical changes initiated by the onset of puberty, they readily become preoccupied with their appearance and acutely sensitive to how they are viewed by their peers. They are often self-involved, hypersensitive to criticism, prone to feelings of humiliation, and thus emotionally vulnerable, just like the full-blown narcissistic adult. Shame often dominates their feelings about bodily functions and sexuality. These narcissistic concerns, in more extreme cases, play a part in the development of anorexia-bulimia in some teenagers. Generally, narcissistic adolescent bodily and social preoccupations will fade with the passage of time, but in the teenager who has experienced emotional deprivation as a child, they may carry over into adulthood as another aspect of narcissistic pathology.

MANAGEMENT OF THE INTERVIEW

The narcissistic patient is often reluctant to seek professional help because to do so threatens his grandiosity. The precipitating reason for the consultation is often because his spouse demands that he obtain help if the marriage is to be saved or because he has become depressed after some job or career crisis. Another common presentation is the conviction by the patient that he is not appreciated by his colleagues or peers, who do not recognize his brilliance and unique contribution to their profession or organization. Unconsciously, the patient expects that the clinician will show him how to change the perception of others to admire his achievements. Another precipitant that brings the narcissistic patient to the clinician may be a profound midlife crisis. This results from a bitter awareness that his grandiose fantasies and goals for himself have not been and may never be met. This awareness often leads to a feeling of being disconnected from others and deeply dissatisfied with life in general.

According to Kohut, there are certain principles that apply to the early interviews with the narcissistic patient. In an empathic manner, acknowledge the phase-appropriate demands of the grandiose self. It is a mistake to tell the patient in initial interviews that his demands on others are unrealistic. It is important to allow an idealizing transference to develop, because it will, in time, lead to a projection of the patient's ego ideal onto the therapist. This process may make the patient feel insignificant by comparison, but it sets the stage for the patient to identify with a figure of authority who does not behave narcissistically. The therapist must be sensitive to every slight or narcissistic injury that he inadvertently inflicts on the patient and must not behave defensively. If an apology is appropriate, it will set an example of something of which the patient is incapable. These exchanges cannot be abstract but must be expressed in real time, using personal pronouns and not labeling them as transference. This recommendation is true even when the patient states, "You are treating me the same way that my mother did."

In initial interviews, some transference indulgence to a limited degree can be useful. It is helpful to link the patient's behavior with underlying feelings, realizing that for this patient only real things have meaning. This includes being able to change an hour or refusing or granting a request. The patient may ask questions about the clinician that initially can be answered, provided the therapist then asks the patient about the significance of what he has learned. This helps to open up a defensive patient. If the patient then shares this information with someone else, the therapist can explore how that made the patient feel. It might be helpful to tell the patient, "It was not my intention that you would share that with someone else." This helps the patient see that he used a shared moment to enhance his status with someone else or to elicit envy. Threats to the *idealizing* transference lead to depression, whereas threats to the grandiose self lead to rage.

> A talented orthopedic surgeon sought psychiatric consultation after he had impulsively resigned from medical center where he had been employed. His resignation, however, had not been preceded by his obtaining another position, and now he was unemployed. He very reluctantly agreed to see the clinician, mainly at the urging of a colleague, one of the few whom he trusted, who was concerned about his friend's excessive drinking and black moods since he had left his job. "They never appreciated me even though I am one of the nation's experts on hip replacement and knee reconstruction. The administration never made my

operating room schedule a priority. They were always shuffling my O.R. nurses around. They didn't realize what I was contributing to their institution." The institution in question was a renowned teaching hospital staffed by a galaxy of prominent physicians, of whom the surgeon had been one among many. The final straw was the hospital annual benefit. "I was given a lousy table, and the Chairman of the Board of Trustees acted like he didn't know who I was."

The feeling that he was not given his proper due extended into his private life. Currently divorced, he had been married three times. "They just didn't get me," he claimed when asked about his previous marriages. "I'm really very sensitive, and they were all self-involved. My last wife wouldn't offer to give me a back rub after an exhausting day of surgery. I had to ask her—unloving bitch. That's why I left her. Honestly, I don't think you can have any idea of what I have been through. I have always given so much of myself and have never really been appreciated or cared about." The interviewer became aware that he was being cast in the role of another in a long line of unappreciative, uncaring people. Using this self-observation the interviewer commented, "There seems to be a consistent history of people not recognizing your emotional needs or your achievements. When did this begin?" "With my parents of course. My father was never home. He was out philandering. My mother was never home either; she was always at one of her ladies' lunches or charity events. The help didn't give a shit about me, and then I was shipped off to boarding school at a ridiculously young age. That was a nightmare. I was bullied and abused. No one cared about me or what I was feeling. I was so little." The patient who had begun the interview in an arrogant and overbearing manner, filled with contempt for other people, had been transformed into the sad, hurt child whom the interviewer could now experience as touching and for whom he felt genuine empathy for his troubled and unhappy state.

TRANSFERENCE AND COUNTERTRANSFERENCE

An underlying fragile sense of self dominates the psychology of the narcissistic patient and dictates the parameters of the clinical interview. Paradoxically, although the narcissist seems so self-involved and oblivious to the feelings of others, he is acutely sensitive to any wavering of the interviewer's attention and reacts angrily to any lapse that may occur. "Why are you looking at the clock? Am I boring you?" exclaimed a narcissistic patient as the first interview approached its end. There was an element of truth in this accusation. Feeling bored in response to the narcissist's egocentricity is a common reaction for the clinician, who may have the feeling that his function is only that of an appreciative audience. There is often no sense of being engaged in a collaborative enterprise designed to bring some understanding to the troubles that brought the patient to request a consultation in the first place. Considerable effort may be required to remain engaged and not drift off into one's own thoughts, reflecting the same self-preoccupation as the patient.

Transference asserts itself in the clinical interview with the narcissistic patient right from the beginning. The patient struggles to avoid a feeling of humiliation concerning his experience consulting a mental health professional. The need for psychiatric evaluation is often perceived by the patient as evidence of a defect or failure of self. This frequently invokes shame and anger at the putative humiliation the consultation represents:

> When asked by the interviewer, "What brings you to see me?" one patient replied, "I think you should see my girlfriend and her mother, not me. They are the problem. Her mother is incredibly intrusive, and my girlfriend is insensitive. Even though she went to Yale, I think she's dumb. They are the issue, not me. I'm only here to humor them." The patient then revealed that his girlfriend, after 5 years of living together, had threatened to break up with him. "It's not easy to reveal these problems," replied the interviewer, empathically acknowledging the feeling of humiliation that consumed the patient. "It's not easy at all, especially since she and her mother should be your patients, not me," the patient responded.

This intervention allowed the interview to go forward and diminished the patient's paranoid feeling of a consultation under duress. He had made the appointment in response to a threat of losing his girlfriend, and he responded with conscious panic and humiliation. Gradually, as the interview progressed, the patient expressed a fear of becoming depressed if he lost his girlfriend, a hopeful sign of human connection that could be brought into play in ongoing therapy.

Hypervigilance and excessive scrutinizing of the therapist are characteristic. This is part of the defensive structure of the narcissistic person, and it is driven by mistrust and fear of humiliation. This behavior is often misinterpreted as a competitive transference. The therapist finds it easier to see the patient in that framework rather than to see that the patient does not wish to accept him as a separate person whom he values. Therefore, it is more accurate to interpret the patient's attitude as devaluing rather than competitive. This is the patient who, when the therapist has to cancel a session, will respond by canceling the following two sessions.

> One patient, who had conscious feelings of superiority and feelings of contempt for others, sent her clinician a bad check. Several sessions passed and no mention was made of the returned check. Finally, after 3 weeks, the clinician showed the patient the returned check. "Oh, that,"

replied the patient. "My bank must have screwed things up; they sent me a notice about a couple of those. I don't know what happened." The therapist remarked, "You haven't brought it up." Now the patient lied and said, "I didn't realize that you got one." The therapist remarked, "You are blaming the bank, I am more interested in how it makes you feel." "Oh," the patient continued, "it's no big deal, one check was yours and the other was to the phone company." The clinician replied, "You sound very defensive. Is there a feeling of embarrassment that you have?" "I would say so; I don't make mistakes like that," the patient responded.

This episode illustrates how shame makes the patient hide. For this person, an apology would have intensified her feeling of humiliation and revealed her fragile self-concept. She did not understand that a genuine apology can bring people closer together through the process of forgiveness and expiating one's guilt. This process was explored with gentle guidance from the therapist. Further discussion of this episode enabled the therapist to point out the haughty, arrogant, defensive position that indicated the patient's inability to expose her deep shame. It was hiding this shame while ignoring her lack of concern for the other person that intensified her feelings of alienation and aloneness.

The narcissistic patient who is better defended and less primitive may not experience the psychiatric consultation as a humiliation. Instead, he is intent on charming and seducing the interviewer. He is delighted to discuss the complexity and difficulty of his life, provided the interviewer remains a *mirror* who reflects but does not disrupt the flow of his narrative. He is not humiliated by being in the clinical situation but sees it as another opportunity to display himself. The transference here is a *mirroring* one. The clinician is merely a reflector. This desire for a mirroring experience continues from infancy, when it would have been appropriate for the caretakers to reflect back to the child their appreciation and love for his exhibitionistic display.

The second type of transference commonly found with the narcissistic patient is the *idealizing* one. Simply by listening to the narcissist's story, the clinician is invested with the grandiosity that permeates the patient's subjective life. "You are so sensitive and brilliant," stated a narcissistic patient in the second interview, startling the clinician, who had been unable to get a word in edgewise or even to interject clarifying questions in the first interview. Rather than challenging this unwarranted endorsement of her brilliance and sensitivity, the clinician kept quiet and listened. Not confronting the idealizing transference in the early interview situation is prudent, because to do so disrupts the patient's fragile sense of self. The urge for the clinician to interpret the idealizing transference out of a sense of guilt or embarrassment may lead to an abrupt termination of the therapy because it threatens the narcissist's fragile sense of self. The clinician's discomfort with the patient's idealizing transference may stem from her own residual unconscious narcissistic wishes to be loved and adored or from a wish to ward off later devaluation.

The countertransference response to the narcissistic patient that requires the greatest vigilance is the tendency to inwardly disparage the patient. Because of his grandiosity, exhibitionism, envy, indifference to the feelings of others, propensity for rage, and sense of entitlement, he may readily engender a hostile and contemptuous response in the interviewer, one that makes the patient seem alien. Such a response does not recognize the underlying and pervasive suffering of the narcissistic patient, which is thinly masked by his egocentricity. The inner suffering is profound and at its extreme includes a fear of self-fragmentation, a panic of falling apart. All narcissistic patients, including those with milder illness, suffer periodically from a sense of inferiority, emptiness, and frightening aloneness. The defensive, compensatory behavior in response to this inner state is ultimately masochistic because it drives people away, confirming their isolation in the world.

The interviewer must tolerate the experience that he does not exist as a separate person in any meaningful fashion for the patient and must be able to use this unpleasant experience as an entrée into understanding the bleak and frighteningly empty inner psychic world of the narcissistic person. Such self-monitoring on the part of the interviewer will engender an empathic and compassionate response to these troubled individuals and enable a therapeutic process to go forward. As an example, after several sessions, an interviewer sensed a moment of vulnerability in the patient as a very brief reaction to an empathic comment. The patient abruptly flushed and excused himself as he rushed into the therapist's bathroom. The clinician heard the water running because the patient had not even bothered to close the door. After a minute or two, the patient returned. He explained, "I felt this sudden flush of tingling in my face, and I just had to splash some cold water on it. Now what were we talking about?" The interviewer got the message and allowed the patient to pursue another topic, hoping to analyze the experience at a later date when the patient felt stronger.

Another narcissistic patient began the second interview with a female clinician by saying, "I don't know why I came back a second time. Sigmund Freud you're not. In fact you seem rather simplistic, not to say dense." "What bothered you so much last time?" responded the interviewer. "You kept challenging my interpretation of the events that led to my losing my job. As if there were any other explanation than mine." The interviewer was in a delicate position. The facts surrounding the patient's dismissal from his job made clear that it was directly related to his high-handed behavior at work and his contemptuous treatment of his superiors as fools in much the same manner that he was now attacking the interviewer. Nonetheless, the interviewer was aware of a failure of her empathy in the first interview. She had been put off by the patient's self-serving explanations and complete obliviousness to his own arrogant and overbearing behavior. He had complained about being surrounded by morons and felt that it was his mission to enlighten his fellow workers concerning their blatant stupidity. He contended that he was infinitely more farsighted and brilliant than anyone around him in the workplace. The interviewer in response had engaged in a dialogue questioning the patient's view of the events that resulted in his dismissal, a direct result of her negative countertransference response. This time the interviewer adopted a more neutral attitude predicated on an awareness of the narcissistic injury and shame the patient had suffered in being fired. "These events have been very hurtful to you, especially as they seem to have come out of nowhere." Without agreeing with the patient's interpretation of these events, or reacting to his personal attack on her, the therapist supported him by understanding his feeling of injustice, shame, and humiliation. This allowed the interview to proceed and led to the patient recounting a long history of personal slights and lack of appreciation from others that he suffered throughout his life—all a consequence, in his opinion, of the envy that his brilliance and perspicacity aroused in those around him.

An alternative approach would be to ask the patient for a detailed account of how he originally obtained this job and his progress with it. Then one can ask, "How were you notified?" and comment in an empathic tone, "What kind of excuse did they give you?" This can be followed by an inquiry regarding the patient's response. This approach allows more details to emerge. A comment about life not being fair is better than one that sounds more appropriate for a small child, in effect, "poor baby."

A patient commented in the second interview that he felt anxious because of an impending social function where he was expected to make a toast. "I really can't speak in front of a group of people. I'm afraid I'll make a fool of myself. I'll say something stupid—or worse, I won't be able to think of anything." The interviewer asked, "Do you feel the people are coming to judge your performance more than to enjoy the celebration of your son's wedding?" With downcast eyes, the patient responded, "I guess I do." The interviewer continued, "Are you pleased with his choice, and are you proud of your son?" "Very much," the patient said. "And are you pleased that people are coming to the party?" the interviewer asked, to which the patient replied, "I appreciate them coming, but it would not have occurred to me to tell them that. I should write this down." The interviewer then replied, "You might want to rehearse it out loud until you like the way you sound." The following week, the patient reported considerable satisfaction with his behavior and his speech at his son's wedding and noted that his son and some old friends asked what had come over him. He felt understood but still surprised by his success.

CONCLUSION

The ongoing psychotherapeutic treatment of the narcissistic patient is beyond the purview of this book, and the reader is referred to standard texts on treatment. Most narcissistic patients, however, can benefit greatly from well-conducted psychotherapy. They are imprisoned by their arrested development, but careful psychotherapy, predicated on a high degree of empathy for their inner anguish, can break the intrapsychic ice and restart the process of emotional growth.

CHAPTER 6

THE MASOCHISTIC PATIENT

Masochism has become a contentious term. Although we believe that masochism and masochistic behavior are psychopathological realities and are pervasive in many patients, there has been a groundswell of social-political opposition to the diagnosis based on the premise that such labeling is a form of "blaming the victim." However, this argument ignores everyday clinical reality and may subvert appropriate therapeutic interventions. Patients who present with a history of unnecessary suffering, self-defeating behaviors, and recurrent self-induced disappointments in life are ubiquitous in clinical practice. The clinician's sophisticated understanding of conscious and unconscious masochism is the first stage in helping such a patient free himself from a destructive dynamic that is predicated on a seemingly paradoxical desire to seek pain.

The term *masochism* first appeared in Krafft-Ebing's treatise *Psychopathia Sexualis*, published in 1886. It contained a detailed description of submissive sexual practices, largely in males, involving humiliation at the hands of a woman as a requirement for sexual arousal. Krafft-Ebing derived the term *masochism* from the name of the nineteenth-century author Leopold von Sacher-Masoch, whose novel *Venus in Furs* (1870) was widely read in Europe. That story began with the narrator having a dreamlike interaction with Venus, a marble goddess, who was wrapped in furs and tormented him with his desire to be sexually humiliated. The narrator talked with his friend, Severin, who then described his own experience with a young woman whom he persuaded to humiliate, beat, and scold him in order to arouse him sexually. Severin eventually signed a contract to become his lover's slave, and they traveled together throughout Europe as slave and mistress. The utter ruin of his life that resulted was compensated for by the constant enactment of his masochistic perversion.

Krafft-Ebing saw masochism as "the association of passively endured cruelty and violence with lust." He further noted, "Masochism is the opposite of sadism. While the latter is the desire to cause pain and use force, the former is the wish to suffer pain and be subjected to force."

Today most clinicians view them as intertwined and speak of sadomasochism. *Sadism* is, like masochism, an eponymous term derived from the name of the eighteenth-century French aristocrat the Marquis de Sade, who, in such works as *The 120 Days of Sodom*, describes in horrifying pornographic detail the cruel and literally murderous abuse of other people for perverse pleasure. It is significant that de Sade proclaims in the above work that "most people are indeed an enigma. And perhaps that it is why it is easier to fuck a man than try to understand him." As Bach has pointed out, the translation is: "it is easier to exploit a person than to relate to him"—a keen insight into the pathology of some sadomasochistic patients and other related character disorders.

Krafft-Ebing emphasized the importance of fantasy for the masochistic patient. He described a desire on the part of the sexual masochistic patient to be "completely and unconditionally subject to the will of this person as by a master, humiliated and abused." Today, themes of humiliation, subjugation, and abuse continue to be important in understanding masochism.

The concept of sexual bondage, which he described as a form of dependence, was of primary importance for Krafft-Ebing. This notion continues to be important today, with masochism also understood as a pathological behavior pattern designed to maintain an attachment to another person. Krafft-Ebing wrote about the masochistic patient's fear of "losing the companion and the desire to keep him always content, amiable, and present."

He also described a second component in masochism that he believed to be *sexual ecstasy*. He saw this as a physiological hyperdisposition to sexual arousal or stimulation, even if that stimulation was mistreatment or abuse. In other words, at both a mental and physiological level of organization, he saw a fundamental tendency toward pleasure in pain for the masochistic patient.

Krafft-Ebing's work exerted a strong influence on Freud. Freud viewed sex as a fundamental biological function that was a powerful motivator of behavior. In understanding the puzzling phenomenon of masochism, which seemed to contradict his "pleasure principle," Freud followed Krafft-Ebing in postulating a primary sexual pleasure in pain and saw this as the basis for both masochistic paraphilias and masochistic character patterns.

The study of masochistic fantasies and behaviors has continued to influence the development of psychodynamic thinking and psychoanalytic theory. Clinicians and theoreticians have struggled with understanding motivations that lead people to pursue pain and to find pleasure in it. Freud defined *moral masochism,* separate from masochistic paraphilia, as the renunciation of pleasure in favor of self-sacrifice as a way of life, leading to emotional suffering coupled with a sense of moral superiority. Many psychoanalysts believe that masochistic sexual fantasies are invariably present in the sexual lives of people with masochistic characters, even if overt masochistic paraphilias are not present. Schafer feels that a diagnosis of masochistic character should not be made without the presence of sexual masochism, because otherwise the diagnosis becomes too inclusive.

One hypothesis is that pain is not pursued for its own sake but rather because all other options seem even more painful. Thus in these situations the pleasure principle is actually preserved. However, this dynamic may be difficult to understand when the clinician is unable to imagine or empathize with the greater pain that the patient envisions (often unconsciously) if he were to pursue alternatives considered by others to be preferable. The pursuit of mental or even physical pain can also be understood as derived from the child's struggle to maintain an emotional connection with an abusive parent. The term *masochistic* is sometimes misapplied to describe *any* self-defeating or maladaptive behavior, even though the self-defeating aspect is an unintended side effect, a "secondary loss," rather than a primary motive of the behavior. The term is also misused when one fails to appreciate that the experience the interviewer views as painful may be one that the patient enjoys. In other words, spending Saturday at a professional meeting is only masochistic if one does not want to do so and finds it painful, yet consciously believes that it is the only possible choice. In order to be considered masochistic, a person must have a conscious subjective experience of displeasure while obtaining gratification at an unconscious level. In this example, the unconscious satisfaction might stem from viewing oneself as dedicated or scholarly.

The masochistic individual is relatively easily recognized. In his work, he typically accepts a job in which he is either overworked or underpaid, or both, and in which there is no prospect of future gain. Apprenticeships or internships do not qualify, because the future potential constitutes a reward. Jobs that offer great internal satisfaction do not qualify either. The person must be doing the job in spite of better choices and feel that he is being exploited. The gratification is at an unconscious level. His personal life is no different; he selects friends and romantic attachments that are inappropriate for him. His relationships end in hurt feelings, disappointment, and resentment. He responds to personal success by feeling undeserving and guilty. This feeling may be acted out through some accident, such as leaving his briefcase in a taxicab. His portrayal of himself as a victim may evoke annoyance and displeasure from others, who may detect that his complaining is really bragging. His affect is usually somber. Even when he does not complain, others are aware that he suffers and perceive him as a "no fun" person. In his attempt to win acceptance from a friend, the masochistic patient will help with his friend's college paper and then be late in completing his own, a fact that he will tell the friend later, thus causing the friend to feel guilty. This is the sadistic component of masochistic behavior, an aspect of which the patient has no awareness.

PSYCHOPATHOLOGY AND PSYCHODYNAMICS

Criteria for Masochistic Personality Disorder

We have identified the following criteria for masochistic personality disorder:

1. Self-sacrificing, accommodating of others, then complains about not being appreciated. Accepts exploitation and selects situations in which he is exploited but then attempts to make others feel sorry for him or feel guilty instead of expressing appropriate assertiveness.
2. In response to overt aggression from others, tries to turn the other cheek but is usually resentful; exploits the role of the injured party, making the other person feel guilty.
3. Somber affect, rarely happy or exuberant—a no-fun person to be with.
4. Self-effacing, politely refusing the genuine efforts by others to meet his needs: "Oh, no, thanks, I can manage it myself."
5. Reliable, overly conscientious, with little time for pleasurable activity; obligation and duty supersede.
6. Avoids opportunities for advancement but then feels resentful for not being chosen. Responds to a promotion with fear of failing or guilt about defeating a rival.
7. Sexual fantasies include themes of humiliation, rejection, abuse, dominance, and submission.

Masochistic traits are often found in association with other character disorders, and interview strategies that are effective for an obsessive character with masochistic features might not apply to the patient with hysterical, phobic, paranoid, borderline, or narcissistic character structure. Masochism is closely related to narcissism and might be thought of as its first cousin. The martyr receives attention and adulation for his suffering, as hundreds of graphic Counter-Reformation paintings attest. The masochistic martyr becomes the center of attention, uniquely "special" and even a "saint," characteristics that overlap those of the narcissistic patient with his grandiose inner world and exaggerated sense of self-importance.

Feminist groups have opposed the inclusion of this diagnosis in the official nomenclature, claiming that it will be used against female victims of abuse by suggesting that they bring it on themselves. To address that problem adequately is beyond the scope of a book on psychiatric interviewing, but it should be noted that the diagnosis does not appear in DSM-5 and that the list that appeared earlier reflects our criteria for the diagnosis and is not official nomenclature.

Masochistic Characteristics

Suffering and Self-Sacrifice

The masochistic character immediately impresses one with his investment in suffering and/or self-sacrifice, manifested in his constant readiness to subordinate his apparent interests to those of the other party. It is easy for him to accept exploitation from others, and he continually seeks out people who will exploit him. He has a job that does not pay him adequately either for his qualifications or for the amount of time he devotes to the work. He has the less attractive room in a shared apartment, goes to the restaurant or film preferred by his companion, and gets the less attractive girl on a blind date. Although he feels exploited, he prefers to suffer silently rather than complain to (and risk hurting) his exploiter. When others offer to do something for him, he politely refuses their efforts to respond to his needs. He is always afraid of becoming a burden, and he believes that he does not deserve their help. Typically, he states, "Oh, no, that's all right; I can manage it myself." His constant self-sacrifice leads to feelings of moral superiority, a trait that might be apparent to others but is not to him. His behavior causes those around him to feel guilty. If he becomes aware of this, he apologizes and offers further sacrifice. Sympathy from others is one of his principal means of feeling better, and therefore he always pursues the position of the most hurt party.

The clinician must also bear in mind that the masochistic individual does not seek any random pain. In order for pain to provide conscious and unconscious gratification, it must be a specific pain applied in a specific way and at least to some extent be under the patient's control. For example, one patient said, "I want you to beat me, humiliate me, and yell at me; I never said I wanted to feel ignored or rejected."

The diagnosis should not be made in situations in which the patient is a captive with no apparent means of escape, when adaptation to unavoidable pain is healthy. Submission to abuse and humiliation may be the only means to adapt to the situation and thereby increase the chance of survival. If the person has the means to escape and does not exercise it, or if he successfully escapes and then voluntarily returns, the diagnosis of masochism is possible. The diagnosis should also not be made when the patient has a clinical depression or during the recovery period from depression, a state in which it is virtually impossible to discern the masochistic trait.

Masochistic Sexual Fantasies as a Diagnostic Criterion

The masochistic patient's sexual life is, in the opinion of some theorists, the underlying source of the character disorder. Sexual arousal occurs in response to fantasies, pictures, or stories depicting themes of humiliation, punishment, rejection, belittlement, or coercion in which the "victim" can deny all responsibility. In spite of Freud's term *feminine masochism*, males are commonly interested in masochistic sexual scenarios.

The centrality of sexual fantasies as a diagnostic criterion for masochism is unique in the diagnosis of character disorders. The capacity for excitement or sexual arousal in response to sadomasochistic themes is an integral component of this character type. The overt acting out of more severe versions of these fantasies occurs only in a sicker group of patients with borderline or overtly psychotic psychopathology. Healthier individuals may have excitement in response to masochistically titillating themes such as a burlesque of a leather-clad female dominatrix subjugating a passive man, but that experience is foreplay to more typical forms of gratification. Nevertheless, when a patient describes such arousal, it is useful to inquire whether it remains central to his fantasy as he is engaged in the culminating sexual experience.

If the diagnostic criterion of masochistic sexual arousal were required, the diagnosis would be made much less frequently, because many patients are too ashamed to admit to such interests, and others are too inhibited even to entertain such fantasies consciously. For example, a female patient typified all of the criteria for masochistic personality disorder except that she denied masochistic sexual interests. Upon the clinician's pursuing this subject, the patient asserted that she had no sexual feelings or interests or fantasies of any sort. In the course of treatment, she became less inhibited and allowed herself to develop sexual interests in which themes of humiliation, pain, rejection, and coercion became present.

The prevalence of masochistic fantasies is reflected in the successful market strategies of publishers of sexually oriented magazines in which masochistic acts are often graphically portrayed. However, most of the people who are titillated by this material never engage in an overtly perverse sexual act but, as described earlier, may think about it during their sexual experiences.

> A masochistic male patient in his 30s denied being aroused by typical sadomasochistic scenes during his evaluation. However, a year into his psychotherapy he reported a fantasy: He assumed a dominating role, issuing orders and instructions to his partner, requiring that she respond to his every whim. Although his overall adaptation was that of a high-level masochistic character, in his sexual fantasy he placed himself in the sadistic role, not an unusual phenomenon in masochistic characters. In response to a question about how the fantasy usually began, he added, "It always starts with the woman being cold, aloof, and unresponsive—perhaps even rejecting." When the clinician asked if he differentiated this from a woman who was in a neutral state of arousal vis-à-vis him, he replied, "Yes, and cold is better." Then the woman was totally overcome by his charm and power to the point of becoming his slave.

This vignette illustrates several points. First, the phenomena of masochism and sadism are positive and negative images of the same theme. The scene involved some form of pain, rejection, or submission, with humiliation a prominent feature and a relative absence of feelings of tenderness, love, closeness, and equal sharing. Second, it is difficult to elicit accurate sexual material. There is no other area in clinical work in which the conscious feelings of the interviewer may so distort his capacity to elicit objective and accurate data. There are also the unconscious conflicts in the interviewer that may further add to the complexity of the challenge. Obtaining an accurate history of a patient's sexual behavior and fantasy is one of the most difficult areas facing the interviewer, partly because of feelings of embarrassment, voyeurism, and intrusion that may be aroused. Nonetheless, gleaning such information is critical. Third, it is of interest that this man acted out this same role in other situations in life. For example, he only played his best tennis when his opponent had taken a commanding lead. As he began to feel he was being humiliated, he experienced a sadistic desire to turn the tables and to humiliate his opponent. In his work he felt humiliated when his boss criticized him. At that point he experienced narcissistic rage and performed at his best, hoping to shame the boss. The interviewer inquired,

"Don't you want your boss to like you?" The patient appeared puzzled and said, "I want him to respect me, maybe even fear me." "Fear you?" the clinician responded. "Yes, that is the ultimate sign of respect," the patient said.

This exchange illustrates the delicate intertwining of sadomasochistic, narcissistic, and obsessional features. The masochistic component is in his entering into a feeling of humiliation by not playing tennis at his best; he then turns sadistic in his wish to humiliate his opponent. The narcissistic component is in his preoccupation with himself; he is putting on a show for the benefit of an invisible (unconscious) audience that exists only in his mind. The obsessional component is in his need to always feel in control.

Superego Relief

For some, pain becomes a necessary prerequisite for pleasure. The superego is assuaged and guilt is expiated either for past offenses or to pay in advance for future pleasure. In the masochistic patient's childhood experience, abuse, pain, or sacrifice was usually followed by love, just as in society fasts are followed by feasts. An example is that of the talented young attorney who had been abandoned by his father at the age of 4.

> He had been brought up by his mother and an assortment of aunts and had no subsequent contact with his father, who became an "unmentionable" in the household. The patient unconsciously felt profoundly guilty about his father's disappearance, feeling, as children often do in cases of divorce or parental death, that he was responsible and that he had achieved an "oedipal triumph," but it was a Pyrrhic victory that distorted his character and gave it a masochistic bent. He proclaimed in the initial interview, "I hate my father. He was irresponsible, selfish, and cruel. How could he leave a little boy who loved him?" Behind this angry statement lay a deep longing and a profound sense of guilt.
>
> Further discussion revealed that the patient regularly engaged in sadomasochistic interactions with senior partners in his law firm. He would be late preparing an urgent brief and would gratuitously and provocatively tease his superiors. The result was that he would be attacked and humiliated in firm meetings. His legal ability was such that he was not actually fired, but the drama that he created would continue in one form or another. As treatment progressed, he became aware of the pleasure he took in being attacked. "It doesn't bother me. Weirdly, I feel better when it happens." He acknowledged enjoying the negative attention, and far from feeling guilty, he took pleasure in these altercations. A number of unconscious dynamics were at work. He had the "sadistic" attention of the father-surrogate, was no longer abandoned, and felt less guilty for his unconscious crimes. His superego was appeased by the beating.

Maintaining Control

Other mechanisms of defense in the masochistic patient are the feeling of safety provided by the familiar and a desire to maintain omnipotent control of the universe. The person who does not try cannot fail. By not competing, one wards off frustration and retains the unconscious fantasy of control of one's universe. For example, if one does not seek a promotion, one does not feel passed over.

In a sadomasochistic dyad, the subtle control of the sadist by the masochist is often a major theme.

> An accomplished graduate student recounted her passionate romantic involvement with a female colleague. Although the sexual excitement factor was intense, this patient's day-to-day experience with her lover was one of regular humiliation, verbal and physical abuse, and constant denigration. She recognized the pathological nature of her involvement with this woman who, alongside her sadistic behavior, was a binge drinker and recurrently unfaithful. "How could I fall head over heels in love with someone who takes such pleasure in treating me so horribly?" the patient lamented. Her history revealed that her mother had had recurrent psychotic breakdowns, usually precipitated by her father's absence on business trips. This left the patient alone with her disintegrating parent, who occasionally subjected the patient to life-threatening situations, such as crashing the family car when the patient was a passenger.
>
> It became apparent to the interviewer that the patient's current lover was a direct stand-in for her mother, someone who was unpredictable, prone to explosive outbursts of rage, occasionally frightening, and, when drunk, dangerous. The patient's masochistic surrender and suffering provided an unconscious attachment to her mother whom, consciously, she pitied. Her moral superiority to her lover was apparent—she was never cruel or unfaithful; she suffered her lover's abuse out of love. She was the forgiving one who, no matter how badly she was treated, would never abandon her lover. Her all-accepting attitude tended to induce further paroxysms of rage and overt cruelty in her partner. Toward the middle of the first interview, the patient commented insightfully, "It's a pretty perverse love, isn't it?" She was correct. Regular beatings formed a central part of their love-play and were sexually exciting for her. In the second interview, it became clear that her flagrant masochism was a subtle means of control. Her lover often threatened to leave her but never could, stating: "You are so forgiving and understanding of my craziness. I need you because you make me feel human after I have behaved like a lunatic." This sadomasochistic interaction provided considerable gratification for both parties and bound them together. The sadistic partner thought she controlled the masochistic one and could abuse her at will, but in fact she was equally controlled by the masochistic partner's submission, suffering, and forgiveness.

Developmental Psychodynamics

The future masochistic patient often grows up in a household where one parent is masochistic, depressed, or both. The following is an example of the enduring impact of this childhood experience:

> A masochistic female patient, when upset at the psychological injuries she recurrently suffered in her professional life through lack of recognition, appropriate advancement, and so on, would become preoccupied with suicidal ideation. She consciously felt on such occasions that she was "worth nothing" and would be better off dead. She contended that her therapist had been of no help to her, and he too would be better off if she were not around to bother him. Her rage and fury at her colleagues and her therapist remained out of awareness as she adopted the role of a martyr, one who was unappreciated for her Herculean efforts on behalf of others.
>
> When the patient was little, her mother had exhibited virtually the same behavior in response to what she saw as a "lack of appreciation." The patient had clear recollections of her mother threatening, "I am going to kill myself." Her mother's behavior on these occasions had sufficiently alarmed the family that she was twice hospitalized. The patient remembered feeling profoundly guilty, abandoned, and agitated at these times. The patient prayed to God to save her mother and made a pact that she would suffer in her place. In this she had succeeded, and she now replicated her mother's psychological maneuvers.

This was a primary identification with a masochistic parent, a common pathological mechanism in the developmental history of the future masochist. It served two unconscious purposes. First, it was adopted competitively to gain the love of the other parent, that is, her father. Second, it maintained a powerful psychological tie through identification with the emotionally unavailable mother.

As a child, the future masochistic patient overemphasizes passivity and submissiveness, expecting that this will lead to approval and affection from others as well as protection from their wrath. When his submissiveness fails to win the parents' warmth and love, the child feels resentful and is given to sulking as an expression of dissatisfaction. Commonly the parents may offer some comfort or affection when the "poor child is unhappy," thereby reinforcing the development of pain-dependent behavior. The child brings that paradigm to his contacts with the outside world and behaves submissively toward other children who seem to take advantage of him. The affection he seeks is not forthcoming, and resentment is experienced toward others. If he returns home having given away his allowance or some other possession, he is scolded by an angry parent, which further fans his mistrust and disappointment in others.

The future masochistic patient develops a model of personal suffering as a means of obtaining attention and affection. Actual abuse by a parent or parental surrogate is translated by the child into "This is how love and attention occur." This becomes the template for future relationships. Illness and the attention and caring this brings from otherwise remote and unaffectionate parents may also reinforce the "pain is pleasure" paradigm.

Fairbairn, in his work with delinquent teenagers raised in abusive households, observed that they were reluctant to admit that their parents were "bad" even though they had regularly been abused by them. They were much more ready to confess that *they* were bad. He surmised that these children were taking on the "badness" that resided in their parents by internalization and making them "good." This seemingly paradoxical mechanism had the effect of inducing "that sense of security which an environment of good objects so characteristically confers." Fairbairn framed this in religious terms:

> It is better to be a sinner in a world ruled by God than to live in a world ruled by the Devil. A sinner in a world ruled by God may be bad: but there is always a certain sense of security to be derived from the fact that the world around is good—"God's in His heaven—All's right with the world!" And in any case there is always hope of redemption. In a world ruled by the Devil the individual may escape the badness of being a sinner: but he is bad because the world around him is bad.

This subtle metaphorical analysis is relevant to the psychodynamics of the masochistic patient who has often been abused in childhood and sees himself as bad. Fairbairn observed that the child internalizes aspects of his bad parents "because they force themselves upon him and he seeks to control them, but also and above all because he needs them." This unconscious dynamic continues to be played out in the adult relationships of masochistic patients who have been raised in unempathic or abusive childhood settings.

Masochism frequently has a secret agenda, namely the control of another person who is bound by suffering in a sadomasochistic drama. As a child, the future masochistic patient often experiences an excess of shame and humiliation from his parents. He responds with a special unconscious defense: "My parent cannot hurt me because I will enjoy the injury. I am more powerful than they are. I will control them with my suffering." This dynamic can come to dominate the clinical situation, and the masochistic patient enacts a negative therapeutic reaction by lamenting, "You are of no help to me," a refrain that tempts the therapist to angry retaliation. This is a re-creation of the childhood situation in which suffering provided power to dominate the parent and expressed the masochistic aggression and vengeance.

Differential Diagnosis

One of the more difficult issues in the differential diagnosis of masochism is the distinction from altruism, an important value in our civilization. A person who risks his life for his country or the parent who sacrifices pleasure for the welfare of a child is not masochistic. The altruistic person experiences conscious and unconscious pride and an elevation of self-esteem from such sacrifices, whereas the masochistic person may experience moral superiority but needs pain as well as the positive effect on the world. The masochistic person derives no conscious elevation of self-esteem from his sacrifices because they are not motivated by love. The masochistic patient feels exploited and unappreciated by others. The gratification derived from his behavior largely stems from the unconscious alleviation of guilt. His sacrifices result from fear, fear that he is not lovable, fear that others will find him selfish and greedy, and so on. In this manner he attempts to buy love from others whom he unconsciously resents. The mechanism is self-defeating because his behavior causes others to feel guilty so that they resent him and respond with avoidance. If the masochistic patient becomes aware of this reaction he is quick to apologize and to offer further sacrifices.

Another major differential diagnosis is with the self-destructive patterns of the borderline patient who shows more aggressive paranoid trends as well as impaired impulse control. For example, the borderline person has a greater tendency to provoke others and then counterattack with a conviction that they deliberately mistreat him. Masochistic sexual fantasies are more likely to be acted out by the borderline patient.

There is a group of patients with dysthymia whose clinical presentation can mimic that of the masochistic patient. This group of depressed patients can be preoccupied with inadequacy, failure, and negative events to the point of morbid "enjoyment." They can be passive; self-derogatory and worried; hypercritical–complaining, conscientious, and self-disciplining; preoccupied with inadequacy, failure, and negative events; pessimistic; and incapable of having fun. This strong overlap has led some psychiatrists to feel that the masochistic patient has an affective spectrum disorder rather than a character disorder. The differentiation from the masochistic patient, however, can be made on the basis of the mood state, which in the dysthymic patient is that of mild depression. The masochistic patient is often gloomy and pessimistic about the future but usually not depressed. When present, masochistic sexual fantasies can also be particularly useful in distinguishing masochistic personality disorder from affective disorders. The sexual fantasies of the masochistic patient have generally crystallized by middle to late adolescence.

The dependent patient is lower functioning and more infantile, lacks the masochistic person's pathological conscience, and is gratified by other people making decisions for him. The passive-aggressive patient is more angry and defiant, thereby suffering greater work impairment than the masochistic patient. He is more likely to arrive late for the appointment, offer little apology, and elicit anger in the clinician.

The compulsive patient who speaks of how "hard he works" is really bragging rather than complaining. His self-esteem is elevated by his capacity to postpone pleasure. He is much more assertive and is able to accept recognition for his accomplishments. He is more directly controlling of others who should "do it his way" because he knows best and is unashamed of this unless it backfires. The avoidant patient, compared with the masochistic patient, is more phobic and more anxious and able to make demands on others that are related to helping him avoid his fears. In addition he tends to avoid situations that cause him anxiety, and thereby he rarely is exploited by others.

MANAGEMENT OF THE INTERVIEW

Inner and Outer Views of Masochism

There is a great discrepancy between how the masochistic patient perceives himself and how he is seen by others. He wishes to see himself as a modest, unassuming, altruistic, noncompetitive, accommodating, generous, shy, unintrusive person—one who is forgiving of others, places responsibility before pleasure, and puts the needs of others before his own. His ideal role model would be Job. However, each of these characteristics ceases to be adaptive when it no longer wins the love and admiration of others. Instead, others are driven away, either as the trait is carried to excess or because the unconscious coercive motivation to control and evoke guilt becomes apparent to the other person.

For example, a therapist receives an emergency telephone call during the masochistic patient's appointment. The patient offers to leave the room. He says, "I feel so insignificant when you have so many people who really need you." If the therapist tries to interpret the patient's wish to court the therapist's favor with that offer or suggests that it might be designed to cover up latent resentment, the patient responds by feeling misunderstood and hurt. It would be preferable to accept the offer at face value or perhaps interpret it as another example of the patient's feeling of unworthiness.

Excessive Modesty and Self-Righteousness

The traits of excessive modesty and self-righteousness often provoke the therapist to attempt to show the patient that he is bringing his troubles on himself or sometimes to feel irritated, with resulting boredom and withdrawal. Interpretations of this dynamic make the patient feel totally misunderstood. The patient's being not openly competitive leads to his losing through default, with resulting diminished self-esteem. The therapist is tempted to encourage the patient to assert himself or be more competitive. This makes the patient feel worse because he believes he will alienate people through such behavior and incur their wrath. His accommodating cooperative trait leads to his accepting abuse from others and then complaining about the unfair treatment he receives. The therapist again is tempted to push the patient to fight back and to stand up for his rights. This tactic usually has poor results. It is difficult for the therapist to understand that the patient believes that acquiescing to others is the way to be accepted.

The patient defers to the wishes of others. This constant self-sacrifice makes him feel others do not care about his wishes. The clinician may encourage the patient to make his wishes known but often subtly abuses him just like everyone else. This is the first patient one asks to shift the time of his appointment to accommodate someone else because he is most likely to acquiesce, suffering but stifling his complaints and submitting to avoid disappointing the therapist. A closer examination reveals the following: The patient has two standards of behavior, one of which is acceptable for others and provides a margin for error, and the other that is reserved for himself, to which he can never measure up adequately. However, in reserving a higher standard by which to judge himself, he develops a compensatory feeling of moral superiority to others. Other people, including the therapist, find this attitude offensive and may reject the patient because of it. However, if it is challenged, the patient feels that the therapist wants to destroy one of his few virtues.

The patient's shy, unobtrusive nature is often perceived as aloofness with an unwillingness to participate in the real give-and-take of a relationship. As seen by others, he is a somber, self-righteous, guilt-provoking, self-effacing, aloof, morally superior martyr who cannot accept or give love and who complains about his misfortunes.

Treatment Behavior

The masochistic patient responds to interpretations by feeling worse. He complains about the treatment and how the therapist is not helping him. This occurs for a number of reasons. The patient is unconsciously highly competitive, resents what he considers the clinician's superiority, and expresses his hostility by defeating the therapist. Interpretations are a blow to the patient's self-esteem, confirming his subjective experience of imperfections and unworthiness.

The masochistic patient often develops a negative therapeutic reaction. This can be interpreted as, "You seem to search for evidence that you are bad, and you overlook or diminish evidence to the contrary." The same is manifested with regard to the patient's progress during the course of treatment. The patient counts only failures and not successes. Masochistic therapists tend to get caught up in this same pattern and share the patient's belief that nothing constructive has happened.

Interpretations are experienced as personal rejections. The patient states, "You don't like me" or "I must be a real pain to you." Although craving love, the patient never misses an opportunity to feel rejected. When the patient experiences a brief feeling of relief signaling the possibility of change or improvement, this activates neurotic fears accompanying the threat presented by success, such as the anticipation of being crushed by rivals or fear of the envy of others. This is a largely unconscious process, in contrast to the dynamic in the narcissistic patient, which occurs in conscious thoughts.

The patient anxiously solicits advice from others, including the clinician: "I just can't decide; I wish you could make the decision for me." The stage is now set. If the interviewer replies, "Well, it sounds like a good opportunity," the patient will state, "Oh, I'm so glad you think so because I'll have to take a pay cut." The interviewer is faced with unattractive alternatives of withdrawing the initial advice, inquiring why the patient withheld crucial information, or keeping quiet. The first may undermine the patient's confidence both in himself and in the clinician. The second is experienced as a criticism. The third increases the danger of the patient acting out and then blaming the clinician. If the therapist does not answer questions like this, the patient states, "I'm sorry I asked you. I know I'm supposed to work these things out for myself." If the therapist attempts to interpret the patient's feeling angry for not getting the advice, the patient will berate himself further, stating, "It's just another example of how infantile I am."

When the masochistic patient tries to free-associate, he typically states, "Nothing comes to mind" or "Nothing has happened since I saw you last" or "I'm trying to think of something to talk about." The patient has a constricted subjective life. His fantasies tend to be concrete and deal with reality problems and his own failures and guilt concerning his feeling of inadequacy. He likes to find nondynamic explanations for behavior and will bring in articles about biological or genetic explanations. At the same time, his ubiquitous response to interpretation is, "You are right; it's all my fault."

Empathy

Masochistic character traits have positive adaptive value that is usually the only aspect of the behavior consciously recognized by the patient. If the therapist does not relate to these positive adaptive aspects, the alliance is endangered and the interview will be unsuccessful. The patient views his martyred attitude as a function of altruism, an admirable trait. His self-effacing stance means that he is noncompetitive—a likeable trait. The patient confuses his acceptance of abuse with being cooperative and accommodating, and he does not see the unconsciously motivated pain-seeking aspect of this behavior. His pervasive moral superiority, which the therapist encounters early on, is experienced by the patient as his being forgiving of other people. He is unaware that this surface forgivingness conceals his unconscious pleasure in registering their deficiencies. The patient considers himself generous and does not realize that he uses giving in order to manipulate others and then deprives them of the opportunity to give to him in return. He cannot understand why others perceive him as aloof when he himself feels shy and nonintrusive.

> A successful businessman complained in an initial interview, "My children are such ingrates. I have set them up, basically given them a comfortable annuity. But they don't even make an effort to celebrate or even acknowledge my birthday. I care about my birthday." Raised in Europe during World War II, he had experienced many deprivations as a child. He had devoted himself to his parents and rescued his father's business from insolvency. It had become the basis of his considerable fortune. His parents had never acknowledged either his achievement or his devotion but remained critical of him until their death. He replayed this scenario with his children. He was simultaneously generous to a fault and highly critical of their attempts to achieve independence and financial autonomy. He regularly used money to manipulate them and then was hurt when they withdrew and did not "acknowledge my birthday." He felt that he was "good," and they were "bad." His aggression was denied, and he was bewildered by their "insensitive" behavior. "I'm sick of suf-

fering," he complained. Gradually, with treatment, be began to understand his need to suffer and that his generosity had a hidden masochistic agenda—namely, to control and yet feel unappreciated and rebuffed.

The clinician should avoid premature interpretation of the patient's enactment of the role of being a clinging, helpless, dependent child. It is necessary to answer the patient's questions or requests for guidance and be interactive early in the treatment but not to make real-life decisions for the patient. If the patient asks, "Do you want to hear more about my mother?" or says "I hope I'm not boring you," one should initially deal with those comments directly, concretely, and without interpretation. The clinician should avoid asking the patient, "Why do you want me to make the decision?" Instead, early in the contact the interviewer could interpret that the patient cannot decide because each choice appears fraught with potential disaster. When the patient agrees, the clinician can then review the negative consequences of each decision and ask the patient which pain he can live with better. Later, the clinician can point out, "Up to now, we have largely considered the negative factors involved in making decisions. Let's try and consider the positive aspects as well." It is only after the patient's unconscious aggression has been somewhat neutralized by the development of loving and tender feelings that the masochistic character can tolerate exploration of his repressed rage.

Initially, the clinician should provide a concerned, holding, and supportive environment. Considerable transference gratification is necessary for this patient in the early phase of treatment. The clinician is advised to avoid silence, a deprivation poorly tolerated by the masochistic patient. The clinician should allow more time for history taking in the initial phase of treatment. This provides an opportunity to develop an appreciation of some of the patient's strengths and areas of healthier functioning. Interventions that tend to alleviate the patient's unconscious guilt are helpful, for example, "Haven't you suffered enough?" or "Haven't you punished yourself sufficiently?" It is often necessary for the clinician to strengthen the patient's motivation for expressive psychotherapy. The masochistic patient is not interested in broadening his self-knowledge because he anticipates that each new discovery will confirm his inadequacy and unworthiness. This pattern may be explored in the early phase of therapy.

The clinician must listen carefully for evidence that the patient reacted to the interviewer's comments as criticism; this must be brought to the patient's attention empathically or the patient will simply transform it into another criticism, responding, "I'm sorry I took it as a criticism; I never can get anything right." The masochistic interviewer may be tempted to say, "Oh, no, it's my fault." Such a stance will only reinforce the patient's masochism.

It is essential to intercede when self-destructive acting out is anticipated and then later analyze the patient's reaction to the intervention. This is often accomplished with a question rather than by direct advice. A financial executive proclaimed, "I'm going to resign" because he felt that his commission was not commensurate with what he had achieved for his firm in the previous year. In reality, his performance had been mediocre, and he had still been handsomely recompensed. The interviewer inquired, "Do you have an offer for another position? You told me it hadn't been a great year." The patient then retreated from his threat of resignation, which would have been a masochistic acting-out, bringing considerable suffering upon himself. However, further discussion revealed that he had experienced the interviewer as suggesting that he had performed poorly, and he felt criticized. The interviewer pointed out that this was not the only possible meaning of his comments.

After the patient has developed some awareness of his angry feelings toward others, the clinician can point out how apparent self-punishment actually punishes others as well as the patient. If the patient accepts the interpretation without becoming depressed, the therapist can then interpret the patient's need to punish himself for having felt so angry at the other person. If the patient responds with depression, it is necessary to interpret the patient's disappointment in himself that he is not more tolerant as well as his fear of losing the other person's love. The patient can then be shown how in his depression he is expiating his guilt and seeking to regain the approval of the offended other by means of his suffering. The clinician then explains that the patient expects the other person to see how much the patient suffers and to feel sorry for him, a basic emotional paradigm that the patient confuses with love. In some instances, the patient has gone through all of these steps with no alteration of his behavior pattern. In those situations it may be necessary for the clinician to say, "All right, haven't you punished your mother enough?" This is *not* an early intervention. It is important to avoid the use of humor with the masochistic patient. The patient will invariably feel ridiculed and respond negatively.

Recognizing that the masochistic patient has great difficulty in accepting or acknowledging feelings of anger, the clinician accepts the patient's label of "disappointment" as the acceptable emotion closest to anger. The clinician must exercise caution in encouraging the patient to express anger toward significant others until he is able to cope with the counter-anger that this evokes, along with the patient's subsequent guilt. Masochistic patients in ongoing treatment often refer repeatedly to being a "disappointment" to their therapist. One patient stated, "I crave your admiration and affection, but I know you are disappointed in me as a patient. So I don't deserve it." This provides an opportunity for the clinician to show the patient that the "disappointment" goes two ways. If he believes the therapist is disappointed in him, he also secretly feels disappointed in the therapist for his "disappointment." The therapist responded, "You are actually disappointed in me because I have not conveyed my respect and appreciation for your efforts or my affection for you. Hence you don't feel you deserve it." This led the patient to recall that he felt he was a disappointment to his father while inwardly feeling disappointed in his father for not showing his love for the patient, a cycle that had come to dominate his relationships with other people. Masochistic patients tend to have a conviction that they are not loveable. They have great difficulty in telling another person "I love you," thereby avoiding a situation in which the possibility exists they will be told they are not loved in return, which is their secret conviction.

Later in treatment the clinician can address the patient's challenges to the psychological explanations of his behavior and interpret his questions and comments regarding genetic and hormonal theories of behavior as a fear of being to blame, something the patient cannot separate from the concept of responsibility for one's actions. The clinician should also recognize the patient's dissatisfaction with the slowness of psychotherapy and his fear that it will not work.

The masochistic patient acts out unconscious guilt and fear and feelings of inadequacy in the form of self-defeating behavior.

A middle-aged masochistic woman came for a session during a snowstorm wearing her boots but no shoes. After removing her boots, she hid her feet under her skirt instead of sitting in her usual position. The clinician remarked on this, and the patient confessed with some embarrassment that her feet had a mild deformity so that she refused to wear sandals or go to the beach. The flow of the material allowed the clinician to associate previous discussion concerning that patient's displaced feelings of castration. She seemed to understand the interpretation and was able to relate it to her inhibitions at work. However, on the way back to her office, she left her briefcase in the taxicab, and that night she bumped into her bedroom door in the dark, cutting her head. It was necessary first to interpret the patient's emotional reaction to the interpretation before connecting the behavior to the interpretation itself. The feelings of shame and inadequacy were defensively displaced to the self-punitive behavior.

A sadomasochistic relationship is encapsulated in the story of one couple:

> The wife asked her husband, "Should I take my raincoat and umbrella to the theater party tonight?" He replied, "No, I don't think you'll need them. I'm not taking mine." When they left the theater that evening, there was a tropical downpour. Their friends had umbrellas, and cabs were scarce. By the time they arrived at their apartment, they were both thoroughly drenched, and she was in a rage. She berated him unmercifully, accusing him of not taking care of her, she did not know why she remained married to him, and so on. He told the interviewer how miserable she made him feel with her complaints about his total incompetence; picking up on her tirade he said, "I don't know what's wrong with me; I can't seem to do anything right."
>
> The interviewer pointed out that this was a classic sadomasochistic story except that each considered him- or herself to be the suffering party and the other to be the sadist. The patient responded, "I guess that's right." The interviewer then asked if it would be possible to have answered her inquiry about the weather by making some joke about himself, such as "You know I'm not a very good weather forecaster. Let's turn on the TV and find out what they predict. Besides, I don't care that much about being wet, but I'll carry the umbrella if they predict rain." "Not in a million years would this have occurred to me," the patient responded. At this point the patient appeared downcast and perplexed. It was time for an empathic recognition of his unconscious sadism. With a slight gleam in his eye, and a smile in his voice, the interviewer asked, "So how did she look dripping with rain? Like a drowned rat?" The patient burst into laughter and then reflected, "I guess I secretly enjoyed her misery, but I had not realized it until now!"

This vignette summarizes the story of their 25-year marriage. She wanted him to be her protector and to take care of her and was furious with herself for being so needy, dependent, and helpless. He found her neediness a burden. He was angry at himself that he had not done more with his business life and that they lived largely on his trust funds. He felt she loved him for his money, much of which he had put in her name. They had not had sex with each other in 15 years. In that way they each suffered deprivation while at the same time they punished each other.

The next example illustrates how the masochistic person's unconscious narcissistic grandiose wishes and fantasies can reinforce his guilt.

> An adult male patient arrived at his appointment overwhelmed with feelings of guilt intermixed with deep sadness concerning his elderly dog who was dying a slow, suffering death. The veterinarian had advised him there was nothing more that he could do. The patient believed that if he put the dog to sleep, he would feel guilty, and if he did not, he

would still feel guilty, so he asked what he should do. To interpret the patient's fear of assuming the responsibility, although correct, would make the patient feel worse and furthermore ignore the patient's sorrow. The therapist began by empathizing with the sadness of the occasion and followed by stating, "It seems that the problem is not really what is in your dog's best interest but rather how to manage your guilt, whatever you do. Does the guilt have to do with the expectation that there *must* be something else you could do?" "Yes, I feel that way," the patient responded. The clinician replied, "Everyone wishes for the power to make such things right. Sad though it is, we have limitations."

At the end of the session, the patient thanked the therapist, shaking his hand, and went straight home and took his dog to the veterinarian. He held the dog's head in his lap while the doctor put her to sleep. He later reported that the experience was one of love, tenderness, and closeness rather than guilt and self-doubt. Later, when he told the story to his mother, she replied, "You should have put that dog to sleep 6 months ago."

In time the clinician explores the maladaptive aspects of the patient's character traits. While doing so, one must be careful to recognize the adaptive components as well.

A young female college student's mother asked her, "You don't mind if we don't come to your college graduation, do you? It is a 3-hour trip each way!" The patient responded, "Oh, no, it's quite all right!" She then expressed her hurt feelings to the therapist, who asked, "Have you considered calling your mother back and telling her, 'I've been thinking it over and I really want you to come. It would mean a great deal to me'?" The patient said the thought had crossed her mind, but she did not want to cause her mother any inconvenience. The patient appeared perplexed. The clinician then suggested, "Your mother may have the same problem that you do and feel that her presence is unimportant to you. She may be looking for reassurance that you really care whether she attends. She may feel hurt if you do not insist." The patient responded, "I would never have considered that in a million years. I'll call her when I leave." She discovered that her mother had the same problem and was delighted to be wanted, and it was a milestone for both of them.

This was an opportunity to help the patient, whose hurt feelings and repressed rage about her mother's absence from her graduation would only further add to the years of accumulated anger for which she had yet to forgive either herself or her mother. The clinician can later analyze any resulting feelings the patient may have of obligation to the therapist or anger at herself that she had not come up with this idea on her own. Therapeutic instances such as this provide a cognitive/affective template that is used to answer future questions from the patient concerning "What should I do?"

TRANSFERENCE AND COUNTERTRANSFERENCE

The masochistic patient's initial transference is clinging, dependent, and apparently cooperative, but later it alternates with anger and unreasonable demands. The patient wants the clinician to replace some frustrating object, usually the emotionally unavailable parent, and become a substitute. The patient fears this will not occur, and the actual frustration of the transference confirms this fear. If the patient's wish is gratified, then he feels dependent, obligated, and ashamed of his childishness, confirming his feelings of incompetence. He resents the feeling that he has become an extension of the clinician just as he had been with his family. Gratification makes him feel his anger is inappropriate, which makes him feel more guilty. If the clinician withholds advice and support, the patient feels frustrated, unloved, helpless, hopeless, and coerced. It is vital that this paradigm be played out in the transference and that the clinician become involved on both sides before attempting to interpret it. The therapist must do this with a feeling of empathy for the patient's no-win situation rather than irritation over his own no-win situation. Masochistic clinicians do not do well with these patients' failure to progress, experiencing it as a proof of their own inadequacy as therapists. The emergence of the patient's conscious envy in the transference signifies progress. This is indicated by statements such as "I wish I could be more like you" or "You have a much better time with life than I do."

Countertransference dangers abound with the masochistic patient. The frequent negative therapeutic reaction in these patients can have an undermining impact on the clinician, making him adopt the patient's feelings of hopelessness and fail to recognize the patient's aggressive sadistic desire to make him feel inadequate and inept. The self-pitying quality of the masochistic patient can easily lead to a feeling of contempt in the therapist and a failure to recognize the patient's genuine misery. The pathology of the masochistic patient is designed to arouse a sadistic response in others, and this is heightened in the clinical situation. Constant self-scrutiny by the clinician of his aggressive feelings toward the patient's subtle and overt provocations is crucial. A typical example of such a provocation is the failure by the patient to pay his bill on time, so that the clinician is forced into the role of a collection agency and is experienced by both as venal: "You only care about my check, not me," declares the patient self-righteously. Such an occurrence provides a rich field for psychological exploration, provided the clinician does not succumb to his own indignation. Injustice-collecting is the stock-in-trade of the masochistic patient; the clinician must constantly monitor his own aggression toward the patient because when it is acted out, for example, by a sarcastic comment, the patient is confirmed in his self-view as a victim mistreated by all, including his therapist.

Other common countertransference responses include assuming the role of an omnipotent parent making decisions for the patient or excusing his guilt. This was dramatically illustrated when a psychiatric resident who was also a Jesuit priest was interviewing a masochistic patient in front of a class. He told the Catholic patient that he was a priest and, after hearing the patient's painful and self-critical story, granted him absolution during the interview. The patient briefly felt better. The other residents were enraged at their colleague's behavior. The class teacher empathically interpreted their envy of their colleague's magic power and how his manipulation concealed his feeling of inadequacy in the role of fledgling psychiatrist.

Another manifestation of countertransference is the clinician suggesting medication when there is no clinical indication. This is an example of responding to the patient's negativity with a feeling of helplessness and a desire to overcome it. Beginning clinicians must resist the temptation to respond to the patient by being nice. It makes the patient feel worse because he believes that he does not deserve it or that he is unable to reciprocate. Excessive support or encouragement can elicit such a response.

Encouraging the patient to assert himself or to compete more actively without interpreting the defensive pattern may also represent an overidentification with the patient's unconscious rage and be harmful. The clinician's overactivity with the patient represents an attempt to deal with the feelings of helplessness and passive inadequacy that the patient engenders. Using the feeling of inadequacy that the patient generates in the clinician is an opportunity to have a shared experience. It is an entrée into the psychology of the patient. Empathically commenting on what progress has been made in understanding the patient's plight while not succumbing to the patient's complaints of "So much remains to be done" can be highly therapeutic.

CONCLUSION

Regardless of the eventual evolution of the official classification of masochistic patients, their existence is apparent, and they frequently pose a considerable challenge to the interviewer. The interviewer must use his knowledge of masochistic character structure as well as his empathy and his self-analysis of the countertransference. The clinician's awareness and understanding of the inner aspects of the patient's character will allow him to establish rapport with the patient by recognizing the ego-syntonic aspects of the patient's view of himself. Each time the clinician explores a negative aspect of a particular character trait, he also supports the patient's need to maintain the positive component of that trait. With that protection of his self-esteem, the patient can best accept his inner anger that he so readily directs against himself.

The masochistic character is one of the most difficult patients to treat successfully because of his tendency to turn the treatment situation into another sadomasochistic relationship. Nonetheless, a consistent empathic position that presents reality to the patient and uses the countertransference constructively and not sadistically carries with it the possibility of therapeutic change that will free the patient from an endless cycle of self-defeating behavior.

CHAPTER 7

THE DEPRESSED PATIENT

The word *depression* is synonymous with *sadness* to the general public. This is not the case for the mental health professional, who views *sadness* as a normal affective response to loss, and *depression* as a symptom or maladaptive syndrome that frequently, but not always, includes the subjective experience of sadness as one of its components. Depressive syndromes were described by Hippocrates and are among the most consistent, stable, and reliably recognized conditions in medicine.

The most common complaints of psychiatric patients relate to the painful affects of anxiety and depression. Some patients develop syndromes or disorders that have these affects as their central theme. Depressive disorders are among the most prevalent in psychiatry. The lifetime risk of a depressive disorder is about 8%. Some individuals have a single episode that lasts from weeks to months, but a larger number have chronic and/or recurrent depressive episodes. A subgroup has bipolar disease—a disorder marked by alternating episodes of depression and mania. Suicide is a complication of depression and a major cause of mortality among psychiatric patients. In addition, depression is associated with a number of medical comorbidities, with the etiological mechanisms not fully understood. Depressive disorders are frequently comorbid with anxiety disorders, substance abuse, and personality disorders.

DSM-5 provides criteria for the diagnosis of a major depressive episode (Box 7–1), the core component of major depressive disorder, and also for persistent depressive disorder (dysthymia) (Box 7–2), the less severe but more chronic condition that has largely replaced the previous diagnostic category of depressive neurosis and represents a consolidation of DSM-IV-defined chronic major depressive disorder and dysthymic disorder.

BOX 7–1. DSM-5 Diagnostic Criteria for Major Depressive Episode

A. Five (or more) of the following symptoms have been present during the same 2-week period and represent a change from previous functioning; at least one of the symptoms is either (1) depressed mood or (2) loss of interest or pleasure.

Note: Do not include symptoms that are clearly attributable to another medical condition.

1. Depressed mood most of the day, nearly every day, as indicated by either subjective report (e.g., feels sad, empty, hopeless) or observation made by others (e.g., appears tearful). (**Note:** In children and adolescents, can be irritable mood.)
2. Markedly diminished interest or pleasure in all, or almost all, activities most of the day, nearly every day (as indicated by either subjective account or observation).
3. Significant weight loss when not dieting or weight gain (e.g., a change of more than 5% of body weight in a month), or decrease or increase in appetite nearly every day. (**Note:** In children, consider failure to make expected weight gain.)
4. Insomnia or hypersomnia nearly every day.
5. Psychomotor agitation or retardation nearly every day (observable by others, not merely subjective feelings of restlessness or being slowed down).
6. Fatigue or loss of energy nearly every day.
7. Feelings of worthlessness or excessive or inappropriate guilt (which may be delusional) nearly every day (not merely self-reproach or guilt about being sick).
8. Diminished ability to think or concentrate, or indecisiveness, nearly every day (either by subjective account or as observed by others).
9. Recurrent thoughts of death (not just fear of dying), recurrent suicidal ideation without a specific plan, or a suicide attempt or a specific plan for committing suicide.

B. The symptoms cause clinically significant distress or impairment in social, occupational, or other important areas of functioning.
C. The episode is not attributable to the physiological effects of a substance or to another medical condition.

Source. Reprinted from American Psychiatric Association: *Diagnostic and Statistical Manual of Mental Disorders,* 5th Edition. Arlington, VA, American Psychiatric Association, 2013. Copyright 2013, American Psychiatric Association. Used with permission.

BOX 7–2. DSM-5 Diagnostic Criteria for Persistent Depressive
Disorder (Dysthymia)

This disorder represents a consolidation of DSM-IV-defined chronic major depressive disorder and dysthymic disorder.

A. Depressed mood for most of the day, for more days than not, as indicated by either subjective account or observation by others, for at least 2 years.

   Note: In children and adolescents, mood can be irritable and duration must be at least 1 year.

B. Presence, while depressed, of two (or more) of the following:

   1. Poor appetite or overeating.
   2. Insomnia or hypersomnia.
   3. Low energy or fatigue.
   4. Low self-esteem.
   5. Poor concentration or difficulty making decisions.
   6. Feelings of hopelessness.

C. During the 2-year period (1 year for children or adolescents) of the disturbance, the individual has never been without the symptoms in Criteria A and B for more than 2 months at a time.

D. Criteria for a major depressive disorder may be continuously present for 2 years.

E. There has never been a manic episode or a hypomanic episode, and criteria have never been met for cyclothymic disorder.

F. The disturbance is not better explained by a persistent schizoaffective disorder, schizophrenia, delusional disorder, or other specified or unspecified schizophrenia spectrum and other psychotic disorder.

G. The symptoms are not attributable to the physiological effects of a substance (e.g., a drug of abuse, a medication) or another medical condition (e.g. hypothyroidism).

H. The symptoms cause clinically significant distress or impairment in social, occupational, or other important areas of functioning.

Note: Because the criteria for a major depressive episode include four symptoms that are absent from the symptom list for persistent depressive disorder (dysthymia), a very limited number of individuals will have depressive symptoms that have persisted longer than 2 years but will not meet criteria for persistent depressive disorder. If full criteria for a major depressive episode have been met at some point during the current episode of illness, they should be given a diagnosis of major depressive disorder. Otherwise, a diagnosis of other specified depressive disorder or unspecified depressive disorder is warranted.
Note: For specifiers, see DSM-5, p. 169.

Source.   Reprinted from American Psychiatric Association: *Diagnostic and Statistical Manual of Mental Disorders,* 5th Edition. Arlington, VA, American Psychiatric Association, 2013. Copyright 2013, American Psychiatric Association. Used with permission.

With the advent of antidepressant medications, the focus of interest in the treatment of depressed patients has shifted from psychological understanding to symptomatology and phenomenology. Clinicians quickly try to classify the type of depression in order to prescribe the most effective medication. This is in spite of the fact that pharmacotherapy and psychotherapy have been shown to be of roughly equal efficacy in the treatment of mild to moderate depression and that most patients respond best to a combination of medication and psychotherapy.

Depression refers to a symptom as well as the group of illnesses that often present with that symptom and have certain other features in common. As a symptom, depression describes a pervasive feeling of sadness accompanied by feelings of helplessness and personal impoverishment. The depressed individual feels that his security is threatened, that he is unable to cope with his problems, and that others cannot help him. Every facet of life—emotional, cognitive, physiological, behavioral, and social—is typically affected.

PSYCHOPATHOLOGY AND PSYCHODYNAMICS

In early or mild depressive syndromes, the patient actively attempts to alleviate his suffering. He solicits aid from others or attempts to solve his problems by magically regaining a lost love object or enhancing his emotional strength. As the depression becomes more chronic or more severe, the patient relinquishes hope. He feels that others cannot or will not help him and that his condition will never improve. The clinical syndromes of depression range from mild neurotic and adjustment reactions to severe psychoses.

The depressed person not only feels bad but typically is his own worst enemy, and he may use that specific phrase in describing himself. Self-destructive or masochistic and depressive tendencies frequently coexist in the same individual. Suicide, a dramatic complication of serious depression, is a phenomenon of crucial importance in the understanding of the psychological functioning of the depressed person.

A patient does not think of himself as depressed unless he is aware of subjective feelings of sadness. However, the psychiatrist refers to some individuals as having "masked depressions" or "depressive equivalents." These patients have the other signs and symptoms typical of depression, but the affective component is warded off or denied. The diagnosis is justified, however, by symptoms other than the patient's conscious affect and by the frequency with which depression is uncovered if the patient's psychological defenses are penetrated. One common syndrome involves prominent somatic symptoms coupled with denial of affective disturbance, and these patients are often seen by nonpsychiatric health professionals.

Cross-national studies have revealed that subjective affective distress is particularly common in Western European countries, whereas somatic complaints, fatigue, and emotional depletion are prominent in many other cultures.

This chapter considers the clinical and psychodynamic aspects of depression and their relation to masochistic behavior and suicide as well as the developmental origins of depressive patterns of adaptation.

Clinical Features

Depressive syndromes involve a characteristic affective disturbance, retardation and constriction of thought processes, slowing and diminished spontaneity of behavior, withdrawal from social relationships, and physiological changes that are magnified by hypochondriacal preoccupation.

Affect

The depressed person feels a lowering of his mood. He describes this as sadness, gloom, or despair or uses any of a number of other words. Laymen who use the word *depression* are referring to this mood with or without the other clinical features of depressive syndromes. The patient may emphasize one particular aspect of depressive feeling, talking of anguish, tension, fear, guilt, emptiness, or longing.

The depressed patient loses his interest in life. His enthusiasm for his favorite activities diminishes, and in mild depression he goes through the motions of eating, sex, or play but with little pleasure. As his depression progresses, he becomes increasingly indifferent to what had previously been major sources of enjoyment. The patient may smile slightly and sadly at someone else's humor, but he has little of his own, unless it is a cynical or sardonic mask covering his self-contempt.

Anxiety, a common symptom in some depressive syndromes, is the psychological response to danger and is often seen when the individual unconsciously believes that there is an ongoing threat to his welfare. At times anxiety, and the closely related picture of agitation, may become a chronic feature, as in the so-called involutional depression. In severe or chronic depression, the anxiety may disappear and be replaced by apathy and withdrawal. This is the common picture in patients who have given up and feel hopeless. The apathetic patient is unable to help himself and elicits less sympathy or assistance from others. However, his withdrawal does protect him from the pain of his own inner feelings as chronic hopeless surrender replaces the anguish of acute despair.

Depersonalization may play a similar defensive function in more acute depressive conditions. The most familiar aspects of the patient's personal identity seem strange. He no longer experiences his body or his emotional responses as part of his self, and he thereby protects himself from the painful feelings of depression. However, the sense of emptiness and feeling disconnected from oneself is also experienced as painful. Depersonalization is a complex symptom that is also seen in other conditions and does not always have defensive significance.

Anger is also prominent in the affect of depressed patients. It may be expressed directly, as the patient complains that he is unloved and mistreated. In other cases it is more subtle, and the patient's suffering makes the lives of those around him miserable. For example, a woman would constantly tell her husband what an awful person she was and how difficult it must be for him to put up with her. Her self-abuse was far more disturbing to him than the faults for which she berated herself. Furthermore, if he failed to reassure her that her self-accusations were not true, she would complain that he too must feel she was awful.

Thought

The depressed person is preoccupied with himself and his plight, worrying about his misfortunes and their impact on his life. He ruminates about his past and is filled with remorse as he imagines magical solutions to his current problems that involve the intervention of some omnipotent force, although he has little hope that these solutions will come about. His repetitive or ruminative thoughts lend a monotonous coloration to his conversation. The mildly depressed individual may fight his depression by consciously directing his thoughts elsewhere, a defense that is particularly common in obsessive-compulsive patients. However, this usually becomes another self-preoccupation as his previous ruminations are replaced by new ones: "How can I get my mind off my problem?" instead of "Why did it happen to me?" or "What have I done to deserve this?"

The psychotically depressed patient may brood over minor incidents of his youth, which are recalled with guilt and fear of retaliation or punishment. One middle-aged man thought that the local newspapers would expose an adolescent homosexual episode, humiliating him and his entire family. In the final stages of psychotic depression, the patient attempts to explain his feelings by finding a hidden meaning in them. This may involve projection, as in the patient who interpreted his plight as a punishment inflicted by a distant relative who was jealous of him. For other patients, the explanatory delusional systems reflect grandiose displacement, such as world destruction fantasies or nihilistic delusions that the universe has come to an end. Another patient employed concrete symbolization, becoming convinced that his body was diseased and rotting away, although he denied emotional distress. These defensive patterns are related to those seen in the paranoid patient and are discussed in detail in Chapter 13, "The Paranoid Patient."

The topics that do not enter the patient's mind are as important as the thoughts with which he is preoccupied. He has difficulty remembering the joys of the past; his view of life is gray with periodic spells of black. The interviewer must bear in mind that there is considerable retrospective falsification as the patient describes his life. It is not unusual for him to portray his mood as long-standing and gradual in onset, whereas his family describes the symptoms as relatively recent and abrupt. In one sense the patient may be correct; he has been concealing his depression from others and perhaps from himself. As he improves, this process may reverse itself; in the early phases of recovery, the depressed patient sometimes sounds much better than he really feels. This may lead to premature optimism on the part of the therapist and is one of the factors that contributes to the increased risk of suicide as the patient starts to improve.

Not only is the thought content of the depressed patient disturbed, but his cognitive processes are distorted as well. His thoughts are diminished in quantity, and although he may be responsive, he shows little initiative or spontaneity. He answers questions but does not offer new data or topics, and his mental life has little variety. He understands what is said and replies appropriately; nevertheless, his thinking and responses are slowed, and his speech may be halting or uncertain. The cognitive disturbances of more serious depressions are so severe that the resulting clinical picture has been termed "pseudodementia." The differential diagnosis includes true dementia, and although the condition is largely reversible, it is believed that brain abnormalities are involved in its etiology.

Behavior

Slowness characterizes the depressed patient's entire life as well as his thought processes. His movements and responses take longer, and even if he seems agitated and hyperactive, purposeful or intentional behavior is diminished. Thus the patient who paces the floor wringing his hands may require many minutes to dress himself or carry out simple tasks. For the behaviorally retarded patient, the change in tempo may be almost bizarre, and in extreme cases it is as though one were watching a slow-motion film.

The patient may participate in life if he is urged, but if left to his own devices, he is likely to withdraw. Those activities that he does select are passive and often socially isolated. One man with an early depressive syndrome first tried to seek social contact with friends. As this failed to alleviate his suffering, he retreated to sitting alone and reading, but in time even this required energy and attention that he could no longer command, and he simply sat staring at the television screen, scarcely noticing whether the set was on or off.

Physical Symptoms

The depressed person's preoccupation with himself is often expressed concretely as a concern with his body and physical health. Hypochondriasis or frank somatic delusions are a more serious manifestation of the same process. These symptoms are related to those seen in paranoid syndromes and are discussed in Chapter 13. Depression is also associated with actual changes in physiological functioning. The patient's metabolic rate is lower, his gastrointestinal functioning abnormal, and his mouth dry, and there are shifts in almost every bodily function that is under neurohormonal control. Depression is accompanied by a significant increase in morbidity and mortality from physical illness.

The most common physical complaints include insomnia with difficulty falling asleep or early morning awakening, fatigue, loss of appetite, constipation (although, occasionally, early depressive syndromes are marked by diarrhea), loss of libido, headache, neck ache, backache, other aches and pains, and dryness and burning of the mouth with an unpleasant taste. The specific somatic symptom has symbolic meaning to the patient. The common symptoms concerning the mouth and digestive system are associated with the importance of oral motives and interests in depressive individuals. Other symptoms may have more individual significance. The headaches of the college professor or the pelvic pain of the menopausal woman may be closely related to the patient's self-concept. One man complained of an "empty gnawing" in his bowels; further discussion uncovered the feeling that he was being eaten up from within by a tumor. Somatic symptoms of unrelated etiology may also become the focus of hypochondriacal concern.

Social Relations

The depressive person craves love from others, but he is unable to reciprocate in a way that rewards the other person or reinforces the relationship. He may become isolated, feeling unable to seek out others, or he may actively search out friends and companions only to alienate them by his clinging and self-preoccupation.

Fearing rejection, the patient makes exaggerated efforts to win the favor of his acquaintances. One man always brought gifts to friends when he visited them and remembered the birthdays of even casual acquaintances. Unfortunately, the message he conveyed was more of self-sacrifice and desperation than of spontaneous warmth and comradeship. Similar behavior may be seen in obsessive-compulsive individuals, because both obsessive-compulsive and depressed persons are concerned with concealing their aggression and winning the favor of others. However, each often alienates others by the very behavior with which he hopes to attract them.

In early or mild depressive states, there may be an increase in social activity, with the patient seeking out others to ease his pain. In his eagerness to be accepted and loved, the mildly depressed person can be a faithful, reliable companion, one who subordinates his own interests and desires to those of the other person. Although he has feelings of envy and anger, he does his best to conceal them, usually by turning them inward, deepening his despair.

As the depression worsens, the patient loses more energy and drive. He cannot face his friends and consequently withdraws into himself. Anticipating that he would be a burden to others, he suffers in bitter silence and guilty self-reproach. The patient's inability to respond to the attempts by others to cheer him up leads him to feel helpless and rejected. This leads others to avoid him, which confirms his feeling that he is unlikeable and unwanted.

Melancholia and Atypical Depressions

A particularly severe depressive syndrome characterized by an almost total loss of the capacity for pleasure and marked vegetative changes is called *melancholia*, a term that means "black bile" and goes back to the ancient Greeks. This is a specific syndrome with distinct clinical features that requires specific somatic treatment. Unfortunately, in our opinion, melancholia was not delineated as a distinct mood disorder in DSM-5. An editorial by Parker et al. in the *American Journal of Psychiatry* in 2010 made a compelling case for such a delineation. The clinical features enumerated in that editorial are listed in Table 7–1.

The patient with an *atypical depression* presents with a reversed vegetative pattern. He often has a long-standing history of sensitivity to interpersonal rejection and a high degree of mood reactivity (e.g., sen-

TABLE 7–1. Clinical features of melancholia (as enumerated by Parker et al.)

1. Disturbances in affect disproportionate to stressors, marked by unremitting apprehension and morbid statements, blunted emotional response, nonreactive mood, and pervasive anhedonia—with such features continuing autonomously despite any improved circumstances. The risks for recurrence and for suicide are high.
2. Psychomotor disturbance expressed as retardation (i.e., slowed thought, movement, and speech, anergia) or as spontaneous agitation (i.e., motor restlessness and stereotypic movements and speech).
3. Cognitive impairment with reduced concentration and working memory.
4. Vegetative dysfunction manifested as interrupted sleep, loss of appetite and weight, reduced libido, and diurnal variation—with mood and energy generally worse in the morning.
5. Although psychosis is not necessarily a feature, it is often present. Nihilistic convictions of hopelessness, guilt, sin, ruin, or disease are common psychotic themes.

Source. Reprinted from Parker G, Fink M, Shorter E, et al.: "Issues for DSM-5: Whither Melancholia? The Case for Its Classification as a Distinct Mood Disorder." *American Journal of Psychiatry* 167(7):745–747, 2010. Copyright 2010, American Psychiatric Association. Used with permission.

sitivity to environmental stimuli). Instead of insomnia, sleep is excessive, both at night and during the day; appetite is increased and weight gain occurs. This pattern is often associated with personality disorders that persist even when the patient is not depressed; it is more common in women and is said to have a different spectrum of response to pharmacotherapy. The atypical symptoms and associated personality characteristics frequently lead these patients to seek psychotherapy and to be diagnostically confusing. The DSM-5 atypical features specifier is presented in Box 7–3.

BOX 7–3. DSM-5 "With Atypical Features" Specifier

With atypical features: This specifier can be applied when these features predominate during the majority of days of the current or most recent major depressive episode or persistent depressive disorder.

A. Mood reactivity (i.e., mood brightens in response to actual or potential positive events).

B. Two (or more) of the following:

 1. Significant weight gain or increase in appetite.
 2. Hypersomnia.

3. Leaden paralysis (i.e., heavy, leaden feelings in arms or legs).
4. A long-standing pattern of interpersonal rejection sensitivity (not limited to episodes of mood disturbance) that results in significant social or occupational impairment.

C. Criteria are not met for "with melancholic features" or "with catatonia" during the same episode.

Note: "Atypical depression" has historical significance (i.e., atypical in contradistinction to the more classical agitated, "endogenous" presentations of depression that were the norm when depression was rarely diagnosed in outpatients and almost never in adolescents or younger adults) and today does not connote an uncommon or unusual clinical presentation as the term might imply.

Mood reactivity is the capacity to be cheered up when presented with positive events (e.g., a visit from children, compliments from others). Mood may become euthymic (not sad) even for extended periods of time if the external circumstances remain favorable. Increased appetite may be manifested by an obvious increase in food intake or by weight gain. Hypersomnia may include either an extended period of nighttime sleep or daytime napping that totals at least 10 hours of sleep per day (or at least 2 hours more than when not depressed). Leaden paralysis is defined as feeling heavy, leaden, or weighted down, usually in the arms or legs. This sensation is generally present for at least an hour a day but often lasts for many hours at a time. Unlike the other atypical features, pathological sensitivity to perceived interpersonal rejection is a trait that has an early onset and persists throughout most of adult life. Rejection sensitivity occurs both when the person is and is not depressed, though it may be exacerbated during depressive periods.

Source. Reprinted from American Psychiatric Association: *Diagnostic and Statistical Manual of Mental Disorders,* 5th Edition. Arlington, VA, American Psychiatric Association, 2013. Copyright 2013, American Psychiatric Association. Used with permission.

Psychotic and Neurotic Depression and Normal Grief

The psychotically depressed individual's relationship with the real world is impaired. His social withdrawal may seem grossly inappropriate; his mental preoccupations interfere with his registration of the external world and with normal cognitive functioning. When delusions occur, they are likely to contribute to his pain by embodying his self-condemnation and punishment, although some measure of comfort may be gained if he can avoid the painful realities of the world because of distraction by his delusional substitute.

The distinction between neurotic and psychotic depressive disorders often seems to be a quantitative one. The clinician considers the external precipitants, the duration of the patient's symptoms, and their severity in making his diagnosis. The interviewer feels more estranged from the psychotically depressed patient. He finds himself observing the symptoms with a feeling of emotional distance rather than participating empathically in the patient's suffering.

Psychotic depressive syndromes are frequently subclassified as "agitated" or "retarded." These terms refer to familiar clinical pictures. The agitated patient paces the floor, wringing his hands and bemoaning his fate. He approaches every stranger, pleading for help in a stereotyped and often annoying way. He may sit down at the table for a meal but immediately gets up and pushes his plate away. He creates an overall impression of intense anxiety, but the lines in his face and the content of his thoughts reveal his depression.

The patient with a retarded psychotic depressive syndrome, on the other hand, shows inhibition of motor activity that may progress to stupor. He sits in a chair or lies in bed, head bowed, body in a posture of flexion, eyes staring straight ahead, indifferent to distractions. If he does speak or move, the act is slow, labored, and of brief duration.

The neurotically depressed patient continues to function in the real world, and his depressive feelings are mild or at least seem proportionate to the external precipitants. If the depression is severe, the precipitating trauma has been extreme, and the interviewer can empathize with the patient's distress. The patient recognizes the realities of the world around him and often improves over a span of weeks or months. For example, a neurotically depressed young widow who had recently been bereaved felt that she could never enjoy her life alone, nor could she conceive of remarriage. However, she was able to take solace in her relationships with her children and in her job. A year later, she looked back on her husband's death with sadness, but she had begun to date other men, was enjoying life, and was contemplating the idea of remarriage. Another woman, who developed a psychotic depression following a similar precipitant, quit her job, was unable to care for her children, and withdrew to her bed, certain that a terrible physical illness had developed. She became morbidly preoccupied with her widowhood, and although after a year her pain was less intense, she had become constricted so that she only left her home to seek treatment for her various medical problems.

There is a spectrum from normal grief reactions through neurotic depression to psychotic depression. The grieving individual responds to a real and important loss with feelings of sadness and a temporary withdrawal of interest in other aspects of life. His thoughts are focused on his loss, and it may be weeks or months before his interest in the world returns to its former level and he is able to renew his relationships with others. There are several features that differentiate this normal syndrome from pathological depression. The grief-stricken individual does not experience a diminution of self-esteem. He is not irrationally guilty, and it is easy for the interviewer to empathize with his feelings. He may have some insomnia, but somatic symptoms are mild and transient. He may *feel* that his world has come to an end, but he *knows* that he will recover and cope with his problems. He is able to respond to comforting gestures from family members and good friends. Finally, grief is a self-limited condition, rarely lasting more than 6–9 months and often less. If the reaction is disproportionate to the loss, either in terms of severity or duration, or if the person feels self-critical, guilty, or personally inadequate, we think of a depressive syndrome.

Precipitating Factors

Biological and Psychological Theories

Depression is often a response to a traumatic precipitating experience in the patient's life, although at the same time it reflects a genetically or constitutionally determined predisposition.

It is often helpful for the depressed patient to understand his symptoms in psychological terms. The discussion of the trigger for the episode does not suggest that it is the most important etiological factor but rather offers an opportunity for the patient to better understand himself. Most depressive episodes, particularly early in the course of the disorder, are related to some external precipitating cause.

Genetic or constitutional models of depression were long seen as being in tension with psychodynamic concepts, but there is no contradiction between these two frames of reference. Today there is little question that most depressive episodes affect individuals with constitutional predispositions who have been affected by precipitating life stressors. The ability of depressive syndromes to communicate helpless dependency and to elicit nurturing care suggests that depressive mechanisms may have adaptive value and that the capacity to develop them may have been selected in the course of evolution. This is in contrast to most evolutionary models of schizophrenia, which emphasize the maladaptive aspects of the illness. For depression, biological and psychodynamic explanations are not only compatible but interdependent.

Specific Psychological Stressors

Loss.   The loss of a love object is the most common precipitant of depression. The prototypic loss is the death of or separation from a loved one. It may also be an internal psychological loss resulting from the expectation that one will be rejected by family and friends. The loss may have actually occurred or it may be imminent, as in the depressive reactions that appear in anticipation of the death of a parent or spouse. Of course, not all losses precipitate a depression. The loss must involve someone important to the patient, and there are certain predisposing characteristics of the patient's psychological functioning and his relationship to the lost object that are discussed later.

There is sometimes an interval of days, weeks, or even years between the actual loss and the depressive response. In these cases the patient may have denied the loss or its impact on him and therefore avoided his emotional response. When something—often an event that symbolizes or exposes the initial trauma—renders this denial ineffective, depression follows. One woman showed relatively little response to the death of her husband but became deeply depressed 2 years later when her cat was killed in an accident. She explained, "I suddenly realized that I was really alone." Mourning can also be delayed as part of normal psychological development, as occurred in an adolescent boy who seemed relatively unaffected by his father's death. Five years later, on the night before his graduation from college, his mother found him crying in his room. When she asked what was wrong, he said, "I keep thinking how Dad would have enjoyed it if only he were here." When he later related this event, his therapist asked, "What did your mother do?" The patient responded tearfully, "She hugged me and said 'He'll be there in our hearts.'" The patient was moved further when the therapist responded, "It is a touching story; it will always be one of your treasures."

So-called anniversary depressions are based on a similar mechanism. A specific season or date is unconsciously associated with a loss in the patient's earlier life. The anniversary of a parent's death is a common example. Depressions during Christmas holidays are in part related to the common feeling of being left out and impoverished at a time when others are together and happy. The child whose emotional deprivation seemed worst at times when his friends were happiest finds himself in later years to be inexplicably depressed during holiday seasons.

In a sense, all adult depressive reactions are delayed responses, with the immediate precipitant in adult life exposing feelings that can be traced to early childhood. Since every child experiences loss and feelings of inadequacy and helplessness, every adult needs to have adequate psychological resources, including loving relationships, in order not to respond with depression when experiencing life's losses.

Threats to self-confidence and self-esteem. Every individual has internal mental representations of the important people in his life, including himself. Self-representation, like representation of others, may be highly accurate or grossly distorted. We use the term *self-confidence* to describe one aspect of this self-representation, a person's image of his own adaptive capacity. In other words, someone who is self-confident perceives himself as able to obtain gratification of his needs and to ensure his survival.

In addition to this self-representation, or mental image of what he is like, each person has an image of what he would like to be or thinks he ought to be—his ego ideal. The degree to which his self-image lives up to that ego ideal is a measure of his self-esteem. If a person feels that he is close to the way he would like to be, he will have high self-esteem; conversely, if he falls short of his own goals and aspirations, his self-esteem will be lower.

Diminution in self-confidence and in self-esteem are cardinal symptoms of depression. The self-esteem of many depression-prone individuals has been based on the continuing input of love, respect, and approval from significant figures in their lives. These may be figures from the patient's past who have long since been internalized or real external figures of current importance. In either event, the disruption of a relationship with such a person poses a threat to the patient's source of narcissistic supplies, love, and dependent gratification. This endangers the person's self-esteem and therefore may precipitate a depression. Depression may also follow the disruption of a relationship with a person who, while not a source of these narcissistic rewards, had become a symbolic extension of the patient's self-image. In this case, the loss of the person is equivalent to an amputation of part of the patient's own ego. The loss of a child frequently has this meaning to a parent.

It is possible for the patient's self-image and self-esteem to be shattered by blows other than the disruption of object relationships. For many individuals, self-esteem is based on self-confidence—that is, as long as they feel able to cope with their own problems independently, they have a good opinion of themselves. A direct threat to this person's adaptive capacity, such as a major injury or illness, may render him helpless and destroy his self-confidence and therefore self-esteem. This is the basis of some depressions seen in association with incapacitating traumatic injuries or chronic illness.

The direct threat to one's adaptive capacity and the loss of love and respect from important people are closely related clinically. For example, the college student who fails an examination may revise his image of his intellectual capacity sharply downward, and for this very reason he may feel that his parents will have less love and respect for him.

Success. Paradoxically, some people become depressed in response to success. Occupational promotion, or any reward that carries increased responsibility and status, may lead to a depressive syndrome. When these paradoxical depressions are studied, one of two underlying dynamics is commonly found. In the first, the patient feels that he does not deserve this success, in spite of objective evidence to the contrary. He believes that the increased responsibility will expose him as inadequate, and therefore he anticipates rejection from those who have rewarded him. For example, a physician who had an outstanding record was asked to direct a clinical program. He first rejected the offer and then accepted it, but he became increasingly mistrustful of his clinical judgment and administrative skills. When he spoke to his superiors about this, they reassured him, but this only made him more convinced that they did not really understand him. Finally, in order to escape from the danger of injuring his patients because of his fantasied incompetence, he made a serious suicide attempt. When provided an opportunity for success, he feared that he would be expected to function independently and would no longer qualify for dependent care.

The second psychodynamic theme underlying depressive responses to success stems from the fear of retaliation for successful achievement that the patient unconsciously associates with assertion and aggression. This patient has often struggled to get to the top, but successful assertion is equated with hostile aggression, and he feels guilty about any behavior that furthers his own advancement. He views competition in terms of oedipal or sibling conflicts, and success implies a transgression for which punishment will follow. He escapes by regressing to a dependent level of adaptation rather than risking the danger of retaliation.

Psychodynamic Patterns

The depressed patient has suffered a blow to his self-esteem. This can result from the disruption of a relationship with either external or internalized objects or from a direct blow to his adaptive capacity. In either event, the patient experiences a deflated self-image and attempts to repair the damage and to defend himself from further trauma. This section discusses several psychodynamic mechanisms that are related to this sequence: identification, the relation of anger to depression, the role of isolation and denial, manic syndromes, the relationship of depression and projective defenses, and suicide.

Identification and Introjection

When death or separation leads to the loss of a loved one, the emotionally charged mental representation of the lost one remains a permanent part of one's inner world. This mechanism is called *introjection*, whereas *identification* is a less global and more subtle process in which the individual modifies his self-image in accordance with his image of the important person whom he has lost, but only in specific selected areas. Both of these processes serve to recapture or retain the lost object, at least in terms of the patient's psychological life. They are crucial in normal development. The child's character is molded by his identification with parents and parental surrogates from his early years, and the oedipal complex is resolved by the introjection of the parent, with this introject forming the basic core of the adult superego.

Clinical manifestations of identification as a defense against grief are common. One young man who had been born and raised in the United States developed speech and other mannerisms similar to those of his recently deceased father, a European immigrant. A woman developed an interest in religion, for the first time in her life, after her deeply religious stepmother died. A woman whose husband was away in the armed forces began to attend baseball games, his favorite pastime, in which she had previously had little interest. Both women reported feelings of closeness to their lost loved ones while engaged in those activities.

Introjection is vividly illustrated when the depressed person's anger toward his lost love object continues after that object has been introjected. We speak of "ego introjects" when the patient attacks himself with accusations that bear little relation to his own faults but that clearly refer to the faults of the lost person. The introject has become allied with the patient's ego and is being attacked by his punitive superego. "Superego introjection" is demonstrated when the voice and manner of the patient's self-criticism can be traced to criticisms that originally had been expressed by the lost loved one but now originate in the patient's superego.

Depression and Anger

Depression is a complex emotion, and it commonly includes admixtures of anger. Perhaps the simplest psychodynamic basis for this is the patient's anger at the lost love object for abandoning him. This is dramatic in small children, who frequently attack or refuse to speak to their parents following a separation from them. It is also demonstrated by the man who, following the death of his mother, destroyed all of her photographs and letters, rationalizing this as a desire to avoid painful reminders of his loss.

The depressed patient displaces his anger to substitute persons who he hopes will replace his loss and continue to gratify his needs but who inevitably fail to do so. This coercive hostility is frequently expressed toward the therapist. The patient unconsciously wants the therapist to replace the loss personally, not merely to facilitate the healing process. When the clinician fails to gratify this craving, the patient becomes disappointed and bitter.

The patient feels guilty about his hostile feelings toward others and is afraid to express his anger directly. He feels inadequate and is convinced that he cannot survive without the love and care of others. Thus any outward expression of hostility is dangerous—he might destroy what he most needs. He therefore may turn it against himself in the form of self-accusation and condemnation, a cardinal feature of depression. The self-love and self-respect of the normal person protect him from destructive self-criticism. These supporting factors are seriously deficient in the depressed person, and he may torture himself mercilessly, suffering shame and guilt.

Isolation and Denial

The depressed individual often struggles to keep his feelings out of awareness and to ignore the events and people in the outside world to which they are a response. These defensive maneuvers protect him from psychological pain. When the patient is successful, one sees depression without depression— that is, the clinical syndrome but without the subjective affect. Usually some aspect of the emotional complex remains. Often, the somatic symptoms are most apparent, and some psychiatrists speak of "somatic equivalents" of depression. These patients look and act depressed. They come to the doctor because of physical symptoms and hypochondriacal complaints that are usually refractory to treatment. When asked if they feel depressed, they say, "No," but add that they have been run-down, tired, and worried about their physical health. Others reserve the term *depression* for conditions in which the subjective clinical affect is present and see these "equivalent" symptoms as premorbid conditions.

Isolation and denial are characteristic defenses of the obsessive personality, and an underlying depression is commonly exposed as one analyzes the defenses of the obsessive-compulsive patient in psychotherapy. This patient has high expectations of himself, and he often feels that he cannot live up to them. He maintains his self-esteem by turning his neurotic traits into highly regarded virtues. When this is interpreted, the patient's underlying feelings are brought into the open; he feels that he is a sham and a failure and becomes depressed.

Manic Syndromes

The interview with the seriously manic patient is discussed in Chapter 14, "The Psychotic Patient." However, an understanding of manic syndromes is important for interviewing depressed patients. There is strong evidence for a genetic and constitutional component to the etiology of bipolar or manic-depressive disorders, and pharmacotherapy is essential in their clinical management. Nevertheless, there are important psychodynamic issues in manic states.

The manic patient superficially appears to be the opposite of the depressed one. His affective display is elated or euphoric, and he is overly active, physically and mentally, as he races from one topic to another, unable to keep his mind on a continuous train of thought. In spite of this surface elation, mania was once understood as a defense against depression, reflecting denial and reversal of affect. Today, although this is not seen as explaining the etiology of the condition, it is still helpful in understanding its psychological meaning.

There is often clinical evidence that the patient's underlying feelings are not as cheerful as they first appear. The manic patient's humor is infectious, unlike that of the autistic schizophrenic patient, but it is often barbed and hostile. If he is being interviewed in a group, he may make embarrassing and provocative comments about the others, perhaps focusing on one person's unusual name or another's physical defect. Although the group may laugh with the patient at first, the discomfort of his victim will quickly win their sympathy. The patient seems to have little compassion, although he may switch to a new target. This behavior reveals his defensive projection; he focuses on the weaknesses of others to avoid thinking of his own. At times, his underlying depression may emerge openly, and in response to warmth and sympathy he may lose control and break into tears.

If depression can be conceptualized as the reaction to a feeling of narcissistic injury and loss, with the ego fearing the punitive and disapproving superego, mania can be seen as the ego's insistence that the injury has been repaired and the superego conquered, that the individual has incorporated all of the narcissistic supplies that he might need and that he is immune from injury or loss. There is a feeling of triumphant omnipotence; because the ego has defeated the superego, it is no longer necessary to control or inhibit impulses. The manic patient insists that he has no restraints, that he is exactly what he wants to be. He is supremely self-confident, undertaking projects and acquiring possessions that would normally seem out of reach. In spite of this apparent victory, his underlying uneasiness is readily apparent. Superego fears may persist in the manic episode, and the patient's frantic, driven quality in part represents his flight from punishment.

This psychodynamic constellation is related to the hallucinatory wish fulfillment with which the hungry infant soothed himself when his cries did not lead to feeding. The cyclic periodicity of mania and depression has been compared with the infantile cycle of hunger and satiation. The manic patient has gratified his appetite by ignoring reality and insisting that he has what he so dearly craves. However, this illusory gratification is only transient, and the feeling of depression returns, just as the fantasies of oral gratification failed to quiet the hunger pangs of the infant.

Projection and Paranoid Responses

Patients frequently alternate between paranoid and depressive states. The depressed patient feels that he is worthless and tends to blame himself for his difficulties. He looks to others for help and may be angry and resentful if it is not forthcoming. If he utilizes the defense of projection to protect himself from his painful self-condemnation, he feels not only that others are failing to help him but also that they are the cause of his difficulty. It is as though the patient said to himself, "It is not that I am bad; it is only that he says I am bad," or "My unhappiness is not my fault; it is what he did to me." Projection is accompanied by shifts from sadness to anger, from looking for help to expecting persecution. The patient's diminished self-esteem changes to grandiosity as he thinks, "I must be very important to be singled out for such abuse."

However, one pays a heavy price for paranoid defenses. This patient's ability to appraise the outer world realistically is impaired, and his social relationships are disrupted. Although his self-image may be inflated, his actual adaptive capacity is often more seriously impaired than it had been while he was depressed. These changes serve as precipitants of a new depressive reaction, and the cycle continues.

The interview with such patients may be marked by shifts from one pole to the other in response to the therapist's interventions. The relationship between paranoid and depressive syndromes is one reason that paranoid patients present suicidal risks—sudden intervening depressions can occur. It is also related to the prominent paranoid features in manic states.

Suicide

The exploration of suicidal thoughts and feelings not only is of critical importance in the practical management of a depressed person but also provides one of the most valuable routes to understanding him. The discussion of suicide, like that of any complex act, can be separated into a consideration of the motives or impulses and of the regulatory and controlling structures that interact with these motives.

The motivations for the seemingly irrational act of taking one's own life are complex and varied. Some patients have no intention of killing themselves, and if the behavior is consciously intended as a dramatic communication rather than a self-destructive act, we speak of suicidal "gestures." However, these are subject to miscalculation and may lead to death. They also may be followed by more serious suicidal behavior, particularly if their communicative purpose is not successful. The distinction between a suicidal gesture and a suicide attempt is somewhat arbitrary, and most suicidal behavior involves both communicative and self-destructive goals. The interview with the depressed patient is designed to provide other channels of communication, and this in itself may reduce the pressure for suicidal behavior.

The self-destructive aspect of suicidal motivation is manifold. For some depressed persons, suicide may provide an opportunity to regain some feeling of mastery over their own fate. There are schools of philosophy that suggest that it is only by taking one's own life that an individual can truly experience freedom. Some depressed people feel they are unable to control their own lives in any other way. They are able to regain a sense of autonomy and self-esteem only by recognizing that the decision to live or to die is up to them. The often-observed clinical phenomenon of an improvement in the patient's mood after he has decided to take his own life is related to this mechanism.

An impulse to commit suicide may be related to an impulse to murder someone else. Suicide can serve as a means of controlling one's own aggressions, as a turning of aggression against the self, or as a means of murdering another person who has been psychologically incorporated by the suicidal individual. Although these mechanisms are quite different, their effect is similar. A person who unconsciously wants to kill someone else may try to take his own life.

Life may seem intolerable under certain circumstances, and suicide can provide a means of escape from a painful or humiliating situation. This is often the case with culturally or socially sanctioned suicide. This motivation is the most comfortable one for a patient's friends, family, or even his physician to accept. However, in our society, culturally sanctioned suicidal behavior is relatively uncommon, even in those who have painful terminal illnesses and are familiar with their diagnosis and prognosis. When it does occur, it is most often associated with some psychiatric disorder, depression being the most common. The clinician must be careful not to convey to the patient consciously or unconsciously that suicide is a reasonable act in view of the patient's problems, a message that may reflect countertransferential discomfort with the patient's anguish or despair.

No one has any personal experience with his own death; thus the psychological meaning of dying varies from person to person and is related to other experiences with which it is symbolically associated. Death may mean separation, isolation, and loneliness; peaceful and permanent sleep; or a magical reunion with others who have already died. More elaborate ideas may be based on religious or spiritualist convictions concerning life after death. Each of these meanings may be attractive under certain circumstances, and the motive for suicide may have more to do with these symbolic equivalents of death than with death itself. At the same time, most patients retain some realistic awareness of the meaning of taking their own lives side by side with their unconscious symbolic elaboration of death. This dichotomy is culturally reinforced by those religions that emphasize the pleasant aspects of the next world but at the same time strictly forbid suicide as a sinful act.

The specific method of suicide that the patient contemplates or attempts often sheds light on the unconscious meaning of the act. For example, the person who takes an overdose of sleeping pills may be equating death with a prolonged sleep, and the use of firearms often suggests violent rage. Dramatic modes of death such as self-immolation usually involve attempts to communicate dramatic feelings to the world. The patient who uses multiple methods simultaneously, such as pills and drowning, is often struggling against a conflicting desire to live and is trying to ensure that he will not be able to change his mind at the last moment.

The strength and nature of suicidal impulses are only two of the factors that determine whether an individual attempts suicide. Most individuals have internalized strong prohibitions against murder, and furthermore, narcissistic self-regard serves as a specific deterrent to suicide. However, if an individual has identified with a parent or other significant figure who himself committed suicide, the situation is different. The incidence of suicide in the children of parents who themselves committed suicide is several times higher than in the general population. There are certainly genetic factors included in this, but these individuals also may have failed to develop the usual inner restraints, and they cannot judge suicidal behavior negatively because to do so would be to reject their own parents.

If an individual simply and unambivalently wanted to take his own life, he would probably not be sitting and talking to a clinician. Some patients seem to want to place their lives in the hands of fate, acting in a way that courts danger but allows the possibility of escape. The behavior associated with such feelings ranges from playing Russian roulette to taking overdoses of pills when one is likely to be discovered, driving dangerously under hazardous conditions, or conveying an ambiguous message that the clinician may or may not interpret correctly. In some respects this is the opposite of the desire for a sense of autonomy and mastery mentioned earlier. The individual denies all responsibility for his continued existence, thereby relieving himself of a weighty burden. If he is saved, he may interpret this as a magical sign that he is forgiven and will be cared for, and the intensity of his suicidal impulses will diminish. The patient who survives a serious attempt and says, "I guess God wanted me to live" is a typical example.

Individuals who are prone to impulsive behavior in general and particularly to impulsive aggression are also more likely to act on suicidal impulses. The combination of depression and impulsiveness is related to the high incidence of suicide in alcoholic patients and in those with acute brain syndromes. In evaluating a patient's suicidal potential, his general impulsiveness, as well as his depression, is an important factor.

The inquiry about suicidal thoughts with a depressed patient includes questions such as "What will be the impact of your death?"; "Who will be affected by it?"; "Have you consulted them about your decision?"; and "What do you imagine their response will be?" These questions not only assist in the evaluation of suicidal risk; they also place suicidal thoughts in relational or interpersonal context and direct the patient's attention to considerations that commonly counter suicidal impulses.

The patient who has suicidal thoughts and impulses has often evaluated his potential for acting on them himself, and he is usually willing to share his conclusions with the interviewer. These can provide an important source of information, but they cannot simply be accepted at face value. Patients can change their minds, and psychological characteristics that seem to be reassuring must be assessed as to their stability and the possibility of change. The patient's intention of maintaining a separation between impulse and action is also assessed by the extent to which he has elaborated concrete plans for suicide and made preparations for carrying out those plans.

Developmental Dynamics

The depressed patient frequently comes from a family with a history of depression, and high aspirations and low self-image have often been transmitted from generation to generation. The death of or separation from a parent early in the patient's life is a common feature in the history. The patient not only experiences the separation and loss but also lives with the remaining parent through a period of grief and despair. The patient has often been the bearer of more than the usual amount of parental hopes and fantasies. Typically, the parents felt themselves to be unsuccessful, and they wanted their child to succeed where they had failed. The child becomes a vehicle for their hopes, and he feels that their love is contingent on his continued success. For example, the syndrome is common in the oldest child born of upwardly mobile immigrant parents. The overt climate of family life is usually one of protective and loving concern. As a consequence, the patient must suppress and deny any hostile feelings. He is pushed hard, not provided with the basis for self-confidence, and not allowed to complain. A similar result can occur in the child who is praised excessively for being "good" and reprimanded or criticized at the slightest sign of disobedience, rebelliousness, or even a suggestion that he is striving for autonomy, all of which are equated with being "bad."

The origins of depressive psychodynamics can be traced to the first year of life. The young infant is the center of his own psychological universe. He feels he is controlling his environment. Nevertheless, even if his parents attempt to gratify all of his needs as quickly as possible, thereby maintaining his narcissistic state, frustration is inevitable. Reality forces him to modify his initial picture of the world and to accept his actual helplessness and dependency on others. This is a normal developmental process, but it also provides the template for future depressions. As an adult, a challenge to the patient's self-esteem re-creates the feelings of the infant who realizes that he needs his mother and discovers that she is not available, triggering a depressive reaction.

The primordial mental state of the infant does not yet include an awareness of self. The infant's experiences are regulated by the mother's biorhythms, voice, movements, and so on, starting *in utero*. The mother–infant bond already begins before their earliest contact. As the infant's sense of self begins to develop, it soon involves some recognition that although he may be helpless, as long as his mother is available, his needs are gratified and his life is secure. Separation from mother is the most dangerous possible threat. Clinical studies suggest that depression-like pictures appear in infants who are separated from their mothers as early as the second half of the first year of life. These infantile depressions result from the separation from a love object, which leads to a threat to security with which the infant cannot cope by himself. His primitive notions of object constancy and of time leave him uncertain that this threat will ever end. If mother does not appear, he first becomes anxious; if this does not elicit caretaking, he soon becomes helpless, apathetic, and fails to thrive.

This primordial depressive state is complicated by further developmental experiences. The child's oral fantasies include incorporative and destructive components. Making the mother part of himself involves cannibalistic or symbiotic impulses that threaten her continued existence as a separate individual. The child becomes fearful that his need for her will lead to her destruction. This mixture of dependent love and hostile aggression is the beginning of the ambivalent relation to objects that characterizes the depressive individual.

There is a developmental pressure for mastery and independence, initially of the infant's neuromuscular apparatus and later of his emotions. Family pressures may also push toward the denial of dependency desires and the achievement of competence and independence. However, his craving for security and warmth from parent figures continues. The child develops close psychological ties to his parents and loved ones, in effect making them part of himself. They become internalized sources of love, but also inner critics and censors, and the patient's ambivalence continues in relation to these introjected objects. When this pattern has been laid down, subsequent losses are followed by sadness, grief, and the internalization of the lost object. One of the earliest psychodynamic models of depression suggested that when the lost object was regarded with particularly intense ambivalent feelings, grief was more likely to turn into depression.

When the parental introject is harsh and critical, the patient has little joy in life and is prone to depression. His superego is punitive and sadistic, stemming from both the incorporation of demanding and perfectionistic parents and his own aggressive fantasies. He allows himself little pleasure and measures his performance to determine whether he has lived up to his inner standards, finding himself lacking. Life is an examination, and if he takes time to enjoy himself, he feels guilty and knows that he will fail. Self-esteem depends on a combination of support from his own internal objects, maintenance of his adaptive capacity, and protection from unusual demands or expectations from others. If the balance among these is fragile, recurrent disruptions are inevitable, and life becomes a series of depressions.

MANAGEMENT OF THE INTERVIEW

The interview with the depressed patient requires active participation by the interviewer. The patient wants to be taken care of, and it is often helpful for the interviewer to do so by providing the structure for the interview as well as to gratify the patient's dependent needs in other ways. It is not enough to help this patient to help himself; he wants more, and subtly or overtly he communicates this to the interviewer. The very nature of his illness makes him pessimistic about the outcome of treatment, and he is more likely to be a passive observer than a willing partner. In addition, his characteristic patterns of relating lead to technical problems in the interview. The clinician must make strategic decisions concerning the mode of therapy earlier than is necessary with most other patients, and he may have to do so while feeling that an error could be not only antitherapeutic but disastrous.

This section considers the chronological development of the interview with the depressed patient, his initial presentation, problems in communication, and the exploration of symptoms, including suicidal thoughts. Some basic principles of psychotherapy are presented, with particular emphasis on their early impact on the patient. The interview with the family of the depressed patient and the characteristic transference and countertransference problems that emerge in interviews with depressed patients are also discussed.

Initial Presentation

The seriously depressed patient usually does not come to the clinician's office alone. He lacks the energy and initiative to get there, and his friends and family feel sorry for him because he seems unwilling or unable to care for himself. When the clinician enters the waiting room, it is the friend or relative who looks up first, greets the clinician, and introduces the patient, who may observe what is happening but does not participate unless invited. The person who has accompanied the patient often speaks to the clinician as though the patient were unable to communicate. The daughter of an elderly depressed woman started by saying, "I guess I'd better do the talking. My mother is hard of hearing, and she doesn't like to talk anyway." The patient's companion expresses the urgent wish that the clinician do something to find out what is the matter. This introduction emphasizes the patient's role as an incapacitated person, an attitude that the clinician should avoid reinforcing. The clinician should arrange to speak to the patient both with and without the companion during the initial interview. Important data concerning the precipitants of the problem, suicidal communications, and the severity of the depression are often obtained from the third party.

The less severely depressed patient may come alone, but his posture, grooming, facial expression, movements, and the physical qualities of his voice reveal his problem before he has completed his first sentence. Initially, the patient's sadness and gloom are usually most obvious, but his anger may also emerge in the interview. His dependent attitude is reflected by his asking for instructions before selecting a chair. The clinician is advised to respond realistically to such a request and to avoid interpreting its deeper meaning, because this patient would experience any such interpretation as a rebuff and rejection.

Some patients conceal their depression, and the first suggestion of the patient's condition comes from the interviewer's own empathic response. This type of response is discussed later, under "Transference and Countertransference."

As the interview continues, the severely depressed patient will wait for the clinician to speak first. He lacks spontaneity and may stare blankly into space or down at the floor. With this patient it is preferable to begin the interview by commenting on his retardation and lowering of mood rather than routinely inquiring about his reason for seeking help. This nonverbal behavior has already provided a chief complaint. The interviewer can translate this into words by saying, "You seem quite depressed."

The patient is slow in answering, and his replies are brief and repetitious, revealing the constriction of his thought processes. In addition, his remarks are either complaining or self-flagellating and are often worded in a rhetorical fashion; for example, "I can't go on; I'm no good to anyone. Why must I suffer like this?" The clinician replies, "I know you feel badly, but if I can learn more about it, perhaps I will be able to help." This patient answers, "What's the use? Nothing can be done for me." The patient has stated his feeling, and the clinician can show concern and continue with the interview. He might ask, "How did it begin?"

The clinician's general manner should be serious and concerned, supporting the patient's mood rather than challenging it. Cheery or humorous comments, too rapid or energetic a pace, or even a smile may give the patient the feeling that the clinician will not tolerate his gloom. The entire interview will be slow, and the clinician must allow extra time for the patient to respond.

The patient with a milder or masked depression may speak spontaneously and will respond to the interviewer's initial inquiry. He often begins with a comment on his emotional pain or a time when things were different and better. He might say, "I don't feel like my old self anymore," or "I've lost interest in everything." At times the patient's self-deprecating tendencies will appear in his first words, as they did with the woman who said, "I feel so old and ugly." It is important to recognize that the patient who says "I don't feel like my old self" has not yet described his feelings. The depressed patient wants to express his unhappiness, and the clinician must provide an opportunity for this before exploring his healthier state. After he has elicited the patient's description of his depression, he can ask, "What were things like before you became depressed?" or "What was your old self?"

The withdrawn, depressed patient does not become emotionally engaged with the interviewer. His outward participation seems marginal to his inner thoughts and feelings, and he may sit staring at the floor, answering questions monosyllabically in a voice that suggests reflex responses. This barrier is extremely difficult to overcome, and continuing with routine queries about the patient's symptoms or his living arrangements will only heighten it. The clinician can start by calling attention to the problem, saying, "Talking seems to be a great effort for you." The patient's conscious desire to be cooperative and agreeable is already demonstrated by his attempt to answer questions, and he may be able to participate more fully if he senses the clinician's sympathetic interest. On rare occasions, sharing silence with the patient will be helpful, but depressed people usually experience the interviewer's silence as a form of disinterest, dissatisfaction, or frustration.

Exploration of Depressive Symptoms

The clinician reaches out more than halfway in the first interview with the depressed patient. The patient is more comfortable when the interviewer leads him, and it is important for the clinician to organize the interview and to provide the patient with continual support and approval for his participation.

If the clinician adopts a passive attitude in an attempt to promote a more active role for the patient, the patient will feel lost, abandoned, frustrated, and, finally, more depressed. On the other hand, if the clinician gives the patient the feeling that, by answering questions, he is doing a good job, the interview will be therapeutic from the start.

The clinician must accept the patient's slowed sense of time in pacing the interview. The interval between comments is longer than usual, and topics that are usually discussed in the first few minutes of contact may be delayed for many hours. If the patient becomes unable to talk or loses the thread, the clinician can sympathize, review what has occurred so far, and try to continue at a slower pace.

Depressed people often cry. This is particularly true with the moderately depressed person early in the course of the illness. The more severely or more chronically depressed patient cries less. If the patient cries openly, the clinician waits sympathetically, perhaps offering a tissue. However, if the patient seems to ignore his own tears, the interviewer can refer to them, encouraging the patient to accept his feelings. A quiet

"You are crying" or "What is it you feel bad about?" is usually suffi-cient. Sometimes a patient tries to conceal his crying. The clinician can comment on this without challenging or interpreting it by asking, "Are you trying not to cry?" The interviewer permits the emotional display and treats it as an appropriate means of expressing feeling. He gently continues the interview when the patient seems able to participate; waiting too long can lead to further tears without any feeling of under-standing, and proceeding too rapidly may leave the patient feeling that the clinician has no interest or patience. If the patient looks up at the interviewer or gets out his handkerchief in order to blow his nose, it is usually time to continue.

The patient has established dependent relations with other individuals, and it is helpful to explore these early in the interview. Disruption of such a relationship is a common precipitant of depressive symptoms, and the pattern that they follow is indicative of the transference that may be antic-ipated. For example, the interviewer asked a depressed woman, "Who are the important people in your life?" She replied, "I'm all alone now. I moved to the city last year when I realized that I was in love with my boss and that nothing could come of it. He was married and had a family." The clinician has acquired information about a possible precipitating cause and might anticipate that similar feelings will develop in the therapeutic relationship.

The depressed patient may begin by talking about how unhappy he feels, or he may discuss what he sees as the cause of his unhappiness. For example, one patient said, "I can't stand it any longer—what's the use in trying? Nobody cares anyway." Another tearfully related how she had learned that her husband was having an affair. The clinician can accept the patient's initial emphasis, but later in the interview it is nec-essary to explore other aspects of the problem. A middle-aged woman explained, "My life is over. My husband discovered that I was seeing another man. He became enraged and threw me out. Neither of my chil-dren will talk to me, and I have nowhere to go." The interviewer asked how this had come about. She explained, "My lover is my high school sweetheart. I hadn't seen him since we went to different colleges, but last fall I tried to contact my best friend from high school. I couldn't find her, but I discovered his phone number and decided to call him." The theme of searching for a lost object from her past was pervasive—along with her despair at the emotional emptiness of her current life, and par-ticularly of her marriage. The interviewer commented, "It seems that the acute crisis may only be the tip of the iceberg—that the depression you have been fending off for years is much greater than what has devel-oped this week." The patient came to agree, and within a few sessions she stated, "In many ways this has been a godsend. I don't know how it will be resolved, but at least we are talking about what we avoided for so long. I am in pain, but for the first time in years I feel like I am alive."

Physical Symptoms

Although the depressed person may not relate his physical symptoms to his psychological problems, he is usually quite concerned about them, willing to discuss them, and grateful for any advice or assistance that the clinician may have to offer. Frequently the interviewer must actively pursue them, because the patient does not think they will be of interest. For example, a man sought psychiatric assistance for his depressed feelings after his divorce but neglected any mention of his insomnia and weight loss. When he was asked about disturbances of sleep, appetite, sexual drive, and so forth, the patient realized that these all formed part of a complex illness that the clinician had seen before. This raised the patient's hopes and enhanced his confidence in the clinician. At times the patient may not realize that he has had a change in physical functioning until the clinician inquires directly about it, and he may deny the extent of its impact unless detailed data are obtained. For example, a 50-year-old man with a moderately severe depression did not spontaneously mention sexual difficulties. When he was asked, he replied, "I'm not as interested in sex as I used to be, but of course I am getting older." The interviewer persisted, "When was the last time you had contact with a woman?" The patient somewhat reluctantly disclosed, "It is almost a year." The clinician inquired further, and the patient reported, "My wife has been troubled by menopausal symptoms and is afraid to take hormones. She feels that I want sex for my own pleasure, without any concern about her. Maybe she is right. At any rate, the problem is solved for now." It took time to get to his anger and resentment that she was indifferent to his feeling of rejection and abandonment. He had treated his loss of libido as a sign of aging in order to avoid facing the marital conflict from which it protected him.

The discussion of physical symptoms provides an opportunity for exploring the patient's style of coping with problems and their impact on himself and his family. If the clinician merely obtains a catalogue of physical complaints, this opportunity is lost, and the patient will feel that the focus is on establishing a diagnosis rather than understanding him. For example, a middle-aged depressed man said, "I haven't been able to sleep in weeks." The interviewer asked, "Is the trouble falling asleep, getting up during the night, or both?" The patient replied, "I seem to be able to go to sleep, but I wake up every morning at 4:30 or so, and I lie in bed and can't go back to sleep." The interviewer inquired further, "What goes through your mind when you are awake in bed?" The patient responded, "I worry about my business, how badly it is doing, and how I've let my family down. My wife blames me for not being able to help the boys get started." The interviewer continued, "Do you do anything to help you get back to sleep?" The patient, somewhat reluctantly, admitted, "I get up and make myself a glass of scotch mixed with milk. It makes me less tense, but then I worry because I drink too much and maybe I should be more careful. If my wife knew what I was doing, she would kill me." The interviewer has delineated the patient's sleep pattern but has also done much more. He has gotten to know him better; learned about his marriage, family, business, and substance abuse; and helped the patient feel listened to and understood in the process.

The depressed patient who is preoccupied with physical symptoms fears that they may be manifestations of a serious physical illness. If the clinician inquires about these symptoms and makes no further comment about them, the patient is likely to become more alarmed. A simple "That problem is common when someone is depressed" or "That will get better as you start to feel like your old self" is often reassuring.

The interviewer does more than elicit the description of the patient's symptoms and their impact on the patient's life; he also provides the patient with some understanding concerning their relation to his psychological problems. If the patient is severely depressed, this will be deferred until later interviews, but even then the clinician can lay the groundwork in his initial inquiry into the symptomatology. For example, in speaking with the depressed man who had lost his sexual interest, the interviewer inquired, "How did you feel toward your wife during this period of time?" This apparently simple question suggests that the patient's loss of sexual interest not only is a physiological side effect of his depression but also is related to his emotional reactions to important people in his life.

The depressed person is likely to discuss his hypochondriacal feelings as he does everything else, in a hopeless and self-demeaning way. One woman sighed and said, "I guess it's all my change of life. I'm just getting old and withered." A man suggested, "My bowels just don't work anymore. They're making me weak all over and giving me terrible headaches. It's affecting my whole body." Further exploration revealed that he was convinced that he had or was about to develop rectal cancer, a conviction that was later traced to his childhood misinterpretation of his father's recurrent complaints of hemorrhoids. The interviewer commented, "Worrying about bowels and what bowel problems might mean goes all the way back to childhood for you. When you saw that you were having bowel trouble, thoughts of your father and of cancer must have seemed natural."

The Need for Active Inquiry

The depressed patient actively tries to conceal some aspects of his behavior from the clinician. The most prominent of these is aggression. The man mentioned earlier who became depressed after his divorce was able to discuss his mood and his physical symptoms in considerable detail. Nevertheless, it was a later session before he revealed his violent temper outbursts, which had contributed to his wife's decision to leave. When he finally described them, he quickly became tearful and began to berate himself for driving his wife away.

It is often easy for the experienced clinician to ascertain that a patient is depressed, to evaluate the depth of the depression, and to trace the clinical picture through the precipitating events in the patient's life to the underlying premorbid personality. In general, one of the most valuable allies in exploring a patient's life is his interest in and curiosity about anything he might learn about himself. However, this may be difficult with the depressed patient, whose preoccupation with himself centers on feelings of guilt and blame. He has little interest in broadening his self-knowledge, because he anticipates that each discovery will only confirm his inadequacy and unworthiness. In addition, he lacks the energy necessary for a project of self-discovery. This means that the interviewer has to assume a larger than usual share of responsibility in mobilizing the patient's motivation. Interpretations around the patient's defensive lack of interest in understanding his problems are generally ineffective and will be perceived only as criticism and rejection.

The so-called parallel history is frequently valuable. After obtaining the chronology of the illness, the interviewer inquires about the rest of the patient's life and develops a longitudinal picture of the patient's experiences during the period in which the illness developed. Links that are obviously important and that were not mentioned by the patient are common. For example, a middle-aged woman who was mildly depressed said, "I have no right to feel so bad. I have no real problems." Later, in describing her recent life, she revealed that her youngest daughter had left for college and that she had moved to a new apartment shortly before she began to get depressed. The interviewer later said, "It must be lonely with your daughter gone." This comment has the effect of an interpretation, but it is gentler and less disturbing to the patient than a direct confrontation, such as "You must have been more upset about moving and your daughter going off by herself than you realized."

The clinician notes to himself that the patient's reaction of severe loneliness reveals problems in her relations with her husband and friends, but he avoids commenting on this early in the interview. In retrospect, he is also aware that her initial denial—"no real problems"—reveals that she has some beginning insight into her difficulty, but she does not feel entitled to respond in the way that she has. It is common for the depressed person initially to deny knowledge of the precipitant of his depression and later, when questioned, to claim that it is too minor or trivial a problem to justify so serious a reaction. The patient is ashamed of what he feels is a weakness and tries to conceal it.

Another example is the businessman who complained of several months of mild depression, with no awareness of the precipitant. Later, when discussing his occupational history, he mentioned that his immediate superior recently announced his retirement and that the patient was asked to replace him. When this was explored further, it became apparent that the patient began to feel depressed shortly after he learned of his pending promotion. This paradoxical response resulted from the patient's guilty reaction to having been chosen over his competitors as well as his fear that he was not adequate and that the promotion would result in his failure.

Discussion of Suicide in the Interview

The discussion of suicide is crucial in gauging the severity and danger of the patient's depression and is essential to enlist the patient's participation in planning a treatment program. It also offers a unique but often overlooked opportunity for understanding the basic structure of the patient's personality.

The experienced interviewer knows that the discussion of suicidal thoughts aimed at increasing understanding of the patient is often the most effective therapeutic measure against suicidal impulses. The clinician tries to help the patient to gain insight into the meaning of his suicidal wishes and to express the same emotions in the interview that would be represented by a suicidal act. This enables the patient's own controls to operate more effectively and reduces the pressure he experiences to end his own life. Often the clinician's concern and his response to the urgency of the situation are themselves therapeutic. A common sequence is illustrated by the young woman who came to a hospital emergency room because she was thinking of jumping off a bridge. An inexperienced first-year resident spoke with her and felt that immediate hospitalization was imperative. The patient objected, but he told her that there was a definite risk and insisted that she accept his plan. He then summoned a more experienced colleague, who arrived to find the patient comfortable, in relatively good spirits, and convinced that her suicidal thought could not possibly lead to any overt behavior. The patient's statements seemed convincing to both physicians, and she was sent home to return for an appointment the following day. The young resident was thoroughly confused and felt that he had missed some basic feature of the case. In fact, both clinicians' initial impressions were accurate: The younger resident's response had been highly therapeutic, and his interest and concern had supported the patient through an acute crisis.

Suicidal behavior is a final common pathway growing out of many types of thoughts, fantasies, and impulses. The clinician inquires about suicide from two points of view. First he wants to know how seriously the patient has considered it, what plans he contemplated, what steps he has taken toward actualizing them, and his attitude toward these impulses. These questions consider the way in which the patient treats the idea of killing himself. At the same time, the clinician inquires into the meaning of suicide to this specific person. What are the unconscious significances of the suicidal act? What is its expressive or communicative function? For example, a woman in her 50s came to see a psychiatrist because of multiple somatic symptoms that several physicians had told her were psychological in origin. She cried during the first interview, saying, "Why does it all have to happen to me? I haven't slept for days; all I do is cry. Doesn't anyone care? Won't anyone do something?" She admitted that she was depressed but insisted that this was a reaction to her physical problems, not the reverse. The clinician asked her, "Have you ever thought of suicide?" She replied, "Yes, sometimes I think that it's the only way out, but I know that I'd never do anything like that." She had spontaneously provided a clue to the basic meaning of suicide to her (a "way out") and her current attitude toward it (a thought that she could contemplate but not act upon). However, the clinician knew from other material in the interview that she tended to be impulsive, so he inquired further, "Have you ever felt that you might do something like that?" She hesitated and then replied, "Well, yes, once. My back pains got so bad I felt it must be cancer, and before I went to see the doctor, I promised myself that if it turned out to be the worst, I would spare both myself and my family the pain." The patient had again suggested that suicide is an escape from certain problems, and she had given a suggestion as to the kind of problems she had in mind. At the same time, it was clear that the controls that were apparently effective at that moment might break down if she felt that severe pain and sickness were imminent. She had also provided the clinician with an important clue as to a route for therapeutic intervention in this area should it later be necessary; she wanted to spare her family any suffering. He asked, "How would it affect your family?" and the patient started crying again. Between tears she explained, "My husband and I live with my mother. My brother died in the war, and I am the only one she has left. She needs me." In this episode the clinician learned something of the patient's attitude toward suicide and the meaning it had for her and enlarged his view of her as a person. It became clear that there was no immediate suicidal risk, but he had some knowledge of the circumstances in which such a risk might appear (including not only a change in her condition but also her mother's death) and the steps that would be required to prevent such an occurrence.

Experienced clinicians always introduce the subject of suicide into the interview with a depressed patient. The beginner fears that he may give the patient an idea or that the patient may take offense at the question. A carefully phrased but direct inquiry such as "Have you thought of taking your own life?" or "Have you felt that you want to kill yourself?" can be of great value even if the answer is "No." It shows the mildly depressed person that the clinician takes his problem quite seriously, and it can lead to a discussion of the positive features of his life, his hope for the future, and his areas of healthy functioning.

Every depressed patient has considered suicide, even if only to reject it. In fact, it is the rare individual who has not thought of the idea of suicide at some moment in his life, but most people do not realize this. They are ashamed and want to hide what they think are strange feelings. A simple direct question about suicide can alleviate this anxiety. If the clinician treats the subject as serious but not bizarre, the patient will feel less ashamed. The patient can also be helped to trace the historical development of his ideas about suicide, giving him more sense of continuity with his past experiences. For example, when a patient indicates that he has been considering suicide, the clinician can at some point inquire, "Have you ever thought of suicide in the past?" If the patient answers "No," the clinician can pursue this further, saying, "What were your feelings concerning the idea of suicide?" This shift from "suicide" to "the idea of suicide" allows a shift in the patient's mind from admitting impulses to contemplating abstract ideas. The patient may reply, "It always seemed horrible to me, such a cowardly thing to do." This will allow the clinician to inquire as to when the patient first had these thoughts, what his mental image of suicide is, and how it developed. Suicidal feelings do not arise *de novo* in adult life but can be traced to earlier roots: important figures who talked about killing themselves or about the advantages of death and family attitudes to which the patient was exposed as a child. For example, one woman revealed that her mother frequently said, "Someday it will all be over," obviously looking forward to death. Another patient's mother would say, "Someday I'll be gone and then you'll be sorry for how you treated me." The discussion of suicide can help to reveal the origins of the patient's problems in his earlier life.

The average person who has suicidal thoughts and comes to see a clinician is intensely ambivalent and struggling to control his behavior. The clinician allies himself with the healthy portion of the patient's ego and thereby keeps the conflict within the patient's mind rather than between the patient and the clinician. The clinician is concerned and involved but maintains his role of a neutral, understanding figure rather than immediately trying to convince the patient to act in a particular way. An anxious and uncertain patient responds to an authority trying to push him toward a specific course of action by pushing back. For example, if a patient indicates that he has considered killing himself and the clinician replies, "That wouldn't solve any of your problems," the patient is likely to reply with an argument. However, if after discussing the suicidal feelings the clinician asks, "What are the reasons that have kept you alive?" the patient will be presenting the arguments that restrain his impulses. When appropriate, the interviewer can inquire, "Have you considered the problems that you create for people you love and care about?" This opens another area for exploration and understanding.

For some individuals, death is not the end of life but only the entry into another state that may be more comfortable than this one. The patient anticipates gratification of dependent needs or the reunion with lost loved ones. This kind of denial and magical thinking is reinforced by popular myths and religious beliefs. Some patients offer these beliefs as rationalizations in favor of suicide. In treating such patients, the clinician should not challenge the patient's conviction of life after death. Rather, he explores the prohibitions against suicide that are usually associated with such beliefs and the patient's own doubt and ambivalence. It is helpful to inquire into the immediate reason for the patient's plan and to point out that because his philosophical views have been long-standing, some more concrete event must have led to his suicidal thought. For example, a middle-aged woman became severely depressed after her husband was killed in an automobile accident. She spoke of killing herself and said, "When I think that I could be with him again, I feel alive!" She had been active in a Fundamentalist religious sect and believed in a concrete life after death, and her suicidal feelings were combined with near-delusional episodes in which she felt that she communicated with his soul. The clinician did not challenge her religious beliefs, or even her communication with the dead, but rather asked her what she felt her husband would have wanted her to do and what course of action her religion prescribed. The patient was able to give up her idea of suicide with the feeling that she was honoring her husband's wishes.

PRINCIPLES OF TREATMENT

The treatment of depressed patients aims at two fundamental goals. First is the alleviation of suffering, anxiety, and painful affects, including guilt; the stimulation of hope; and protection from self-injury. Second is modifying both the biological and psychosocial context, with the aim of both resolving the immediate precipitant and preventing recurrence. Supportive psychotherapy, medication and other somatic therapies, and exploratory psychotherapy can be helpful in achieving each of these goals.

Supportive Psychotherapy

The first goal in the treatment of depression is to alleviate the patient's pain and suffering. This can be done by psychotherapeutic and/or pharmacological methods. The psychotherapist attempts to improve the patient's defensive functioning and provide substitute gratifications, enhancing denial, projection, repression, reaction formation, or whatever defenses are most effective in protecting the patient from his painful feelings. The therapist's patient and caring attitude allows the patient to lean on him emotionally as a replacement for the patient's lost love object, providing transference gratifications that temporarily substitute for the frustrations of reality.

The depressed patient feels hopeless and may have little motivation for treatment. Initially it may be necessary to stimulate and reinforce his hope and to seek out latent motivations where none seem readily apparent. When the patient can visualize a future in which he is not depressed, the clinician can begin to enhance the therapeutic alliance. The interviewer attempts to convey hope from the initial contact. For example, although a depressed college student reported that he had been unable to attend classes, the clinician carefully scheduled future appointments so that when the patient was ready to return, he would not have a time conflict with school. The message was that the clinician expected the patient to be able to resume his activities. In other situations, the clinician might advise the patient to defer an important decision "until you are feeling better." This phrase is used rather than "because you aren't up to it." The patient is told not only that he is sick but also that he will get well.

A related principle of treatment is the protection of the patient from self-injury. The most dramatic aspect of this is the prevention of suicide, but there are subtler forms of self-destructive behavior that are common in depressed patients. The law student who wants to quit school and obtain a lower-status job as a legal secretary and the businessperson who plans to relinquish an opportunity for promotion as a result of depression are both examples. Initially, the clinician's role is to identify the problem and use his authority to prevent the patient from doing serious or irreparable harm to himself. Later, he offers the patient insight into the meaning of this behavior and interprets its psychodynamic origins. For example, a woman who became depressed after her husband indicated that he planned to seek a divorce told her clinician, "What's the use; nobody cares about me anyway. I'm tired of working so hard for other people. I'm going to quit my job, and when I use up my money, I'll go on welfare." Her depression was mixed with conscious anger, which suggested a relatively good prognosis for the depressive symptoms. The clinician noted this and realized that once she left her job, she might have difficulty obtaining a comparable one. He told her, "You're angry at the world, but right now you're mad at yourself too. I'm afraid if you quit your job, you might suffer more than anyone else. Perhaps you should wait until we can talk about it more and you can decide exactly what will be in your best interest."

This type of intervention may create a problem, since the clinician does not want to assume responsibility for the patient's executive ego functioning, thereby diminishing the patient's self-confidence and self-esteem and adding to his depression. In order to minimize this, the clinician clarifies that his offering of direct advice is only a temporary role. For example, another woman sought psychiatric help after a separation from her husband. Her psychiatrist asked about the practical legal aspects of the impending separation. She said, "I told my husband to do whatever he wanted and just give me the papers to sign. I'm no good to anyone else; I might as well help him." The clinician indicated concern at her failure to protect her financial and legal interests, but she said she just did not care. He explored her feeling that she did not deserve anything and finally said, "It seems clear that you would be acting differently if you weren't depressed. I don't think you're ready to deal with the reality of the situation yet." If she had been less severely depressed, he might have explored her failure to act in her own best interests, uncovering her defensive inhibition of assertion.

In addition to stimulating the patient's hope and protecting him from self-injury, the clinician tries to reduce the patient's guilt by addressing the expiatory aspects of the patient's behavior. The suffering of depressive illness is associated with the unconscious hope that forgiveness will follow. If the interviewer comments, "You have suffered enough" or "You deserve a better life," he may be able to alleviate some of the patient's guilt.

Conscious guilt is often related to the secondary effects of depression. The patient may say, "I am such a bother to everyone. They'd be so much better off without me." He is guilty because he is unable to perform his work or provide for his loved ones. The clinician can reply, "You're sick. You've done so much for them; now it's their turn to take care of you." Occasionally it is necessary to invoke the patient's guilt about the anger that he unconsciously discharges through his symptomatology. This manipulation utilizes guilt about expressing aggressive impulses to help suppress depressive withdrawal and encourage the patient to function more adequately. For example, the clinician can say, "I understand that in your present condition you don't really care what happens to you, but your family still cares, and it causes them pain to see you suffer. Even if you can't make the necessary effort to feel better for yourself, think about doing it for your children." Even in the case of the depressed patient whose loved ones are deceased or otherwise absent, the interviewer can reach back into an earlier time in the patient's life to identify some loved one who now remains as an important person in this patient's past.

Although the depressed patient needs considerable support, he becomes uncomfortable if the interviewer is overly warm or friendly. He feels unworthy and is unable to reciprocate. Beginning psychotherapists are sometimes overeager in their expression of positive feelings. When their depressed patients withdraw, they become even nicer, with the result that the patient becomes even more anxious and guilty rather than comfortable. He may experience the therapist's positive support as an attempt to reassure him because he really is bad.

The use of humor is a problem in the interview with the depressive patient. If the patient demonstrates any remaining sense of humor, it is better to encourage and respond to this than for the clinician to initiate humorous interchanges himself. The depressed person is likely to respond to the clinician's spontaneous attempts at humor as evidence that he is misunderstood or even that he is being ridiculed.

The clinician often uses the term *depressed* when he summarizes the patient's description of his problem. He may offer it in his own formulation, saying, "It sounds as if you have been quite depressed for some months." This is in contrast to the frequent avoidance of diagnostic terms. The same clinician would not say, "You are suffering from hysterical symptoms." There are several reasons for this difference. One, which was discussed earlier, is the dual meaning of the term *depressed*, which refers both to a clinical syndrome and to a related affective state. Although it may be unusual for the clinician to employ diagnostic labels in the interview, he frequently identifies the patient's emotions, and "You seem depressed" may be seen as analogous to "You seem angry." However, this does not tell the whole story, because it is common for the clinician to say, "You are suffering from a depression," clearly referring to the clinical entity. The reason for this can be understood if we consider the principle behind the usual avoidance of diagnostic labels. Patients often employ such labels in order to support their projective defenses. Thus they claim, "There's nothing I can do about it; it's my neurosis," as though a neurosis were a foreign agent, such as a virus, that is the cause of their problems. An important issue in treatment is to help that patient to experience neurotic behavior as being under his control as a preliminary step to exploring methods of changing it. Any phraseology that suggests that the patient has a disease will work counter to this goal and will therefore be antitherapeutic.

With the depressed patient, and occasionally with some others, this problem is reversed. The patient not only accepts responsibility for his difficulties but also exaggerates his own role and tortures himself with guilt and self-condemnation. His self-accusations may also torture others or may conceal an underlying denial, but nevertheless the initial problem in treatment is often to dilute the patient's conviction that he is to blame. Phrases that suggest that he has an illness assist in this attempt. At the same time, the thought that the patient is sick suggests that he may get better and challenges the depressed person's view of his situation as hopeless and eternal.

Somatic Therapies

Pharmacological and other somatic treatments are important therapeutic methods. They are considered here only in terms of their impact on the interview. Regardless of their neurobiological mode of action, these treatments always have psychological meaning to the patient. The clinician may want to enhance this or interpret it, but he should keep it in mind. The placebo effect of medication can be increased if the clinician suggests that the pharmacological regimen is potent and will alleviate the patient's symptoms. It is preferable to encourage the patient to associate this placebo reaction to the treatment as a whole rather than to any specific drug, because it may be necessary to change medication during the course of therapy. The clinician can say, "We have several effective drugs, and we may want to switch from one to another." Comments such as "We'll see if this does any good, and if not, we'll try something else" dilute the placebo effect. If there is a latent period before the drug has a therapeutic effect, it is well to advise the patient in advance, or he will feel that the treatment is not working. The placebo reaction is a psychobiological response, and its effect on the patient is "real," including some of the same side effects as those of active drugs.

The patient may introduce the discussion of somatic treatment by questions such as "Is there any medication that could help me?" These questions often reflect the fantasy of intervention from an omnipotent external force in the form of either magical assistance or punishment. The clinician can learn more if he delays his reply and instead asks, "What did you have in mind?" One patient said, "I understand there are some new pills that will make this all go away." Another replied, "You can do anything you want to me if only it will help. I don't care if it has side effects." The first person was hoping for the intervention of a good parent, whereas the second had to atone for his sins before he could feel better. The clinician does not interpret these wishes early in the treatment, but nevertheless they are important. The first patient may well respond to psychological suggestions that the treatment will be potent and effective. The second experiences his depression as punishment, and excessive reassurance about the safety of the treatment might actually have a negative effect.

Electroconvulsive therapy (ECT) is an effective treatment for depression that is most often employed if the condition is unresponsive to medication and psychotherapy. It is occasionally discussed in interviews with depressed patients, because either the clinician or the patient has become aware of the patient's lack of therapeutic response. ECT is explained and discussed like any other form of therapy, but the clinician should recognize that the phrase "electric shock" implies magical power and danger. Patients often indicate fears of what this treatment will do to them, and they often unconsciously equate it with early traumatic experiences and physical punishment. In contrast, they usually have early life experiences with pills and medicines that lead to feelings of trust and security. The clinician can ask about the patient's fears. Pain, loss of memory, death, change of personality, and infantile regression are all common ones, and reassurances should be as specific as possible. The patient will feel more comfortable if he is prepared for what he will experience, such as the pretreatment injections. However, it is not helpful to discuss the technical details of the treatment that will not affect the patient's subjective experience. The patient should be prepared for the organic mental syndrome that follows, and the more matter-of-factly this is discussed, the more easily he will accept it.

When the clinician describes any somatic treatment, he should provide as clear and specific a statement as possible. He should discuss not only the practical aspects of the regimen but also the anticipated therapeutic effects. For example, it is preferable to say "These pills will help your spirits to improve" rather than "This should help the problem." There are aspects of depression that are not helped by drugs, and it may be helpful to spell these out. The clinician can say, "Of course the medicine won't help you get your husband back" or "The pills will help you feel better, and then you will be able to deal with the financial problem more effectively." The patient will feel more self-confidence and self-esteem if he sees the treatment as enabling him to solve his own problems rather than having to rely on the clinician to resolve them for him.

Exploratory Psychotherapy: Interpretation of Psychodynamic Patterns

If the patient is severely depressed or so despondent that he is unable to talk to the interviewer or to participate in the routine of everyday life, the only psychological treatment is supportive. In the interview, the clinician will listen to the patient's concerns and will try to reassure him about his fears. He will search for islands of adaptive functioning that are relatively intact and try to focus on them, expressing little interest in the developmental roots of the patient's character if the patient himself is not preoccupied with them. For some patients, this type of therapy is adequate to eradicate depressive symptomatology, and there may be no motivation or indication for deeper psychotherapy.

For those patients who are to be treated in exploratory psychotherapy, the clinician shifts his basic clinical strategy after the immediate crisis is under control, although always recognizing the risk of transiently aggravating the symptoms. This approach in the treatment of depressed patients requires more active participation on the patient's part. Unlike the first mode of treatment, which is aimed at alleviating symptoms, it offers the possibility of influencing the course of the patient's life, possibly decreasing the likelihood of future depressions and moderating his depressive character pathology. Clarifications and interpretations are designed to explore the unconscious psychodynamic factors that maintain the symptoms. The clinician interprets the defenses in order to uncover thoughts and feelings that the patient is trying to avoid.

In the initial interview with the depressed patient, the interviewer may offer interpretive comments that are designed to test the patient's ability to deal with insight. For example, a middle-aged man became depressed after moving to a new city. He told the clinician of his wife's unhappiness with the new community, his children's difficulty in adjusting to their new school, and his constant rumination that everything had been fine until he uprooted their home because of his professional ambition. His wife had refused to furnish or decorate their new home. He finally broke down crying and said, "If there were only some way to escape, to get away from it all. I just can't take any more." The clinician listened and then said, "You must get pretty angry with her." The patient immediately began to berate himself, saying, "I've been an awful husband. My whole family is upset, and it is all my fault." The clinician's interpretation was accurate, but the patient's response revealed that at this point, his reaction to such knowledge was to become even more depressed. The clinician decided that even this tentative exploration of the patient's repressed rage should be deferred until later in the treatment.

At times, what the clinician thinks of as uncovering exploratory therapy is experienced by the patient as supportive. One common pattern observed in the interview with the depressed patient is for the patient to start slowly, have difficulty talking, and seem somewhat retarded. As the clinician reaches out, inquires about symptoms, and explores the origins of the patient's difficulties, the patient becomes livelier and more animated, participates well, and seems to search actively for the meaning of his behavior and to explore it in the interview. The clinician feels pleased and reassured and then tells the patient that the interview is drawing to a close. The patient lapses back into hopeless gloom; the insight of a moment earlier has become irrelevant. He was responding to the supportive relationship implicit in the interview process, and the content of the uncovered material was of little therapeutic significance.

The psychodynamic aspects of depression are often apparent to the interviewer long before awareness of them can be of any conceivable value to the patient. Beginning clinicians are often eager to practice interpreting, and when something is clear to them, they want to share it with the patient. The depressed person provides a willing audience. He is glad to listen and rarely challenges what the clinician says. However, the therapist must remember that insight is a means, not an end, in treatment. If the patient uses the clinician's comments to verify that he is worthless, the clinician is interpreting prematurely, no matter how accurate and insightful his observations. Denial is an important defense against depressive feelings, and interpretations of denial may work counter to supportive therapy.

The tendency of depressed or masochistic patients to take the clinician's interpretation and use it as a weapon against themselves has been termed a "negative therapeutic reaction." When it becomes a problem in the interview, the clinician either alters his interpretative approach or tries to deal with the patient's response as a form of resistance. He might say, "You seem to search for evidence that you're bad."

Direct interpretations of the patient's anger are more likely to be disturbing than supportive. However, euphemistic phrases such as "You are very disappointed in him" may be acceptable. The clinician takes care not to challenge the patient's right to feel the way he does. Usually this neutrality will be interpreted as active support for the patient's feeling. Some therapists have been taught that depression results from anger directed against the self and therefore openly encourage the patient to direct anger at key figures in his life. Although this is occasionally effective, the results are often disastrous, because the patient becomes frightened that his controls may not be effective and that all of the dangers that he fears from expressing his rage will occur. The result is commonly a loss of confidence in the clinician and a flight from treatment, especially when a spouse says, "I think I liked you better depressed."

The patient who raises the question of a chemical or hormonal basis of his depression is usually challenging the clinician's discussion of psychological factors or attempting to deny them. The patient feels that it is bad to be depressed, that somehow it is his fault, and he feels less culpable if he can find a physical cause. His desire to defend himself from feeling that he is to blame for his troubles is a positive sign and should not be challenged by the clinician. If the patient is utilizing biological explanations in the service of psychological denial, the overall strategy of therapy should determine whether this is to be interpreted or supported. Usually, rather than interpreting this as a defense, the clinician simply indicates that there is no contradiction between the psychological meaning of the patient's depression and any physical basis that it might have. This explanation must be adjusted to the patient's level of sophistication. For example, a relatively uneducated person who has asked if he might just be run-down physically could be told, "There is no question that you feel run-down, and that is part of your problem. At the same time, I think you are worried and upset about what has happened and feel disappointed in yourself. I suspect that makes things worse." It is useful to explain to the patient that he has been under stress and that stress has both a physical and a mental component, that it affects both his body and his personal feelings.

The preceding discussion of psychotherapy has been relatively superficial, but as mentioned earlier, this is intended to counteract the tendency of beginning clinicians to go too deep, too fast, in treating depressed patients. Major clinical improvement and extensive diagnostic information are often obtained by a simple supportive approach.

Interviewing the Family

Family members of the depressed patient are often seen by the clinician, whether they accompany the patient to the initial interview or come later in treatment. They may be sympathetic and concerned about the patient, angry with him, or more often both, although one emotion may be concealed. The clinician is interested in obtaining information from the family, in modifying their behavior as part of the treatment for the patient, and in exploring the interaction between the patient and his family.

A few clinical illustrations may highlight some characteristic problems.

A female adolescent sought help because she was despondent and contemplating suicide following the disruption of her relationship with a boyfriend. A psychiatrist advised treatment, but she was sure that her parents, who lived in another city, would refuse to support such a plan. The psychiatrist offered to see them, and the patient called a few days later, saying that her mother was coming to the city, and arranged an appointment. When the mother arrived, she was obviously angry at both the patient and the psychiatrist. She started the interview by speaking of the overindulgence of contemporary adolescents and the need for willpower and self-discipline with respect to emotional disturbances. The clinician asked, "What has your daughter told you about our talk?" The mother replied that the girl had described the disruption of her relationship with her boyfriend, her subsequent visit to the psychiatrist, and their extensive discussion about suicide. "Furthermore," she added, "I think it's terrible that you talked to her so much about suicide. You're likely to put ideas into her head." The clinician half-turned toward the patient while asking her mother, "Did she tell you why we talked so much about suicide?"

At this point the patient interrupted, sobbing loudly, and telling her mother for the first time of a suicide attempt she had made some months earlier. The effect was dramatic; the mother was insistent that the clinician arrange for immediate treatment and questioned him about the advisability of the girl remaining in school. This concern had been concealed by the mother's need to deny her daughter's difficulty, but the clinician had enlisted the girl's aid in a confrontation that had broken through her mother's denial. At the same time, the clinician had challenged the girl's distorted image of her parents' attitude toward her welfare and had laid the groundwork for later interpretations concerning the patient's role in their apparent indifference to her difficulties.

A depressed middle-aged woman was accompanied to the initial interview by her husband, a successful attorney. He spoke of his concern about her condition and bewilderment about what to do. He said that she had been so worried that he felt that she needed a rest, a vacation, and urged the clinician to prescribe one. He made it clear that money was no object where his wife's health was concerned. At the same time, he indicated that business pressures made it impossible for him to go with her. His wife sat through this discussion silently, staring at the floor. The clinician responded by turning to her and asking, "Do you feel he's trying to get rid of you?" The husband protested vehemently; his wife looked up with a flicker of interest. Later, when speaking to the husband alone, the clinician was able to explore his conscious irritations and dissatisfactions with his wife, which he had concealed lest he aggravate her problems. When the interviewer again pointed out the hostility that had emerged in the husband's therapeutic suggestion, he became quite distraught. He then revealed that he was having an affair with another woman and that much of his anger at his wife covered feelings of guilt that he was the cause of her problem. When these were discussed, his attitude shifted to a more realistic acceptance of her illness. He was still dissatisfied and angry with her, but no longer angry because she was sick.

It is not unusual for the family to provide crucial information concerning precipitants or stresses in the patient's life that the patient has not revealed in the early interviews. One middle-aged man said that there were no problems at home, but later, when his wife came in with him, she revealed that their son was flunking out of high school. The patient interrupted, saying that he felt that his wife was exaggerating the problem, but when it was discussed more fully, it became apparent that he had refused to accept it.

In each of these episodes, the clinician's interview with the family served to facilitate treatment. Members of the patient's family had developed fixed attitudes that contributed to the patient's difficulties and that were perpetuated in part because the patient was unable to question or confront them. The clinician assumed the role that would otherwise be played by the patient's healthy ego and thus reversed a vicious cycle that had contributed to the depression and the increasing rigidity of the family conflict.

The family of the depressed person may prefer that he remain depressed. This is often related to the patient's inhibition of aggression and his masochistic willingness to tolerate his family's exploitation. If this is the case, they will be opposed to any treatment that threatens to lead to change, and the clinician will find that they are more accepting of a poor prognosis and a stable hopeless situation. This may provide an indication for family therapy. It is not unusual for this family to interfere with treatment just as the patient shows signs of improvement.

Depressed people feel deprived and rejected, even without a realistic basis. It is usually an error for the clinician who is treating a depressed person to treat another member of the patient's family, because it will contribute to the patient's feeling of rejection and deprivation. Of course, this does not apply to family sessions that include the patient, which may be helpful in treatment.

TRANSFERENCE AND COUNTERTRANSFERENCE

In response to his feeling of helplessness, the depressed patient may develop a clinging, dependent relationship, with the expectation that his therapist has the magical omnipotent power to effect a cure. He tries to extract nurturant care through his suffering, cajoling, or coercing the clinician into helping him. He may become openly angry or more depressed if he fails at this attempt. This mixture of dependency and anger characterizes the transference. On the surface he is hopeless, but his unconscious hope is revealed by his feeling that the clinician has the capacity to help him.

The patient's dependent feelings emerge as he reveals his inability to make even simple decisions. Usually he does not directly ask for the clinician's help, but his obvious helplessness elicits the clinician's sympathy and concern. Without realizing it, the clinician may find that he is guiding not only the interview but also the patient's life and that he is, implicitly or explicitly, offering advice about practical problems, family relationships, or anything else. Silent requests for the clinician's aid are often combined with tributes to his wisdom and experience. For example, a young woman said, "I don't know whether to call the guy I had coffee with last Saturday. I wish I could make my own decisions, like you do." The therapist was placed in the position of either suggesting a course of action or depriving her of valuable advice and guidance. If he declines to give advice, saying, "I think that you should make that decision yourself, but we can certainly discuss it" or "I don't know what you should do, but let's talk about the questions you have about it in your own mind," the patient reacts as though she were deprived and rejected. She feels that the therapist could provide direct help but for some reason has refused. On the other hand, if the clinician did make a suggestion, it is common for new information to emerge that makes it clear that it is wrong. For example, if the therapist says, "Well, you seemed to like him Saturday," the patient might reply, "Good, I'm glad you said that. I wasn't sure, because my roommate said he has taken advantage of every girl in town." The therapist is now on the spot: Does he withdraw his statement, explore the patient's withholding of critical data, or simply keep quiet? None of these alternatives is satisfactory; the first leaves the patient wondering whether the therapist feels inadequate, the second is experienced as an attack, and the third creates the danger that the patient will accept the clinician's suggestion and further escalate the problem.

This pattern reveals the close relation between the patient's dependency feelings and her anger. She wants something, but she assumes in advance that she will not get it and is angry as a result. When the frustration actually occurs, it only confirms her feelings. If, on the other hand, her wishes are gratified, she still has difficulty. She feels even more dependent and is ashamed of her childishness. To receive what she craves is to relinquish any view of herself as an independent, competent person. Furthermore, she resents any suggestion that she is in some way an extension of the therapist, a relationship that is felt as similar to that she had with her family.

The patient often finds frustration and rejection more comfortable than gratification because when his wishes are gratified, his anger is exposed as inappropriate and guilt follows. One depressed woman called the clinician at home on a Sunday afternoon, saying that she was upset and asking if he would see her right away. To her surprise, he agreed. By the time she came to his office, she was contrite and apologetic, fearing that she had disturbed him for something that was not truly an emergency. Her guilt about assuming that he would not help was more prominent than her original concern. Her reaction was also based on her fear of obligation: If one accepts a favor, the other person owns your soul!

In time, the therapist must interpret this entire pattern, pointing out the risks of gratification with its consequent enslavement as well as the danger of frustration and disappointment in the patient's mode of relating to potential sources of dependency gratification. However, before such an interpretation is possible, the clinician has usually gone through this sequence many times and has erred on both sides of the dilemma. Perhaps one of the most critical aspects of treating the depressed patient is to respond to such experiences with understanding rather than irritation. This is discussed further later in this section.

The discussion of suicide often becomes a vehicle for the patient's transference feelings. Allusions to suicide are sure to elicit the clinician's concern, and at times the patient may be primarily motivated by this goal. As the patient becomes involved in therapy, suicide may also become a vehicle for angry or competitive transference feelings. The patient may learn that the most effective way to challenge the clinician's self-esteem is to demonstrate how impotent he is in stopping the patient's self-destructive behavior. One young woman who had been hospitalized after a suicide attempt became angry when her therapist would not permit her boyfriend to visit her. She would appear for each appointment with a razor blade or some sleeping pills, repeatedly exposing the hospital's inability to protect her adequately. The patient who informs the therapist that he has a cache of sleeping pills at home "just in case" is demonstrating similar feelings. The inexperienced therapist feels that his grandiosity has been challenged and tries to get the patient to give up the supply or to promise not to use it. The patient experiences this as the clinician's attempt to disarm him and render him helpless. Any outpatient who wants to kill himself can, and the therapist who accepts the patient's power in this situation has taken a step toward analyzing the underlying transference feelings.

Discussions of suicidal behavior that are motivated by transference feelings may become an important resistance. However, talking about suicidal feelings is a much preferable form of resistance to acting them out, and premature interpretations may provoke the patient to prove that he really means it. The suicidal patient usually acts out in other ways as well, and interpretation can often be attempted in less dangerous areas of behavior before it is applied to suicide.

In addition to the patient's dependent, angry, and guilty transference feelings, the patient often evokes anger or guilt in the interviewer. His suffering itself tends to make others feel guilty, and this may be accentuated by comments such as "I hope you had a nice weekend; it's nice that some people can enjoy life." Early in treatment, it is best not to interpret the aggression in such remarks. Later, when the envy and anger are closer to the surface, the interviewer may comment on them. The therapist's vacations are particularly important in the handling of the depressed patient's transference feelings. The patient's dependency needs and his anger at the clinician's inability to gratify them are accentuated, and his powerlessness to control the clinician's behavior is underlined. Suicidal behavior may appear as a means of either holding onto the clinician or punishing him for going. Often this whole constellation is denied until the doctor has actually left. Emergency department psychiatrists are familiar with suicidal behavior that occurs just after psychotherapists have gone on vacation. Forceful and repeated interpretations may be necessary in the weeks preceding the vacation. With the seriously depressed patient, it is always a good idea to let the patient know where the clinician is going, how to get in contact with him, and who will be available for emergencies.

The patient's masochistic trends sometimes seem to invite sarcastic or frankly hostile comments by the clinician. These are rarely helpful, although it may be useful to interpret the way in which the patient attempts to provoke them.

The depressed person elicits strong feelings in those who have close contact with him. Most prominent is the empathic depression that can be such an important diagnostic tool in the interview with a patient who denies his own depression. Whenever the clinician feels his own mood lowering during an interview, he should consider whether he is responding to the patient's depression. This response reflects an identification that the skillful interviewer always experiences with his patient.

In addition to this empathic reaction, the clinician may respond in a less useful way. For example, the dependent transference discussed earlier may elicit a complementary omnipotent countertransference. The patient acts as if to say, "I'm sure you have the answer," and the therapist responds with agreement. A paternalistic or overprotective style is the most common manifestation of this problem. One clinician suggested that his patient, a middle-aged depressed man, read certain books and encouraged him to learn tennis for recreation. The patient at first responded positively but then began to complain that he did not have the energy to pursue these activities, and he felt that the clinician was disappointed in him. The depressed patient is initially pleased by active interest and encouragement, but his dependent craving is always greater than the therapist can possibly gratify, and the patient often comes to feel frustrated and rejected. The therapist who has actually played the role of the omnipotent parent finds it difficult to interpret the transference aspect of these feelings. This common pattern of countertransference is related to the universal desire to be omnipotent, if only in the eyes of others. Many psychotherapists have an unusually strong wish for power to control the lives of others.

One of the most dramatic manifestations of omnipotent countertransference is the clinician who assures the suicidal patient, "Don't worry, we won't let you kill yourself." This statement can never be made with certainty, and the patient realizes that the clinician is promising more than he can deliver. At the same time, any responsibility that the patient may have felt for his own life is diminished. One patient later reported that his inner response to this assurance was "We'll see!"

Another pattern of countertransference with depressed patients involves the clinician's feelings of guilt and anger. The patient conceals his angry feelings and often expresses them by using his suffering to make others guilty. The clinician who does not understand this process may respond to it nevertheless. A depressed man did not appear for an appointment during a heavy snowstorm but did not call to cancel it. When the clinician called, the patient answered the phone and said, "Oh, I thought you'd realize I wouldn't be in, but don't worry, I'll put your check in the mail today." The implication was that the therapist was calling because he was concerned about payment, not because of his interest in the patient. The clinician started to defend himself, protesting, "No, that's not it," but the patient interrupted, saying, "I shouldn't have said that. Anyway, I'll see you next week." The clinician felt that he had been misunderstood and at first worried that he shouldn't have called. This type of guilty response to the patient's covert aggression is common. When the pattern has been repeated a few times, the clinician is more likely to become angry. Clinicians sometimes express their anger at depressed patients openly, often rationalizing their reaction as an attempt to mobilize the patient or to get him to express his feelings. The clinician's guilt or anger may also be a response to his feeling of helplessness in the face of the patient's overwhelming demands. It is difficult to tell a hopeless, crying patient that the session is over, and it is an annoying imposition to extend the time beyond the end of the patient's hour.

Another manifestation of countertransference is the boredom and impatience commonly felt while treating depressed patients. This serves as a defense against the clinician's concealed feelings of depression, guilt, or anger. It usually occurs after several sessions; the first interview with a depressed patient typically causes less anxiety than usual in the clinician. The decrease in normal anxiety results from the patient's preoccupation with himself, which prevents him from taking an active interest in the therapist. However, the clinician's initial comfort rapidly shifts to boredom as the patient's constricted interests and painful feelings become apparent. The clinician who wants to be entertained by his patients will have little success treating depressed patients. Disinterest and indifference are far more destructive to the treatment than more obviously negative feelings of anger or guilt, since the latter reflect an emotionally charged relationship. They are usually closer to consciousness and are easier to work through. The clinician who feels bored with a depressed patient may subtly try to drive that patient out of treatment without being aware of it, and the patient's feelings of rejection will reinforce his depression and may even precipitate a suicidal crisis.

It is easy to exploit the depressed person. He submits masochistically, and his slowness to respond and inhibition of aggression make him a ready victim. If the clinician finds that there is a patient upon whose time he is likely to intrude, or whose appointments he often changes, it is usually someone who is depressed and masochistic. The reader is referred to Chapter 6, "The Masochistic Patient," for a further discussion of these issues.

Medication is important in the treatment of depressed patients and provides a theme for the countertransference. The clinician may initiate pharmacotherapy or switch to a new drug, not because of clinical indications but because he is tired of the patient's symptoms. The patient may correctly feel the physician's impatience and react by feeling rejected and more depressed. The clinician is more comfortable if he thinks that it is the patient rather than his treatment that has failed.

Depressed people want to be cared for, but a central aspect of their pathology is that they drive away the very thing they crave. If the clinician recognizes the inevitability of this pattern, he is less likely to overreact to the patient's needs and also less likely to reject the patient for having them. This intermediate position allows him to respond appropriately, interpret effectively, and play a truly therapeutic role.

CONCLUSION

Interviewing the depressed patient requires sensitivity and a capacity for empathic understanding of severe psychological pain. The clinician will find few clinical situations that so test his basic humanity as well as his professional skill. However, the stakes are high. Depression often affects productive and potentially healthy individuals who have an excellent prognosis for recovery. Treatment may strongly influence the outcome, and here, as nowhere else, the clinician is in the traditional medical role of healer and saver of lives.

CHAPTER 8

THE ANXIETY DISORDER PATIENT

Anxiety is a universal emotional experience precipitated by ordinary concerns and worries. Pathological anxiety is the most common clinical presentation in psychiatry either as the primary symptom or as a major accompaniment of many psychological disorders ranging from the neurotic to the psychotic. Anxiety disorders, phenomenologically united by the subjective experience of overwhelming and disabling anxiety that appears to have little basis in reality, have been classified into various discrete entities in DSM-5. However, this taxonomy may be more illusory than real because "pure" forms of these disorders are not common, and comorbidity studies have shown that one type frequently overlaps with another. Unlike illnesses in which depressive affect is dominant, the classification of the anxiety disorders seems more like the charting of unstable and shifting islands in a sea of anxiety.

Some differentiate *fear* as an evolutionary adaptive response to *conscious* real dangers (the phylogenetically determined *fear–flight* response) from *neurotic anxiety,* which is seen as a reaction to *unconscious* dangers. Freud addressed the latter and used the term *anxiety neurosis* to encompass acute anxiety attacks (modern panic disorder), chronic anticipatory anxiety, and phobia. He observed that all three could lead to *agoraphobia,* a constriction of everyday life designed to prevent exposure to situations that would lead to crippling anxiety. His century-old classification anticipated aspects of the modern taxonomy of the anxiety disorders. Freud's early theory of the cause of neurotic anxiety was essentially a physiological model in which he postulated that anxiety resulted from a damming-up of undischarged libido (his *actual* neurosis, so-called because he thought it was based on a somatic process). Later he developed a psychological theory of anxiety as a *signal* of unconscious conflict heralding the dangers of a forbidden instinctual wish being expressed and acted on. In this construction, *signal anxiety* represents unconscious conflict between sexual or aggressive wishes and the countervailing forces of the ego and superego. The ego mediates the limitations of external reality while the superego arouses fears of retaliation and punishment if forbidden impulses are acted upon. The patient with neurotic anxiety often has no conscious awareness of this psychodynamic mechanism.

Freud's model of the origins of anxiety is an ego-psychological one. Modern thinking also encompasses constitutional factors and the object relations of childhood development. The innate capacity to manage everyday anxiety is thought to be highly dependent on the biologically based temperamental disposition of the infant. Some newborns are more reactive and agitated by both external and internal stimuli than others. Those who are high-reactive may go on to show greater stranger anxiety and more persistent separation anxiety. *Separation anxiety*—the fear of the loss of the caretaker on whom the child is dependent—is a universal aspect of development and in the temperamentally vulnerable person can persist beyond childhood. Separation anxiety disorder is now delineated as a separate diagnostic entity in DSM-5 (Box 8–1). Neuropsychological irritability combined with separation anxiety continuing into adulthood is posited by some to be at the core of panic disorder.

BOX 8–1. DSM-5 Diagnostic Criteria for Separation Anxiety Disorder

---

A. Developmentally inappropriate and excessive fear or anxiety concerning separation from those to whom the individual is attached, as evidenced by at least three of the following:

1. Recurrent excessive distress when anticipating or experiencing separation from home or from major attachment figures.
2. Persistent and excessive worry about losing major attachment figures or about possible harm to them, such as illness, injury, disasters, or death.
3. Persistent and excessive worry about experiencing an untoward event (e.g., getting lost, being kidnapped, having an accident, becoming ill) that causes separation from a major attachment figure.
4. Persistent reluctance or refusal to go out, away from home, to school, to work, or elsewhere because of fear of separation.
5. Persistent and excessive fear of or reluctance about being alone or without major attachment figures at home or in other settings.
6. Persistent reluctance or refusal to sleep away from home or to go to sleep without being near a major attachment figure.
7. Repeated nightmares involving the theme of separation.

8. Repeated complaints of physical symptoms (e.g., headaches, stomachaches, nausea, vomiting) when separation from major attachment figures occurs or is anticipated.

B. The fear, anxiety, or avoidance is persistent, lasting at least 4 weeks in children and adolescents and typically 6 months or more in adults.

C. The disturbance causes clinically significant distress or impairment in social, academic, occupational, or other important areas of functioning.

D. The disturbance is not better explained by another mental disorder, such as refusing to leave home because of excessive resistance to change in autism spectrum disorder; delusions or hallucinations concerning separation in psychotic disorders; refusal to go outside without a trusted companion in agoraphobia; worries about ill health or other harm befalling significant others in generalized anxiety disorder; or concerns about having an illness in illness anxiety disorder.

Source. Reprinted from American Psychiatric Association: *Diagnostic and Statistical Manual of Mental Disorders,* 5th Edition. Arlington, VA, American Psychiatric Association, 2013. Copyright 2013, American Psychiatric Association. Used with permission.

Generalized anxiety disorder, panic disorder, and phobia all possess a common theme, namely a low, probably biologically based, threshold for the toleration of anxiety. Hence, they are clinically interrelated and may overlap. Phobia and panic disorder are especially intimately connected and are often aspects of the same clinical syndrome. The experience of frightening panic attacks leads to a constriction of life, an avoidance of specific situations—agoraphobia—that might potentially lead to the precipitation of such attacks. Agoraphobia is now delineated as a separate diagnostic entity in DSM-5 (Box 8–2). Agoraphobia and specific phobia can be viewed as, in part, a defensive reaction on the part of the patient. The choice of phobia and its symbolic meaning have important psychodynamic elements.

BOX 8–2. DSM-5 Diagnostic Criteria for Agoraphobia

A. Marked fear or anxiety about two (or more) of the following five situations:

1. Using public transportation (e.g., automobiles, buses, trains, ships, planes).
2. Being in open spaces (e.g., parking lots, marketplaces, bridges).
3. Being in enclosed places (e.g., shops, theaters, cinemas).
4. Standing in line or being in a crowd.
5. Being outside of the home alone.

B. The individual fears or avoids these situations because of thoughts that escape might be difficult or help might not be available in the event of developing panic-like symptoms or other incapacitating or embarrassing symptoms (e.g., fear of falling in the elderly; fear of incontinence).

C. The agoraphobic situations almost always provoke fear or anxiety.
D. The agoraphobic situations are actively avoided, require the presence of a companion, or are endured with intense fear or anxiety.
E. The fear or anxiety is out of proportion to the actual danger posed by the agoraphobic situations and to the sociocultural context.
F. The fear, anxiety, or avoidance is persistent, typically lasting for 6 months or more.
G. The fear, anxiety, or avoidance causes clinically significant distress or impairment in social, occupational, or other important areas of functioning.
H. If another medical condition (e.g., inflammatory bowel disease, Parkinson's disease) is present, the fear, anxiety, or avoidance is clearly excessive.
I. The fear, anxiety, or avoidance is not better explained by the symptoms of another mental disorder—for example, the symptoms are not confined to specific phobia, situational type; do not involve only social situations (as in social anxiety disorder); and are not related exclusively to obsessions (as in obsessive-compulsive disorder), perceived defects or flaws in physical appearance (as in body dysmorphic disorder), reminders of traumatic events (as in posttraumatic stress disorder), or fear of separation (as in separation anxiety disorder).

Note: Agoraphobia is diagnosed irrespective of the presence of panic disorder. If an individual's presentation meets criteria for panic disorder and agoraphobia, both diagnoses should be assigned.

Source. Reprinted from American Psychiatric Association: *Diagnostic and Statistical Manual of Mental Disorders,* 5th Edition. Arlington, VA, American Psychiatric Association, 2013. Copyright 2013, American Psychiatric Association. Used with permission.

PSYCHOPATHOLOGY AND PSYCHODYNAMICS

The Phobic Patient

Phobic behavior is found in a wide variety of neurotic, characterological, and psychotic syndromes (Box 8–3). Phobias and panic attacks can be differentiated from generalized anxiety disorder and posttraumatic stress disorder, although they have many features in common. The distinctions are considered in the section on "Differential Diagnosis." The phobic person copes with his inner emotional conflicts and anxiety by attempting to repress his disturbing thoughts and impulses. When this repression fails, he displaces his conflict to a place or situation in the outside world and tries to confine his anxiety to that situation. The external situation now symbolically represents his inner psychological conflicts; if he can avoid this situation, he can decrease his anxiety and obviate the possibility of a panic attack. It is this avoidance that is the essence of the phobia. The specific symptom may be a symbolic condensation that includes aspects both of a forbidden wish or impulse and of the unconscious fear that prevents its direct gratification. Other unconscious determinants may include threats to attachment and a chronically impaired sense of safety. Phobic defenses lead to a general constriction of personality as the patient relinquishes freedom and pleasurable activity in order to avoid conflict and anxiety.

BOX 8–3. DSM-5 Diagnostic Criteria for Specific Phobia

A. Marked fear or anxiety about a specific object or situation (e.g., flying, heights, animals, receiving an injection, seeing blood).

Note: In children, the fear or anxiety may be expressed by crying, tantrums, freezing, or clinging.

B. The phobic object or situation almost always provokes immediate fear or anxiety.

C. The phobic object or situation is actively avoided or endured with intense fear or anxiety.

D. The fear or anxiety is out of proportion to the actual danger posed by the specific object or situation and to the sociocultural context.

E. The fear, anxiety, or avoidance is persistent, typically lasting for 6 months or more.

F. The fear, anxiety, or avoidance causes clinically significant distress or impairment in social, occupational, or other important areas of functioning.

G. The disturbance is not better explained by the symptoms of another mental disorder, including fear, anxiety, and avoidance of situations associated with panic-like symptoms or other incapacitating symptoms (as in agoraphobia); objects or situations related to obsessions (as in obsessive-compulsive disorder); reminders of traumatic events (as in posttraumatic stress disorder); separation from home or attachment figures (as in separation anxiety disorder); or social situations (as in social anxiety disorder).

Specify if:

Code based on the phobic stimulus:

300.29 (F40.218) **Animal** (e.g., spiders, insects, dogs).

300.29 (F40.228) **Natural environment** (e.g., heights, storms, water).

300.29 (F40.23x) **Blood-injection-injury** (e.g., needles, invasive medical procedures).

> **Coding note:** Select specific ICD-10-CM code as follows: **F40.230** fear of blood; **F40.231** fear of injections and transfusions; **F40.232** fear of other medical care; or **F40.233** fear of injury.

300.29 (F40.248) **Situational** (e.g., airplanes, elevators, enclosed places).

300.29 (F40.298) **Other** (e.g., situations that may lead to choking or vomiting; in children, e.g., loud sounds or costumed characters).

Coding note: When more than one phobic stimulus is present, code all ICD-10-CM codes that apply (e.g., for fear of snakes and flying, F40.218 specific phobia, animal, and F40.248 specific phobia, situational).

Source. Reprinted from American Psychiatric Association: *Diagnostic and Statistical Manual of Mental Disorders,* 5th Edition. Arlington, VA, American Psychiatric Association, 2013. Copyright 2013, American Psychiatric Association. Used with permission.

The term *phobia* is sometimes misused. The "cancer phobic," for instance, has an obsessive fear, or perhaps a hypochondriacal idea, but not a true avoidance. Another misuse is illustrated by the phrase "success phobia," which refers to a psychodynamic formulation explaining an unconscious fear of success. The patient with "cancer phobia" may avoid going to hospitals, and patients with "success phobia" may avoid vocational advancement because of unconscious fears, but these are not true phobias in the traditional sense.

Phobic Symptoms

The phobic individual is characterized by his use of avoidance as a primary means of resolving problems. In the classic phobic reaction, neurotic symptoms dominate the patient's existence. His mental life centers on unrealistic and distressing fears (open spaces, heights, subways, elevators, traffic jams, and so on). The phobia usually involves something that the patient can and does encounter frequently. He offers rational explanations for his fear, but usually recognizes that these only partially account for his feelings. Nevertheless, although he often perceives his fear to be inappropriate, he feels that avoidance of the phobic situation is the only reasonable choice in view of his intense fear. The patient will agree that it is irrational to be afraid of the subway, but he is convinced that because he is afraid, he has no alternative but to keep away! The interviewer can often uncover hidden meanings by empathic inquiry concerning the imagined consequences of forcing himself into the phobic situation.

> A patient with an overwhelming phobic fear of enclosed spaces such as elevators remembered a frightening experience of being smothered with a pillow by an older sibling while playing on the bed with her. She thought she was going to die and lost control of her bladder. When her sister lifted the pillow from her face, she made fun of the patient for wetting herself. The patient felt humiliated. The murderous aggression, terror, and subsequent shame embodied in this episode became symbolized and encapsulated in her phobia.

Phobic symptoms frequently progress and extend from one situation to another. A woman who first is afraid of buses becomes fearful of crossing streets and finally even hesitates to venture outdoors. A man who is frightened of eating in restaurants overcomes this fear but is then unable to ride on subways. Patients will not readily volunteer the details of their initial symptoms, and it may require many interviews to uncover the fear that precipitated the first episode. Such persistence is worthwhile, because it is in the original context that the major psychodynamics will be exposed. This, of course, accounts for the patient's propensity to obscure the matter.

The typical phobic patient attempts to conquer his fear. As he does so, shifts in symbolization or displacement result in the substitution of new phobias for the old ones. The new symptoms may be less distressing to the patient or may involve more secondary gain, but they are always aimed at avoiding the same basic conflict.

Phobic Character Traits

Far more common than the symptomatic phobia is the use of avoidance and inhibition as characterological defenses. This is present in all patients who have phobic symptoms, but it is also widespread in other individuals. The psychodynamics of phobic character traits are similar to those of phobic symptoms. In both, the patient avoids a situation that represents a source of anxiety, but in the phobic character the fear is usually unconscious and the avoidance is explained as a matter of taste or preference. Often, interest or intrigue is mixed with fear, representing the emergence of the forbidden wish, and the patient envies people who can comfortably enter the phobic area. To illustrate, a young woman who did not like speaking in front of groups envied her husband's ability to do so and felt that this ability meant that he was totally free of all anxiety. Other patients may be unaware of the neurotic basis of their avoidance, but accompanying symptoms of anxiety will reveal the underlying emotional conflict. An attorney who avoided all athletic activity was a devoted follower of newspaper accounts and television broadcasts of sports events. On occasion he would feel palpitations and faintness during the violent moments of football games. The anxiety that prevented him from participating in his childhood emerged directly when he was a spectator in adult life. If the denial is more extensive, there is simply a lack of interest in the entire area. This is recognized as defensive avoidance only when the person's life situation exposes his inhibition as maladaptive. For example, a woman living in the center of a large city can explain her inability to drive a car as a reasonable choice, but when she moves to the suburbs and still refuses to drive, the neurotic basis of the preference is exposed.

Phobic traits can be basic to character structure. The individual is preoccupied with security and fears any possible threat to it, constantly imagining himself in situations of danger while pursuing the course of greatest safety. This person is familiar as the man who spends his vacations at home, pursues the same interests, reads the same authors, and works at the same tasks year in and year out. He has a limited number of friends and avoids new experiences.

A common example of phobic character traits is the young woman who is married to an older man. She lives near her mother and speaks to her by telephone several times daily. Her children have also developed phobic symptoms and are excused from school gym classes because of minor physical difficulties. The family members are familiar visitors to their general practitioner's office. She looks younger than her age and is quite charming with men, although not quite as popular with her female friends. At times she may seem impulsively exhibitionistic as her seductiveness emerges in protected social settings. The man with a similar defensive pattern is more prominently concerned with assertion than with sexuality. His boyishness is often mixed with so much bravado that he may seem more foolhardy than frightened. This defensive assertiveness is more likely to be aimed at a powerful superior than at a peer, and he hopes he will be seen as a self-confident and promising young man but unconsciously does not expect to be seen as an adult.

The phobic individual usually values sexual behavior primarily for the accompanying sense of warmth and security. He is often reluctant to initiate sex, thereby hoping to avoid any responsibility for acting on forbidden impulses.

Differential Diagnosis

Phobic defenses are often seen in patients whose personality types are predominantly obsessive or histrionic. The resulting clinical picture reflects both the phobic avoidance and the more basic character structure. This patient's conflicts are revealed through exploration of his phobic defenses. He often has no awareness of their content, which basically involves dependency, with admixtures of sexuality or aggression.

The obsessive-phobic individual is most often concerned with the avoidance of aggression. He may be fearful of using knives or driving a car. These fears may extend to symbols of control and power. A successful businessman with a strongly obsessive character refuses to touch any money, a symbol of social power. The obsessive person spends hours ruminating about his phobia, and his constant preoccupation is often more disabling than the actual symptom itself. Every obsessive patient, even if he does not have phobic symptoms, will reveal some characterological inhibitions that involve defensive avoidance. For example, one may see an aversion to competitive sports rather than a symptomatic fear of handling knives or sharp objects. In this case, aggressive impulses are avoided through an inhibition of activity rather than by a neurotic symptom relating to symbols of aggression.

The conflicts of the histrionic patient with phobic defenses are most likely to involve sex or dependency. Symptoms are frequently elaborated and dramatized. It may require many interviews to determine the content of the patient's phobias. To illustrate, in an initial interview a woman described her fear of walking on the street alone. She denied awareness of what she feared, admitting only that she might become "upset." Several interviews later, she added that she feared that a man might make sexual advances. Her fear that she might not decline such overtures was only revealed after a year of treatment. The histrionic phobic patient is frightened by her own emotionality and avoids experiences that produce overwhelming emotions. Either her sexual responses are inhibited or her sexual behavior is almost nonexistent. Some fears involve physical sensations that are similar to those of sexual excitement, such as being in a sailboat that is heeling over in the wind.

It is common for several conflicts to be represented symbolically by a single phobia. An agoraphobic woman who insists on being accompanied on the street by her husband avoids sexual temptation, and her husband's presence also reassures her that he has not been injured and is available to care for her. Her interest in other men and her fears for her husband's welfare are both related to her repressed anger toward and dependence on her husband, and this anger is more directly expressed by her excessive demands, which restrict his life as well. Her phobic symptom enables her to obtain gratification of infantile dependent wishes while avoiding direct expression of her sexual and aggressive feelings. The denial and avoidance of these impulses stem from an early fear of the parental disapproval that would result from their recognition and gratification.

Phobic defenses are only partially effective, and the phobic individual continues to experience anxiety. Therefore, phobic patients typically experience the emotional and physical symptoms of anxiety, such as palpitations, dyspnea, dizziness, syncope, sweating, and gastrointestinal distress, depending on how their autonomic nervous system is constituted. These may form the basis for hypochondriacal preoccupation or panic attacks in more severely phobic patients.

The clinician's reassurance and simple explanation of the psychological basis of these physiological symptoms may seem to be readily accepted by the phobic person. However, he is prone to continue his worries about somatic illnesses and often pursues other medical treatment without telling the clinician. When he obtains evidence of an organic disease, or when some medical treatment leads to improvement, he has further support for his own belief that his problem is really physical and that emotional conflicts are of little importance.

Generalized anxiety disorder is characterized by excessive worry of one form or another that is present most of the time and is difficult to control, leading to impairment of normal life activities. The manifestations of this worry are protean—concerns about health, occupation, social capacities, the possibility of harm occurring to oneself or loved ones, and so on. It has a pervasive, chronic quality unlike the acute attacks of panic disorder or the specificity of phobias, and it permeates everything, making life miserable for the patients and others around them, including the clinician. Major depression coexists in two-thirds of these patients, suggesting a shared biological origin. The clinician must approach these patients empathically and not succumb to the countertransference irritation that their irrational concerns can arouse. The underlying psychodynamics of these patients' all-encompassing worry often revolve around persistent expectations that they will be found inadequate and irritating, a self-fulfilling prophecy that can be usefully addressed in the transference.

Mechanisms of Defense

Displacement and symbolization. For avoidance to be effective, the conflict within the mind of the patient must be displaced to the outside world. The patient shifts his attention from an emotional conflict to the environment in which that conflict occurs. For example, the child who is fearful of competitive relations with his classmates avoids going to gym. More elaborate displacements may be based on symbolic representation. Every mechanism of symbolic representation may be involved, and the interpretation of phobic symptoms is as complex as the interpretation of dreams. Displacement can also be based on some accidental connection between the emotional conflict and a particular place or situation. In most clinical phobias, all of these mechanisms are involved. For example, the fear of subways in young women is often traced to the symbolic sexual significance of the subway, which is a powerful vehicle that travels through a tunnel and vibrates in the darkness.

Projection. Phobic avoidance often involves projection as well as displacement and symbolization. The analysis of a subway phobia may first reveal a fear of attack, then a fear of sexual attack, and finally an unconscious fear of loss of control over sexual impulses. The patient's impulses are projected onto the other riders in the subway, and this projection allows the patient to rationalize the fear.

The link between phobic defenses and projection relates to the link between phobic and paranoid traits. Like the paranoid patient, the phobic patient uses relatively primitive defenses, with denial playing a prominent role. He thinks concretely, focuses on the external environment rather than his inner feelings, and keeps secrets from the interviewer. However, in contrast to the paranoid patient, the phobic patient maintains reality testing. He denies the inner world of emotions more than the outer world of perception. The phobic patient displaces his anxiety to the environment and projects his impulses onto others, but rarely onto anyone emotionally important to him. He maintains firm human relationships in order to ensure continued gratification of his dependent needs. Therefore, the initial interviews are conducted with an aura of goodwill. The patient represses his hostile or negative feelings, and he typically has no interest in exploring his inner mental life. He often exhibits an infantile confidence in the clinician's magical ability to alleviate his distress.

Avoidance.   The defensive utilization of avoidance is the essential characteristic of the phobic individual. The ancillary defenses of symbolization, displacement, and rationalization serve to make the avoidance possible. Phobic defenses are effective only when anxiety can be confined to a specific situation that the individual is able to avoid so that his psychological conflicts will no longer disturb him. This sequestration of anxiety to an external situation is rarely completely effective, and therefore the phobic individual must also avoid thinking about his internal conflicts. It soon becomes apparent in the interview that a phobic individual does not, cannot, or simply will not discuss certain topics. The central problem in interviewing or treating a phobic patient is to lead him, even at times to urge him, to move into the areas of action in his daily life. The patient must be encouraged to do something that he does not want to do, but the interviewer must not make the patient phobic of the interview itself. This usually means allowing the patient to establish a dependent relationship and then using it to reward him for entering frightening situations.

The phobic patient shows a striking intolerance for anxiety, and it is this fear of anxiety that usually motivates him to seek help. He may be able to avoid the object of his phobia and even avoid thinking of his conflicts, but he is not able to avoid the anticipatory anxiety of what would happen if he were to enter the phobic situation. His usual goal in treatment is to become immune to anxiety, even in circumstances that would frighten anyone. During the treatment, the clinician must inquire not only into what is so frightening about the phobic situation or the forbidden impulses but also into the patient's intolerance of anxiety.

The phobic partner.   The patient's fear of anxiety is highly contagious, particularly for other individuals with unconscious phobic tendencies. The partner of the phobic patient, who accompanies her whenever she ventures outdoors or across the street, has accepted the patient's belief that anxiety must be avoided at all costs. If the patient improves with treatment, the partner can become a major obstacle to therapy as his latent phobias become more manifest. The prototype for this role is to be found in the interaction of the overprotective mother and the anxious child. Questions such as "Are you sure she's ready to try it by herself?" are common. The patient will often attempt to enlist the interviewer into the partner role. She does this by dramatizing her anxiety and suggesting that the interviewer's help is all that is needed to conquer the problems. This infantile magical orientation toward treatment may feed the interviewer's omnipotent fantasies, but it only reconstructs the pattern of relationships that created the phobia.

Counterphobic behavior.   Counterphobic patterns are an interesting developmental variant in which the patient denies his phobias. His behavior dramatizes his disregard of realistic fears, and he seems to prefer situations in which there is a potential for disastrous consequences. This patient has also displaced his anxiety to these external situations and has symbolized his unconscious fear by mastering the realistic external danger. However, whereas the phobic person then avoids the external situation, the counterphobic individual accepts the realistic danger as a challenge and thus conquers his unconscious fear. Both defensive patterns involve magical thinking. The phobic patient usually selects a situation in which there is mild realistic danger, however slight, and then magically believes that it will certainly happen to him. The counterphobic person selects a setting in which danger is possible, or even probable, but never certain. His magical feeling is, "I am completely in control here, so there is no reason for fear." The individual who is fearful of asserting himself with women and yet participates in extreme sports is a common example. He enjoys the admiration he receives as being brave, or adventurous, or fearless.

Mixtures of phobic and counterphobic defenses are common, and detailed investigation of counterphobic persons often reveals widespread patterns of inhibition in other areas of life. For example, the same individual who risks life and limb racing cars might be uncomfortable speaking in public. Counterphobic defenses may provide greater secondary gain and social usefulness, and as with all symptoms, it is necessary to separate their adaptive value from their neurotic origins. They may also allow relatively direct gratification of the forbidden impulses, but with little flexibility or spontaneity of behavior. The counterphobic individual rarely seeks help for this pattern, but the daring aspects of his behavior may alarm others.

For example, it would seem totally incongruous that a Navy jet fighter pilot would be afraid of heights. When the incongruity was pointed out, the man replied, "It's about control. When I land at night on an aircraft carrier, I am in control. I know exactly what I'm going to do and how to do it. I've trained to do this." The interviewer asked, "What about the observation platform on the Empire State Building? Can you look out at the horizon?" The reply was affirmative. "How about looking straight down?" "Forget it" was the answer. The interviewer continued, "Let's lower the wall down to your knee level." The man interrupted, "Don't even go there!" The interviewer continued, "Are you afraid you might be tempted to jump?" The former pilot replied, "That's it; you've got it." It is difficult to find a more illuminating illustration. Who among us is not awed by the prospect of a night carrier landing in a jet fighter? Nevertheless, this man had been trained thoroughly in stages and had developed confidence in his *self-control* in that situation. He had internalized his teachers as part of a professional identity. The roof of a building or a high rock ledge was a different story. Here, his most primitive wish to fly with the ease of a bird was stimulated. His confidence in his ability to control this grandiose wish was not solidified. It is like the dream of young men to fly magically like Superman. Not many older men still have that dream because reality has, over the years, chipped away at their feelings of grandiosity. A survey of some of our psychiatric residents revealed that some of the young women have also had that dream, but they reported much more fear of falling than the feeling of exhilaration described by the male residents.

The Panic Disorder Patient

In panic disorder (Box 8–4), the characteristic attacks, although often brief (usually less than 1 hour, often 5–10 minutes in duration), are intensely disabling. With emergence of the attack, apparently out of nowhere, the individual is overwhelmed by sudden, acute anxiety accompanied by frightening somatic symptoms, such as breathlessness, sweating, rapid heartbeat, shaking, nausea, dizziness, choking, chills, and the terrifying feeling that death is imminent. Panic attacks tend to be recurrent and often lead to secondary fear of venturing out of the home because the person dreads being in a situation that he cannot readily leave if an attack takes place; he thus becomes conditioned to fear the place where the panic attack occurred or places that resemble it.

BOX 8–4. DSM-5 Diagnostic Criteria for Panic Disorder

A. Recurrent unexpected panic attacks. A panic attack is an abrupt surge of intense fear or intense discomfort that reaches a peak within minutes, and during which time four (or more) of the following symptoms occur:

Note: The abrupt surge can occur from a calm state or an anxious state.

 1. Palpitations, pounding heart, or accelerated heart rate.
 2. Sweating.
 3. Trembling or shaking.
 4. Sensations of shortness of breath or smothering.
 5. Feelings of choking.
 6. Chest pain or discomfort.
 7. Nausea or abdominal distress.
 8. Feeling dizzy, unsteady, light-headed, or faint.
 9. Chills or heat sensations.
10. Paresthesias (numbness or tingling sensations).
11. Derealization (feelings of unreality) or depersonalization (being detached from oneself).
12. Fear of losing control or "going crazy."
13. Fear of dying.

Note: Culture-specific symptoms (e.g., tinnitus, neck soreness, headache, uncontrollable screaming or crying) may be seen. Such symptoms should not count as one of the four required symptoms.

B. At least one of the attacks has been followed by 1 month (or more) of one or both of the following:

 1. Persistent concern or worry about additional panic attacks or their consequences (e.g., losing control, having a heart attack, "going crazy").
 2. A significant maladaptive change in behavior related to the attacks (e.g., behaviors designed to avoid having panic attacks, such as avoidance of exercise or unfamiliar situations).

C. The disturbance is not attributable to the physiological effects of a substance (e.g., a drug of abuse, a medication) or another medical condition (e.g., hyperthyroidism, cardiopulmonary disorders).

D. The disturbance is not better explained by another mental disorder (e.g., the panic attacks do not occur only in response to feared social situations, as in social anxiety disorder; in response to circumscribed phobic objects or situations, as in specific phobia; in response to obsessions, as in obsessive-compulsive disorder; in response to reminders of traumatic events, as in posttraumatic stress disorder; or in response to separation from attachment figures, as in separation anxiety disorder).

Source. Reprinted from American Psychiatric Association: *Diagnostic and Statistical Manual of Mental Disorders*, 5th Edition. Arlington, VA, American Psychiatric Association, 2013. Copyright 2013, American Psychiatric Association. Used with permission.

One of the first descriptions of what would later be called panic disorder is to be found in Freud's *Studies on Hysteria*. In "The Case of Katharina," Freud in 1890 described an 18-year-old adolescent with recurrent episodes of acute anxiety accompanied by severe breathlessness. Katharina recounted, "It comes over me all at once. First of all, it's like something pressing on my eyes. My head gets so heavy, there's a dreadful buzzing, and I feel so giddy that I almost fall over. Then there's something crushing my chest so that I can't get my breath." She further described, "My throat's squeezed together as though I were going to choke" and "I always think I'm going to die—I don't dare to go anywhere; I think all the time someone's standing behind me and going to catch hold of me all at once." In a penetrating interview (by modern standards, perhaps too "penetrating"), Freud quickly established that the onset of her disorder was precipitated by sexual advances that had been made by her father when she was 14 years old. The symptoms—the pressure on her throat, and so on—symbolized his sexually aroused body lying on her. Given the traumatic nature of these incestuous advances, Katharina's recurrent anxiety episodes could just as easily be classified as an example of posttraumatic stress disorder, which is emblematic of the fluid and interchangeable nature of the anxiety disorders.

Donald Klein's pharmacological treatment studies in the 1960s led to the modern delineation of panic disorder as a clinical entity distinct from generalized anxiety disorder. Klein used tricyclic antidepressants in the treatment of panic disorder and agoraphobia with considerable success. The symptoms of acute panic, with its palpitations, sweating, trembling, dyspnea, fear of imminent death, and so on, and secondary inhibitory agoraphobia were often effectively interrupted and prevented by this pharmacological intervention. This therapeutic discovery spawned considerable important clinical research into the biological nature of the anxiety disorders and their possible genetic relationship to depressive disorders. (Two-thirds of panic disorder patients experience an episode of major depression in their lifetimes.) Klein posited a theory of exaggerated separation anxiety as the psychological core of panic disorder.

Developmental Psychodynamics of Phobia and Panic Disorder

Phobic symptoms are universal in children. In fact, although initially they are frequently denied, the existence of childhood phobias will eventually emerge in the history of almost every neurotic patient. The widespread phobic symptoms of children no doubt reflect the normal tendency toward primitive and magical thought in the developing child.

Very young children show definite tendencies toward risk taking or harm avoidance. The terms *inhibited* and *uninhibited to the unfamiliar* have been used by developmental psychologists to distinguish these two groups of children. These behavioral patterns correlate with the *high-reactive* and *low-reactive* temperamental dispositions identified in 4-month-old infants. The high-reactive infants were more likely to become shy and timid children. The low-reactive infants were more risk-taking and sociable and less disturbed by the unfamiliar. These studies indicate genetic factors that predispose one to problems with anxiety, risk, and danger and to individualized views of what constitutes safety.

Anxiety in the appropriate context is a universal signal of external danger. The first external danger in life is the presence of a person who is not the "mothering" person. Infants vary enormously in this degree of stranger anxiety. Next, when a healthy bond is established with the mothering person(s), the stage is set for separation anxiety. This, too, serves a major adaptive role because it protects the young child from wandering out of the sight and sound of the mother. This mechanism can be observed in a family of ducks in a pond. The little ducks follow the mother in an order that is established soon after hatching and is maintained. The last one in line has the greatest chance of being eaten. This metaphor applies to human young as well.

The situation is further complicated by the development of a sense of self early in childhood. Through interaction with caregiving, loving parental figures, the developing self learns that some behaviors please the caregivers, whereas others displease them. The child learns to conceal displeasing behavior by not doing it when the caregivers are present. The caregivers discover this and express disapproval. This is the essential paradigm for beginning to internalize parental values. When the wish to obey and win love supersedes the wish to defy to the degree that the child loses his conscious awareness of the latter, we speak of repression. The stage is now set in children with an appropriate predisposition to develop an anxiety of their own forbidden impulses and wishes, which still exist at an unconscious level.

The phobic individual learns as a child that the world is a frightening and unpredictable place. His parents may reinforce this view through either their timidity or their explosive or violent outbursts. In some families, the mother is herself somewhat phobic, and the father is unpredictable, irritable, and angry. This is a not uncommon story in the history of the patient who may later develop posttraumatic stress disorder in response to a real-life trauma. The whole family is frightened of the father's episodes and tries to avoid them. Other patterns are common; for example, the father may share the mother's fearfulness, and the threat of aggression may come from outside the family circle. There is an important difference between the typical childhood experiences of the paranoid patient and those of the phobic patient. Both involve the fear of rage and even violence, but the family of the phobic patient offers some hope of safety, so that the child develops a sense of potential security, although at the price of anxiety and diminished self-confidence. In contrast, the paranoid person learned that the only security from external dangers that his family could provide involved a total loss of the sense of identity and that his only chance for both independence and safety resided in constant lonely vigilance.

The phobic person overestimates both the dangers of the outside world and the inner emotional danger of anxiety. Often the fears of outer dangers have been learned directly from his parents. At times these may be reinforced by actual increases in danger, either because the child is vulnerable, as in the chronically ill, or because the family lives in a setting that presents realistic dangers. The exaggerated fear of anxiety is related to the mother's inability to perceive her child's emotional state and her consequent defensive overprotection. The infant needs both adequate exposure to external stimuli and protection from overstimulation. The appropriate balance between these is a function of the mother's sensitivity to her child's signals of distress. If she responds indiscriminately as though all signals mean distress, the child does not have an opportunity to develop a normal tolerance for anxiety. In other words, the mother's anxiety and consequent difficulty in responding to the child can lead to the later development of intolerance to anxiety in that child.

The mother's insensitivity to and overevaluation of the child's anxiety continue throughout the subsequent stages of development. She responds to the child's normal separation anxiety by refusing to allow him out of her sight, she handles his stranger anxiety by limiting his contacts with new people, and she teaches him to deny sexual or aggressive impulses that may lead to conflict with his parents or with his developing superego. At each stage of development, the child fails to conquer his anxiety and must learn to deal with it in some other way. He identifies not only with his parents' fears of the world but also with their unusual sensitivity to fear and their mode of coping with it. This is seen most clearly in school phobias in which the mother's separation anxiety is at least as great as that of the child.

The developmental history of the phobic patient typically reveals that he was afraid of the dark, of being alone in his bedroom at night, of nightmares and demons. The door to his room was left open or his light was left on. He was comforted by these reassurances that his family was close at hand. His parents emphasized the dangers of traffic in the street, bullies on the playground, evil men lurking in the park, or the hand of fate in the form of terrible illness. He was warned never to cross the street or to ride his bike after dark, although his peers had long engaged in these activities. Parental prophesies about bullies were accurate, because his timidity provoked bullying behavior from his classmates. If he did not want to go to camp or became frightened of school, his family reacted to these fears by allowing him to avoid the situations that caused them.

The phobic patient frequently utilized one of his parents as a partner during his childhood. By agreeing to accompany and protect the child and thus mitigate his separation anxiety, the parent not only encouraged the development of phobic defenses but also revealed his own underlying phobic character. The child was led to feel that his own adaptive skills were inadequate and that magical reliance on his parent would somehow help to compensate for this. If he was helpless, his parents might be able to protect him.

The panic disorder patient often has a history of traumatic childhood experiences based both on their constitutional vulnerability and on family environment. Normal separation anxiety is not well tolerated. This may reflect a biologically based low threshold for an inborn fear response to the unfamiliar, with an accompanying high autonomic arousal. Simultaneously, actual frightening behavior by a parent or caretaker may lead to insecure attachment and a chronically impaired sense of safety. The combination of these two, constitutional and environmental, may lead to an avoidance of situations that are unfamiliar and could be mastered by experience, particularly in the presence of a comfortable, calm, reassuring parent. One psychodynamic theory of panic attacks posits that threats to attachment in adulthood trigger regression to the childhood experience and become physiologically manifest in the autonomic fear reaction of the panic attack.

The combination of little self-confidence, low toleration for anxiety, a dependent mode of adaptation, a tendency for magical thinking, early exposure to models who use phobic defenses, and the use of symptoms and suffering as a means of dealing with authorities leads to the development of the phobic character.

MANAGEMENT OF THE INTERVIEW

The phobic and panic disorder patient relates easily during the initial portion of the interview. He comes seeking relief and is polite and eager to talk about his problems. Silence and resistance arise later in the interview, but the opening moments are marked by an aura of goodwill. As the interview progresses, it becomes apparent that the patient's agreeableness continues only if the interviewer cooperates with the patient's defenses—that is, if he helps the patient avoid anxiety by not pursuing certain topics and by offering magical protection. The task of the interviewer is to direct the discussion into these forbidden areas but at the same time to maintain the rapport necessary to sustain the relationship through the painful exploration of the patient's psychological problems.

Early Cooperation

The phobic patient is frequently accompanied to the first appointment. He may come with a member of his family or with a friend. If he comes alone, he often expects to be picked up afterward, or his companion is waiting in the car. If the interviewer has reason to suspect that the patient is phobic, it is advisable to see the patient alone, speaking to his companion only afterward, if at all. If the diagnosis is not apparent until both are in the clinician's office, the clinician should use the first convenient opportunity to tactfully dismiss the companion in order to speak with the patient alone. The companion's presence protects the patient from anxiety by inhibiting thoughts and feelings that are disturbing. Because the clinician wants to explore these thoughts and feelings, he is more likely to be successful if the companion is not present. There is no purpose in interpreting the defense at this point, and a simple "Could you wait outside while I speak with your brother?" or "Can we talk alone while your husband waits outside?" will suffice. The request should be addressed to the individual who the interviewer senses is least likely to object.

Some phobic patients have an almost exhibitionistic eagerness to relate their distress and describe their inability to overcome irrational fears. Others are more ashamed of their problems and may conceal their symptoms. The interviewer will learn to recognize the latter group by the overt anxiety and the extensive use of avoidance in the patient's life and in the interview itself. Whether the patient presents his symptoms as a chief complaint or reveals them only reluctantly, he is more eager to obtain the clinician's reassurance than to investigate his own emotional life. The interviewer, however, wants to discuss the patient's problems and symptoms and thereby gain some understanding of the patient's psychological conflicts. In view of these discrepant goals, the natural starting point for the interview is a discussion of the symptoms.

Early in the interview the patient may ask, "Will you be able to help me?" The timing of the question suggests that it is a request for magical reassurance. The interviewer can use this as a lever to initiate a more thorough investigation of the problems, replying, "I can't give you an answer to that until you've told me more about yourself." He offers the promise of future help in return for enduring present anxiety. Although many patients experience relief from simply talking about their problems, this process makes the phobic patient more anxious. He needs a direct promise of the benefit before he will participate in the treatment process.

Exploration of the Symptoms

The problems encountered in interviewing a phobic or panic disorder patient are often encapsulated in the exploration of his symptoms. (Obsessive and histrionic patients also have symptoms, but their discussion is seldom a central focus of resistance, although the obsessive-compulsive disorder patient often conceals his symptoms.) The phobic patient responds differently. His characteristic defenses often emerge in the discussion of his symptom, just as they did in its formation. When the interviewer tries to talk about the patient's behavior, the patient shifts the discussion to a neutral topic or asks the clinician for help while avoiding exposure of his problems. His displacement of inner conflicts to the outside world may appear as a concentration on the external world rather than his inner feelings.

The phobic patient's symptoms are associated with considerable anxiety, and some phobic patients offer them as the chief complaint or mention them early in the interview. The clinician asks for a detailed description of the symptoms, the situations that evoke them, the history of their development, and the therapeutic measures that the patient has attempted on his own behalf before coming to the initial interview.

> In an initial interview, a single 30-year-old professional woman described the onset of her panic attacks: "It was so bizarre. It first occurred during my lunch break 10 days ago. I went into a deli to buy a sandwich. The store was crowded, and I had to wait in a long line. I suddenly felt extremely anxious and became cold and clammy." The interviewer asked how she was passing the time as she waited in line:
>
>> Now I remember: I was reading a story in a newspaper about a woman who stabbed her boyfriend. My heart started to race. I thought to myself, "I'm having a heart attack. I have to get out of here." I fled

into the street, called my office on my cell phone, and told them I was sick and had to go home. I raced back to my apartment, closed the blinds, popped a Valium, and lay down on my bed. That helped, but I continued to feel this sense of dread. I've gone back to work, but it hasn't been easy. My office is on the 35th floor, and now the elevator scares the shit out of me. I can't get in if it's crowded. Sometimes I think I'm going crazy. I've been to see my internist. He said I'm in perfect health, but I'm not; I'm on the edge of a nervous breakdown.

The interviewer clarified what she was experiencing: a psychological disorder expressing itself through frightening physical symptoms. Naming what she had experienced—a panic disorder—and indicating that it was treatable had a calming effect.

Such delineation of the illness is an important part of any clinical interview. Telling the patient that the syndrome is clinically recognized, that many people have it, and that it is treatable is a therapeutic intervention that diminishes anxiety. Anxiety is exacerbated by the patient's feeling that the experience is outside the realm of human knowledge and is incomprehensible.

The same patient had a successful career in the financial world and was ambitious and hardworking. She had broken up with her boyfriend 2 weeks before the onset of her symptoms over his refusal to get engaged. The interviewer asked about this relationship. "What is he like? How did you relate to one another? What were your similarities and differences?" This inquiry revealed that she had been unusually dependent on him to make decisions, such as where they would go on vacation and how they would spend their weekends. Given the patient's forthright and independent attitude in her professional life, her constant deferral to her boyfriend seemed paradoxical.

Such a story is not uncommon in the panic disorder patient and speaks to the underlying discomfort that many such patients possess concerning their assertive strivings in intimate relationships.

The patient's father was described by her as a frightening figure during her childhood. He was irascible and frequently lost his temper. She characterized her mother as "infantile": "She always acted like a little girl who needed to be taken care of and pampered. She wasn't too good at taking care of me. I'm not sure she should have been a mother." As a child, the patient was shy, fearful, and constantly worried. Separation issues were a problem during her early development. She had difficulty when her mother left her at school and had to come home from summer camp because she was inconsolably homesick.

The interviewer asked about her feelings concerning her boyfriend's reluctance to commit to the relationship and its subsequent breakup. "I was furious. I wanted to kill him. I don't tolerate anger well. It frightens me. Then I feel guilty. At the same time I felt so alone. I needed him. That weakness made me feel more angry. It was a vicious cycle. I became depressed, guilty, and angry." This productive interchange allowed the interviewer to explore her fear of anger and its connection to the childhood anxiety that her father's outbursts had engendered. She continued, "I feel so insecure when I'm alone and not in a relationship. I'm not even sure the actual person is so important. I just need someone there to make me feel comfortable. Sort of pathetic isn't it?" This confession enabled the interviewer to explore her insecure attachment to her mother, whom she had experienced as more like a demanding sibling than a protective and comforting parent, and her childhood desire for someone she could count on to comfort her and relieve her anxieties and worries. These themes, combined with the appropriate use of medication, were further explored and developed in the therapy and led to a successful treatment.

Unraveling the Details

The interviewer listens to every aspect of the patient's description of his symptoms in order to understand their psychological significance. For example, one woman who is afraid of crowds may emphasize her concern about the people "who brush against me," whereas another will speak of her feelings of being "alone in the midst of strangers." The first description would suggest concern about sexual feelings; the second connotes anxiety over separation from the sources of dependency gratification. Of course, the interviewer would not interpret this to the patient until later in the treatment.

The consequences that a patient fears, were he to enter the phobic situation, may involve the projection of a repressed wish or the fear of its expression and the retaliation that would ensue. The patient may be able to elaborate detailed fantasies of what he fears, with no awareness that he is describing an unconscious wish. This is valuable information for the clinician, but again, it should not be shared with the patient early in treatment. For example, a woman who was afraid to go out on the streets was able to portray in some detail the sexual events she feared. However, it was many months before she was aware of her own sexual desires. The phobic symptom represents the unconscious fear far more clearly than the forbidden wish.

A woman described her fear of restaurants, and the clinician inquired, "What would happen if you did go into a restaurant?" The patient replied, "I would get upset," expecting the interviewer to stop at this point. Instead he asked, "And what would happen if you did get upset?" The patient was surprised and answered with annoyance, "I might faint and have to be carried out on a stretcher." The interviewer continued, "And what if that happened?" Now the patient felt justified in her anger, and she replied, "How would you like to be carried out on a stretcher?" The interviewer answered, "We both know that you have a dread of such a situation that is different from the distaste that the predicament would hold for others, and I would like to help you with it." The patient relaxed, saying, "Well, my dress might come up—people might notice the rash on my legs, or they might say, 'Look at that one; she must be on her way to the mental hospital.'"

The interviewer had uncovered the patient's fear of going crazy as well as her shame about her appearance. Further exploration revealed a mixture of exhibitionistic and aggressive impulses, and her self-punitive need to be controlled and humiliated in retaliation for them.

The Initial Episode

The initial episode of the symptom is particularly enlightening. A middle-aged woman who was afraid of eating meat could offer no explanation for this behavior but was able to recall that it had first occurred at the dinner table during an argument between her husband and daughter. She later revealed that a frequent battle in her childhood centered on the religious proscription against eating meat on Fridays. The symptom was related to her fear of the open display of defiant aggression both in her current life and in her childhood.

Physiological Symptoms

In describing their symptoms, some phobic and panic disorder patients discuss their subjective sense of anxiety, whereas others, utilizing more extensive denial, emphasize the physiological concomitants of anxiety, such as trembling, palpitations, or chest pain. The interviewer can lay the groundwork for future interpretations by linking these physical responses to the appropriate subjective states. He might say, "When you get giddy and feel faint, there must be something frightening you," or "That tightness in your chest is the kind of feeling people get when they are anxious." Some individuals experience anxiety as a diffuse bodily sensation that borders on depersonalization. If hyperventilation plays an important role in the production of symptoms, the patient may loosen his collar, complain that the room is stuffy, or ask to have the window opened. Now the interviewer makes a difficult choice. If he remains quiet, the patient will likely feel he is insensitive to the complaint. On the other hand, if he accommodates the patient, the patient will expect more indulgence. If the room is indeed stuffy, there is no harm in opening the window. The chances are that the patient was reacting to a topic under discussion. By opening the window and continuing the exploration of the uncomfortable topic, he has an opportunity to ask, "Do you feel better now?"—but only if the patient continues the discussion. The phobic patient might ask, "Can't we talk about something else?" or an equivalent. Now the interviewer can comment, "Perhaps there is something inside you that made the room feel stuffy, something that this topic has triggered." This exchange typifies the continuing negotiation that exists between the clinician and the phobic patient's fears.

A common physiological manifestation of anxiety, which the phobic patient tries to ignore, is the gurgling of his stomach. When this occurs during the interview and the patient reacts with discomfort, the interviewer can remark, "It seems as though you're embarrassed about the noises your body makes." This indicates that the interviewer is comfortable discussing such matters and that the patient's feelings about his body are an appropriate topic for the interview.

Identification

If the patient has ever known anyone with a similar symptom, the exploration of this relationship can offer further insight. Phobic patients frequently employ relatively primitive modes of identification, and phobic symptoms are often based on a specific model. It is unusual not to uncover a phobic parent or grandparent or some other individual who offered a phobic pattern with which the patient could identify. Furthermore, the patient usually has great empathy for other phobic persons and may have surprising insight into the dynamic significance of the other person's symptom, although he is quite unable to see the same mechanism in his own behavior.

Changes in the Symptoms

It is revealing for the interviewer to detail the shifts and developments in the history of the symptoms. A specific conflict that is difficult to identify in any given symptom becomes obvious when this historical pattern is viewed as a whole. For example, a man presented a fear of eating in restaurants. When more details were elicited, he revealed that this was a recent symptom and that previously he had been afraid of flying. The history soon revealed a long string of apparently unconnected phobic symptoms, all of which occurred in situations in which he was out of contact with his mother. He had counterphobically refused to give her his cell phone number because "She's so intrusive." He harbored great unconscious resentment of his mother, and his aggressive impulses toward her were manifested by a fantasy that she would become ill and be unable to contact him. His resulting guilt and anxiety were controlled by the phobic symptoms.

Avoidance

The Patient's Sensing of Danger

At some point, the interview progresses to a more general discussion of the patient's life. The interviewer may ask, "What are your other worries?" or inquire into the patient's mode of dealing with problems in his life. The patient is skillful at shifting the topic to comfortable subjects, and the interviewer's task is to frame the questions so that the patient cannot escape dealing with the real issues. When this is successful, the avoidance mechanism will be seen in its purest form as the patient says, "I'd rather not talk about that"; "That is very upsetting to me"; or "Can we change the subject?" This is a critical point in the interview, for it allows the interviewer to establish that anxiety is not a valid reason for avoidance. He can reply, "I appreciate that it is difficult for you, but I know that you want help, so let's go ahead and see what we can do," or "Try to do the best you can. I will try to make it easier." In this way, he bargains with the patient, withholding the promise of help until the patient is willing to move into the phobic area, at least in his thinking.

It is difficult to provide the needed reassurance and at the same time to avoid condescension or the suggestion that the patient is an infant. However, with sicker or more dependent patients, the interviewer's direct assurance of protection from anxiety may be necessary: "I've treated other patients with this symptom, and I don't think that any harm will come to you." This is a magical maneuver, and it encourages a dependency adaptation on the part of the patient. It allows the patient to establish a positive transference that facilitates the treatment. The complications are dealt with later, but with a severely phobic patient the exchange of avoidance for magical dependency may represent a major improvement.

The Patient's Search for Treatment

Phobic patients actively seek treatment. They consider it a form of insurance and may collect therapies and remedies in the same way that other people collect insurance policies. There is a feeling of security that stems from having a therapist, and it is this security, rather than therapeutic effect, that seems to motivate the patient's search.

Often the patient conceals his treatment from others, and it is helpful to ask the phobic patient who knows that he is seeing a mental health practitioner. He may feel that he will get more support and reassurance from other people if they are not aware that a therapist is caring for him. He does not trust the clinician to provide adequate assistance and therefore feels safer if he is able to keep other channels open. At times this patient may see two clinicians simultaneously, keeping one a secret from the other. Hence a careful exploration of the patient's prior and current attempts to seek psychiatric help is critical. The patient may already be taking medication prescribed by another clinician, and this may only emerge when the interviewer broaches the subject of psychopharmacological treatment. The patient may experience guilt over this dual treatment. The clinician can then ask, "Were you afraid that I would be offended if you preferred another doctor's prescription?"

Phobic patients try to treat themselves. They develop magical rituals that partially alleviate their difficulties, and they frequently conceal these from the clinician until they find out whether his "magic" is an adequate substitute. It is necessary to systematically but sympathetically explore the treatment techniques that the patient has utilized before coming to treatment. Useful questions include "What do you do when you get anxious?"

The patient's self-treatment often involves the substitution of one phobia for another, trying to maximize secondary gain and minimize realistic inconvenience and secondary pain but still defending himself from anxiety. He may report with great pride that he has forced himself to ride in an airplane, provided it is a short flight, or to go out in crowds, as long as it is not at night. By bargaining with himself in this way, he achieves a subjective sense of trying to deal with his problems while continuing to avoid their psychological roots.

The issue of the clinician's vacation often presents a dilemma with the phobic patient who in response to this upcoming separation may request medication if it has not previously been prescribed. The contemporary psychiatrist has generally given a phobic or panic disorder patient medication well before an impending break in the treatment. Such a decision should be made early in the treatment and not in response to the patient's anxiety about an impending separation during which there will be no opportunity to monitor the drug's therapeutic impact and possible side effects.

Secondary Gain

For example, with a woman who reveals discomfort while describing her need to be accompanied to the neighborhood store by her husband, the interviewer can comment, "You are unhappy about asking him to go with you." The patient will respond either with further expression of her guilt or with an attack on her husband for his exploitation of her dependency on him, thereby justifying her own behavior. In either event, the comment has led to a shift from a discussion of the overt behavior to its emotional significance. It is true that the symptom may reflect hostility toward her husband, but this is too strongly repressed to be interpreted in an initial interview. It is more useful to reinforce the patient's conscious unhappiness with the secondary effects of her symptoms. This also avoids repeating the struggles with friends and family that every phobic patient has had before he comes to the clinician and begins to cement an alliance between the therapist and the healthy portion of the patient's ego.

The secondary gain is important to the interviewer because it aids in understanding the patient's psychodynamics and because it provides one of the strongest resistances to change. The interviewer can ask, "What can't you do because of your symptoms?" This may seem to be a blunt inquiry into an aspect of his psychological function, but there is usually sufficient denial that the patient has no awareness that the answer reveals emotional conflicts. Other useful questions include "What is the effect on your family if you are unable to go outdoors? or "How do you manage to get things done if you can't take the subway?" The patient often reveals discomfort in describing the impositions that he makes on his family and friends. The interviewer can use this opportunity to sympathize with the embarrassed portion of the patient's mature ego.

Those social acquaintances who recognize a psychological basis for the patient's difficulties usually interpret the secondary gain as providing the basic motivation. Their view is that the patient is manipulating his environment in order to obtain certain benefits. The patient responds with injured indignation, feeling that he is accused of enjoying painful symptoms over which he has no control. The interviewer can avoid this unfortunate struggle by maintaining his position of neutral inquirer into the patient's behavior, attempting to understand rather than to judge it. For example, if a patient's family thinks that she acts frightened of going outside in order to avoid her responsibilities, the interviewer can ask, "How do you feel when they say things like that?" If she reveals anger, he can support it, and if she denies it, he can give her permission to express her feelings by commenting, "It must be annoying to be blamed for something over which you have no control."

Avoidance in the Interview

The defensive avoidance that characterizes the phobic symptom is also a critical resistance in the interview. It may appear as an inadvertent omission, a tendency to steer the conversation away from certain subjects, a request for permission not to talk about uncomfortable topics, or an outright refusal to speak. This patient frequently omits crucial data about important areas of his life and then denies responsibilities for this omission. A phobic Caucasian woman spoke at great length about her plans for marriage, but only inadvertently revealed that her fiancé was Asian. She explained, "You never asked me about that," a characteristic phobic response. The interviewer replied, "Did you think I might have something to say about it?" He thus addressed himself to the avoidance behind the patient's denial. Another patient, a young psychologist with phobic character traits, first revealed that he had congenital heart disease when, after months of treatment, the therapist pursued a reference to his scar. The patient explained that the scar resulted from a childhood surgical procedure to correct the defect. The surprised therapist inquired, "Why have we never discussed this before?" The patient explained, "I didn't realize that it had any psychological significance." The interviewer responded with a direct confrontation, "It is hard for me to accept that, with your training, you could think that such a childhood experience was unimportant."

PRINCIPLES OF TREATMENT

The Need for Reassurance

After relating his difficulties, the phobic patient will seek reassurance. He may ask, "Do you think you can help me?" or "Is there any hope?" Other patients may seek the same reassurance more indirectly, asking, "Have you ever treated any cases like mine?" The interviewer translates the meaning by responding, "I guess you wonder if I'll be able to help you." The phrasing of the patient's question has prognostic significance; the patient who is more optimistic and who expects to play an active role in his own treatment has a more favorable prognosis.

The clinician can reply to these requests for reassurance by saying, "The more we talk about your problems, the more I will be able to help you deal with them." This answer shifts some responsibility for the cure to the patient while offering the clinician's assistance and indicating the first step that the patient must take.

The phobic or panic disorder patient also characteristically asks, "Am I going crazy?" His fear of anxiety leads him to perceive his symptoms as evidence of total emotional collapse, with the loss of all control over his impulses. He wants the clinician to take over, to tell him that he is not going crazy, and to assume the responsibility for his emotional controls. The question about going crazy provides an opportunity for exploring the content of the patient's fear. The interviewer asks, "What do you mean, crazy?" or "What do you think it would be like to be crazy?" He can further inquire whether the patient ever knew anyone who was crazy, and, if so, how that person behaved. Finally, he can offer reassurance coupled with an initial interpretation of the patient's inner psychological conflicts: "You must be frightened about the feelings you have bottled up inside. You've never lost control in the past, so why should it happen now?"

Often the patient will not be reassured by the content of what the clinician says, but he will detect the clinician's calm and lack of anxiety. Phobic patients frequently try to provoke anxiety in others, particularly in parental surrogates such as mental health practitioners. The way in which the clinician handles his own anxiety and his attitude toward his patients will serve as a model for the patient and, particularly in early interviews, is more important than any interpretation of the patient's behavior.

Educating the Patient

The phobic patient avoids far more than he is aware of, and one goal of the early interview is to explore the scope of the avoidance and to educate the patient about it. The initial interventions are aimed not at providing the patient with insight into his symptoms but at expanding awareness of his neurotic inhibitions. The therapist might comment, "It is striking that you haven't said anything about the sexual aspects of your marriage" or "Do you ever feel angry at anyone?" The patient will probably reply that he has no problems in these areas, that he has nothing to say about them, or that this has no bearing on his symptoms, but the groundwork for future interpretations is established.

One goal of treatment is to facilitate understanding of anxiety. Phobic patients often think that other people do not experience anxiety, and their goal is to become immune from it themselves. Early attempts to interpret this are bound to be superficial and ineffective. In time, the interviewer can indicate that anxiety is a normal emotion and that the patient's anxiety is often appropriate, but only disproportionate to the stimuli that trigger it. Frequently it is the patient's fear of future anxiety (so-called anticipatory anxiety) that is the major problem.

Questions concerning the patient's perception of other people's reactions are useful in increasing the patient's knowledge about anxiety.

> After a patient reported a panic attack following a "near miss" accident in which a friend was driving, the interviewer asked, "How did your friend feel at the time?" The patient answered, "He was a little upset, but not as upset as I." This provided an opportunity to explore the patient's overevaluation of his anxiety and the fact that his responses were qualitatively similar to those of others. The interviewer replied, "Could it be that you were just more aware of your own feelings than you were of his, and you were not in control of the car?" The patient answered, "No!

He doesn't feel like I did. He isn't afraid of fainting or having a heart attack or feeling 'way out.'" The interviewer then said, "It sounds as if
you and your friend were afraid of different things, and his anxiety was
only related to the danger and the potential accident." This provided an
avenue for the exploration of the unconscious determinants of the patient's fear. The issue involved control and who almost lost it. If he had
been driving he would have felt to blame. Because he was not, he felt he
was risking his life with someone else in control. He had experienced similar feelings as a child with his mother, feeling he needed her for his safety
but recognizing that she was also sometimes reckless, which made him
feel in danger.

The phobic patient often needs assistance in recognizing his emotions. This has already been discussed in relation to anxiety, but it is also
true of other feelings. Feelings are replaced by symptoms, and in time the
clinician will learn the pattern this follows. When the patient describes a
headache, the clinician can point out, "The last few times you complained
about a headache, you were angry at someone. Are you angry now?"

Medication

The appropriate use of medication is a crucial component in the effective treatment of the phobic or panic disorder patient. As with the depressed patient, the combination of psychopharmacological treatment
and psychotherapy is therapeutically synergistic in the anxiety disorder
patient.

The psychological meaning of medication with any patient should
never be ignored. This is especially true with the anxious-phobic patient.
The patient does not just want a pill; he wants assurance that the clinician
has powerful magic that offers protection from anxiety and can provide
safety and security. Paradoxically, some patients are reluctant to consider
medication even when it is clearly indicated. "It is such a sign of weakness. I don't want drugs," asserted a phobic patient when the clinician
said that medication was an important part of the treatment. Exploration
of this issue led to an uncovering of an aspect of the patient's childhood
experience: "My mother was always popping pills or drinking when she
was upset. I don't want to be like her." The clinician was able to point out
that the appropriate use of medication for her condition did not mean
that she would turn into her mother or that she would become dependent
on drugs. He clarified that medication would dampen her anxiety and facilitate her ability to achieve mastery of her phobic fears. He commented,
"We will explore their psychological meaning together, and the use of
medication will help us to do that. Overwhelming anxiety, like pain, is
disabling and dominates your mental world. We have to reduce its inten-

sity so that we can address its psychological origins." This intervention enabled the patient to accept the use of medication, which, after psychotherapeutic work, she was ultimately able to dispense with, although she kept an unfilled prescription in her handbag as a reassuring talisman.

The Role of Interpretation

The early activity of the interviewer is aimed at encouraging the patient to tell his story, to describe the details of his symptoms, and to discuss his personal life. The patient does not want to talk about his sexual, aggressive, dependent, or competitive feelings, but it is important that he be urged to do so. The interviewer demonstrates that he is not phobic in these areas of life and that he expects the patient to follow his lead.

In these early phases of contact, it is seldom helpful to challenge the patient's avoidance in the outside world, but the clinician quickly interprets the avoidance that appears in the interview, such as the omission of important material or the refusal to discuss some area of life. Premature direct suggestions or interpretations concerning the psychological meaning of a phobic symptom will increase the patient's defensiveness and interfere with the interview. The interviewer characteristically understands far more than he interprets to the phobic patient.

When a phobic symptom or panic attack is analyzed, anxiety and avoidance are discussed before symbolization or displacement. The patient must first realize that he is anxious and that he avoids the source of his anxiety before he can begin to explore the conflicts that underlie it. Projection is usually interpreted after the other defenses have been thoroughly analyzed.

The specific secondary gains associated with the patient's symptoms may offer clues as to what type of bargain will be most effective in getting the patient to relinquish his phobia. In time, the clinician will offer to replace these secondary gains but will require as a precondition that the patient enter the feared area. Medication, magical reassurance, and supportive interest and concern can be used as substitutes for the secondary gratifications that the patient obtains from his symptoms. For example, if the secondary gain involves the gratification of dependency needs, the clinician may develop a relationship in which the patient can obtain this gratification within the transference. The clinician can also support the direct expression of the patient's aggressive feelings, particularly when they occur without the rationalization provided by the symptom. For example, when the patient becomes angry and then makes a guilty apology, the therapist could say, "You seem to feel that you don't have the right to get angry" or "Aren't you allowed to feel angry?"

The bargaining aspect of treatment occurs when it is necessary to associate the therapist's support and gratification explicitly with the patient's relinquishing his symptom. Needless to say, this is a technique that is employed only after extensive treatment. An example occurred when a phobic man arrived for his session and stated, "I know I won't be able to talk about anything today; I'm just too anxious." The therapist, who knew from previous experience that the man meant what he said, smiled and replied, "Well, shall we stop now?" The patient became quite angry, but he did not want to leave, so he was forced to talk about his feelings.

When the phobic patient seeks help from others, he often seeks rules for life, formulae that will serve as safeguards against anxiety. This emerges in the psychiatric interview as an interest in general formulations that suggest guides for conduct without involving the details of his life. The phobic patient will ask if he needs more rest or suggest that his trouble is that he worries too much. He wonders if he should just take it easy and clings to any suggestion from the clinician in this area. The clinician can reply to these requests by interpreting the patient's avoidance. He can say, "I guess that you don't like the idea that your symptoms are related to your own thoughts and feelings." On other occasions the patient may ask, "Do you think I should try to take the subway?" The therapist could reply, "Are you wondering whether I'll push you before you're ready?"

After the meaning of a phobic symptom or panic attack has been explored in detail, it still may seem necessary for the clinician to play an active role in encouraging the patient to enter the feared situation. However, this clinical problem may represent the patient's fear of assuming the responsibility for acting on his new insight—in a sense, he is phobic of giving up his phobia. He is fearful of the new and unknown feelings and also of the mature adult role involved in deciding to make a major change in his behavior. Frequently, the patient will accuse the clinician of becoming impatient or fed up with him, projecting his own self-contempt onto the therapist. The clinician now shifts from analyzing the dynamics of the specific symptom to discussing the transference relationship and the patient's attempt to avoid any personal responsibility for his own improvement by attributing it to the clinician's power. If this is successful, the clinician's active intervention may no longer be necessary.

Depression

Phobic patients often become depressed during treatment. They fear that giving up their symptoms will necessitate relinquishing infantile dependency gratifications. Depression may be a sign that treatment is

progressing, and the therapist should provide the support and encouragement that the patient needs at this phase. It is often a critical point in
treatment, because the patient is not asking the clinician to protect him
from imagined danger but to help him with the problems he has when
he faces the real world.

> One of us treated a middle-aged woman who happened to be a trustee
> of the hospital where he worked. Her worries focused on her own health
> (she was healthy) and the health of those she loved. She visited multiple
> specialists and enjoyed the status of "the special patient." She began a
> session by discussing a friend whom she described as "fortunate" be-
> cause of her devout religious faith, and she expressed envy for the sense
> of security that it provided her friend. "I wish I had something like that
> to comfort me in my moments of insecurity." The psychiatrist replied,
> "You have something similar in your belief system that provides you
> comfort; it is medicine, and you have surrounded yourself with highly
> qualified physicians who represent a team in which you have placed
> your trust and faith. You endow them with great power, and you are in-
> clined to see them as omniscient. Like most religious persons, you occa-
> sionally question their power to help you."
>
> The patient listened intently and appeared mesmerized, gently turn-
> ing her head from side to side in amazement. She said, "It is so obvious;
> it's been there right in front of my face all these years. Why didn't I fig-
> ure that out myself?" The psychiatrist said in a joking tone, "I guess
> that's what you pay me for." They both laughed.

COUNTERTRANSFERENCE

The phobic patient elicits three major countertransference problems: omnipotent idealization (the benevolent omniscient, omnipotent parent);
condescending infantilization; and frustrated anger. The patient seems to
want to be treated as a helpless child. If the therapist goes along with this,
he often adds the condescension that reflects his feelings about adults
who want to be treated as infants. The presence of this response may reflect the therapist's difficulty with his own feelings of dependency, but it
may also suggest that he is overresponding to the patient's demands.

If the therapist initially accedes to the patient's demands, accepting
omnipotent idealization as reality rather than transference, he may eventually grow irritated and angry. If the clinician then reveals this anger, the
patient will feel that his transference fears have been confirmed and that
treatment is another strange and frightening situation in which he is
helpless when confronted with a powerful and arbitrary parent.

The anxiety disorder patient has more overt anxiety and often elicits
responsive anxiety in the interviewer. This anxiety often leads to contra-

dictory short- and long-range goals—the immediate soothing, calming effects of reassurance and support may be antitherapeutic in the long term. The problems of sensing the amount of anxiety that the patient can tolerate at any given stage and of timing interventions appropriately are a major challenge to the art of the therapist.

CONCLUSION

The anxiety disorder patient is responsive to a number of therapeutic approaches. This is true with all the anxiety disorders. Cognitive-behavioral therapy, psychodynamic psychotherapy, and the judicious use of medication all potentially have a part to play in the effective treatment of the anxious patient. An awareness of the patient's individual psychodynamics should inform the application of these differing treatment modalities in order to enhance therapeutic response.

CHAPTER 9

THE BORDERLINE PATIENT

"**B**orderline" is an old concept that reflects the confusion engendered in clinicians confronted by these distraught, impulsive, upset, and disturbing patients. They are not psychotic, although they can sometimes manifest psychotic features and for brief times become overtly psychotic. Most of the time they seem well enough to be regarded as neurotic, but with these added features on the "border."

Most psychiatric syndromes are described in terms of presenting psychopathology. The borderline syndrome is distinctive because it was discovered in the office of the dynamically oriented psychotherapist. The concept is clinically derived; it was first recognized because these patients seemed to become worse when treated with intensive psychotherapy and revealed far more serious psychopathology than was suspected in the initial evaluation. They were viewed as more well-integrated neurotic individuals at assessment but manifested impulsive, self-destructive, and demanding behaviors when dynamic psychotherapeutic treatment was initiated. The transference rapidly became intense, filled with anger or with inappropriate expressions of love or intense erotic feelings. Often extreme idealization alternated with massive devaluation. Simultaneously the patient was resistant to taking any perspective on his or her self, constantly employing externalization and denial.

Reflecting the clinical confusion caused by these patients, a welter of terms have been applied to their condition in the past: pseudo-neurotic schizophrenia, ambulatory schizophrenia, preschizophrenic personality structure, "as-if" personality, psychotic character, and hysteroid dysphoria. Each of these attempts at classifications captured some aspect of the borderline patient, but it was not until the second half of the twentieth century that more comprehensive and inclusive clinical descriptions emerged.

Falret, in France in the 1890s, published a vivid clinical description of the borderline patient. He used the term *folie hysterique*. He observed that these patients showed extreme changeability in ideas and feelings, that they could shift abruptly from excitement to depression, and that their intense love for someone was quickly transformed into hate. Although some of Freud's case studies published in the early part of the twentieth century, especially the Wolf-man, would be seen as borderline patients today, it was not until the 1930s that Adolph Stern asserted that there existed a large group of patients who fit neither the psychotic nor the neurotic category. He found that they were extremely difficult to manage by any psychotherapeutic method. He discerned that these patients announced themselves by what occurred in the course of dynamically oriented treatment, namely a near-psychotic transference. In the 1940s, Helene Deutsch described a group of patients whose emotional relationships to the outside world and their own egos appeared impoverished or absent. She coined the term *as-if* to describe the personality of these patients who superficially appeared "normal" but lacked genuineness so that even the naïve observer experienced something missing in them. Deutsch accurately described the identity disturbance and the inner emptiness that characterize the borderline patient. Around the same time, Hoch and Polatin delineated a group of hospitalized patients initially thought to be schizophrenic but who did not fit that diagnosis because even though they were manifestly psychotic at times, the episodes were of short duration and would disappear. They considered the essential clinical features to be pan-neurosis, pan-anxiety, and chaotic sexuality and classified them as *pseudo-neurotic schizophrenia*. John Frosch introduced the term *psychotic character*. He felt that it was a distinct counterpart to the well-described neurotic character and emerged during the course of psychoanalytic treatment. Although psychotic symptoms could readily appear in these patients, the symptoms were transient and reversible. He suggested that this symptomatology was an integral part of their character structure and not a way station to or from psychosis.

In the 1950s, Robert Knight denoted *borderline* as an entity unto itself, no longer linked to psychotic illnesses such as schizophrenia. He viewed the borderline patient as someone in whom normal ego functions were severely weakened. In the late 1960s, Otto Kernberg used the term *borderline personality disorder* to describe what he regarded as the salient feature—a specific, stable, but grossly pathological personality organization. His description was predicated on a psychodynamic formulation. Like Knight, he emphasized ego weakness, especially poor impulse control and impaired frustration tolerance. In addition, he described the use of primitive defense mechanisms, pathological internalized self and object relations, and intense unmodified aggression. Somewhat later Michael Stone criticized the purely psychodynamic model for its implied causation and suggested that there were powerful genetically determined biological components to the disorder relating it to bipolar disease.

The integration of the phenomenological research of Grinker and Gunderson with the psychodynamic models of earlier investigators led to the DSM-III and DSM-IV diagnostic criteria for borderline personality disorder.

The DSM-5 criteria for borderline personality disorder (Box 9–1) are designed to enhance diagnostic reliability and therefore present a narrower concept of the disorder than that employed by many clinicians.

BOX 9–1.   DSM-5 diagnostic criteria for borderline personality disorder

---

A pervasive pattern of instability of interpersonal relationships, self-image, and affects, and marked impulsivity, beginning by early adulthood and present in a variety of contexts, as indicated by five (or more) of the following:

1. Frantic efforts to avoid real or imagined abandonment. (**Note:** Do not include suicidal or self-mutilating behavior covered in Criterion 5.)
2. A pattern of unstable and intense interpersonal relationships characterized by alternating between extremes of idealization and devaluation.
3. Identity disturbance: markedly and persistently unstable self-image or sense of self.
4. Impulsivity in at least two areas that are potentially self-damaging (e.g., spending, sex, substance abuse, reckless driving, binge eating). (**Note:** Do not include suicidal or self-mutilating behavior covered in Criterion 5.)
5. Recurrent suicidal behavior, gestures, or threats, or self-mutilating behavior.
6. Affective instability due to a marked reactivity of mood (e.g., intense episodic dysphoria, irritability, or anxiety usually lasting a few hours and only rarely more than a few days).
7. Chronic feelings of emptiness.
8. Inappropriate, intense anger or difficulty controlling anger (e.g., frequent displays of temper, constant anger, recurrent physical fights).
9. Transient, stress-related paranoid ideation or severe dissociative symptoms.

Source.   Reprinted from American Psychiatric Association: *Diagnostic and Statistical Manual of Mental Disorders,* 5th Edition. Arlington, VA, American Psychiatric Association, 2013. Copyright 2013, American Psychiatric Association. Used with permission.

In the broader view, patients with a variety of personality disorders, such as histrionic, narcissistic, obsessional, and paranoid, who are at the more disturbed end of a continuum are considered borderline. In addition, borderline phenomena are ubiquitous and can be found in many patients who are not diagnostically borderline.

There is also a continuum of clinical severity within the borderline category. The more extreme patients make frequent appearances in psychiatric emergency departments, are hospitalized, and have recurrent acrimonious encounters with legal and social authorities through their propensity for domestic violence, drug abuse, reckless driving, and other impulsive behaviors. Many less disturbed borderline patients presenting in an ambulatory setting, however, can initially appear quite charming, sympathetic, and basically neurotic. The underlying disturbance will only manifest itself in an ongoing treatment situation, although hints of borderline pathology may be found when a careful history is taken.

The protean elements of borderline psychopathology do not have a single theme except what can be termed *stable instability* of emotions, relationships with other people, ego functions, and identity. This fluid and volatile state of so many aspects of psychological structure and function results in astonishingly sudden transformations of personality. The greater percentage of patients diagnosed as borderline patients are women between the ages of 20 and 50 years. The relative rarity of the diagnosis in older populations may suggest that the condition subsides over the course of the life cycle. This may reflect the diminution of drive intensity and emotional energy that occurs in the course of aging. Some have suggested that it may also reflect clinician bias and diagnostic prejudice.

PSYCHOPATHOLOGY AND PSYCHODYNAMICS

Borderline Characteristics

Affective Instability

In more serious cases, the common eruption of wild and uncontrolled emotions characterizes the borderline patient. In the midst of one of these episodes, the borderline patient can seem frightening, demonic, or repugnant to others. He would seem to be "possessed." Borderline patients have a low emotional flashpoint together with an "excess" of affect that they draw upon and that fuels these episodes. Relatively innocuous minor misunderstandings with another person can precipitate outpourings of rage. When seized by anger, the borderline patient enters an altered state of consciousness in which reasoning, reality testing, and an awareness of the feelings of other people no longer exist. These episodes resemble the temper tantrums of a small child whose developing ego is overwhelmed by a suffusion of angry frustration. Affective instability in the borderline patient is not confined to outbursts of anger but can also manifest itself in intense, although often unrequited, feelings of love and sexual desire. These can occur early in a relationship when the other person is barely known. These intense excessive romantic longings for the other person are an expression of a type of emotional "hunger" that plagues the borderline patient. Initially, the fact that the love is not returned has little impact on these feelings. However, the patient becomes increasingly demanding and impatient, insisting that there be some reciprocal demonstration of love. A sexual encounter early in the relationship, frequently initiated by the borderline patient, often catalyzes these overwhelming romantic feelings and may be interpreted as "proof" that they are reciprocated and as justification for demands on the other.

The less-disturbed borderline patient, when not overtaken by a state of wild emotion, can be experienced as quite sympathetic by the interviewer. However, relatively stable emotional periods are interrupted by episodes of intense emotional display when real or perceived slights occur or an erotic fixation develops. Healthier borderline patients are capable of maintaining a long-term relationship or marriage, albeit one often punctuated by affective storms and crises. They can also have relatively productive vocational or professional lives, although their career paths tend to be inconsistent because of their outbursts and impulsivity.

In addition to the marked emotional reactivity of the borderline patient with episodes of anger or demands for intimacy, there are also more pervasive underlying disturbances of mood. Episodes of depression and dysphoria, usually of short duration (days or even hours rather than weeks), are also common and may often occur in response to some minor disappointment or perceived rejection such as a friend being late for an appointment or a casual remark by a friend, lover, or therapist that the patient regards as insensitive or uncaring. The borderline patient may become acutely anxious concerning some aspect of her health and assume that a minor ailment such as a cold or dysmenorrhea is an early manifestation of a life-threatening illness. When this happens, her internist or gynecologist will be barraged with telephone calls and demands for immediate medical appointments or other reassurances. The doctor's attempts to reassure the patient may be ineffective and may only lead to a never-ending search for a more concerned caretaker. Eventually the anxiety will dissipate, but not before the borderline patient's physicians have been left exasperated and exhausted by incessant demands for reassurance or further medical evaluation.

Borderline patients usually have far more control over their affect in the initial interview than they possess later in treatment, when they may be prone to what have been called *affect storms*. These emotional outbursts are characterized by an intensely aggressive and demanding quality directed at the therapist, who will feel psychologically assaulted. The therapeutic approach to this phenomenon is to set clear boundaries at the beginning of treatment. The reader is referred to Kernberg's paper on this issue concerning ongoing therapeutic management of affect storms in the treatment of the borderline patient.

Unstable Interpersonal Relationships

Tumultuous interpersonal relationships are typical of the borderline patient's life. There is a hyperdramatic, theatrical quality to his involvement with other people, exemplified by extremes of alternating positive and negative emotion permeating feelings about everyone in his world. In contrast to the histrionic patient, whose often-appealing emotionality is attention-seeking, the emotional outbursts of the borderline patient are expressions of uncontrolled affect that are often irritating to the recipient.

Initial idealization of another person by the borderline patient will often be followed by devaluation and denigration. Intense involvement after a relatively superficial encounter with another person is typical.

> "This is the best friend I have ever had," stated a borderline patient after sharing a cup of coffee with a fellow college student whom she had met only the day before. "We have this amazing understanding, instant empathy. We are soul mates." Two weeks later, this best friend was regarded as shallow and tawdry. When the interviewer inquired how this transformation had taken place, the patient replied: "She didn't return my telephone calls for over a day and she had my cell phone number. Completely unreliable and uncaring." The interviewer replied, "That's quite a change in your feelings—from best friend to worthless." Realizing that this is common with childhood "best friends," the interviewer proceeded to explore the patient's early history of best friends who then disappointed her and her experience of her parents' role in helping her integrate these episodes.

The emotional hunger of the borderline patient can lead to the rapid idealization of the other person soon after meeting. The new friend or lover is "perfect," compassionate, and completely involved. This idealization is a manifestation of the craving to be loved and adored by the other person, an experience lacking in the borderline patient's memories of childhood, which are often marked by feelings of neglect or frank emotional and physical abuse. The idealization can also be seen as the representation of a desire to be idealized in return. When inevitable flaws appear in this projected fabric of perfection, an inescapable aspect of the vagaries of any relationship, the idealization turns into its opposite and the friend or lover is seen as uncaring, mean, and rejecting. The relationship comes to a stormy end, with angry recriminations on the part of the borderline patient. Rarely does the borderline patient recognize that his behavior, impossible demands, and unrealistic expectations may have contributed to this outcome. It is always the other person's fault. The borderline patient will often reveal a history of romantic relationships, all of which have foundered in his opinion because of some appalling inadequacy, insensitivity, or disappointing behavior on the part of his lovers. These experiences are perceived by the patient as abandonments or rejections.

In the more disturbed borderline patient, anger can quickly escalate into physical violence. Knockdown battles with partners or brutal beatings of children for minor infractions may lead to involvements with the law and social agencies and appearances in psychiatric emergency departments. The capacity to delay gratification or inhibit impulsive anger is drastically impaired in the severe borderline patient and is at the core of his dysfunctional interpersonal relationships. At times, these rage attacks in the severely disturbed borderline patient may extend to homicidal behavior.

Sexuality

The borderline patient can often be sexually appealing and easily attract partners. Sexuality is not inhibited as it often is with histrionic patients, and the borderline patient may be very sexually active and orgasmic. The borderline patient is frequently the protagonist in a seduction. The process begins with slightly too long eye contact or a flagrant flirtation. The exaggerated sexuality may, for a time, bind the partner as passionate physical intensity compensates for the emotional storms that punctuate other aspects of the relationship. A young man commented about his borderline girlfriend: "My friends are furious with me for staying with her. She's a lunatic, a wild woman they tell me. They are right, but she's so fantastic in bed. I don't want to give that up." The interviewer replied, "Her ability to disinhibit you seems more important than a happy, loving relationship." Eventually, he did give her up when her episodes of uncontrollable rage escalated to frightening proportions as she tore up his papers and destroyed his property. The sexuality of the borderline patient, like other aspects of their relationships, is object-connected, albeit of a primitive nature, colored by alternations of idealization and devaluation. Intense erotic feelings concerning the therapist appearing very early in a consultation or treatment are clues that the clinician is dealing with borderline pathology. Idealization and devaluation also occur in the narcissistic patient, but the narcissist is less personally involved and can terminate a relationship much more easily with less anger and more contempt. People are more expendable. The narcissistic attachments are more shallow and therefore more easily transferred to a new person.

Identity Disturbances

An unstable identity is characteristic of the borderline patient. Most people have a stable inner feeling of self that remains consistent even in the face of the fluctuations in mood, emotional stresses, personal losses, and so on that occur in everyday life. This consistent personal identity, which forms early in childhood and continues to consolidate throughout adolescence, is unstable in the borderline patient. As one patient expressed it, "I never know who I am from day to day." The borderline patient may feel both to himself and to others like a different person from one day to the next. For example, a borderline patient who was aggressive, demanding, indignant, and self-righteous in his first interview session was plaintive, passive, and childlike in the second session, stating that he felt he was hopeless. This vulnerable hurt "child" was in striking contrast to the formidable person who had arrived for the first session.

The borderline patient often seeks identity based on the responses of others. It is as though the other person's response provides a temporary representational structure that consolidates who the patient is for that moment. This need for the outside world to provide psychic structure is at the root of the borderline patient's incessant craving for emotional responses from other people. Borderline patients thus appear healthier in structured interview situations than in unstructured ones in which they may seem more disorganized and disturbed.

This unstable sense of self will often extend to sexual and gender issues. "Am I gay or straight? I don't know. I do know I can have sex with men or women, enjoyable sex, but I don't know whom I prefer. It's very confusing and makes me feel crazy," lamented one borderline patient. Another pondered a sex change operation, without understanding or learning what it would entail. Sudden, impulsive vocational changes, occurring almost on a whim, can figure in the history of borderline patients, reflecting this unstable sense of self. A borderline physician had pursued training in three different specialties, dropping out of each residency when it lost its appeal. Now he wanted to be a psychiatrist, hoping that this training would provide an answer to the confusion surrounding his professional identity. Buried behind that wish was an unconscious hope for a solution to the dilemma of "Who am I really?"

One clinical manifestation of identity disturbance occurs when the interviewer literally does not recognize the patient at the second visit because he or she seems like an entirely different person. For a deeper understanding of this disturbance in identity and the appearance of different states of consciousness and behavior in the same patient, the reader is referred to Chapter 11, "The Dissociative Identity Disorder Patient." There is often overlap between the borderline patient and the dissociative identity disorder patient, and both usually share a history of recurrent childhood trauma.

Rejection Sensitivity

Borderline patients fear rejection and are hypersensitive to any subtle fluctuation in the interviewer's attention. For example, the interviewer who is tired and stifles a yawn or who glances at the clock to check how much time remains will find the borderline patient responding with anger. This loss of total attention from the interviewer will be experienced as an abandonment that confirms the patient's underlying dread of inevitable rejection. This exquisite fear of rejection is often a self-fulfilling prophecy. The volatile and difficult behavior of borderline patients frequently drives people away from them, confirming their worst fears and plunging them into depression.

The borderline patient typically responds to being alone with fear and confusion. Hence, there is a desperate need for the presence of another person, which provides an external bulwark against experiencing inner chaos. For the clinician, ending sessions and planning vacations will pose particular difficulties with borderline patients. The normal end of a session is often experienced by the borderline patient as a rejection and abandonment. As a session was coming to a close, a patient stated, "I need another minute. We can't stop right now. It would make a big difference to me if I could just finish talking about this issue." As the therapist prepares to go on vacation, the borderline patient will often become increasingly symptomatic, make covert or overt threats of suicide, and demand contact with the clinician when he or she is away. "Where will you be? How can I reach you? Can I have your phone number?" are typical responses by the borderline patient to the therapist's imminent summer vacation.

Impulsivity

Impulsive behavior, often self-destructive or even life-threatening, is typical of the borderline patient. Unprotected sex with partners who are barely known is an example. Although the borderline patient may have an awareness that this could place her at risk for venereal disease or pregnancy, this will not prevent dangerous, impulsive sexual behavior. Intemperate and excessive use of alcohol or illicit drugs in dangerous settings is another example of the impulsive behavior of the borderline patient. The use of drugs and alcohol is often driven by a desire to feel more "alive" or "real" through the intense experiences that these substances induce. This need to feel more "real" is motivated by a wish to escape the profound inner emptiness that plagues the borderline patient. Borderline impulsivity naturally extends into their interpersonal relations and vocational situations. Friends can be dismissed without reason: "I don't care about her anymore. I can't explain it." Jobs can be resigned without an alternative in sight: "It just wasn't right for me. I couldn't stand it. I have nothing else in the offing and I don't know how I'm going to live, but there will be a way." Frequently the borderline patient expects that such a display will cause the other person to feel guilty. The narcissistic individual, in contrast, has no further use for the other person. His attachments are more exploitative than manipulative. This becomes apparent when the other person fails to respond favorably and sympathetically to a petulant display. The borderline patient will be hurt by the lack of response; the narcissist will look for a more effective strategy. Reckless behavior, untempered by rational thought concerning its consequences, is typical of the borderline patient.

Self-Mutilation and Suicidality

Suicidal gestures and behaviors are often prominent in the histories of borderline patients and may pose grave dangers. When confronted with rejection by a romantic partner or inflamed with anger at family or therapist, the more disturbed borderline patient will often resort to potentially fatal actions such as medication overdose or wildly reckless driving. A history of such behaviors, usually beginning in adolescence, is an indication of the severe nature of the disorder and the imperative need to establish an alliance with the clinician, who can provide a forum for the expression of such impulses before they are put into effect.

A history of self-mutilative behavior, especially cutting the skin with a knife or razor or burning or scarring, is common. There is a malignant cast to these acts too, because such self-mutilative behaviors in the history of a borderline patient double the likelihood of a successful suicide in the future. It has been posited that the cutting of the skin and its associated pain and bleeding are concrete manifestations of the patient's inner psychic pain as well as an attempt to overcome feelings of mental numbness. Such episodes often take place in a dissociative state in which the borderline patient is watching herself cutting her skin but does not feel present in her body.

Paradoxically, self-mutilative behavior such as cutting or burning is often accompanied by little physical pain. These episodes provide an experience of intense feeling that the borderline patient does not otherwise experience. Such self-generated intense experiences counteract the inner feeling of deadness. They also highlight the experience of the boundary between the self and the outside world, reassuring a person who may not have a firm sense of such boundaries. It is common for borderline patients in psychiatric hospitals to conceal their self-mutilation from the staff and then suddenly reveal it, taking apparent satisfaction in the staff's distress and surprise. Often this behavior is misunderstood as manipulative when it is more importantly linked to the patient's attempt to reaffirm possession of control of her body; no one else knows what she has done until she chooses to inform them.

Paranoid Ideation and Dissociation

Paranoid thinking is common in borderline patients. A woman with borderline personality disorder, after her university failed to grant her tenure, complained, "It's all part of a larger hostile organized conspiracy against me because I'm a lesbian and outspoken faculty member." The interviewer knew from the patient's earlier sessions that certain elements of her tenure application were weak and replied, "Did you consider any alternative explanations?" The lack of recognition from the outside world is a blow to the borderline patient's fragile self-esteem and can readily lead to quasi-delusional thinking. The borderline patient's belief that he is being cruelly mistreated defends against an even more painful inner feeling of inadequacy. Misperceptions of cues and misunderstandings of other people's intentions are common. Casual behaviors of others such as being accidentally bumped on a crowded bus can lead to paranoid outbursts: "Why are you pushing me?" Real external stresses can lead to paranoid convictions. "My editor gave me this impossible assignment so that I would fail and then she can fire me," concluded an accomplished magazine writer when faced with a pressing deadline.

Dissociative episodes, as well as depersonalization or derealization, are common in the borderline patient. *Depersonalization* is a loss of feeling of one's own reality, whereas *derealization* is the experience of finding the outside world strange and different. Depersonalization includes seeing parts of one's own body as unfamiliar or changed or feeling fatter or thinner or shorter than usual. These experiences are usually transient and occur in response to stress, and they will often respond when the clinician reassures the patient that the state is temporary and, when possible, links it to identifiable precipitating events. The episode of depersonalization defends the patient against awareness of the link. A borderline patient had a furious argument with her husband over their son's failure to complete a homework assignment. She promptly entered a dissociative state and called her therapist, announcing, "I am in mental fragments; pieces of me are scattered through the universe. The 'me' of me doesn't exist. I am no one." The therapist responded by reviewing the events that preceded the episode with her and added empathically, "It is a painful way to control your anger." The patient was then able to recover from her fragmented state.

Differential Diagnosis

The boundaries separating borderline personality disorder from more severe forms of other personality disorders are often unclear, and the categories may well overlap. The more primitive variants of histrionic, narcissistic, and paranoid personality disorders often merge with borderline personality disorder and make for a comorbid diagnosis. In general, however, the relative lack of self-destructiveness, impulsivity, and exquisite sensitivity to abandonment separates the narcissistic, paranoid, or histrionic patient from the borderline patient. Both borderline and narcissistic patients idealize and then devalue others. The differences in the manner in which they do so are important in distinguishing the two personality disorders and are elaborated later. The antisocial patient also often overlaps with the borderline patient. Most borderline personality disorder patients are female, whereas most antisocial personality disorder patients are male, and a proportion of patients with either diagnosis will meet criteria for the other, sharing extreme aggressivity and impulsivity. Gunderson has suggested that these two diagnoses may be highly related forms of psychopathology and that the distinctions are gender-related. Bipolar spectrum disorders can easily be confused with borderline personality disorder because they may both present with mood lability and impulsivity. A distinction can be made, however, by a carefully conducted history that will reveal, in the bipolar patient, a history of early onset of depression, episodes of hypomania, and genetic predisposition in a positive family history.

Comorbidities

There is a high rate of comorbidity between borderline personality and depression. The depression is often associated with feelings of emptiness, unrequited dependency needs, and anger along with the depressed mood. Feelings of guilt, preoccupations with perceived personal failures, and vegetative symptoms are less common than in other depressed patients. Repeated and potentially fatal suicidal gestures often occur in borderline patients with concomitant depression. Alcoholism and other substance abuse are other common comorbidities. The high rate of comorbidity with bipolar illness has led to speculation that borderline conditions are milder variants of bipolar II disorder. Bipolar II illnesses in the hypomanic phase share characteristics with borderline disorders, including irritability, impulsivity, reckless behavior, heightened sexuality, and a propensity for furious outbursts over minor misunderstandings.

Borderline Versus Narcissistic Devaluation

Borderline and narcissistic patients both idealize and devalue others. However, there are important differences in the ways in which they do so. The borderline patient alternates between idealization and devaluation like a young child who changes best friends and whose frustration tolerance and capacity to delay gratification have not matured. Nevertheless, the borderline patient cares about the other person, even though the alternating attitudes may lead to a slow deterioration of the relationship. The narcissistic patient is more exploitative; the idealization is related to an idealized projection of an omnipotent self. If the other person fails to manifest this delegated omnipotence for the patient's benefit, the other is cast aside as no longer of use to the narcissistic patient, who then shifts to a new person who is expected to enhance the patient's grandiose fantasy. The narcissistic patient's rage is more of a contemptuous nature when manipulation of and extraction from the other are no longer possible. The borderline patient's trigger is usually a threat to the patient's dependency needs rather than a threat to the patient's grandiosity. The narcissistic patient's idealization is related to power, influence, glamour, and status that will further self-aggrandizement and carries little evidence of human caring. The narcissistic patient "borrows" a friend's car with a feeling of entitlement and without permission, whereas the borderline patient does so from a boundary problem—that is, not distinguishing between "mine" and "not mine."

Developmental Psychodynamics

The developmental origin of the borderline patient's lability and intensity of emotions, fluctuating reality testing, and unstable relationships is complex and controversial. Genetic endowment and early experience are probably both involved. Infants exhibit variation in irritability and anxiety from birth. The propensity for easily aroused anger and low frustration tolerance that lie at the heart of the borderline patient's tempestuous interpersonal relations is probably genetically determined. Disturbed interpersonal relations are also possibly genetically determined, although at this stage of our knowledge there is no definitive evidence for this.

Just as the parents shape the infant's behavior, the infant elicits and shapes parental responses. The result depends on the interaction between the two. An irritable, crying infant creates a stressful experience for any parent. The empathic parent with a high degree of patience responds by providing a soothing, comforting environment. This may lead to gradual acquisition of emotional and healthy ego development. A stable sense of self and an integrated internal image of the caretakers are contingent upon experiencing consistent empathic responses from the parenting persons. The parent has to acknowledge the emotional needs of the child. "You are hungry," "You are angry," and "You are sad," when empathically experienced and tenderly voiced by the caregiver in a manner that accurately reflects the child's emotional state, lead to a growing mental representation of inner states and desires. Mirroring of the infant's state by the mothering person is integral to the child's development of reality and of a mental awareness of his or her inner self. It is also central to the development of an integrated inner image of the caretaker. When the caretaker is gratifying the child's basic needs for food, comfort, physical closeness, and so on, she or he is experienced as "good." When these basic needs are not met—the child is hungry, uncomfortable, angry, or frightened—and there is no immediate comfort or empathic response from the outside, the caregiver is experienced as "bad." Over time, with sufficient gratification and the experience of "good-enough" mothering, the child fuses the representations of both the gratifying "good" mother and the frustrating "bad" mother into an integrated internal image.

This process of development appears to be distorted in the future borderline patient. The derailment may reflect a highly irritable and difficult-to-comfort infant, a self-preoccupied and narcissistically impaired parent who does not have a natural capacity for maternal empathy with a reservoir of nurturing emotion for the child, or both. This interactive process between a volatile infant and an empathically limited parent may lead to a fragmented sense of self and distorted "split" internal images of other people. Important individuals in the adult borderline patient's world remain all-good or all-bad, reflected in the often bewildering alternation of the adult borderline patient's view of someone as initially "wonderful" and shortly thereafter as "terrible" (a frequent experience directed at the clinician engaged in the treatment of the borderline patient). The sense of self of the borderline patient is fluid and unstable, reflecting how the external empathic acknowledgment of the individual's internal state as a child was never internally registered. In essence, the borderline patient has never felt confident in knowing who she or he really is. An organized sense of self is contingent upon the experience of empathic parental mirroring. (See Chapter 5, "The Narcissistic Patient," for a more extensive discussion of parental mirroring.)

The borderline patient will often provide a history not only of childhood neglect and emotionally absent parents but also of frank abuse, both physical and sexual. A history of beatings and sexual molestation is frequent in borderline patients' accounts of their childhood and adolescence, suggesting a further understanding of their feeling of fragmentation of their already fragile sense of self. The theme of being a victim, a prisoner in an abusive household, carries over into the borderline patient's adult world and frequently colors the treatment situation. The therapist will commonly be experienced by the borderline patient as just another in a long series of emotional abusers.

The normal attachment of the child to the parent facilitates the capacity to perceive mental states in the self and others. The borderline patient who as a child has been subject to recurrent abuse tends to lack this capacity. An inconsistent, abusive parent of a borderline patient will, by his behavior, grossly inhibit the development of this ability to reflect on the mental state of self or others. The developing child is unable to consider the mental state of the parent who is mistreating her so egregiously. The capacity to consider the feelings of others develops only when a child has experienced sufficient love and sensitivity from caregivers and can identify with them, incorporating their goodness as part of the child's developing sense of self. The lack of stable, predictable connectedness becomes an important factor in disturbed interpersonal relations.

Adolescent borderline patients are prey to uncontrollable emotions exacerbated by the onset of puberty, are still trapped in a neglectful and abusive household, and are unable to reflect on their own mental state or connect to that of others, and thus they often engage in wildly self-destructive actions. Substance abuse, promiscuity, eating disorders, school truancy, petty crime, fights, and self-mutilation run like a red thread through their teenage histories. Typically, the parent, even if abusive, is not all bad but may provide some warmth, love, and protection, albeit inconsistently. It is the guilt of the abuser following the abuse that leads to the abuser acting warm, tender, and caring. In that way, a pattern is laid down associating abuse with love. The desperate and impossible search to find someone who will satisfy emotional hunger in this self-destructive manner is a consistent feature of the borderline patient's subsequent relationships, including those with therapists.

Superego formation is distorted in the borderline patient. Recurrent abuse and mistreatment in childhood lead to the child's identification with the abuser, who is perceived as "strong": "The world has mistreated me; therefore the world owes me—my behavior is justified because I have been treated badly" is the underlying subtext behind much borderline behavior. Boundaries, both mental and physical, were often transgressed by the borderline patient's parents. It is this transgressive, abusive, inconsistent behavior that interferes with the normal process of superego development.

In contrast, the parental failure in the development of the narcissistic patient is more one of the exploitation of the child for the narcissistic needs of the parent. "My child is the best, the brightest, the most everything." Implicit is the idea that this is because of the parent's perfection (or unconsciously as a compensation for feeling a lack thereof). "Of course you don't have to wait in line, or take turns, because you are so special." When the child does not receive this recognition from others, the parent says, "They are just jealous of your greatness." The child receives repeated rebuffs. The parent fights the teacher to change a B grade into an A. The parent boasts about the child's specialness in front of the child. The child cannot understand why others do not perceive him in the same grandiose way as the parent. This is different from the abuse experienced by the borderline patient, but it also impairs the child's capacity for warm and caring interpersonal relations.

Unlike the narcissistic patient, the borderline patient feels guilt, but it does not have much influence on her behavior. The experience of transgressive behavior in the borderline patient's childhood will often lead to a desire to reexperience it in later life situations and in treatment, where the borderline patient will often make attempts to seduce the clinician. This unconscious desire to relive a traumatic incestuous experience is motivated by the guilty pleasure that it originally invoked and a wish to master the desire, to turn passive into active and not be helpless in the face of remorseless yet stimulating abuse. These developmental dynamics are expressed in the treatment situation, where the patient may unconsciously recapitulate his or her traumatic and troubled history in the interactions with the therapist.

MANAGEMENT OF THE INTERVIEW

The borderline patient is often the most challenging and taxing patient that the mental health professional will meet. The reasons for this include both the complexity and gravity of the illness and the intense, often negative and disturbing, countertransference responses that the borderline patient evokes. The patient is more disturbed than the more typical neurotic character, but not so disturbed as to feel "different" and easily be "objectified" by the therapist.

The less disturbed borderline patient, like the histrionic patient, often seems easy to interview. To the inexperienced clinician, the patient can, at first glance, seem like an "excellent" psychotherapy patient. There is easy access to the unconscious; conflicts and fantasies are freely articulated. Borderline patients resemble the dramatic patients described in the early days of psychoanalysis—sensitive, complex, and compelling, with apparently deep psychological awareness. Colorful, enticing descriptions of their lives and both normal and perverse sexual fantasies emerge in the interview situation. The usual barrier to the unconscious seems porous. There is so much fascinating clinical material that they are obviously quite special, ready and often eager for intensive psychotherapy that, especially to the beginning therapist, clearly seems the treatment of choice. The patient implies that insight-oriented therapy will provide therapeutic solutions to difficult but tractable problems. The interviewer is cast in the role of rescuer.

The more experienced clinician, however, will see more serious pathology in this facile presentation of apparently "deep" psychological access. Healthy defenses are not adequate; too many emotionally charged and profoundly conflictual issues are permeating the clinical situation well before a treatment alliance has been established. The apparent easy access to the unconscious suggests the lack of normal filtering barriers and reflects the unstable psychic functions of the borderline individual. This latter characteristic explains why the borderline patient looks much healthier in structured settings than in unstructured ones, where they may seem fragmented. Borderline patients look normal on structured psychological tests such as the Wechsler Adult Intelligence Scale but psychotic on projective tests such as the Rorschach.

Exploration of the Presenting Issues

A borderline patient claimed in an initial interview, "My boyfriend is a jealous lunatic. If I look at someone, he accuses me of wanting to seduce him. It happens all the time. Men do make passes at me, and sometimes I respond. It's true that I have slept with other men since I've been going out with him—they are attracted to me—but his jealousy leads to terrible fights. He's paranoid. I don't understand why I stay with him."

The interviewer in this situation is in a delicate situation. The patient's externalizing style and denial of responsibility for her provocative behavior require sensitive exploration. The danger is that the interviewer can easily be cast in the role of moralizing accuser, which will undermine any possibility of a therapeutic alliance. The interviewer may reply, "Tell me the details of a recent instance." The patient may not start at the beginning of the "scene" but instead begin with the boyfriend's angry outburst. The interviewer can listen and then proceed with further exploration. "How did it begin? Where were you, and what was happening?" The patient may then reveal that she flirted with someone else in front of the boyfriend or perhaps described such a scene to him. The interviewer can ask, "What reaction did you expect him to have?" The patient may seem stumped and pensive. She then might say, "I guess that he thinks that I am beautiful, that he is lucky to have me, and he's glad that other men agree." Now the interviewer has tactical choices: He can either say nothing and wait, perhaps with a raise of eyebrows, or less subtly reply, "Did you think that flirting in front of him was the best way to achieve that?" One could wait for further reactions from the patient, acknowledge her wish for a more demonstrative boyfriend, or suggest that her boyfriend, in his own way, was quite responsive and that his jealousy provides the evidence that he cares in a way that she may consciously find painful but at the same time unconsciously satisfying.

"Men do find you attractive" is another possible response by the interviewer to the borderline patient's lament about her boyfriend. It acknowledges the patient's often-desperate need to be found desirable and yet is not condemnatory. "Do you find me attractive?" may be the patient's reply. The interviewer can say: "Being found attractive is important to you," which acknowledges the wish but does not compromise the clinician into a collusive agreement. The borderline patient's incessant desire to receive reinforcing confirmation of her attractiveness, tragic life history, constant mistreatment by the world, and poignant personal condition may place difficult demands on an interviewer during the initial interview. The interviewer's desire to maintain an empathic stance constrains him from contradicting the borderline patient's view of the world, which is often marked by externalizations, contradictions, and denials of personal responsibility. The interviewer's rising sense of indignation at the increasingly preposterous constructions of life events that the patient relates, casting herself as innocent while denying her aggressive, provocative, and demanding behavior, has to be carefully monitored. As with the paranoid patient, empathically recognizing her sense of hurt or distress without joining the patient in agreement can be an appropriate and therapeutic response. "I have been so abused and misunderstood," says the patient. The interviewer replies, "That must be very painful for you to talk about. It sounds like life has been disappointing to you." These interventions help to maintain an empathic alliance so that exploration and discovery can continue.

> In an initial interview, an attractive young professional woman revealed a long history of physical and emotional abuse by her mother but remained comparatively dispassionate as she described this traumatic upbringing. When the interviewer asked about her romantic life, however, she became vituperative. She had broken off her first engagement in college, explaining, "He was everything to me, my dream, but I could tell his family wouldn't accept me. I broke the engagement before he could reject me—I was so hurt." Shortly thereafter she became engaged again. When this second fiancé was transferred because of his work to a town 100 miles distant from where the patient was in graduate school, she said, "I couldn't take the distance, the loneliness; I started another relationship with a classmate." She felt that her fiancé was abandoning her and told him of this new relationship. "He said he would forgive me and wanted to work it out, but I could see how angry he was and I broke it off." The interviewer commented, "You are quite sensitive to the feeling of rejection." In response, the patient recounted other, more transient relationships. She became emotionally labile in the interview as she proceeded to describe her many boyfriends, alternating between being tearful and furious. She complained, "They always disappoint me. They are ingrates, just using me sexually."
>
> A consistent pattern emerged of the patient acrimoniously ending every romantic relationship as she became more emotionally involved. Though highly intelligent, she viewed the problems in her star-crossed romantic life as lying outside herself, explaining her mistrust of men in general. In a bitter tone she stated, "Men are all like my father: selfish, pathetic, obsessed with sex." The interviewer inquired, "Tell me about your father." She replied with vehemence, "He abandoned my mother and me when I was only 6 months old. I have never seen him since. Can you believe that?" The interviewer answered, "It's understandably painful for you to believe that he wouldn't want to see you. All the men in your life now seem to have his traits—selfish and uncaring." The patient replied, "That's so right. You understand. You're very insightful."

Now the interview has entered a perilous phase in the clinical engagement of the patient. The interviewer is cast in the role of the all-understanding, all-good person who has been so absent from her life. He should remain dispassionate and not be taken in by this flattery because as the therapeutic enterprise progresses, it will inevitably turn into its opposite, when the borderline patient will become devaluing in response to the therapist's failure of empathy or refusal to violate clinical boundaries: "You know nothing; you don't understand me. You are incompetent and unfeeling."

> A young borderline woman began her third interview by saying: "I hate you. I'm not better; I'm worse since I began seeing you. I'm so depressed

and unhappy. I've gained weight; I can't fit into my clothes." At this point she was weeping and yelling in fury. "I want to smash something, break up your office, hit you." She began pounding the chair in which she was now writhing and screamed, "Don't you know anything? You can't help me. I want to die; I feel so bad." The rage emanating from the patient was overwhelming, arousing anxiety in the interviewer and the fear that she would indeed do something violent. Paradoxically, the interviewer was also aware of being unmoved by her distress and thought to himself, "I've only seen her twice before and yet she feels I should have cured her." Recognizing that this would be a sarcastic reprisal, a sadistic reaction to the patient's accusations, the interviewer instead first acknowledged the patient's conscious affect and then explored deeper fears: "You're frightened that nobody can help you. You seem frustrated and very angry. Have you had disappointing experiences with other therapists?" The interviewer was then able to elicit a history of recurrent disappointments and abandonments, including those with previous clinicians, that occurred whenever she became close to someone. This intervention calmed the patient down. The tempest passed away as quickly as it had appeared. Much later in the treatment, she developed an awareness of how her volatile behavior and outbursts of fury drove people away. Prior to this hard-won insight, she had seen herself as blameless in a sequence of acrimonious romantic breakups that had left her despairing and suicidal.

Early Confrontations

Because of the borderline patient's tendency toward impulsive and frequent self-destructive behaviors, it is essential that the interviewer explore those aspects of the borderline patient's life that imperil personal safety. Reckless, unprotected sexual encounters; alcohol and substance abuse; and entering risky social situations are examples. The interviewer, without being condemnatory, can elicit this history and try to place it in a context that gives it meaning. The borderline patient will say, "When I'm angry and upset, I need relief. Sex gives me that. I often don't care who it is with." The interviewer can reply, "You don't seem to care enough about yourself to worry whether it's safe or whether you will get pregnant. It is as though you want to take risks." This type of intervention allies the interviewer with the healthy elements of the borderline patient's ego rather than prematurely focusing on the impulse-ridden, angry, and self-punitive themes.

A careful history of drug use is essential in the interview of the borderline patient. Although many borderline patients avoid illicit drugs, knowing that their use may precipitate unpleasant and even frankly psychotic states, others seek them out because of the high that they provide. When intoxicated, they feel more intensely alive, in contrast to the emptiness and inner deadness that often constitute their baseline state. Problems with drug abuse may require specific treatment. Such multifaceted treatment approaches are often necessary with borderline patients. Making the drug-abusing borderline patient a partner in a multiple therapeutic approach to his disorder is central if this endeavor is to be successful. The interviewer can state, "You give a clear history of regularly using heroin as a way of dampening down your inner anguish. We need to address the treatment of your heroin use, since it has taken on a life of its own, one that threatens your chances for recovery."

Borderline patients do commit suicide! This danger frequently hovers over the interview situation and arouses anxiety in the interviewer. The borderline patient will recount, "I was just so furious I wanted to end it all. I swallowed all the pills I could find. If my roommate hadn't come home and taken me to the emergency room, I would be dead rather than talking to you." The interviewer must confront this situation head-on. He can respond, "When you are really upset, you feel the solution is to annihilate yourself. You and I have to work on this together, looking for ways of dealing with being angry other than destroying yourself."

Self-mutilative behavior is common in the sicker borderline patient. Cutting the skin with a knife or razor and burning the flesh with a cigarette are typical examples. These may occur in micropsychotic episodes. Often, early in the treatment, the patient will coyly announce: "I burned myself today" while swathed in covering garments that conceal these self-induced lesions from the clinician. The interviewer can respond, "I would like to see the burns; would you show them to me?" This intervention brings the hidden masochistically and erotically induced behavior into the light of day in the consulting room. Now, not secretly hidden, this symptomatic assault on the self can be looked at objectively and its meaning explored. The interviewer inquires, "What was going through your mind as you did this?" or "What were you feeling that led to this behavior?" The observing ego of the borderline patient is now brought into play, and the therapist and patient can begin to try to understand this action. "I was so angry at you for what you said last time we met. You seemed so cool and aloof. I don't believe you really care about me. This seemed to be the only thing I could do." The interviewer can respond, "Do you feel that you had no alternative but to burn yourself to get through to me? You can talk to me about how you feel without burning yourself to show how I have failed you." The therapeutic intent is to bring thought and verbal expression into the clinical situation instead of acting out the feelings in an impulsive, self-destructive way.

This brings up the subject of limit setting in the interview with the borderline patient. This is the patient who violates the clinician's boundaries. He picks up a piece of mail from the office desk; stands by the desk and reads something on it; takes a book off the bookshelf and leafs through it; sits in the chair that has the pad and telephone beside it; stands at the window instead of taking the proffered seat; or says "Can I use your phone?" while picking it up. Many years ago, one of us came from his office into the waiting room to meet his new male patient. He had heard the patient enter the waiting room but could not find him. Suddenly he realized that someone was taking a shower in his bathroom. "Mr. A?" he called out. From the shower came the reply, "I'll be right out, Doc. I'm just finishing my shower." The patient had structured the contact so that he had angered the interviewer before they had met. "I hope you don't mind, "said the patient as he entered the office. The interviewer replied, "You decided to do it even though you thought I might mind. Is this your way of beginning a relationship?" Much to the interviewer's relief, there was no second interview. This less-than-ideal outcome, including the interviewer's sense of relief, speaks to the powerful unconscious countertransferential enactment that the borderline patient can elicit from the interviewer. The patient's showering in the interviewer's office was provocative and elicited a furious response from the clinician that was acted out by directly confronting the patient with his aggression. If the interviewer had self-monitored his countertransference, he could have realized that a drama was unfolding that was key to understanding the patient. A tempered, interested, empathic response by the interviewer would have made it more likely that the patient would have returned for a second visit.

The male borderline patient most commonly uses nonsexual means to express his lack of boundaries, employing money, tips on the stock market, or other temptations for the interviewer. One incident occurred at the end of a consultation when the patient offered to pay in cash. The interviewer replied, "I would prefer that you pay by check." The patient insisted, adding, "But I'm carrying the cash; I could be hit over the head and mugged," in a plaintive tone. "Oh," said the interviewer, "would it be better if *I* got hit over the head and mugged?" Both parties smiled, and the interview ended. In a subsequent session the patient expressed his relief that the interviewer did not accept cash and had not colluded with the patient in a mutual enactment. It was too early in the relationship to explore the patient's veiled suggestion that the therapist might want to join in a conspiracy to evade income taxes.

In another common scenario the patient makes reference to his investing prowess and how he has doubled his money in a short time.

One can justify, clinically, an inquiry into the manner in which the patient accomplished this, but it is a trap for the young clinician who has education debts, a family to support, and so on. The minute the interviewer asks, "What did you say the name of that stock was?" the trap is sprung and the patient concludes that the clinician is more interested in easy riches than in his problem. Should the interviewer use that information, he has violated professional ethics. Instead the interviewer could comment, "I really don't need business information to help with your problem, but it seems that you are eager to provide it to me. What is that about?" This way he both sets limits and emphasizes the theme of the therapy—exploring the motives that underlie impulses rather than acting on them.

The same principle applies to the sexually aggressive borderline patient. A powerful seductiveness is often prominent in the interview situation. An attractive borderline woman used the male clinician's first name in an initial interview and announced, "I enjoy talking to you. It would be nice if we could go out for a cup of coffee instead of being locked up in here." At this point the interviewer has heard all he needs to predict an interview that will be controlled by the patient and in which both content and process will verge on the pornographic. The longer this is allowed to continue, the more uncomfortable the situation becomes for both parties. The patient in this example has already crossed the boundary. The interviewer could have replied, "You have just given me the most recent example of how you get into predicaments that end up unhappily for you. Do I need to explain further?" If the patient blushes, sits up, and proceeds, it is easy for the interviewer to follow up, "Now, let's review some basic data about your life." If instead the interviewer is intimidated and titillated by the patient's seduction, a drama will unfold. She will display that she is not wearing underpants under her miniskirt and launch into a graphic account of her sexual adventures: "I'm a great lover. I believe the body and all its orifices should be used to find ecstasy." She may recount the story of her many lovers and their sexual predilections, drawing the interviewer into an almost fantastic, pornographic, and titillating world. Sexual fantasies, erotic situations, polymorphous perverse behaviors, and a mixture of heterosexual and homosexual encounters may take the interviewer's breath away. Inwardly, the interviewer can acknowledge the success of the patient's wish to sexually arouse him, a wish predictable from her state of undress and her flamboyant narrative. The graphic sexual history may be compelling, but behind it lays the desperate emotional hunger that fills the patient's life and is alive in the interview. If the patient says, "Let's get out of here and have a drink," the interviewer can reply, "It feels like you think I am more interested in your sex life than in your fear of being alone. You seem to have been disappointed by your lovers even though you feel willing to give them everything you have. It may well be that I won't satisfy you either, but by trying to understand your wishes and my failure to satisfy you, we may have a chance to help you change." The gentle assertions by the interviewer that this situation is different, that he will not be seduced, that he has the patient's best interests at heart, and that he is committed to try to understand what has transpired all convey the hope of therapeutic change.

The turbulent personal relationships of the borderline patient will quickly infuse the interview situation and help to establish the diagnosis. An early desire by the borderline patient to discuss transference-based dreams such as "I dreamed last night that we were having sex; it was so fulfilling" suggests that the interviewer is dealing with a borderline patient. The borderline patient's determination to talk about erotic fantasies and transference responses right from the beginning represents the absence of normal boundaries. The easy expression of embarrassing material is a clue. It is part of a wish to seduce the therapist as well as a manifestation of the fluidity of the sense of self and others. Boundaries are permeable and interchangeable. The interviewer's appropriate role in such situations is to maintain an even, empathic, and supportive posture. Deep interpretations based on apparently "insightful" early material presented by the borderline patient are potentially disastrous because the borderline patient does not possess the ego strength to integrate such interpretations and may have a paranoid and rageful response. A borderline patient in a first interview described her relationship with her mother following her father's death in a car accident when she was 4 years old: "She beat me regularly, saying it was my fault he died. He was going out to get orange juice and milk for me when he crashed. She kept beating me every time I said I missed him." The patient had a long history of involvement with physically abusive men who also beat her. The interviewer, in the second interview, connected these aspects of her history and commented, "You seem to be recapitulating your life with your mother in your relationships with men." The patient erupted, "Are you a complete idiot? My mother was doing her best; she didn't want to be reminded of my father's death. It was my fault. In many ways she's a saint. The men I have been involved with are pigs, and I think you're one too." Although the interviewer's reconstruction may have been valid, it did not allow for the fact that the patient was desperately clinging to an internal comforting image of the good mother, the "saint," so that she would not have to confront the reality of the abusive evil mother. Combined with her primitive sense of guilt concerning her own destructiveness, the potential loss of this comforting image of her "good" mother was overwhelming. The therapist became the evil, unfeeling parent.

The early management of the interview with the borderline patient necessitates an empathic, supportive, but in many respects noninterpretive posture. Over time, consistent empathic responses to the patient may allow the patient to identify with the interviewer and thereby increase his curiosity for more understanding of himself. In the early interview situation with the borderline patient, even though there may be patently obvious unconscious dynamics driving the patient's behavior, it is more prudent to remain on the surface and not indulge in clever, deep interpretations. Of course, dangerous or self-destructive behavior must be confronted directly from the very beginning of the relationship. This will come to be seen by the borderline patient as empathic caring. Dynamically based deep interpretations of unconscious motivation, however, will often be seen as the opposite—intrusive, condemning, and unfeeling.

Borderline patients are often "veterans" of multiple attempts at psychopharmacological treatments. This reflects the wide breadth of their basic disorder, which can include brief psychotic episodes, depression, anxiety, and impulsivity. Psychotropic interventions may help to make the treatment less stormy, but a discussion of medication goes beyond the scope of this book. The reader is referred to one of the standard texts of psychiatric therapeutics. However, it is important to note that the relational context in which the medication is prescribed and monitored is more important with these patients than almost any others and that there is no medication that can itself treat the complex characterological structures that inevitably are superimposed on these patients' core deficits.

TRANSFERENCE AND COUNTERTRANSFERENCE

Manifestations of intense transference may appear from the moment the borderline patient arrives for the first appointment: "I didn't imagine you would be so cute"; "What a wonderful office, so tasteful"; "You seem so distinguished"; "It's such a relief to be here in the hands of someone I know can really help me." Such effusive opening gambits based on the intense transference craving of the borderline patient are diagnostically significant. The patient develops this emotional hunger in response to parents who were experienced as expressing little interest in her inner life. The borderline patient insists on an immediate emotional connection to assuage the emptiness and inconsideration that persist in his or her memories of childhood. Romantic and frankly sexual fantasies about the clinician will enter the treatment situation early. A rapid idealization of the clinician is common and is potentially seductive if it is taken at face value. "You are so understanding. You must be an extraordinary therapist. Your patients are very fortunate"—such affirmations of intense longing based on little or no prior knowledge of the therapist speak to the wish to be given special consideration and caring, a desire to be appreciated and nurtured. The interviewer cannot dispel this fantasy with a dismissive "You don't even know me." Instead, he may respond, "You really need to be understood. That is our task together, to try to understand you, so that we can attempt to change things in your life that seem to give you so much grief."

The transference with the borderline patient will inevitably become turbulent; an initial idealization will usually turn into its opposite in a manner that is often perplexing to the clinician. "You don't seem to understand me at all. I don't think you get it," the borderline patient says, a statement that seems to come out of nowhere. The clinician responds, "What did I say or not say that made you feel that way?" "You didn't hear how hurtful it was for me when my mother did not like her Christmas present. She always rejects what I give her. You took her side by saying 'That's her way.' She's an abusive, unappreciative bitch. How could you say, 'That's her way'? How could you defend her when she hurts me over and over again, no matter how nice I try to be to her?" The clinician finds himself cast in the role of the abusive, unappreciative parent. Anger roils the treatment situation. Suddenly the patient sees the therapist as another in a long line of uncaring, stupid, and abusive people. This alternation from being adored to being despised has to be seen as a manifestation of the borderline patient's inner world in which there is no integrated sense of other people with all their virtues and failings combined into one image. This alternation of idealization and devaluation of the therapist offers an opportunity to explore the defense of splitting within the transference. A sustained, empathic, supportive posture offers the possibility that over the course of time the borderline patient will experience an emotionally important individual, the therapist, as possessing both virtues and faults. This will help to diminish the constant oscillation between the all-good person who quickly transforms into the all-bad, a process that never seems to stop.

The powerful emotional arousal that borderline patients evoke in the clinician lies at the center of the therapeutic experience. These feelings can range from a hostile dread of what the patient will do next or demand to an erotic or anxiety-ridden preoccupation with the patient that can easily fill the clinician's waking life and emerge in her dream world.

Self-monitoring of one's countertransference reactions to the borderline patient right from the initial encounter is crucial to maintaining the parameters of the clinical situation and will obviate the boundary violations that can so readily occur with these patients. Countertransference can be a valuable vehicle for understanding the borderline patient's mental world. The intensity of feeling stimulated by the borderline patient carries with it many perils, including the temptation to actually engage in subtle or blatant boundary violations or even unethical behaviors. Borderline patients often possess an exquisitely sensitive emotional radar that enables them to hone in on the clinician's vulnerabilities. They will frequently sense the distaste and sadistic impulses that their impossible behavior and importunate demanding for special treatment are provoking in the clinician. "I can tell you hate me because I called you at home at 2:00 A.M. But I was desperate. I had to speak to you." This type of accusation, because it is sometimes correct, will evoke guilt in the interviewer and, in reaction, may lead to inappropriately solicitous behavior such as extending the time of sessions, making special treatment arrangements, and bending over backward to accommodate the patient. Borderline patients often have a history of sexual and physical abuse in childhood combined with parental emotional neglect. Thus they may portray themselves in a compelling manner as helpless victims, which in turn can arouse rescue fantasies in the interviewer. The therapist then has the fantasy that he will make up for what the borderline patient did not receive emotionally as a child and thus undo the abuse. Because many borderline patients may be highly seductive and sexually arousing, these rescue fantasies combined with the patient's incessant demands for "true intimacy" can, at the extreme, devolve into the worst type of boundary violation, sexual involvement with the patient. Although relatively uncommon, this extreme form of boundary violation represents the most malignant corruption of the interview situation and is, naturally, an ethical, psychological, and often legal disaster for clinician and patient alike. It is crucial that the interviewer honestly acknowledge to himself the noxious or erotic feelings the borderline patient is stimulating. This conscious awareness enables the interviewer to step back and not be swept away. It is often useful to seek supervisory consultation with an experienced colleague when countertransference feelings reach a fever pitch.

CONCLUSION

Patients with borderline personality disorder are often the most difficult and vexing patients to treat. The emotional roller coasters that they create in the clinical situation place great demands on the interviewer's capacity for objectivity, compassion, and tolerance. The clinician will directly experience the stormy tempests, blurring of ego boundaries, desperate emotional hunger, erotic stimulation, and fluid self-states that plague the borderline patient and cause him so much chaos and unhappiness. This inner whirlwind experienced by the clinician is a potentially valuable entrée into the borderline patient's world. If understood as such, and not reacted to by overt anger or subtle reprisals, the therapist's subjective and often painful experience can be a vehicle to clinical understanding and the maintenance of a healing therapeutic alliance. An even, empathic, and supportive posture in the early phase of treatment of the borderline patient can consolidate the development of a more stable sense of self in the patient, lead to a more integrated internal view of other people, diminish self-destructive behavior, and open the way for more directly interpretive work. Most important, it can lead to a better, less fragmented life for the patient. In essence, the clinician has to be able to withstand the emotional abuse that the borderline patient has herself experienced and not succumb to the despair and rage or incestuous seduction that was her lot. Notwithstanding the immense strain that the borderline patient exerts on the clinician's psyche, successful psychotherapeutic and psychiatric treatment is eminently possible with these profoundly troubled individuals, and such effective treatment can be deeply rewarding for the therapist.

CHAPTER 10

THE TRAUMATIZED PATIENT

ALESSANDRA SCALMATI, M.D., PH.D.

Trauma is common in everyday life. It can take many forms, from the unexpected loss of a loved one to a serious motor vehicle accident, the diagnosis of a life-threatening illness, or being the victim of an assault. Popular attention has focused on the aftermath of severe trauma such as civilian disasters, industrial explosions, natural catastrophes, terrorist attacks, life-threatening combat situations, rape, and childhood sexual abuse.

Many people respond to a traumatic event with an acute stress reaction or an increase in anxiety of short duration that resolves spontaneously without need for treatment. Some people develop a more chronic traumatic stress response that becomes impairing and disabling.

Being the victim or witness of a traumatic event does not imply a pathological response or enduring psychological trauma. In fact, even though close to 90% of people will be exposed to some kind of traumatic event during their lifetime, according to a survey conducted in the early 2000s to establish the prevalence of psychiatric disorders in the population, the lifetime prevalence of posttraumatic stress disorder (PTSD) was 6.8%.

From the beginning, an essential question of traumatic studies has been what differentiates between people who develop a disabling response to trauma and those who are more resilient in response to similar tragedies.

Traumatic events and their effect on the human psyche occupy center stage in the current psychiatric landscape, and it is easy to forget that until 1980 PTSD was not an acknowledged diagnosis. Even though trauma, war, misfortune, loss, death, illness, and suffering are and have always been common, for many millennia the stories of sorrow and heartbreak, of soul-sickness and madness, caused by life tragedies, fate capriciousness, and human cruelty were mostly the province of poetry and art, not of medicine and science.

It has been suggested that the interest of science in the psychological effects of trauma only became relevant when life expectancy in Western societies grew to a length that allowed for concerns other than mere physical survival. It is possible that a more comfortable lifestyle, afforded by the industrial revolution, the Enlightenment—with its focus on reason—and a decrease in fatalism and the will of God as an explanation for human events, also played a role. However, by the middle of the nineteenth century, psychiatrists and neurologists started describing with more interest and consistency symptoms that seemed to have their origins in past traumatic events in the patient's life.

What makes the study of the psychological effects of trauma different from the study of any other mental illness is the necessity of an event outside of the human psyche to occur in order for the disorder to exist. PTSD (and acute stress disorder) is the only diagnosis that requires the clinician to determine that exposure to "a traumatic event" has taken place.

Starting with the American Civil War, doctors reported more systematically cases of acute distress experienced by soldiers during and after combat. However, military authority and society at large were quick to accuse the sufferer of cowardice, unless a medical explanation could be devised. The cultural moral standard expected men to be capable and willing to fight for their country and their cause. Soldiers who refused to fight or escaped from the battlefield were accused of desertion and court martialed. Although it might be easy for us to scorn the preoccupation with honor of European countries at the beginning of the 1900s that allowed the unspeakable slaughter of the trenches, it is important to remember that similar ideals of masculinity, strength, and heroism still play a role in modern military culture and contribute to the obstacles veterans encounter even today in accessing and receiving care. During this era, with the exception of a few studies that investigated the effects of trauma in victims of railway accidents, and in survivors of an earthquake in Southern Italy, outside of military hospitals, the other main area of investigation in the traumatic neurosis was the study of hysteria. Patients suffering from hysteria, mostly women, presented with a host of confounding symptoms and many somatic complaints. Contrary to war, neither sexual violence nor the abuse of children had been per se the focus of literature. However, any superficial reading of fairy tales, legends, and mythology from any culture and tradition cannot fail to detect rather accurate descriptions of early life loss, abandonment, neglect, and abuse. Of course, it is a matter of debate whether this is a representation of the inner fantasies of the child, and a projection of our worse fears, or a fair appraisal of what we know to be all too common. The two explanations do not need to be mutually exclusive; fantasies can be not only projected but also enacted with tragic consequences. At the beginning of the nineteenth century, the Bronte sisters, along with Charles Dickens, offered some interesting descriptions of child abuse and neglect that were quite revolutionary for the time, particularly in a society that considered children the property of their parents and male and religious authority unquestionable. However, notwithstanding some sensationalistic reporting in the news of the time, and some increase in the literature of more realistic descriptions of violence and abuse, society was not ready to accept the reality of sexual violence or child abuse as commonly occurring events.

Controversies surrounded the work of Jean-Martin Charcot, who had suggested that the cause of hysteria in his patients was a traumatic event, most likely a past sexual trauma. After Charcot's death, Joseph Babinski, who took over the directorship at the Salpêtrière Hospital in Paris, declared that the cause of hysteria was a preexisting suggestibility in the patient and that women suffering from hysteria, when forced to, would abandon the symptoms. These principles were embraced by French and German physicians and applied with a rather extreme level of cruelty to "treat" French and German soldiers suffering from war neurosis during World War I. The "treatment" used involved the application of electric shock and was in general so painful and brutal that the soldiers preferred to go back to the trenches.

Pierre Janet was also a student of Charcot but followed the initial course of research and maintained the belief that hysteria was caused by a past traumatic event that had caused a "vehement emotion" that created a memory that could not be integrated into personal awareness and was split off into a dissociated state. This state was not accessible to voluntary control, and the person was not able to make a "narrative of the event." This state of affairs caused a "phobia of the memory" that failed to be integrated, but it left a trace, or *idée fixe* ("fixed idea"). These fixed ideas were constantly reoccurring as obsessions, reenactments, nightmares, somatic symptoms, and anxiety reactions. Janet also described the patient's hyperarousal and reactivity to triggers and reminders of the traumatic event. The patient was not better until he or she could integrate the traumatic memory into consciousness.

Sigmund Freud studied with Charcot at the Salpêtrière, and in his early writing he initially agreed with the interpretation of hysteria symptoms as caused by an early seduction or sexual trauma. However, as

Freud started focusing on infantile sexuality, he changed his view and reinterpreted hysterical symptoms as being a reaction to the fantasy of a seduction and, therefore, a defensive response to a conflict between an unconscious wish and a prohibition, not the somatic response to a trauma. As far as war neurosis was concerned, Freud recognized the similarities between the symptoms of World War I veterans and those of patients with hysteria. His hypothesis was that the conflict at the core of war neurosis was between a wish to survive and a wish to act honorably. Freud initially hypothesized that the soldiers' symptoms would improve once the war was over, eliminating the threat to their life and therefore resolving the conflict and rendering the symptoms obsolete.

Charles Myers and William Rivers are the two psychiatrists best known for their work with World War I soldiers in Britain. Myers was the first to use the term *shell shock*. Both were advocates for a more humane treatment of soldiers and a recognition of their suffering as real and not a result of cowardice or a preexisting moral weakness.

Abram Kardiner, an American psychiatrist, worked with World War I veterans between 1923 and 1940. He carefully described his patients' symptoms and reported that many of these veterans had been admitted to psychiatric and medical hospitals and had received multiple diagnoses (including malingering) before a connection was made between their symptoms and the history of trauma. Kardiner was the first to focus on the physiological hyperreactivity associated with traumatic reactions. He described the patients' chronic state of hypervigilance, irritability, explosive anger, and recurrent nightmares. Kardiner's descriptions include veterans reporting an overwhelming sense of futility; most of them were socially withdrawn, and intent on avoiding any possible recollection of the trauma.

The work of Kardiner was applied and expanded upon by a group of American and British psychiatrists working with servicemen during World War II. John Spiegel, William Menninger, and Roy Grinker confirmed many of Kardiner's observations about the state of hyperarousal and Janet's observations about the lack of a narrative memory, even though the patients maintained a very precise somatosensory memory of the trauma that could be easily triggered. Hypnosis and narcosynthesis were used to help the patients to abreact the traumatic memories. However, it was noted that abreaction without integration did not result in resolution of the symptoms.

Studies on the psychological symptoms of Holocaust survivors started to appear almost a decade after the end of World War II and were prolific in the 1960s and 1970s. The survivors were afflicted with a variety of symptoms: somatic symptoms, nightmares, hyperarousal, irritability, social withdrawal, and extreme grief reactions (sometimes associated with the hallucinated images of dead relatives). It is important to note that this last symptom, which has been confused with psychosis as recently as the Vietnam War, is rather common in victims of massive trauma, particularly when the trauma is associated with the traumatic loss of loved ones. Holocaust survivors, and veterans, who have lost beloved companions in action will speak of these visions or ghostly visitations, but they will have no other symptoms to indicate a psychotic disorder. William Niederland was the first to coin the term *survivor syndrome* to describe the decline in function and chronic stress reaction of survivors who suffered not only psychologically but physically from a host of stress-induced maladies. Henry Krystal, who was himself a survivor, described the experience of the concentration camp victim and the victim of massive trauma as one of "giving up": in a situation of inescapable terror, when any attempt to activate the flight or fight response is futile, the mind response "is initiated by surrender to inevitable danger consisting of a numbing of self reflective functions, followed by a paralysis of all cognitive and self preserving mental functions." Krystal also described alexithymia as a consequence of protracted trauma.

During this same period Robert Lifton conducted a remarkable study interviewing survivors of the atomic bomb devastation in Japan, recognizing in them a very similar preoccupation with death themes and a numbing of capacity for enjoyment and intimacy. Lifton compared the reaction of the Japanese survivors with those of Holocaust survivors.

Meanwhile, in the United States, Burgess and Holstrom termed the symptoms of their patients who were victims of rape—and who reported nightmares, flashbacks, and hyperarousal—as *rape trauma syndrome*; they found these symptoms to be similar to those in many other syndromes already described. Andreasen et al. described the stress reaction of a burn victim. Herman and Hirschman worked with victims of incest and domestic violence. Kempe and Kempe published the first well-documented account of the pervasive problem of child abuse. Shatan and Lifton started "rap groups" with Vietnam veterans who were tormented by nightmares, flashbacks, rage, and a growing sense of alienation. Horowitz described the alternating states of reexperiencing and numbing common in trauma survivors.

By the time the committee for the American Psychiatric Association's DSM-III was discussing which disorders to include, there were groups lobbying for the inclusion of a "Holocaust survivors syndrome," a "war neurosis," a "rape trauma syndrome," a "child abuse syndrome," and so on. As Kardiner had written with some frustration in 1947,

"[The traumatic neuroses] have been submitted to a good deal of capriciousness in public interest. The public does not sustain its interest, and neither does psychiatry. Hence these conditions are not subject to continuous study, but only to periodic efforts which cannot be characterized as very diligent. Though not true in psychiatry generally, it is a deplorable fact that each investigator who undertakes to study these conditions considers it his sacred obligation to start from scratch and work at the problem as if no one had ever done anything with it before.

In fact, the fragmentation in the field had not yet reached a level of integration with the incorporation of PTSD as an official diagnosis in the DSM system. PTSD was grouped with the anxiety disorders (because of the high anxiety and hyperarousal state), even though research suggested the important role of dissociation in the disorder. Disputes about the appropriate placement continued for decades; field studies and evidence suggested different criteria to be included in the manual, and controversies continued to surround the diagnosis. It was suggested that a second diagnosis could be introduced, that of "Complex PTSD," to account for the more pervasive disruption in the system of meaning and personality structure observed in survivors of massive trauma. It was also suggested that PTSD be moved to the dissociative disorder category. In DSM-5, the trauma-related disorders occupy a separate category, between the anxiety and dissociative disorders. There is a new criterion, which specifically addresses "a negative alteration in cognition and mood," and there is an option to specify whether the disorder presents with dissociative symptoms.

Controversy most likely will always surround the field of trauma studies, because neither society at large nor the field of psychiatry will ever feel completely comfortable to fully address the problem of responsibility (causality/blame) for the consequences of violence. However, having a diagnostic category legitimized the field, and it provided a language to standardize research and to compare results.

PSYCHOPATHOLOGY AND PSYCHODYNAMICS

Diagnosis

The DSM-5 diagnostic criteria for PTSD appear in Box 10–1. Table 10–1 summarizes the differences between the diagnostic criteria for PTSD in DSM-IV-TR and DSM-5.

BOX 10–1. DSM-5 Criteria for Posttraumatic Stress Disorder

Posttraumatic Stress Disorder
Note: The following criteria apply to adults, adolescents, and children older than 6 years. For children 6 years and younger, see corresponding criteria below.
A. Exposure to actual or threatened death, serious injury, or sexual violence in one (or more) of the following ways:

  1. Directly experiencing the traumatic event(s).
  2. Witnessing, in person, the event(s) as it occurred to others.
  3. Learning that the traumatic event(s) occurred to a close family member or close friend. In cases of actual or threatened death of a family member or friend, the event(s) must have been violent or accidental.
  4. Experiencing repeated or extreme exposure to aversive details of the traumatic event(s) (e.g., first responders collecting human remains; police officers repeatedly exposed to details of child abuse).

   Note: Criterion A4 does not apply to exposure through electronic media, television, movies, or pictures, unless this exposure is work related.

B. Presence of one (or more) of the following intrusion symptoms associated with the traumatic event(s), beginning after the traumatic event(s) occurred:

  1. Recurrent, involuntary, and intrusive distressing memories of the traumatic event(s).

   Note: In children older than 6 years, repetitive play may occur in which themes or aspects of the traumatic event(s) are expressed.

  2. Recurrent distressing dreams in which the content and/or affect of the dream are related to the traumatic event(s).

   Note: In children, there may be frightening dreams without recognizable content.

  3. Dissociative reactions (e.g., flashbacks) in which the individual feels or acts as if the traumatic event(s) were recurring. (Such reactions may occur on a continuum, with the most extreme expression being a complete loss of awareness of present surroundings.)

   Note: In children, trauma-specific reenactment may occur in play.

  4. Intense or prolonged psychological distress at exposure to internal or external cues that symbolize or resemble an aspect of the traumatic event(s).
  5. Marked physiological reactions to internal or external cues that symbolize or resemble an aspect of the traumatic event(s).

C. Persistent avoidance of stimuli associated with the traumatic event(s), beginning after the traumatic event(s) occurred, as evidenced by one or both of the following:

  1. Avoidance of or efforts to avoid distressing memories, thoughts, or feelings about or closely associated with the traumatic event(s).

2. Avoidance of or efforts to avoid external reminders (people, places, conversations, activities, objects, situations) that arouse distressing memories, thoughts, or feelings about or closely associated with the traumatic event(s).

D. Negative alterations in cognitions and mood associated with the traumatic event(s), beginning or worsening after the traumatic event(s) occurred, as evidenced by two (or more) of the following:

1. Inability to remember an important aspect of the traumatic event(s) (typically due to dissociative amnesia and not to other factors such as head injury, alcohol, or drugs).

2. Persistent and exaggerated negative beliefs or expectations about oneself, others, or the world (e.g., "I am bad," "No one can be trusted," "The world is completely dangerous," "My whole nervous system is permanently ruined").

3. Persistent, distorted cognitions about the cause or consequences of the traumatic event(s) that lead the individual to blame himself/herself or others.

4. Persistent negative emotional state (e.g., fear, horror, anger, guilt, or shame).

5. Markedly diminished interest or participation in significant activities.

6. Feelings of detachment or estrangement from others.

7. Persistent inability to experience positive emotions (e.g., inability to experience happiness, satisfaction, or loving feelings).

E. Marked alterations in arousal and reactivity associated with the traumatic event(s), beginning or worsening after the traumatic event(s) occurred, as evidenced by two (or more) of the following:

1. Irritable behavior and angry outbursts (with little or no provocation) typically expressed as verbal or physical aggression toward people or objects.

2. Reckless or self-destructive behavior.

3. Hypervigilance.

4. Exaggerated startle response.

5. Problems with concentration.

6. Sleep disturbance (e.g., difficulty falling or staying asleep or restless sleep).

F. Duration of the disturbance (Criteria B, C, D, and E) is more than 1 month.

G. The disturbance causes clinically significant distress or impairment in social, occupational, or other important areas of functioning.

H. The disturbance is not attributable to the physiological effects of a substance (e.g., medication, alcohol) or another medical condition.

Specify whether:

With dissociative symptoms: The individual's symptoms meet the criteria for posttraumatic stress disorder, and in addition, in response to the stressor, the individual experiences persistent or recurrent symptoms of either of the following:

1. **Depersonalization:** Persistent or recurrent experiences of feeling detached from, and as if one were an outside observer of, one's mental processes or body (e.g., feeling as though one were in a dream; feeling a sense of unreality of self or body or of time moving slowly).
2. **Derealization:** Persistent or recurrent experiences of unreality of surroundings (e.g., the world around the individual is experienced as unreal, dreamlike, distant, or distorted).

Note: To use this subtype, the dissociative symptoms must not be attributable to the physiological effects of a substance (e.g., blackouts, behavior during alcohol intoxication) or another medical condition (e.g., complex partial seizures).

Specify if:

With delayed expression: If the full diagnostic criteria are not met until at least 6 months after the event (although the onset and expression of some symptoms may be immediate).

Posttraumatic Stress Disorder for Children 6 Years and Younger

A. In children 6 years and younger, exposure to actual or threatened death, serious injury, or sexual violence in one (or more) of the following ways:

1. Directly experiencing the traumatic event(s).
2. Witnessing, in person, the event(s) as it occurred to others, especially primary caregivers.

   Note: Witnessing does not include events that are witnessed only in electronic media, television, movies, or pictures.

3. Learning that the traumatic event(s) occurred to a parent or caregiving figure.

B. Presence of one (or more) of the following intrusion symptoms associated with the traumatic event(s), beginning after the traumatic event(s) occurred:

1. Recurrent, involuntary, and intrusive distressing memories of the traumatic event(s).

   Note: Spontaneous and intrusive memories may not necessarily appear distressing and may be expressed as play reenactment.

2. Recurrent distressing dreams in which the content and/or affect of the dream are related to the traumatic event(s).

   Note: It may not be possible to ascertain that the frightening content is related to the traumatic event.

3. Dissociative reactions (e.g., flashbacks) in which the child feels or acts as if the traumatic event(s) were recurring. (Such reactions may occur on a continuum, with the most extreme expression being a complete loss of awareness of present surroundings.) Such trauma-specific reenactment may occur in play.

4. Intense or prolonged psychological distress at exposure to internal or external cues that symbolize or resemble an aspect of the traumatic event(s).
5. Marked physiological reactions to reminders of the traumatic event(s).

C. One (or more) of the following symptoms, representing either persistent avoidance of stimuli associated with the traumatic event(s) or negative alterations in cognitions and mood associated with the traumatic event(s), must be present, beginning after the event(s) or worsening after the event(s):

Persistent Avoidance of Stimuli

1. Avoidance of or efforts to avoid activities, places, or physical reminders that arouse recollections of the traumatic event(s).
2. Avoidance of or efforts to avoid people, conversations, or interpersonal situations that arouse recollections of the traumatic event(s).

Negative Alterations in Cognitions

3. Substantially increased frequency of negative emotional states (e.g., fear, guilt, sadness, shame, confusion).
4. Markedly diminished interest or participation in significant activities, including constriction of play.
5. Socially withdrawn behavior.
6. Persistent reduction in expression of positive emotions.

D. Alterations in arousal and reactivity associated with the traumatic event(s), beginning or worsening after the traumatic event(s) occurred, as evidenced by two (or more) of the following:

1. Irritable behavior and angry outbursts (with little or no provocation) typically expressed as verbal or physical aggression toward people or objects (including extreme temper tantrums).
2. Hypervigilance.
3. Exaggerated startle response.
4. Problems with concentration.
5. Sleep disturbance (e.g., difficulty falling or staying asleep or restless sleep).

E. The duration of the disturbance is more than 1 month.
F. The disturbance causes clinically significant distress or impairment in relationships with parents, siblings, peers, or other caregivers or with school behavior.
G. The disturbance is not attributable to the physiological effects of a substance (e.g., medication or alcohol) or another medical condition.

Specify whether:

With dissociative symptoms: The individual's symptoms meet the criteria for posttraumatic stress disorder, and the individual experiences persistent or recurrent symptoms of either of the following:

1. **Depersonalization:** Persistent or recurrent experiences of feeling detached from, and as if one were an outside observer of, one's mental processes or body (e.g., feeling as though one were in a dream; feeling a sense of unreality of self or body or of time moving slowly).
2. **Derealization:** Persistent or recurrent experiences of unreality of surroundings (e.g., the world around the individual is experienced as unreal, dreamlike, distant, or distorted).

Note: To use this subtype, the dissociative symptoms must not be attributable to the physiological effects of a substance (e.g., blackouts) or another medical condition (e.g., complex partial seizures).

Specify if:

With delayed expression: If the full diagnostic criteria are not met until at least 6 months after the event (although the onset and expression of some symptoms may be immediate).

Source. Reprinted from American Psychiatric Association: *Diagnostic and Statistical Manual of Mental Disorders,* 5th Edition. Arlington, VA, American Psychiatric Association, 2013. Copyright 2013, American Psychiatric Association. Used with permission.

TABLE 10–1. Comparison of the criteria for posttraumatic stress disorder in DSM-IV-TR and DSM-5

PTSD	DSM-IV-TR	DSM-5
	Part of the anxiety disorders	Part of trauma- and stress-related disorders
Criterion A	Includes response of fear, helplessness, and horror	Includes professional responders; no need for reaction of fear, etc.
Criterion B	Reexperiencing	Reexperiencing
Criterion C	Avoidance	Avoidance
Criterion D	Hyperarousal	Negative alteration in cognition and mood
Criterion E	Duration at least 1 month	Hyperarousal
Criterion F		Duration more than 1 month
Specify:		With dissociative symptoms
Specify:	With delayed onset	With delayed expression

PTSD and acute stress disorder (ASD) are now a separate category—trauma- and stressor-related disorders—and they are no longer part of the anxiety disorders. DSM-IV-TR includes the following in criterion A for PTSD: "the person's response involved intense fear, helplessness, or horror" (p. 467). This is no longer necessary in DSM-5; however, the vicarious traumatization and professional exposure suffered by people in at-risk professions is specifically included in the kind of trauma that would qualify for the disorder under Criterion A. Criteria B and C are essentially unchanged, and Criterion D in DSM-IV-TR is now Criterion E in DSM-5. Criterion D in DSM-5 is the new cluster of symptoms—negative alterations in cognition and mood (p. 271)—that is meant to describe a more pervasive deterioration of functioning. A "with dissociative symptoms" specifier has been added, and the acute and chronic specifiers have been dropped.

Box 10–2 contains the DSM-5 diagnostic criteria for acute stress disorder (ASD).

BOX 10–2.   DSM-5 Criteria for Acute Stress Disorder

A. Exposure to actual or threatened death, serious injury, or sexual violation in one (or more) of the following ways:

  1. Directly experiencing the traumatic event(s).
  2. Witnessing, in person, the event(s) as it occurred to others.
  3. Learning that the event(s) occurred to a close family member or close friend. **Note:** In cases of actual or threatened death of a family member or friend, the event(s) must have been violent or accidental.
  4. Experiencing repeated or extreme exposure to aversive details of the traumatic event(s) (e.g., first responders collecting human remains, police officers repeatedly exposed to details of child abuse).

    Note: This does not apply to exposure through electronic media, television, movies, or pictures, unless this exposure is work related.

B. Presence of nine (or more) of the following symptoms from any of the five categories of intrusion, negative mood, dissociation, avoidance, and arousal, beginning or worsening after the traumatic event(s) occurred:

Intrusion Symptoms

  1. Recurrent, involuntary, and intrusive distressing memories of the traumatic event(s). **Note:** In children, repetitive play may occur in which themes or aspects of the traumatic event(s) are expressed.
  2. Recurrent distressing dreams in which the content and/or affect of the dream are related to the event(s). **Note:** In children, there may be frightening dreams without recognizable content.
  3. Dissociative reactions (e.g., flashbacks) in which the individual feels or acts as if the traumatic event(s) were recurring. (Such reactions may occur on a continuum, with the most extreme expression being a complete loss of awareness of present surroundings.) **Note:** In children, trauma-specific reenactment may occur in play.

4. Intense or prolonged psychological distress or marked physiological reactions in response to internal or external cues that symbolize or resemble an aspect of the traumatic event(s).

Negative Mood

5. Persistent inability to experience positive emotions (e.g., inability to experience happiness, satisfaction, or loving feelings).

Dissociative Symptoms

6. An altered sense of the reality of one's surroundings or oneself (e.g., seeing oneself from another's perspective, being in a daze, time slowing).
7. Inability to remember an important aspect of the traumatic event(s) (typically due to dissociative amnesia and not to other factors such as head injury, alcohol, or drugs).

Avoidance Symptoms

8. Efforts to avoid distressing memories, thoughts, or feelings about or closely associated with the traumatic event(s).
9. Efforts to avoid external reminders (people, places, conversations, activities, objects, situations) that arouse distressing memories, thoughts, or feelings about or closely associated with the traumatic event(s).

Arousal Symptoms

10. Sleep disturbance (e.g., difficulty falling or staying asleep, restless sleep).
11. Irritable behavior and angry outbursts (with little or no provocation), typically expressed as verbal or physical aggression toward people or objects.
12. Hypervigilance.
13. Problems with concentration.
14. Exaggerated startle response.

C. Duration of the disturbance (symptoms in Criterion B) is 3 days to 1 month after trauma exposure.

Note: Symptoms typically begin immediately after the trauma, but persistence for at least 3 days and up to a month is needed to meet disorder criteria.

D. The disturbance causes clinically significant distress or impairment in social, occupational, or other important areas of functioning.

E. The disturbance is not attributable to the physiological effects of a substance (e.g., medication or alcohol) or another medical condition (e.g., mild traumatic brain injury) and is not better explained by brief psychotic disorder.

Source. Reprinted from American Psychiatric Association: *Diagnostic and Statistical Manual of Mental Disorders,* 5th Edition. Arlington, VA, American Psychiatric Association, 2013. Copyright 2013, American Psychiatric Association. Used with permission.

There are two main differences between ASD and PTSD in DSM-5. One is temporal: ASD symptoms appear immediately after the traumatic event and persist for at least 3 days and resolve within 1 month; PTSD lasts for more than 1 month, can have a delayed onset and expression, and has a chronic course. Moreover, even though the clusters of symptoms in ASD and PTSD mostly overlap, in PTSD there are stringent criteria about how many symptoms from each cluster are necessary to meet the criteria. In ASD any nine symptoms from any of the five categories will do. Dissociative symptoms are part of the diagnostic criteria in ASD, and not a subspecification as in PTSD, whereas only one of the symptoms of the negative mood cluster is included in ASD compared with the four in the PTSD criteria.

Epidemiology

In the National Comorbidity Survey, the prevalence of lifetime and current (over the last 12 months) PTSD was estimated to be 6.8% and 3.6%, respectively. Even though traumatic events are common, studies support the evidence that there are protective and risk factors for response to traumatic exposure. Data suggest that the risk of developing PTSD is higher following the exposure to interpersonal violence than after natural disaster. Men have a higher lifetime exposure to traumatic events, but women will develop PTSD more frequently after traumatic exposure. It is unclear whether gender is a risk factor or whether the kind of trauma is a risk factor. Women are more often exposed to sexual assault and interpersonal violence, in which they have a high degree of perceived helplessness. Rivers was the first to describe a strong correlation between the experience of helplessness and severity of symptoms in World War I veterans. It is unclear whether this could be a factor in the difference in PTSD prevalence between men and women. Men develop very high rates of PTSD after sexual abuse and assault; however, there are other confounding factors that make comparisons difficult. Identifying as other than heterosexual increases the risk of traumatic exposures for all genders and also increases the risk for developing PTSD. In the United States, Latinos, African Americans, and Native Americans have higher rates of PTSD than Caucasians, whereas Asian Americans report the lowest rate. Twin and family studies seem to confirm a genetic vulnerability. Lower socioeconomic status is a risk factor. As already noted, exposure to some kind of trauma (sexual trauma, genocide, protracted imprisonment, combat) is more likely to result in PTSD. Another risk factor is having participated in atrocities (it is not relevant whether it was done under duress). It is of interest that a family history and a personal history of mental illness, before the trauma, have been suggested as risk factors: in particular, a history of temperaments associated with impulsive and externalizing behaviors is associated with increased risk of traumatic exposure and increased risk of developing PTSD. Some professions are at particular risk for traumatic exposure and for developing PTSD: military personnel, police, firefighters, and emergency medical workers.

Several authors have focused their attention on protective factors and resilience. The ones more consistently reported are good social support and an ability to recruit it in case of need, adaptive coping skills, cognitive and emotional flexibility, optimism, and perceiving one's life as meaningful.

Psychopathology

It is beyond the scope of this chapter to provide an in-depth review of the field of biological and neurophysiological trauma studies. During the last few decades, animal models, neuroimaging, and neuroendocrinological studies have helped map the beginning of an understanding of the way PTSD symptoms develop and persist. Many of the symptoms of PTSD are part of a neurophysiological response to stress that might have been adaptive under acute threat but become maladaptive when it persists in nonthreatening conditions. The two main areas affected are memory and arousal.

Traumatic memories are encoded in a fragmented, unintegrated fashion. Patients report vivid recollections, often accompanied by somatosensory experiences, as if their entire body and all of their senses were remembering; many patients will describe "being back" or "being there." These recollections are also accompanied by intense arousal and usually negative affect (e.g., anxiety, fear, anger). It is important to note that these memories cannot be summoned volitionally and that they are often not connected to a coherent narrative, as in the following example:

> A woman who had been raped as a teenager had only fragmentary memories of the event and during the initial interview was struggling to explain what had happened. She was concerned that I would not believe her and that I would think she was making up her story because the details she was giving me were so vague. However, when I inquired, she acknowledged that she suffered from episodes that made her "feel crazy and out of control," during which she would be suddenly catapulted back and remembered more that she wanted to. She found herself assaulted and retraumatized by her memories, not in control of them. She wanted to be able to remember, to tell a story, to own the story of what

had happened. Instead, the recollections came unbidden, making her doubt her own sanity. When she felt calm, she was too frightened to access the content of the memories, and the fragmentations continued.

For this woman and in most patients suffering from flashbacks and intense traumatic recollections, the memory is usually triggered externally. The patient might not be aware of what the trigger was, and the fear of any sensory stimulation might cause disabling avoidance of any engagement or activity. Nightmares bring the recollections into the night and contribute to sleep disruption, which is now thought to be an important factor in the development of PTSD. One war veteran was so frightened by his nightmares that by the time he came for treatment he had developed a routine in which he would only nap, no more than 90 minutes at a time.

Hyperarousal is not only associated with reexperiencing; patients live in a state of constant alertness. "I am always on guard," a Vietnam veteran explained. "I explode easily; I take everything personally," said an otherwise successful and accomplished lawyer, survivor of a brutal kidnapping during a trip in South America. "I do not trust anybody; you never know what people might want," was the refrain of a survivor of sexual abuse by clergy. I once mentioned to a Holocaust survivor that he had good neighbors after I observed them bring him soup during an illness (I was at his house for a home visit). His reply was, "I had good neighbors in Poland, too." His Polish neighbors had denounced him and his family to the Gestapo. None of these patients could ever relax. They were ready every moment of every day for the unavoidable danger; behind every corner lurked the next threat; every person was a potential enemy. Hyperarousal, when sustained, taints people's lives, probably leading to negative mood and cognition, like the fear of reexperiencing leads to avoidance.

Psychodynamics

Although the work of Breuer and Freud started as work on trauma, and Freud famously claimed that "hysterics suffer mainly from reminiscences," later Freud shifted his attention to privilege intrapsychic phenomena and conflicts. However, he was puzzled by the war neurosis, and "Beyond the Pleasure Principle" is his attempt to make sense of some of the symptoms that did not fit into his theory. He postulated that the death instinct, "the most universal endeavor of all living substance, namely to return to the quiescence of the inorganic world," caused soldiers to be trapped in the horror of nightmares, in an endless repetition compulsion.

In drive theory and ego psychology, trauma came to be seen as mostly linked to preexisting pathology; outside events mattered only when they resonated with internal conflicts and fantasies. Anna Freud expressed doubt that there could be any event that could by itself cause a traumatic response in the absence of an intrapsychic conflict.

Many renowned psychoanalysts worked with trauma victims, Bergmann used superego pathology and the concept of identification with the aggressor in working with Holocaust survivors and their families. Krystal, himself a Holocaust survivor, also spoke of identification with the aggressor, survivor's guilt, and affect tolerance as helpful concepts to consider when working with victims of massive trauma. However, in 1990, in their introduction to the seminal work *Generations of the Holocaust*, Bergmann and Jucovy wrote that psychoanalytic investigation "did not appear sufficient to conceptualize and explain the bewildering array of symptoms presented by the survivors." As demonstrated by many talented experts in the field, the most creative clinical work with trauma victims, done using psychodynamic concepts, requires a flexible application of ideas without rigid adherence to a theoretic framework. Each patient is unique and will experience a traumatic event in a very personal and unique way, colored by his or her personality, temperament, and past history. A psychodynamic approach, with its attention to the details of the patient's emotional life, offers the opportunity to make the patient feel valued again as a human being after the dehumanizing experience of trauma. Intrapsychic fantasies play a role in how anybody responds to any event in his or her life; however, to look for preexisting pathology in the mental life of any person with PTSD will feel invalidating and blaming to the patient. During the last few decades, the areas of child abuse and the treatment of adult survivors of child abuse have received a lot of attention, and much theoretical and clinical work has gone into the conceptualizing their pathology. Often the consequences of early life trauma are more likely to result in personality disorders (see Chapter 9 of this book). Attachment theory also mostly concerns itself with early life trauma. The consequences of attachment trauma are important to remember mostly because poorly attached individuals (i.e., individuals with poor social support and poor ability to recruit their support system in case of need) generally are at increased risk of developing PTSD after trauma exposure.

Trauma and the Life Cycle

For many patients the symptoms of PTSD remit after 3 months, most will no longer have symptoms that meet the diagnosis after 6 months, and even the patients with a chronic course will have periods of improved functioning. However, there is increasing evidence in the literature that, particularly for patients with severe and debilitating PTSD and exposure to massive traumatic events (e.g., genocide, prolonged sexual abuse or intimate partner violence, extended imprisonment, combat), the disease can recur at vulnerable times in the life cycle when normative or stressful events can serve as triggers. For example, there are many reports of Holocaust survivors experiencing a reactivation of symptoms after an acute medical illness, after a death in the family, or after a separation (e.g., divorce, children leaving for college, children getting married). Aging can also be associated with an increased risk for losses, disability, and dependence, all of which can be triggers for reactivation of PTSD. The task of engaging in end-of-life work can bring about unresolved issues for survivors of trauma and can cause significant worsening of symptomatology. Of note, older adults can experience a significant increase in morbidity and lower quality of life associated with a subsyndromal presentation of PTSD.

Comorbidities

Patients with PTSD often come into treatment having received disparate diagnoses, none of which are related to their history of trauma. They are often being treated with multiple medications, with unclear indication, many of them with controlled substances to which they are addicted. It is imperative to conduct a thorough clinical interview and to obtain a careful, even though sensitive, trauma history, and not to diagnose other disorders if the diagnosis of PTSD alone is sufficient to explain the clinical picture.

PTSD is often comorbid with substance abuse; patients will use alcohol and substances to numb their state of hyperarousal, to improve their sleep, to deaden their despair, and to feel alive again after the dissociative haze and numbness of trauma. Patients who abuse substances are likely to engage in reckless, self-destructive behavior, and their suicidality should be closely monitored.

Chronic PTSD is often comorbid with depression; however, if a substance use disorder is co-occurring, no other disorders should be diagnosed until it is clear that the mood disturbance is not purely in the context of the substance use.

Great care should be taken before an anxiety or a dissociative disorder is diagnosed as comorbid to PTSD. This is not impossible, but the likelihood is that most of the anxiety and dissociative symptoms seen in such patients are part of the original clinical picture.

Because people with impulsive and externalizing behavior are at an increased risk for trauma exposure and for development of PTSD, personality disorders can be comorbid with PTSD.

Patients with severe PTSD might be in a state of such disorganizing anxiety, so dissociated and so tormented by flashbacks as to appear psychotic. Exposure to severe trauma can precipitate a psychotic episode, and this should be ruled out if appropriate. Patients with chronic mental illness are also vulnerable to exploitation and often live in impoverished conditions where trauma is more likely to occur; therefore, the possibility that the two conditions might be comorbid should be considered.

Of note, older adults with a major neurocognitive disorder and a past history of trauma might present with episodes resembling psychosis or agitation, often triggered by institutionalization or other environmental disruptions. Such episodes could be symptoms of PTSD, as in the following example:

> A Holocaust survivor in a nursing home became severely agitated for no obvious reason until it was discovered that her place at the table in the dining room had been changed. The patient was unable to explain what the problem was and was unaware that there was any association. When the clinician considered the dining room arrangement, it became obvious that from her previous position, with her back to the wall, the patient had a full view of the room and of anybody who came and went; at the new seat she had her back turned toward the door. The patient was restored to her old seat, and the agitation subsided.

MANAGEMENT OF THE INTERVIEW

The interview of the traumatized patient poses specific challenges. Exposure to traumatic events causes a sense of loss of control, which renders quite daunting the experience of therapy and the vulnerability it evokes for most trauma victims. Moreover, particularly for survivors of massive and extensive trauma, the capacity for trust and intimacy has been impaired, and establishing a therapeutic alliance might require prolonged effort. Under such conditions, even though it is imperative that the interviewer maintain an empathic stance, the therapist's being overly effusive in his or her manifestation of interest and support can be perceived as disingenuous or intrusive. No matter how innocently, the patient should never be touched, regardless of his or her level of distress, as in the following example:

> Mr. A was 15 when he revealed for the first time to a young counselor that, at the age of 10, a priest had sexually abused him. Mr. A was very

distressed during the interview. The counselor put his arm on the young boy's shoulder, probably to comfort him. Mr. A left the interview feeling confused about the intentions of the counselor and did not seek therapy for another 30 years. Most likely such delay in being able to access help in this patient was multidetermined. However, this early episode was one of the first he mentioned in later therapy when he discussed his mistrust of doctors and therapists.

In patients who have already felt exploited and violated, the therapist needs to set clear boundaries and establish the goals of the interview, and the expectations of the therapeutic process, in a respectful way, leaving as much control of the process to the patient as possible. It is also important to remember that many severely traumatized patients might not reveal their history at the time of the initial interview (even when the process will unfold over several sessions); either they do not attribute their symptoms to the trauma, or they feel too ashamed to bring it up before a more solid therapeutic alliance has been established. A thorough exploration of the patient's history, which includes matter-of-fact, nonjudgmental questions about possible traumatic exposure, is most likely to elicit information, but still some patients will require more time.

As clinicians, we encourage patients to talk about personal, painful, shameful secrets and fantasies. We make it possible to broach the most difficult topics by signaling to our patient our willingness to listen and our ability to tolerate what they have to say without being overwhelmed by affect. A history of trauma requires on our part a similar acceptance. Details of the history should never be pursued if the patient is unwilling to give them, but they should always be tolerated, no matter how unpleasant, if the patient needs to share them, as in the following example:

> Mr. B, a 76-year-old Holocaust survivor, was referred for therapy by a social worker at the hospital where he still worked as an administrator. Mr. B had never been in treatment before. He called to schedule the appointment the day after I had accepted the referral; he was pleasant on the phone and flexible about the schedule. He arrived on time, was well dressed, and appeared younger than his age. His demeanor was pleasant, and he was well engaged, well spoken, and slightly anxious.
>
> The initial interview unfolded over the course of two sessions. Mr. B's chief complaint was his inability to control his temper. He described it as a lifelong problem that bothered him but that he could not explain: "I guess I sort of have a short fuse. I feel that people step on my toes and I lose my temper, then I feel bad about how I behaved. I get very angry very quickly. I do not like it. I was always like that, also with my kids when they were growing up. I had to leave the house because I would not know what I could do. Also with my wife, I would not argue with her for fear of losing control. It is not a good feeling." When specifically

asked, he denied ever losing control and hitting either his wife or children or ever having a physical confrontation with anybody. However, he always felt afraid of the possibility. Another complaint was his poor sleep: "I am not a good sleeper. Never have been. But I am used to it. Does not bother me. My doctor gives me something for it. Does not help much. I spend my night moving around the bed. Sometimes I wake up with my head where my feet should be." When I asked him if he ever had nightmares, or if he remembered his dreams, he replied promptly, "Don't remember a thing. And what should I have nightmares about? I had a pretty normal life. Wife, two kids, a job." Without challenging his view of his life as "normal," I inquired about his early life:

A.S.: Mr. B maybe I misunderstood, but I thought Ms. S. told me you were born in Poland?

Mr. B: Yeah, but I was very young during the war, I remember nothing.

A.S.: Can you tell me what happened, or is it difficult for you to talk about it?

Mr. B: No, it does not bother me at all. I never think about it. It really did not affect me. I mean, I remember when they took my parents, but it really did not bother me, I was too young to understand what it meant.

Mr. B was silent for a moment and I waited. He did not appear distressed, rather puzzled by my interest.

A.S.: Can I ask how old you were when your parents were taken?

Mr. B: Six, I was six.

A.S.: It is incredible that you survived. Young children were very vulnerable, particularly without their parents.

Mr. B: My aunt told me I was hidden with different relatives. I remember very little. I remember my uncle. I know he saved my life. He got me out of the ghetto before it was too late. He was a good man. He was my mother's brother. He did not make it. I met up with his son many years after the war. He lives in Israel. He is a couple of years older than me. I did not know he was alive. He found me. He did not want to talk about what happened. Just as well. What's the point? After the war I went to live with my aunt, on my father's side, until I left Poland to come to the U.S., then I met my wife. She was also from Europe. She lost her family in the camps. She died last year.

This recitation of horrors had been given with very little affect. I expressed my sympathy at his wife's death, and he dismissed my concern, saying she had been a sickly woman, as if this fact dispensed with his feelings about her death. Mr. B only could express some affect when talking about his children and grandchildren. He had a son and a daughter and four grandchildren. His demeanor was much warmer and more engaged when speaking about them. He expressed much regret at not having been more involved in their life during their formative years; he blamed his job and his fear of his temper for his estrangement. He was now more involved with the grandchildren. He was aware of some tension, particularly with his son, who he felt was resentful because Mr. B had been "an absent father." His daughter, who lived out of state, would have liked him to move closer to her, but he could not imagine his life without working. At the second meeting, Mr. B described the details of his parents "being taken": while he was playing with other children in the street of the ghetto, Mr. B saw his parents being escorted away by German soldiers, and he remembers the soldiers asking his father while pointing toward the children, "Which one is yours?" and his father answering without looking at Mr. B "We have no children." Mr. B did not follow his parents, and he never saw them again. He described this memory in vivid details, but he claimed it is not associated with any feelings. It is impossible to know if this is the memory of what happened or a condensed memory of different events. However, we can surmise that Mr. B most likely did witness the arrest of his parents, who most likely went out of their way to protect their child. At the end of the second session, I summarized the interview findings, and I explained to Mr. B how many of his symptoms and difficulties could fit a subsyndromal picture of chronic PTSD. I added, "However, you are telling me the war did not affect you. And you would know how you feel better than I do. So maybe in your case, your problems do have a different explanation, and we can look for it together." Mr. B was hesitant at first and asked me if I planned to force him to talk about the war all the time. Once we agreed that we would talk about whatever he felt comfortable talking about, Mr. B was much more open to considering the possibility that the experience of losing his parents might have been more meaningful than he thought.

There are situations when early-life traumatic events might determine later behaviors that cause retraumatization. I have already alluded to the controversy of blaming the victims for their problems, and this is particularly problematic with victims of intimate partner violence and sexual abuse. The unfortunate reality, though, is that women who are raised in abusive households are more likely to marry or live with abusive men, and women who are victims of incest might be unable to protect their children from similar forms of abuse. The dynamic forces that can cause these behaviors are too complex to be explored in detail here; however, it is important for the interviewer to be aware of these possibilities and of the pitfalls of taking sides during the interview, as in the following example:

> Mrs. C was a 40-year-old legal secretary admitted to the inpatient unit after an overdose, precipitated by the discovery that the father of the child her 15-year-old daughter had just given birth to was the patient's 55-year-old boyfriend. Mrs. C was very tearful during the initial interview, and also very angry, both with the boyfriend and with her daughter, who, she believed, had consented to the sexual liaison. Mrs. C kept rumi-

nating about what her daughter had revealed to her about "the affair." She insisted she had no idea this had been going on for over a year, she could not understand why the daughter was angry with her, and she could not understand why the daughter claimed he "had forced himself on to her" and yet she had not complained sooner. After listening to the patient's angry ruminations for a while, the interviewer became aware of her increasing difficulties empathizing with her, and her own desire to shake the patient out of her denial of the obvious role she had played in her daughter's victimization. The interviewer recognized her own aggressive impulses and decided to shift the focus of the interview away from the charged topic of the current crisis to try to understand Mrs. C better. The interviewer said, "This is understandably very distressing for you to talk about. Let's take a break from it now and see if we can cover some other information we need. Then we will get back to it, when maybe you feel a little more composed." It was with some surprise that the interviewer discovered that when Mrs. C was 13, her stepfather repeatedly raped her. She became pregnant, and her mother forced her to leave the house and to live with her aunt, while the mother continued living with the stepfather. Mrs. C gave the child up for adoption and managed to go back to school. After an abusive marriage to the father of her daughter, she had started living with her current boyfriend 3 years before. Both her husband and her current boyfriend had never been able to hold a job, and they were heavy drinkers. Mrs. C was quite successful at her job and took a lot of pride in her ability to support the family. Mrs. C had dreamt of a bright future for her daughter, who had the advantage of "a loving supportive mother." Mrs. C felt her daughter had betrayed her and was unable to see any parallel between her own traumatic adolescence and the tragedy that had just unfolded in her child's life. [*The problem that both Mrs. C and the interviewer faced in such a predicament was that in this tragic reenactment, Mrs. C quite strongly identified both with the victim (the daughter) and with the aggressor (the mother who fails to protect the child). For the interviewer, it is important to maintain a measure of compassion and empathy for both sides, in order for an alliance to be possible.*] The interviewer said, "It sounds to me this is a terrible situation. You had hoped your daughter would have a different life; instead you find yourself back to where you started." Mrs. C began to cry and for the first time she could address her rage unambiguously at the boyfriend. "How could he do it? She is just 15, he is a man, he should know better," Mrs. C said. "You are right. She is a child, he is the grown up. Like you were the child and your stepfather was the grown up," said the interviewer.

The following case illustrates the necessity of avoiding overcharging with meaning early conflicts in areas involving traumatic material, even when this might be accurate and the patient appears to be high functioning and capable of insight. Although intrapsychic conflicts and fantasies happen in the mind, and part of our job as therapists is to make our patients comfortable with the nature of their internal processes, trauma, particularly interpersonal trauma, will prove to victims, witnesses, and perpetrators that feelings and thoughts cannot always be contained. As therapists, we have to be much more humble when we try to convince a trauma victim that people can control themselves and feelings do not necessary translate into behaviors, because they have seen what happens when this does not hold true.

> Mr. D was a 67-year-old successful accountant, never married, and referred for a consultation by his internist who was concerned about a worsening addiction to benzodiazepines and an increased use of alcohol over the last 2 years. Mr. D felt somehow annoyed by the fact that his internist, with whom he had had a rather friendly relationship for years, refused to continue prescribing benzodiazepines for him, unless he accepted the referral. By the time he came to see me he was taking approximately 6 mg of alprazolam daily, 30 mg of temazepam, and 10 mg bid prn of diazepam. Because of his social position he felt uncomfortable shopping around for another doctor, and he had been somehow embarrassed by an attempt he had made. Therefore, even though he told me clearly he was not interested in therapy, he came reluctantly for a consultation. He acknowledged having "a few drinks every night and more on the weekend." He would not be more specific about the number, but he said that he usually drank beer or wine, he had never been charged for DUI or had any other legal problems, and he denied having blackouts or seizures, had no eye-openers, had no episodes of withdrawals, and had no participations in AA or any other treatment modality. He denied his drinking was a problem: "I go to work every day. I have a stressful job. I am not a bum. I am successful, never got into trouble." He did not consider his benzodiazepine abuse a problem either. He claimed that he did not use any other recreational or prescription drugs, neither currently nor in the past. Mr. D was at first a rather vague historian, not very engaged in the process, somehow dismissive and defensive. He presented as a rather polished elegant man, very fashionably dressed and well spoken, and he appeared reluctant to speak of his early life. He made many sarcastic remarks about "therapists wasting their time looking for the source of all evils in childhood." At the end of the two-session interview process, a picture emerged of a deprived childhood in a poor family with an alcoholic, abusive father and a dependent mother.
>
> Mr. D had always been a very bright student. He had gone to Catholic school and hoped to make it out of the poverty and deprivation of his background, but his family neither could afford nor encouraged higher education. In a desperate attempt to escape, Mr. D joined the U.S. Marine Corps right in time for Vietnam, where he spent three tours of duty. He returned highly decorated after having sustained two non-life-threatening injuries. He was determined to use the opportunity the Marine Corps gave him for an education. He selected rigorous courses, networked skillfully, graduated with honors, and he was hired at a prestigious firm. He was now a senior partner at a successful accounting firm.
>
> Mr. D could not quite tell when he had started drinking or when he had started drinking more. His reliance on benzodiazepines had devel-

oped many decades before because of poor sleep and nightmares. He was dismissive of the notion of combat-induced PTSD and considered the idea to be "blown all out of proportion." At first he had stayed in touch with his family. He had provided much needed financial support, and he had also become the emotional support for his mother and younger sister, until during a visit he had a physical fight with his drunken father and he became terrified by his murderous rage. He left and never returned, not even for his parents' funeral. He still financially supported his sister, who had never left their hometown and who was just marginally functioning. He had not spoken with her in more than a decade.

Mr. D had good relationships with his partners at the firm; he loved classical music and regularly attended concerts with two friends, whom he had known since college. He enjoyed traveling, and he often traveled alone. He dated mostly women from disadvantaged backgrounds that he could help financially or socially, but he never "got serious." Whenever the relationship became too intimate, he broke it off. "Can you tell me what caused the breakups?" I asked. "I do not like to feel that I need anybody," said Mr. D. "It is fine if they need me. But I would much rather remain independent." For the last 2 years he was involved in an unstable sexual relationship with a younger woman, who was clearly a much heavier drinker than he. She was quite dysfunctional and was unable to hold a job. Mr. D supported her and was trying to "help her get her life together." "Correct me if I am wrong," I asked, "but if I got the time right, since this relationship started your drinking has been getting worse. Can the two be connected?" Mr. D at first denied the connection, then was quiet for a moment, and said, "Maybe. Maybe. I mostly drink when we are together. I am trying to get her to stop...." "It is important to you to feel that you can be helpful," I said. "I like to help if I can," said Mr. D. "That is commendable," I said. "However, if you are yourself struggling, you won't be of much use to anybody. You might want to think about that." "I believe you might have a point," he said. Mr. D agreed to engage in treatment with the only purpose of decreasing his benzodiazepine use, and he agreed to come in monthly.

This case presents multiple layers of complexities. Mr. D came from a deprived abusive background, and he desired to protect his mother from his abusive father. Probably an unresolved and highly charged oedipal conflict was playing a role in his repeated involvement with women in need to be rescued and that he would not allow himself to marry. It was very tempting to make this connection for him. However, Mr. D also went to Vietnam, where he was exposed to highly traumatic combat situations; he saw many of his friends killed, he risked dying many times, he was injured twice, and he killed many times. The effects of these events on the psyche cannot be underestimated. When he was a young boy, Mr. D had some hope for himself. He believed he might not be like his father; he believed he could make something else of his life, and he had dreamed of an escape. Vietnam deprived him of that hope. Of course, even without the war, we can speculate that a part of him would have been identified with his father and of his fear that he was capable of behaving as brutally. However, after the war, he did not only have to contend with what his father was capable of doing, he had to contend with what he knew himself to be capable of doing.

> At the time of the attack on September 11, 2001, Mr. E was a 31-year-old man who worked as a financial analyst for a consulting firm at the top of one of the towers of the World Trade Center in New York City. He was married and had two daughters, ages 5 and 6. Ten years later, Mr. E was seen at the emergency department after the police found him in the proximity of a bridge attempting to climb the parapet. During the interview, Mr. E was quite detached, and he appeared indifferent to his surroundings and to the process of the assessment. He denied feeling sad or anxious and said, "What's the point anymore?" After some effort, he was able to explain that, more than by hopelessness, he was tormented by a sense of pervasive futility. The morning of September 11 there was a special performance at Mr. E's older daughter's school, and he had planned to go to work late. That was why he was alive, whereas almost all of the other employees of his firm were dead. He had not felt lucky; he had not felt grateful; he had felt numb. He had been unable to feel much of anything since.
>
> For the first year, Mr. E had "gone through the motion of living," found another job, and apparently moved on. He never looked for treatment because he saw no reason: "Nothing had happened to me; I was not even there. I was nowhere near." However, he could not even look at his wife or his children; he was almost angry with them. Then he had "gone crazy." The interviewer asked Mr. E what he exactly meant by that, and Mr. E gave a long list of self-destructive activity in which he had engaged. He had started drinking and using drugs, he had cheated on his wife, he had lost his job, and he had had a car accident while driving drunk. In an impulsive act he had left his family for a young woman he barely knew. His wife had filed for divorce. He had spent the last 5 years drifting, almost completely estranged from his daughters, and barely able to hold a job. He did not see any future for himself, and not much of a point in trying. He could not explain what had happened to him.
>
> Before September 11, his life had been charmed; he had a dream job, a great marriage, and two children he adored. He could not have wanted more. Even on that cursed day, he had been lucky; everybody told him, everybody congratulated him, on his incredible luck. He just could not explain it. He had no history of drug abuse before the attack, no psychiatric history, no obvious problems. "I used to be happy" he kept repeating, puzzled. "I do not understand why I am still alive."
>
> Interviewer: You say it as if you thought you should not be.
> Mr. E: Well I should not. The others are all dead, I should have died too.

Interviewer: But you did not.

Mr. E: Why not? What am I supposed to do with it? I feel I am supposed to do something with it. Do you know how many guys worked at our firm?

Interviewer: How many?

Mr. E: More than 200.

Interviewer: That's a lot of people.

Mr. E: 192 are dead; the rest were either sick or on vacation or shit like that.

Interviewer: So you survived and now you are responsible for the lives of 192 people. Is this the way you see it?

Mr. E: I am not responsible for their lives, but I am alive and they are not. I am supposed to make something of it; I am supposed to deserve it. Instead I feel dead. I fucking feel like I died too. If this is the way it's going to be I might as well get it over with.

Interviewer: Is there anything that you think might make it better for you?

Mr. E: Too late.

Interviewer: Can you explain what you mean?

Mr. E: I really would like for my kids to know I care. I would like them to know I am not just some screwed up loser. But I think they hate me now.

Interviewer: Do you think it is worth a try to sort yourself out for your kids? It is a hell of a legacy to have a parent commit suicide. Are you sure that is the way you want to be remembered?

This last example illustrates the challenge of interviewing a patient who has already been told many times that "he was lucky." Maybe the interviewer also feels this way and finds it difficult to justify the patient's despair and self-destructive downward spiral. However, "survivor's guilt" is a burdensome legacy, which has been described in relation to survivors of the Holocaust and to veterans, and even in the case of children who do better than their siblings when emerging from a particularly brutal upbringing. Its devastating effects should not be underestimated. The meaning of it can be debated. For some patients it is linked to the desire to maintain the memory of the deceased. It is a state of relentless and rage-filled grieving. For others it is a desperate attempt at looking for a hidden meaning in their own survival that is felt burdensome to the point of being unbearable. Some patients find the idea of being chosen—of having been given a second chance—to be exhilarating and liberating. However, it is not up to the interviewer to attribute this uplifting meaning to the experience.

TRANSFERENCE AND COUNTERTRANSFERENCE

As the last case example of the previous section illustrates, meaning is never too far removed from the experience of trauma. Meaning can be personal, social, political, racial, gender-based, religious, and historic. Perhaps in other areas of psychiatry we can nurse the illusion of keeping reality at bay, but not so when working with trauma. Not only will unresolved intrapsychic conflicts—both ours and our patients'—resonate with the dynamic created by the traumatic reenactment, but also the roles that we and our patients identify with in society will play a role in the reenactment and change the meaning of the therapeutic interaction during the interview and the therapy that follows.

Any trauma victim will have internalized, particularly during interpersonal violence, identifications with the main characters in the drama. It is important to remember that any lessons learned by our brain under threat will not be easily forgotten; this is an essential law of survival. The younger the age at trauma exposure, the more devastating will be the impact on the developing personality and the more pervasive the effect of traumatic reenactment on most interpersonal interactions. However, even for people exposed to trauma as adults, the impulse to reenact seems almost irresistible. Substance abuse and engagement in self-destructive behaviors of other kinds (e.g., DUI, high-risk sports, abusive relationships, suicidal behavior) are examples of reenactment. Some choices of very high-risk jobs might also fall into this category.

To be schematic, we could say that the possible roles to reenact are usually fairly established. In most traumatic situations there will be the following: a victim, a perpetrator (in case of interpersonal violence), possibly a witness (maybe an indifferent bystander), and hopefully a rescuer. Even if some of these roles did not exist in reality, they were usually assigned in fantasy, either at the time of the event or in re-elaboration, conscious or unconscious, in the patient's mind. Therefore, when patients come into treatment, most times they have played and replayed these roles themselves. It might be assumed that most patients have at least a partial identification with each role, and it is unwise for the interviewer to take sides in this drama. It is also common for patients to experience the interviewer, at different times during the interview, as a perpetrator, a witness, an indifferent bystander, or a rescuer. Of course, as health care professionals, we will feel much more comfortable with the role of the rescuer, but our desire to rescue the patient is probably one of the most dangerous countertransferential enactments of which we need to be aware, as in the following example:

Mr. A, who has been mentioned previously, was 10 when he was sexually abused by a priest in an orphanage where he had been placed after the death of his mother. His father was an abusive alcoholic and unable to care for him. Mr. A was the youngest of eight siblings, all of whom were significantly older; however, none was able to take care of him. Notwithstanding many years of abuse, neglect, and violence, in his late teens, with the help of a mentor, Mr. A was able to return to school, and eventually he became a fireman. Mr. A had never married and he had no children. He had maintained some relationships with his nieces and nephews, several of whom he had helped through school. All of his siblings were deceased. He had started drinking to excess in his teens, and this remained a problem for him during his entire life. He had several friendships with other firemen, and he had several drinking buddies.

When Mr. A arrived for his first interview, he had just retired after a very serious injury on the job. He had been a fireman for more than 25 years, and he was very proud of his career. He felt unable to imagine himself at home, and his drinking had escalated. It is important to note that at the time of the initial interview he did not mention the sexual trauma or much else about his teenage years. Mr. A was superficially cooperative, pleasant, and almost deferential, yet he seemed to avoid any attempt at deepening the level of the interaction. His level of despair was almost palpable, and yet I felt that Mr. A did not perceive empathic comments as comforting. On the contrary, he seemed to experience any attempt at closeness as intrusive. He said that he just wanted "something to help me sleep" and that he had "never been one for talking." I was tempted to explain all of Mr. A's symptoms to him, including his avoidance, in terms of PTSD, and to offer therapy as a possible solution that could improve his life and provide much comfort in terms of increased social support. I felt very warmly about Mr. A; I found him bright, generous, resilient, and likable. He already had some stable social bonds and had been able to maintain a stable job; there was obvious potential. I then became aware of my rescue fantasy and decided to hold back and reassess the interaction. Once my own role in the reenactment became clear, I could see more clearly the dangers of the present situation: Mr. A was a heavy drinker with very limited social support and significant distressing symptoms, and he had just lost the most adaptive strategy to cope with his problems (his job). I said, "Mr. A you have gone through some pretty rough times, but you did not get discouraged in the past. However, I think that this time might be different. Your job and the pride you took in it meant a lot to you. I am not sure the solution is just a matter of finding you a sleeping pill. I think this is a little more serious than that." He shifted uneasily in his chair and looked clearly uncomfortable. Even though he had already denied being suicidal, I asked again, "Have you been thinking about killing yourself?" For the first time he looked at me directly and replied without hesitation, "I have to tell you that it has crossed my mind. But I think it would be cowardly. My friends would be disappointed. It is not the way I want to go. But if something should happen to me, I would not mind."

The dangers of being too caught up in our own formulation and to lose track of the actual priority are only too obvious in Mr. A's case example. It is important to remember that when we are engaged in a rescue fantasy, we are usually not helping the patient. To help the patient, we need to be vigilant about the source of the fantasies. In this case, Mr. A might have projected on to the interviewer his own desire for a caring mother, but he was also angry at his mother for abandoning him. The risk of enacting the role of the rescuer is that no real rescue happened in Mr. A's life, and each rescue fantasy is doomed to fail: his mother died, his father and his siblings abandoned him, and the priest abused him. There is no happy ending in this story. This was not a story I even knew at the time, and therefore I was at much higher risk of failing, enacting a role for which I did not know the script. My own contribution to the fantasy was my own narcissistic need to feel powerful in the face of the despair and helplessness that I so often experience when working with trauma patients. In order to be able to offer realistic, and compassionate help, I need to keep my narcissistic need and my vulnerability well within my level of awareness:

> Mrs. F was a young teenager when she was transported to the Auschwitz concentration camp with her family. Mrs. F was born and raised in a small village in Poland; the majority of the village inhabitants were Hasidic Jews. Mrs. F herself was raised in a very large, observant family. She was the second oldest and was the only one to survive. Her five younger siblings had been immediately sent to the gas chambers with her mother, together with her older sister and her baby. She had been separated from her father and brother-in-law at arrival; she discovered at liberation that they had both died during the death marches in January 1945. After the war, Mrs. F met her husband in a displaced persons camp; they married and moved to Israel. They immigrated to the United States in the 1950s after the birth of their son, their only child. Mrs. F was referred for treatment of depression a few months after the death of her husband when she was 82.
>
> During the interview, Mrs. F was very forthcoming with the details of her trauma history; she described her childhood and her family of origin in idealized idyllic terms, and she described herself as a very innocent girl who had undergone a terrible ordeal and yet retained her religious faith. She was very proud of her religious upbringing and felt very strongly that the outstanding moral teachings of her parents had allowed her to survive the experience. Up to this point, the interviewer had felt sorry for Mrs. F and overwhelmed by the mind-numbing quality of her trauma, yet she also felt unable to connect with her. The interviewer somehow felt Mrs. F was not really in the room. The interviewer said tentatively, "I cannot imagine that anything could ever make you feel right about what you lost and suffered. However, I am glad to hear that you feel your faith gave you the strength to bear it." "I was lucky that

I was brought up properly by my parents. You have no idea the things I saw; the things that happened," Mrs. F said. "Do you want to tell me what you mean?" asked the interviewer. "Some of the things other girls did for food…you know girls would do anything…with the kapos, with the Germans even, you know…they would do anything. We were always hungry." Mrs. F said all this with a tone of contempt, all the while darting glances at the interviewer looking for approval. "I would never do such a thing. I was raised different. My parents taught me better," concluded Mrs. F with obvious pride. The interviewer was tempted to agree and praise Mrs. F for her high moral standard, but something felt amiss. "Mrs. F, I do not feel I have a right to criticize anything anybody did in order to survive," said the interviewer. "You mean you would not think badly of a girl? I knew a girl who…you know, she just did it for some bread," said Mrs. F. "I really feel I have no right to judge," repeated the interviewer, very aware of her growing discomfort. Mrs. F pressed with a challenging tone, "I mean, if you are not sure, would you have done such a thing?" The interviewer felt quite intimidated; she did not want to start discussing her doubts about her own moral strength, and at this point she was able to regain enough self-reflecting ability to understand that moral strength did not have much to do with this interaction at all. The interviewer was suddenly aware of the reenactment in which the patient had engaged her, with the patient playing the role of the punitive, harsh, perpetrator shaming the victim, blaming her for her degraded state and the interviewer in the role of victim unable to tell the difference between good and evil. We can speculate about the role of an overly rigid upbringing, internalized punitive parents, unresolved conflicts, and so on. However, one might wonder if even the most loving parental images would not have to make room, in the still developing mind of a young teenager, for the sadistic authority figures concocted by the horror of the Holocaust and internalized under such chronic inescapable threat of death. Having regained her composure, the interviewer replied, "I do not know what it is like to be hungry all the time. I do not know what it is like to be afraid of being killed at a whim. I do not know what it is like to have lost everything. I do not know what I would do. I am not sure that normal rules applied in Auschwitz." Mrs. F started to cry and cried silently for a few minutes. When she began talking again, she changed the topic and never spoke about this again. It is impossible to know if she was talking about herself, if she was the girl who had exchanged sex for a piece of bread, or if there were other acts for which she reproached herself. However, the rest of the interview was devoid of any moralistic tirades and felt more genuine and intimate.

There are a few other aspects worth examining in the interview above. First of all, the interviewer did not pursue the issue of sexual exploitation further when Mrs. F changed topic; it should always be up to the patient to decide how many details of the story to share. As interviewers, we want to facilitate the process of the creation of a coherent meaningful narrative; we do not want to elicit a confession. An interview should not become an interrogation. At another point, the interviewer was tempted to go along with Mrs. F, to agree with her in expressing a judgment on the victim's behavior, in blaming the victim for her own degradation. It is important to understand the reasons for this temptation. On one side, we can delude ourselves that in so doing we might avoid painful material (maybe even protect the patient, maintain a defense); however, this would be ill advised, because even though this might work in the short term by stopping any revelation, in the long run, by our having allied ourselves with the "internalized perpetrator," we will always be perceived as dangerous and untrustworthy by the victim. It is also important to identify another mechanism that is at work in this interaction: an attempt to maintain the illusion of the "innocent victim," a fantasy shared by both victim and rescuer. Many victims of trauma feel contaminated by what they did in order to survive, were forced by the perpetrator, or just because of the dehumanizing conditions under which they found themselves. After they reenter civil society, they feel changed and no longer worthy. Their identification with the aggressor places the blame for their behavior on them, not on the traumatic circumstances or on the perpetrator. Many survivors have created a narrative that is fit for public consumption that has been somehow sanitized of most of the acts and behaviors that are all too common in extreme conditions but hard to accept and tolerate in more normal social settings. However, the real narrative, the knowledge of what really happened, is what torments the victims. They feel unable to share it, certain that they would elicit horror, the same horror and blame they elicit in themselves. Unfortunately, this plays against the fact that there is a sort of hagiography that has been created around certain groups of victims, such as Holocaust survivors or veterans: they are viewed as modern-day holy people; they are heroes, and they cannot be criticized. Society wants to believe in the more palatable version of their story, which makes the narrative two-dimensional. However, as Solzhenitsyn said, "If only it were all so simple. If only there were evil people somewhere insidiously committing evil deeds and it were necessary only to separate them from the rest of us and destroy them. But the line dividing good from evil cuts through the heart of every human being, and who is willing to destroy a piece of their own heart." Therapy needs to restore depth and complexity to the narrative; it is therefore imperative that the interviewer does not fall into the trap of expecting the victim to be "pure." As therapists, we also need to be aware of every human being's (including our own) need to maintain a narcissistic fantasy of invulnerability and omnipotence in order to simply go about the business of living. Every interview with a victim of trauma is a challenge to such a fantasy. It is important to become aware of the specific way in which this challenge will express itself in the countertransference to each patient. With Mrs. F, the challenge was to the narcissistic fantasy of being able to maintain moral superiority in the face of degradation. In other cases, it might be more specifically to the fantasy of physical invulnerability. In yet another case, the interviewer found herself unable to pay attention to a woman sobbing after the sudden death of her infant son, and it was only after discussing this case with her supervisor that the interviewer made the association with the fact that she herself had a 6-month-old baby at home.

> Mr. G was a 90-year-old British man who came for treatment after his wife of 60 years died after having Alzheimer's disease for 10 years. During the initial interview, Mr. G spoke about his early life: He was born in London in 1915. He had been in the British Royal Air Force during World War II; he had conducted many missions over Europe and had been shot down, injured, and rescued by farmers in France. He had an affair with the daughter of the family and then had gone back to England, where his girlfriend waited for him. They married in 1945, moved to the United States in 1960 because of a job he had gotten as an engineer, and they had three children. The rest of his life had been mostly uneventful until his wife's illness. The interviewer found herself quite fascinated by Mr. G's early life, which sounded like a romance, but she had to admit that Mr. G did not show any sign of PTSD. He spoke about his war experiences with equanimity and had no interest in lingering over them. He wanted to talk about the loss of his wife: a much more mundane topic, but it was the reason for the interview and the subsequent treatment.

This case example illustrates the need to be mindful of the risk of privileged voyeurism that listening to traumatic narrative can cause in the interviewer. The fact that we elicit a history of exposure to trauma in the patient's past does not mean we should make it the focus of treatment, if that is not the patient's wish, particularly if there are no obvious clinical indications. Moreover, even though some traumatic stories sound like book or movie plots, the horror, the pain, the suffering, the degradation, that our patient has experienced should never be forgotten. When we start looking at our traumatized patient as a source of entertainment, and we feel our interest and curiosity titillated, we need to ask ourselves what is being reenacted in the interaction. No traumatic details should be pursued to satisfy the curiosity of the interviewer, because this will re-create the traumatic condition of objectifying the victim. It is also important for the interviewer to be mindful of his or her ability to tolerate gruesome details and of the necessity to do so. Some patients will in fact engage in the reenactment of torturing their audience with unnecessary excruciating details of their ordeal without much conscious awareness of their sadism. This should not be endured, even though the sadism of the patient should not necessarily be directly confronted. However, the defensive motivation of their behavior, if explored, could help the work of therapy.

CONCLUSION

Working with trauma victims is challenging, and it requires patience, skills, and flexibility. The horror of the patient's story, as in Coleridge's "Rime of the Ancient Mariner," will grip the attention of the clinician who will, by the end of the patient's tale, feel

> ...like one that hath been stunned,
> And is of sense forlorn:

Clinicians will need to pay close attention not only to the patient's distress and emotion, but also to their own responses and reactions in order to manage dangerous traumatic reenactments and to identify vicarious traumatization and prevent burnout. However, once a trusting relationship has been established, psychotherapy can be effective and rewarding for both patient and clinician.

CHAPTER 11

THE DISSOCIATIVE IDENTITY DISORDER PATIENT

BRAD FOOTE, M.D.

Dissociative identity disorder (DID; formerly multiple personality disorder) has a long history in psychiatry. The diagnosis has sometimes been met with skepticism, thought to be induced by the clinician through hypnosis or suggestion and hence in its purported iatrogenic origins not a "real" illness but a manifestation of "hysteria." However, the frequent appearance of possession and trance dissociative states in many disparate cultures has long been observed by anthropologists. Possession states are often found to be an intrinsic part of what the cultural historian Ronald Knox called "enthusiastic" religions. These altered states of consciousness, experienced as possession by a deity of one form or another, can occur in a group setting, which frequently involves dancing, rhythmic singing, and sometimes the use of intoxicants, but they can also occur spontaneously in individuals. The eighteenth-century British artist William Blake, deeply religious, described himself as an "enthusiastic hope-fostered visionary," and his paintings and engravings reflect his recurrent dissociative experiences. The cross-cultural ubiquity of dissociative states, whether group induced or spontaneous, as well as copious research over the last 35 years, speaks to a real syndrome now codified in DSM-5.

Singular feminine pronouns will be used throughout this text because 80%–90% of dissociative identity disorder patients in clinical populations are female.

The nineteenth-century French neurologist Jean-Martin Charcot, who made many seminal contributions to descriptive organic neurology, was appointed physician at the Salpêtrière Hospital in Paris at age 37. While there, he became fascinated by neurotic patients who manifested hysterical convulsive episodes, which he described as "hystero-epilepsy." He was one of the first clinicians to recognize previous psychic trauma as being central to "hysterical" attacks. His clinical conferences, wherein patients under hypnosis would manifest hysterical seizures, became famous and were attended by physicians from all over Europe, one of whom was the young Sigmund Freud. Charcot used hypnosis to access and display extravagant dissociative phenomena in his patients. Later, Josef Breuer, in his collaborative work with Freud, explicated dissociative phenomena in the psychotherapeutic situation, most notably in the case of Anna O. In this case, Breuer noted that two entirely distinct states of consciousness were present and that they alternated: in one state the patient was depressed and anxious, whereas in the other she was "naughty," exuberant, and abusive. This condition appears to have been precipitated by the psychic trauma she experienced on her adored father's sudden death. Freud's interest in dissociative phenomena rapidly waned, however, as he began to develop libido theory to explain the origins of neurotic symptoms. Nonetheless, brilliant phenomenologist that he was, he acknowledged in 1910: "The study of hypnotic phenomena has accustomed us to what was at first a bewildering realization that in one and the same individual there can be several mental groupings which can remain more or less independent of one another." This anticipated the contemporary view that dissociative disorders involve a disturbance in the normally integrated functions of consciousness, memory, identity, perception, and behavior.

In 1932, the psychoanalyst Sándor Ferenczi noted "the almost hallucinatory repetitions of traumatic experiences which began to accumulate in my daily practice." He went on to emphasize the reality of childhood trauma, especially sexual trauma, in many of his patients, disputing Freud's view that fantasy was at the root of most patients' remembrances of trauma in the clinical situation. Additionally, Ferenczi observed that trauma can result in splitting of the personality.

Seen through the eyes of our current nosological system, classic hysteria can be broken down into a long list of DSM-5 diagnoses. However, the phenomena that are most specifically characteristic of hysteria are dissociative and somatoform (conversion) symptoms. The connection between "double consciousness" and hysteria persisted through the psychiatric nosologies of the twentieth century. For instance, in 1968 DSM-II included "hysterical neurosis," with two subtypes, the conversion type and the dissociative type, maintaining the close relationship these entities formerly shared in grand hysteria. However, with DSM-III, "hysteria" was no longer deemed an appropriate psychiatric descriptor; the connection between dissociative disorders and somatoform disorders was sundered, and the dissociative identity disorder diagnostic criteria emerged in a form almost identical to the current criteria. By the time of DSM-5, the traumatic origin of dissociative pathology was well enough established so that a proposal was made to include dissociative disorders under trauma-related disorders; ultimately, however, this connection was represented only by chapter proximity (the chapter for trauma- and stressor-related disorders is followed immediately by dissociative disorders, followed by somatic symptom and related disorders) and by the inclusion of a *dissociative subtype* as a specifier for posttraumatic stress disorder (PTSD).

Today, DID is recognized as an entity distinct from other psychopathological conditions, rooted in childhood trauma. The surprising frequency of DID in the ambulatory setting has been repeatedly demonstrated and speaks to the need to accurately diagnose and treat this often debilitating disorder.

PSYCHOPATHOLOGY AND PSYCHODYNAMICS

The DSM diagnostic criteria for DID are straightforward (Box 11–1): DID is the condition wherein a person manifests two or more discrete personality states that at times take control of her behavior, associated with gaps in memory (amnesia). Before painting a more detailed clinical picture, we must begin by stressing the origin of these symptoms in a *chronically and severely traumatic childhood*. Dissociation is both a spontaneously occurring reaction to trauma and a defense against being psychologically overwhelmed by a traumatic situation from which one cannot physically escape. Two important fundamental principles follow: first, the entire multiple personality system is structured around avoiding traumatic memories and affects, and all interactions with the patient are informed by this knowledge; second, the patient with DID never suffers from DID symptoms in isolation and will display multiple other trauma-related symptoms as well—at the very least, PTSD, coupled with a distorted view of herself and of the world that is full of negative beliefs or *schemas*. This constellation of symptoms is often referred to as *complex PTSD*, and the clinician treating a patient with DID should become familiar with this entity, as it offers a unifying conceptual foundation for work with these polysymptomatic patients. The practical corollary is that when treating a patient with DID, the clinician must expect to be confronting extensive comorbid psychopathology as well, especially PTSD, borderline personality disorder (BPD), and depression, all embedded in a matrix of extremely negative schemas such as hopelessness, the expectation of being exploited, and especially self-hatred.

BOX 11–1. DSM-5 Criteria for Dissociative Identity Disorder

A. Disruption of identity characterized by two or more distinct personality states, which may be described in some cultures as an experience of possession. The disruption in identity involves marked discontinuity in sense of self and sense of agency, accompanied by related alterations in affect, behavior, consciousness, memory, perception, cognition, and/or sensory-motor functioning. These signs and symptoms may be observed by others or reported by the individual.
B. Recurrent gaps in the recall of everyday events, important personal information, and/or traumatic events that are inconsistent with ordinary forgetting.
C. The symptoms cause clinically significant distress or impairment in social, occupational, or other important areas of functioning.
D. The disturbance is not a normal part of a broadly accepted cultural or religious practice.
   Note: In children, the symptoms are not better explained by imaginary playmates or other fantasy play.
E. The symptoms are not attributable to the physiological effects of a substance (e.g., blackouts or chaotic behavior during alcohol intoxication) or another medical condition (e.g., complex partial seizures).

Source. Reprinted from American Psychiatric Association: *Diagnostic and Statistical Manual of Mental Disorders,* 5th Edition. Arlington, VA, American Psychiatric Association, 2013. Copyright 2013, American Psychiatric Association. Used with permission.

Comorbid symptomatology aside, the DID syndrome itself consists of a system of different personality states, coupled with a system of amnestic barriers that separate them. The personality states typically represent different ages, different genders, different memories (especially traumatic ones), and different affects and attitudes. When different personality states take control of the patient's behavior, there is often some degree of amnesia—that is, each personality state will usually remember what occurred when that state was in executive control but often will not remember the activities of other personality states (also commonly referred to as *parts* or *alters*). Patients' experience of this is quite varied—ranging from patients who are aware of the existence of different personality states and can describe them ("That's Ruth; she's the angry one; she usually comes out when my father is around") to patients who understand nothing about their condition other than that they have disturbing experiences of "blanking out" and are later told of things they did that they do not remember. The degree of amnesia is quite variable, but when it is severe, disremembered behavior can be an extremely distressing experience for the patient—for example, finding lacerations that she does not remember inflicting or receiving phone calls from men asking for a repeat of a sexual encounter of which she has no memory.

DID, although usually diagnosed in adulthood, actually begins in childhood, in the context of severe trauma such as extreme, chronic physical and/or sexual and/or emotional abuse. Splitting off the awareness of a traumatic experience (dissociative amnesia) was observed in the nineteenth century by Pierre Janet and Freud; later, acute posttraumatic amnesia was repeatedly described in soldiers on the battlefields of World Wars I and II. In the development of DID, the child begins with a similar process of distancing herself from the trauma, as if it were happening to someone else, and of sequestering it from awareness. However, when the trauma is chronically repeated, and the process of creating internal dissociative barriers occurs repeatedly, these barriers begin to become concretized as psychological structure, and the patient's self-awareness becomes chronically split. This defense at first serves to protect against intolerable experiences of trauma, but eventually, other psychological issues, such as conflicts over anger or sexuality, are also resolved by dissociating, and the patient's personality becomes chronically "multiple," with some personality states that remember certain traumas, other personality states that contain certain affects, and still other personality states that perform certain functions, such as working or mothering. The patient pays the price of lost internal cohesion and continuous sense of self but manages to survive childhood; later, as an adult, the problematic consequences of divided identity and discontinuous memory become manifest. Although there is infinite variability in the personality system of the patient with DID, we describe certain commonly encountered configurations.

The median number of alters in the DID "system" is eight, although the number ranges from the definitional minimum of two to "polyfragmented DID," which has scores of alters. The most frequent types of alters, present in almost every patient with DID, include angry/violent alters, "persecutory" alters, alters who feel suicidal, and child alters. Other commonly encountered types are teenage alters (often rebellious and angry); highly sexualized/promiscuous alters; pleasure-oriented alters, who may use substances and who prefer to deny emotional distress; calm and constructive alters, who may have extensive knowledge of the personality system (sometimes called *internal self-helpers*); alters who perform necessary day-to-day functions (working, mothering, being a wife); abusive parental alters modeled on the abusive parents; comforting alters representing fantasied loving parents; and opposite-gender alters. Understanding the personality system of the patient with DID requires not only acquaintance with the roster of personality states but coming to know which parts of the patient typically present for treatment sessions and which are opposed to treatment; which parts tend to ally with each other or to oppose each other; which parts tend to be "out" under what circumstances; and, finally, the level of awareness that different alters possess about their condition—especially ascertaining whether alters are aware of the reality that they share one physical body and are all part of one person.

Additionally, the patient's psyche is not only divided, it also typically harbors a host of maladaptive attitudes (such as self-hatred) and maladaptive behavior (such as suicidality). The patient's internal reality is painfully confused, with different parts that express diametrically opposed attitudes (e.g., fear of being touched vs. indiscriminate sexual activity) and with posttraumatic confusion between the past and present, with some parts living as if they were frozen in time in an unending flashback of abuse. *Persecutory alters* are personality states that express attitudes vis-à-vis the host self, such as "She's a wimp; she deserves to be hurt for letting herself be abused like that!"—attitudes that are then used to justify behaviors such as self-cutting, which the persecutory alter may experience as if she were cutting someone else's body and not her own. Many of these more "negative" alters voice hostility and contempt for the therapist. Other alters may display behaviors such as substance abuse, promiscuity, or intense anger or may tend to submit passively to victimization. The personality states are arranged in a somewhat stable system whereby the patient manages to compensate for her fragmentation and memory lapses in a way that often permits more or less adequate function while concealing the DID from even close observers.

This last point bears expanding and helps to explain why multiple studies have found that patients with DID typically spend years in the mental health system without their condition being diagnosed. Although the DID diagnosis is defined by the identity fragmentation and amnesia described earlier and although these symptoms may occasionally be reported at the patient's initial presentation, patients with DID have usually been able to hide the symptoms from the outside world and may themselves be only dimly aware of them, so patients with DID typically present with complaints of depression, anxiety, or suicidality, not amnesia or different personality states. Keeping her symptomatology hidden is a high priority for the patient with DID, who has spent years concealing her sexual abuse and who zealously hides her dissociative experiences as well. Auditory hallucinations, which are present in more than 90% of patients with DID and which represent the intrusions of other personality states into awareness, are usually present since childhood, but the patient may never have revealed them for fear of being judged as "crazy." Often the patient's system of personality states and amnestic barriers does not emerge until well into treatment. DID patients are often highly intelligent and may be much more high functioning than one would expect given the symptoms just described.

Psychodynamics

In understanding DID, one touches on several psychodynamic issues of historical and clinical importance. DID is the modern-day heir to classical "grand hysteria," and many of its essential characteristics were spelled out in Breuer and Freud's foundational *Studies on Hysteria*; their formulation was in turn strongly indebted to the work of Pierre Janet and Jean-Martin Charcot, among others. Janet's writings have been resurrected in recent years by scholars of dissociation as constituting an early description of dissociative phenomena that is still relevant today. Between 1883 and 1889, Janet studied several cases of hysteria in detail and described "psychological automatisms," "double consciousness," and "double personality," all of which presage our understanding of the activities of the dissociated states that are at the core of DID. The eminent neurologist Jean-Martin Charcot, in his final major book in 1889 (a book that was translated into German by Freud), discussed cases of hysterical paralysis following accidents and proposed that a sudden trauma could cause a "nervous shock," with an accompanying hypnosis-like mental state, with this state leading to the formation of hysterical symptoms. This traumatic model of hysteria is also central to our current understanding.

Breuer and Freud's 1893 "Preliminary Communication" section of *Studies on Hysteria* contained most of the elements of today's model of DID. They stated that almost all hysteria was caused by psychological trauma; emphasized the importance of "hypnoid states" (a hypnosis-like alteration of consciousness experienced in response to trauma) as the first step in the development of hysteria; described the clinical syndrome wherein two personality states alternate, each remembering only its own pertinent history; and believed that the splitting-off of the traumatic memory and affects was pathogenic and that its reintegration was ultimately therapeutic, saying,

> [W]e have become convinced that the splitting of consciousness which is so striking in the well-known classical cases of "double conscience" is present to a rudimentary degree in every hysteria, and that a tendency to such dissociation, and with it the emergence of abnormal states of consciousness (which we shall bring together under the term "hypnoid") is the basic phenomenon of the neurosis.

In this same monograph, however, Breuer and Freud posit two different pathways to hysteria. The first one, above, resembles our current understanding of dissociative disorders, in which traumatic memories are sequestered from awareness "due to the fact that they originated during the prevalence of severely paralyzing affects," which we would call *peritraumatic dissociation*. In a crucial divergence, however, the authors also outlined a different pathway, still centered on the exclusion of distressing material from awareness, but emphasizing psychological defense, not hypnoid states—"a question of things which the patient wished to forget, and therefore intentionally repressed from his conscious thought." Freud soon came to see the two models—paralyzing affects due to trauma, leading to a dissociative "hypnoid state" and double consciousness, versus defense against psychological conflict, utilizing repression, in which double consciousness is seen as epiphenomenon—as contradictory.

The reader knows that this second view—repression of conflicted material—ultimately prevailed in Freud's conceptualization of psychopathology. Breuer and Freud's original view of hysteria as traumatic in origin (the "seduction theory") is similar to our current view of DID. Eventually, however, Freud came to believe that every seeming hypnoid hysteria was at root a defense hysteria—and now intrapsychic conflict, and repression, took explanatory precedence over traumatic dissociation. In this model, actual childhood sexual trauma was less important than childhood sexual wishes, which were banished from awareness not because of dissociation born out of traumatic paralyzing affect but because the patient "wished to forget" them.

The modern-day observer of DID enjoys another vantage point from which to view this debate. The robust connection between trauma and dissociation has been empirically established beyond any reasonable doubt. In DID, we now know that we do not have to choose between the trauma/dissociation model and the conflict/defense model, because both mechanisms are clearly on display. Exposure to sudden trauma can indeed induce a hypnoid state, which we would now call traumatic dissociation; however, dissociation also clearly serves as a defense as well. When a child develops dissociative amnesia for sexual abuse, the amnesia originates as a hypnoid state but also serves a defensive purpose—although the defense is against intolerable affects, not conflicted wishes. Furthermore, later in the genesis of a typical case of DID it can clearly be seen that dissociated personality states can come into being not only as a response to trauma but also out of a need to process conflicted affects such as rage and sexuality. The phenomenology of traumatic hysteria and of defense hysteria coexist and overlap in the patient with DID. This fundamental understanding—that patients with DID have dissociated in response to overwhelming traumatic affects and that this dissociation has come to serve as the patient's central and ubiquitous defense, against both traumatic memories and conflicted impulses—informs all treatment models and guides all clinical interactions.

Ever since the modern age of renewed interest and research in DID, beginning in the early 1980s, we have relied on a neat two-factor explanatory model for the development of DID: exposure to severe early trauma combines with the individual's innate tendency to dissociate and produces pathological dissociation. In recent years, longitudinal research data have shown disorganized attachment, measured in infancy, to be strongly predictive of later dissociation, independent of trauma exposure. This information, combined with clinical observation, has forced us to exchange our two-factor model for a three-factor model, which includes psychodynamics of attachment as well.

John Bowlby's attachment theory holds that human beings are endowed from birth with the disposition to form an attachment to a caregiving figure when alone or threatened. Although this was evolutionarily necessary for survival, it is also believed that creating a successful attachment with at least one caregiver is essential for healthy emotional and social development. When attachment is measured in infants, *disorganized attachment* refers to a constellation of infant behaviors in which a coherent effort to seek and maintain attachment is lacking. It has been suggested that the parent's own attachment difficulties or past traumas are expressed in a variety of behaviors, such as the parent feeling frightened, or helpless, or angry, which then frighten the infant and which present the infant with the dilemma that she is frightened of the very person to whom she should be turning for reassurance—leading to disorganized attachment. The exact role of attachment issues in the formation of DID is not as well understood as that of trauma. What we can clearly say is that the same childhood environments that are filled with trauma and abuse will also frequently offer an extremely challenging context for the child to find secure attachments. Just as a child may dissociate in the face of overt trauma such as sexual abuse, she may also retreat dissociatively when her efforts to find parental emotional resonance are disappointed by grossly, or even subtly, unresponsive parent figures. Parental abuse or neglect may be rooted in the parents' own difficulties with mental illness or substance abuse, making them less available for reliable emotional connection. Worse still is the situation in which the child must turn her need for attachment toward a parental figure who is also abusing her. One can easily imagine the psychological defensive advantage of splitting the image of the object into two, based on their loving versus abusive qualities, and one can also imagine the difficulty for the child of integrating her own diametrically opposed attachment responses toward these two parental aspects. Dissociative splitting seems at times to hide away, as if for safekeeping, the hope for love that has been repeatedly disappointed—sometimes embodying this hopefulness in a particular personality state. These overwhelming attachment needs, and insecurities about attachment, assume a central role in most DID treatments. They are seen especially in child alters who approach the clinician with an ardent longing for caretaking and appear as well in persecutory alters whose hostility and bravado defend against an intense but unacknowledged desire to feel cared for by the therapist.

Differential Diagnosis

The two disorders that cause the most diagnostic confusion with DID, based in each case on one major symptom shared with DID, are schizophrenia and bipolar disorder. A large majority of patients with DID experience receiving input from dissociated personality states in the form of auditory hallucinations. Whereas these are "psychotic" by definition because they violate consensual reality, the underlying process is not a psychotic one: there is no thought disorder, other associated psychotic symptoms are not present, and the symptoms do not respond to antipsychotic medications. These symptoms could be compared with vivid flashbacks in PTSD, in that there is a break with consensual reality—no one else is able to see the traumatic scene that is being reexperienced—but the symptoms are attributed to PTSD, a psychotic diagnosis is not given, and antipsychotic medications are not used as treatment. However, because the auditory hallucinations in DID are often those of deprecatory voices, or of voices urging dangerous actions such as harm to self or others, they closely resemble the auditory hallucinations of schizophrenia or psychotic mood disorder. In fact, a number of studies have replicated the finding that patients with DID actually display more so-called Schneiderian first-rank symptoms of schizophrenia (e.g., voices talking to each other, "made" actions or feelings) than do those with schizophrenia. Distinguishing the two conditions can be difficult; the presence or absence of other positive symptoms, especially thought disorder, and negative symptoms is a helpful clue, as is the clinical "big picture" (i.e., a patient who reports hearing voices since she was 6 years old, in the context of a traumatic childhood, but whose general level of functioning is much higher than what would be expected with severe childhood-onset schizophrenia, may be suffering from DID). Ultimately, the clinician must determine whether the voice represents a personalized entity (e.g., the patient describes a familiar voice, reports "that's Angel, she's always telling me how stupid I am," and goes on to describe Angel as a blond teenager who wears punk clothes), and whether this entity ever takes over the patient's behavior (e.g. "Kenya's" voice is heard when the patient feels angry, and at times the voice becomes very loud, followed by amnestic episodes during which the patient behaves aggressively). This differential diagnosis is sometimes straightforward, but often it is difficult to clarify, and the clinician may need to tolerate an extended period of diagnostic uncertainty, which may include neuroleptic trials.

Rapid-cycling bipolar disorder shares with DID a dramatic oscillation between emotional states, such as a depressed, responsible persona versus a promiscuous, substance-using, hedonistic one. If these changes are attributable to DID, the switches are instantaneous rather than transitioning over hours or days; there might be amnesia for some of the activities; the different states might be described as having different names or physical attributes; the associated vegetative symptoms would generally not be nearly as pronounced as those of bipolar disorder; and symptoms such as grandiose delusions would not be expected.

The difficulty of diagnosing DID has been well established, with multiple studies confirming that the typical patient with DID has been in the mental health system for 7 years before DID is diagnosed—raising the question of what diagnoses the patients were given during the years of treatment that preceded receiving the DID diagnosis. Therefore, the diagnoses of schizophrenia and bipolar disorder not only represent differential diagnostic possibilities but are also frequently seen as misdiagnoses given to patients with auditory hallucinations or with alternating, dramatically different personae, whose true diagnosis should be DID. The third diagnosis, which is often difficult to distinguish from DID, is BPD. However, whereas diagnosing schizophrenia or bipolar disorder versus DID is usually an either/or question, BPD and DID are often present simultaneously, with 80% of patients with DID meriting a

BPD diagnosis and 50% of patients with BPD eligible for a dissociative disorder diagnosis (DID specifically in perhaps 10%–30% of BPD cases). This is not surprising given the frequent traumatic origins of both conditions; symptoms we think of as "borderline," such as suicidality and emotion dysregulation, are highly prevalent in DID. Most patients with DID qualify for the additional BPD diagnosis; the important question here, when assessing a patient already diagnosed with BPD, is whether the identity disturbance and splitting seen in BPD rise to the level of distinct personality states, with amnesia, that would warrant considering a DID diagnosis.

The amnesia that characterizes DID necessitates diagnostic discrimination between different causes of memory disturbance. When the screening question "Do you ever have periods of time that you can't account for?" is answered with "yes," the two most common non-DID causes are substance use and seizure disorders; confirmatory histories can usually be obtained with relative ease. Another important differential diagnosis contrasts DID with normal forgetting and normal personality state changes. When a patient endorses memory disturbances, most of these will turn out to be of the "I can never remember where I left my keys" variety associated with normal forgetting, versus reporting "At times I find myself someplace and have no idea how I got there," which is more suggestive of DID. Similarly, persons may report feeling like "a whole different person" in a particular setting, but they do not usually mean a person with a different name, age, gender, or physical attributes, and they are not usually amnestic for the activities of this "different person."

Malingered or factitious DID is probably suspected far out of proportion to its actual occurrence, but clues would be the presence of clear secondary gain and a patient's report that emphasizes the symptoms of DID that are commonly known from media portrayals and are thus more likely to be feigned (dramatically different personality states, childhood trauma) and that omits symptoms that are less well known but are in fact epidemiologically just as common (e.g., auditory hallucinations, intrusive thoughts/emotions/impulses/actions, depersonalization).

MANAGEMENT OF THE INTERVIEW

The issues in the management of the interview of a patient with DID are very different at different stages of treatment, and we will give examples to illustrate how the interview changes over time. The differences are especially pronounced when we compare early interviews in which the diagnosis is not yet clear with later sessions, after the diagnosis has been firmly established and agreed on by patient and clinician and there is a shared vocabulary about the existence of different "parts" of the patient. We look first at an example of the kinds of delicate explorations that characterize early treatment.

The Early Phase

Patients with DID seldom present with a clear description of different personality states, instead reporting generic symptoms such as depression, anxiety, or suicidality. There is usually a history of significant childhood trauma, although the patient may avoid the topic, minimize the severity, or say "I don't know—maybe—I don't really remember." The clinician may become suspicious of DID because a patient describes amnestic episodes ("losing time") or dramatic changes in behavior that the patient herself finds puzzling—or because the clinician notices significant gaps in the patient's memory for events that occurred during the week or for the contents of previous clinical sessions. The clinician wonders, "Might this patient have DID?" and sets out to ascertain the presence of symptoms such as the sense of "other people inside," of alternate personality states that control her behavior at times, and of disremembered behavior—as well as to inquire into the presence of chronic auditory hallucinations, representing the intrusion into awareness of disavowed aspects of the personality. The patient's tendency to underreport these symptoms is highly unconsciously motivated. The symptoms of patients with DID developed in childhood, in the context of severe ongoing abuse, and this abuse occurred in secret, or else it would have been stopped and the development of DID possibly averted. Thus, the patient's symptoms arose in the context of a closely held, shameful secret, and the notion of revealing the symptoms carries the same powerful negative emotional valence as revealing the abuse. Patients have deeply held beliefs, which become activated as the clinician begins to make diagnostic inquiries, that disclosure of their long-held secrets (i.e., their abuse and their unusual internal experiences) would be dangerous and are therefore subject to severe internal prohibitions. Additionally, patients with DID usually experience their symptoms as evidence that they are "crazy" and have been trying to "act normal" for many years by concealing them. Any diagnostic inquiry risks upsetting this tenuous equilibrium. Therefore, as the clinician begins to explore DID symptoms, he or she proceeds with a high degree of caution, expecting to encounter strong resistances to revealing them. The clinician moves slowly and carefully and is ready to pause at signs of alarm in the patient, as in the following example.

> A single mother in her twenties presented for treatment after hospital-ization for a suicide attempt; a history of significant childhood trauma was obtained. The clinician first noted that the patient was never able to give a detailed account of the attempt, saying that "It's very hazy," and then began to be aware of subtle discontinuities in conversations in ses-sions in which the patient, who was intelligent and alert, would seem confused as to what was being discussed. Finally, at one of these junc-tures, the clinician asks the patient if she remembered what they had just been discussing. The patient replies "of course," but when the clini-cian follows up by asking her to recount the preceding few minutes of discussion, she admits that she cannot remember. The clinician then in-quires about memory symptoms, and the patient admits, with obvious discomfort, that in fact it was a distressingly frequent occurrence to find herself with no memory for preceding events. The clinician asks for ex-amples, and the patient reveals that this even included finding herself in bed with strange men with no memory of how she had gotten there—in the absence of substance intoxication. At this point, the clinician sus-pects DID but does not want to frighten the patient and is also careful to use language that is compatible with either the presence or absence of DID—language that straddles both diagnostic possibilities. Examples of such straddling language are phrases such as "a part of yourself" or "different aspects of your personality"; inquiries might be phrased "Sometimes a part of you takes over?" "Sometimes you feel like a differ-ent person?" or "You have strong internal conflicts about this—like a war inside?" This language allows the patient to expand on her internal experience without having to declare baldly the presence of DID and without the clinician having to prematurely judge the diagnostic issue. The inquiry continues with the clinician asking whether the patient hears voices; the patient seems ambivalent, at first saying "I don't think so," but after receiving reassurance from the clinician that these are rou-tine diagnostic questions, admits to this symptom as well, adding that she has never told anyone about this before. When the clinician asks for more details about the voices ("What do they say?" "Are they familiar?" "Do the voices feel like another part of you is speaking to you?"), he suddenly notices the patient looking extremely frightened. He quickly hypothesizes that the diagnostic inquiry has gone far enough for that moment and asks, "Are you getting feedback inside that you aren't sup-posed to talk about this?" The patient is clearly surprised at the precise description of her internal experience and nods in agreement. At this point, the clinician knows to provide reassurance and psychoeducation, saying "It is totally understandable that it would be uncomfortable to talk about things that you have been keeping inside all these years," ex-plaining that symptoms such as missing time and hearing voices do not mean that a person is crazy and in fact occur frequently in people who undergo trauma as children. The clinician adds that although he thinks it might ultimately be very useful to the patient to explore these things

further, the choice would be entirely hers, and he will not press her to talk about things she does not wish to discuss.

In the typical treatment of a patient with DID, a session such as this one would be followed by the gradual unfolding, in a markedly stop-and-start manner, of a clearer picture of the patient's internal experience of other aspects of herself. She might retreat from previously described symptoms, saying "I'm really not so sure about what I told you," and might require repeated reassurance that the clinician does not now judge her negatively or think she is crazy. Psychoeducation might be repeatedly delivered, in small doses, along with the consistent message that there is no hurry to explore these matters, that the clinician is willing and interested but all therapeutic work will be based on the comfort level of the patient. Not uncommonly, one or more lengthy discussions of the question "Is it worth it to dig all of these things up?" will be required, with the clinician validating the patient's fear of emotional upset but explaining as well the potential benefit.

In these early phases of treatment, if the patient voices interest in continuing to explore her hitherto-unexamined internal experience, the clinician will be asking a multitude of exploratory questions. The clinician is trying to walk a line between being too inquisitive and spooking the patient versus not inquiring actively, with the attendant risk that the patient's fear will prevail in the form of a passive resistance wherein she simply avoids mentioning these matters.

Approaching the Personality States

A definitive choice point in the clinician's treatment of DID is the approach to the patient's alternate personality states (commonly referred to in the literature as *alters* but often referenced as *parts* when speaking with the patient). This subject has been exhaustively reviewed, and we will not re-create the entire discussion here. We briefly summarize by saying that although there is great variability in the patient's ability to understand and to explain her condition, by definition a patient with DID is living chronically with subjectively separate personality states. These discrete states, which have their own sense of identity, their own characteristic affects and behaviors, and their own often traumatic memories, are experienced by the patient as being different people (the "delusion of separateness," which is, however, not a psychotic symptom and is not responsive to antipsychotic medication). Effective psychotherapy of DID crucially involves the clinician directly engaging the alter personalities on their own terms and entering into their subjective experience of separateness, while consistently purveying the message that they are *not* in fact separate people, they are parts of one person, and that the patient's improvement in therapy requires these parts to become gradually less separate—to improve communication and cooperation between parts, leading to less amnesia, less confusion, and improved function. The clinician will be clear that the specific goal of "integration" (i.e., dissolution of all internal dissociative barriers, with all personality states combining into one) is chosen by some patients but is optional—but that the goal of improved internal cooperation and communication is mandatory if the patient wishes to get better.

From the beginning, once the clinician suspects DID, he or she must proceed with the awareness that although he or she is talking to one person, in the background may be multiple other parts of the patient who may be listening to the conversation, forming their own opinions and judgments and choosing whether to participate in the psychotherapy. The success of the therapy ultimately rests on finding a way to engage these other parts of the patient's personality—for if not engaged, the particular issues that they represent (e.g., anger, sexuality, mistrust, self-hatred) will be sequestered away from the therapeutic process, and therapy will have minimal impact on them.

> A 22-year-old part-time college student had been in treatment for several months, and the evidence supporting a diagnosis of DID had accrued to the point of near certainty; however, the clinician had not yet confirmed this by direct contact with alters. The diagnostic evidence included repeated periods of amnesia with disremembered behavior as well as auditory hallucinations that the patient could characterize familiarly ("That's Jessie. She's always mad. She doesn't like getting pushed around. She's always telling me to fight."). In session one day, the patient feels dismayed that she had spoken angrily and rudely to one of her college instructors ("She must think I'm a total bitch; now there's no way I'm going to pass that class!"). The clinician asks whether she remembers the incident clearly (she does not), and continues, "Do you think maybe that was another part of you?" The patient is thoughtful, eventually replying, "Probably." The clinician asks if she knows which part of her, and after a long pause, the patient replies "maybe Jessie." The clinician attempts to explore further ("What makes you think so?"), but after an even longer pause, the patient answers, "She says I shouldn't be talking to you"—and then voices the wish that Jessie would just go away, because "She's always messing things up for me! Things would be way better if I could just get rid of her!" The clinician asks if the patient would like to hear his thoughts about Jessie; the patient assents, and the clinician provides important information: "First of all, I know this is not going to make you happy, but you can't get rid of

her. I know it feels like Jessie is a different person, and I know this is still hard to understand, but you and Jessie are actually two parts of the same person. And you know, I'll bet if I talked to her, she'd say the same thing as you—she'd probably be mad at you and say that *her* life would be better if you weren't around. And then I would say the same thing to her that I'm saying to you—you can't get rid of her; you are both parts of the same person." The patient responds, "That's messed up!" and the clinician continues, "And you know something else? Even if you *could* get rid of her, you actually *wouldn't* be better off without her. Because you know all of those times that she got mad and got into fights with people? She was actually sticking up for you. That's something she's really good at: being strong, getting angry when you need to get angry—which is something that you find really hard to do, right?" The patient affirms her difficulty in this area, and the clinician continues, "So yes, I know that sometimes it seems like she's overreacting—and I agree, sometimes she probably takes it a little too far—but I will tell you, having heard a little bit about what you went through as a kid, I am 100% certain that she has good reasons to be really angry—and I'm sure if she told me some of the things she is angry about, I would be angry at them too. So maybe she gets a little bit too angry sometimes—but she is actually a totally valuable part of who you are, she carries a lot of your anger and your strength, and you wouldn't be better off without her. What *would* be good is if the two of you could start to figure out a way to work together, instead of being at war with each other all of the time." The patient replies, "That's never going to happen!" and the clinician persists: "I know, it seems like the two of you are really far apart now. But I know you want to feel better, and I'm pretty sure that she'd like to feel better, too—we just have to start to find a way for you *both* to feel better."

The clinician might choose this moment for an additional piece of resistance analysis, as well: "And one more thing? She says that you shouldn't be talking to me? Well, I can understand that, too. I think that when you were a kid, you learned that you had better keep your mouth shut about what was going on, and that if you didn't, bad things happened, right? So she figured out that the safest approach was to not tell people things—so of course, when she sees you talking to me, she tells you not to. You know what? I think that she has been really smart all of these years, not talking to people. But I want to suggest to her that although that was the best policy in the past, it's not going to be the best policy forever. Jessie probably looks at me and thinks, 'Why should I trust that person? It's not safe to talk to him.' So I'm going to invite her to actually look at me, and at the conversations we're having, and not to just assume that because it was dangerous to talk in the past, that that's true here too. She is really good at being a watchdog and making sure you don't get burned by trusting anyone, right? So I'm fine with her being a watchdog here with me, too, and watching me really carefully, and if it seems like I'm up to no good, she can warn you about it or ask me what I'm up to. Because if she's a really good watchdog, that just makes it safer if we try to move ahead in therapy and actually talk about things."

The clinician has been pursuing a number of goals in the above exchange. Throughout therapy, the clinician applies gentle but steady pressure against the patient's experience of dividedness and in favor of the idea that seemingly separate entities are actually parts of one person; similarly, the proposition is steadily advanced that despite their seeming differences, parts can solve the problem not by dissociating ("getting rid of her") but rather by associating ("getting along, working together, working toward the same goals"). Also, all such conversations ("Do you think a part of you was responsible for the angry outburst?") serve the purpose of helping the patient to make connections to different parts of herself rather than simply disavowing them as alien or as beyond her understanding. Here the patient's angry feelings and behaviors have been split off from her usual more cooperative attitude, and these aspects of herself have been posed as being in hostile opposition to each other; the clinician is validating the importance of both aspects of the patient and working to gradually reduce the split. The clinician is modeling fairness and equality ("I would say the same thing to her that I'm saying to you") and positioning himself as an even-handed broker for future negotiations between parts. The clinician is reframing problematic aggressive behaviors as understandable in light of past experience—introducing the idea of childhood schemata, attitudes, and behaviors that made sense in the past but that now need to be modified in the patient's adult life. The clinician is giving the message that the angry part of the patient is *valuable*—usually an extremely important intervention with a patient who most likely feels chronically and severely devalued. The clinician gently models the possibility of emotional modulation and of non–black-and-white views ("She has good reason to be angry but she probably takes it a bit too far sometimes"). The clinician is building a relational foundation that will eventually be used to directly engage with the angry alter—although that part of the patient has not yet presented herself to speak with the clinician, the clinician is assuming that what he says is being heard by all parts of the patient, so he is giving messages of respect, validation, understanding, and willingness to negotiate and is treating the angry part as an equal of the more cooperative part—all of which will hopefully lead up to the point at which the angry and mistrustful alter may be willing to directly engage with the clinician in treatment. Finally, the clinician is directly addressing the resistance (mistrust), framing it as a childhood schema that is perhaps no longer necessary, inviting the patient to examine it in the light of the present, and giving paradoxical permission for the patient to remain mistrustful as a way to allow therapeutic progress. Predictably, the treatment of this patient will include dozens of iterations of similar conversations.

Later Stages

At later stages in treatment, the patient and the clinician both become more familiar with the patient's system of alternate personality states, and other techniques for managing the interview may gradually be employed. The following vignette takes place almost a year into the treatment of Isabel, a 35-year-old married mother of two. The patient's diagnosis of DID has been firmly established, and the patient has committed to its psychotherapeutic exploration; as this has proceeded, the patient has developed increasing awareness of the feelings and behaviors of some of her alters—several who have spoken directly with the clinician and are cooperating with therapy and several who have chosen not to enter the therapy arena, voicing suspicion and hostility.

> Isabel's explorations of her traumatic past and of her other personality states have at times been extremely anxiety provoking, but she has also felt relieved to finally start to unburden herself of these secrets and has made a good therapeutic alliance. In this spirit of optimism, she has overcome considerable trepidation and self-doubt and has returned to work after a 10-year absence. She is performing well at her job and is being considered for a promotion. However, she is beginning to have absences from work because her seizure disorder, which had been well-controlled for a number of years, is becoming symptomatic again—including, on one occasion, a seizure as she was getting into her car. After one such incident, the patient tells her clinician that she was baffled to discover that the pillbox she uses to keep track of her medications showed that she seemed not to have been taking the antiepileptic medications at all—a dramatic change from her normally meticulous behavior. In response to the clinician's inquiry, she says she has "no idea" what is going on, and the clinician asks if she thinks it is possible that some other part of her has been choosing not to take the medications. After a long pause for reflection, she nervously allows that this might in fact be true: "I have a funny feeling that it might be Nobody"—"Nobody" being the name of an alter who is known to be chronically angry and uninterested in participating in therapy and who makes derogatory comments suggesting that the patient is "a worthless piece of garbage" who should kill herself. The patient adds, "I can't tell you any more. She won't talk to me."
>
> The clinician does not typically ask to speak to a particular alter, preferring that the choice of which part of the patient participates in therapy on a given day be left to the patient and that parts will choose to participate as they feel ready to do so and when they have material to discuss. Here, however, the clinician chooses to break this rule, because the behavior in question threatens not only the patient's job but her safety as well. He asks, "Do you mind if I ask to speak to Nobody?" and the patient assents. The clinician says, "I'm hoping to speak with you, Nobody. I know you haven't wanted to talk to me before, but it seems that you have been making sure that Isabel doesn't take her medica-

tions. I'm guessing that you have serious reasons for doing that—and I would really like to hear what your concerns are." After a pause, the patient answers in a somewhat gruff and masculine voice, "Goddamn right I've got reasons! Not that *you* care!" (The clinician registers this last phrase as an opening—the patient is allowing herself to voice her disappointment at his perceived noncaring, which is one step removed from admitting to wanting him to care.) The clinician replies, "Well, you will probably be surprised to know that I absolutely do care—that I think your opinions are just as important and valuable as Isabel's, or anyone else's." The patient pauses, then says, "I figured you were on Isabel's side; you probably thought I was just some asshole who was trying to mess things up." The therapist answers, "I'm not sure about trying to mess things up—all I knew was that you seemed really angry and that you didn't trust me very much. Maybe you heard me tell Isabel that I was sure that you had good reasons for being angry and not trusting people?" The patient replies, "Yeah, that's why I came out to talk to you today—you get *one* chance!"

In response to the therapist's repeated statements of genuine interest, Nobody proceeds to explain that "Isabel is an idiot, trying to work—doesn't she know they're just going to keep piling more and more work on her? They know she can't handle it—then she'll screw up, and everybody will see what a fool she is!" Nobody admitted that, in response to these negative feelings about working, she decided on a course of sabotage: "I come out every night when it's time for her to take the pill, I close up the pillbox, and she thinks she took it." In her plan, the patient's seizure disorder would reemerge and she would have to quit work, "and if she crashes the car, she deserves it anyway for being so stupid." This is ego-syntonic with Nobody's chronic suicidal feelings.

The clinician has two agendas: to ensure safety and to further the therapeutic process. Both can be achieved by empathically engaging Nobody. The clinician addresses the patient (still self-identifying as Nobody at this moment—but the therapist is ever mindful that he is communicating with all parts of the patient) and voices understanding of her concerns, saying that he had not realized the catastrophic expectations that the patient was confronting in the workplace. He suggests that perhaps, rather than approaching the issue through subterfuge, Nobody could express her concerns directly to Isabel. This suggestion is met by a pessimistic "Why bother? She never pays attention to me. No one cares what I think. I'm nobody!" The therapist answers that he is absolutely committed to everyone being listened to and asks, "For example, does it seem like I'm listening to you now?" The patient acknowledges, with obvious surprise, that she *is* being listened to. The therapist continues that he is espousing neither her position nor Isabel's, but that both have valid concerns. He says, "For instance, she really wants to work, but you really don't want her to get in over her head and end up feeling humiliated. Perhaps there is a middle ground where everyone's concerns are respected—where she works but doesn't keep taking on new jobs so quickly?" He points out that whatever solution is chosen, what is important is that all parts of the patient treat each other with respect and learn to work together. He also points out that despite Nobody's reputation as a destructive force, her actions demonstrate that she has actually been acting out of concern for the patient, trying to prevent a negative scenario from occurring.

Near the end of the session, Nobody says, "OK, I'm out of here. But maybe I'll talk to you again. That wasn't so bad." The patient switches, Isabel reemerges, and the therapist asks, "Have you been listening to this conversation?" If she says no, the therapist briefly fills her in. If the patient has been listening, she might say, "I can't believe she's been tricking me about the pills, but now I see where she was coming from." The therapist closes with a safety check, making sure that the patient will not drive if she has not been taking her pills. If the patient claims helplessness in the face of disremembered behavior ("How am I supposed to know if she's taking the pills?"), the therapist strongly endorses the patient's personal responsibility—that although until now the patient has not been aware of this behavior, all parts are responsible for keeping track of dangerous behavior and amnesia does not win her a reprieve from this responsibility. Depending on his judgment of the patient's readiness to hear an interpretation, he might add that "Maybe one reason why she was able to keep you in the dark was that you partly agreed with what she was doing—you also felt nervous about working, so maybe you didn't mind so much that another part of you was sabotaging the work—so you didn't look that closely."

This vignette illustrates several important principles in dealing with the patient with DID. The clinician takes pains to build alliances with all parts of the patient, approaching them on their own terms (their subjective experience of separateness), all in the service of the eventual goal of collapsing these internal divisions. Here, his previous work in validating the perspective of the persecutory alter Nobody is rewarded when Nobody is grudgingly willing to risk direct engagement. The clinician takes a position as the hub of a metaphorical wheel, with the patient's personality states gradually establishing connection through the clinician's central presence.

First, awareness: the clinician unfamiliar with dissociative configurations would not have known to inquire whether another part of the patient might be involved in behaviors that the patient does not remember. Next, the clinician needs to overcome his or her own resistance to seeking direct contact with an alter and recognize the necessity of entering the patient's long-standing dissociative personality structure or else forgo gaining unfiltered access to important aspects of the patient—including, especially, the opportunity to directly address the patient's mistrust and her hostility toward the clinician and toward herself, which is otherwise sequestered away. The clinician hopes that if the mistrust is adequately processed, the defended-against longing for attachment will be able to emerge. The clinician occupies an even-handed stance between warring personality states and elucidates the self-protective intention behind Nobody's seemingly destructive behavior—again working to reduce the split between different parts of the personality, pointing out the more complex reality that even ostensibly pro-employment Isabel harbored mixed feelings. Heinz Kohut postulated that analyzability is present in a patient "whose self—or, to be more exact, a remnant of whose self—is still, potentially at least, in search of appropriately responsive selfobjects." This formulation is illustrated dramatically in the treatment of dissociative patients, with whom the treatment's success often rests on the clinician's ability to access the longing for attachment that is hidden beneath a convincing facade of hostility.

The clinician fully acknowledges the patient's reality of separateness and simultaneously enters it and undermines it. When a part of the patient disavows responsibility for undesirable behaviors ("I don't know anything about that"), the clinician emphasizes that the whole patient must take responsibility for all of her behavior. This is especially important when confronting safety issues, which are highly prevalent with dissociative patients. The clinician may find safety assessment daunting ("The part that I'm talking to says she won't hurt herself, but how can I know about other parts?"). At such times, it is often useful to remember comparable assessments with nondissociative patients—for instance, a borderline patient may promise to stay safe, but the clinician might worry that when she is in another affective state, these promises may not hold. In both instances, the clinician's final judgment as to the patient's safety represents his or her informed weighing of the strength of all aspects of the patient's different mood states and cognitions, both dangerous and protective.

At times, patients with DID can be seen to represent the clearest expression of classic psychodynamic principles. For instance, a psychodynamic formulation of Isabel might postulate that although the patient wants to succeed, she has an unconscious fear of success—on closer examination really a fear of failure—and thus she is unconsciously sabotaging her work efforts. When dealing with a patient with DID, the clinician may have the opportunity to meet and speak directly with these hypothetical "unconscious" aspects of the patient's self, such as the saboteur "Nobody." However, unlike the gradual unearthing of therapeutic material across the "horizontal split" of the classical repression barrier, here the conflicted feelings are personified and separated by a "vertical split"—that is, the feelings embodied in a self-state will emerge instantaneously to full consciousness and then just as abruptly exit awareness.

TRANSFERENCE AND COUNTERTRANSFERENCE

Transference

Transference issues abound in the treatment of the patient with DID—with the potential for countertransference errors seemingly limitless. The typical patient with DID has survived a traumatic childhood that included severely distorted relationships with caretaking figures, laying the foundation for highly negative transference expectations as well as establishing a host of powerful negative cognitive schemas (e.g., unlovability, mistrust). This traumatic background means that patients with DID usually suffer from what has been called *complex PTSD*, which includes severe posttraumatic symptoms as well as the kinds of issues often encountered with borderline patients, such as emotion dysregulation and suicidality. Thus we expect to encounter many of the same transference and countertransference issues described in the chapters on the borderline patient and the traumatized patient, in addition to a large set of issues more specific to DID.

Discussion of transference in DID treatment takes place under the umbrella concept of the *traumatic transference,* which, as Loewenstein points out, contains two distinct components. He uses the term *flashback transference* to refer to the specific phenomenon wherein some aspect of the psychotherapy situation triggers in-the-moment reexperiencing of childhood trauma. At times, the patient is able to articulate this clearly ("When you sit a certain way, when you lean forward in your chair and put your hand under your leg, it makes me feel really scared") and can explain the connection to a specific abuse experience. However, it is probably more frequent for flashback like phenomena to occur without the therapist being aware of it—either because the patient knows it is occurring but fear or shame prevents her from discussing it or because the flashback is being triggered outside of her awareness, without her noticing anything other than increased anxiety. Therefore, the therapist must always be ready to inquire about unexplained anxiety (or dissociation or cognitive disorganization) or about a subtle distancing shift in the therapeutic relationship. This can be quite challenging because the flashback triggers range from expectable (e.g., therapist shares the same gender, age, physical appearance with a past abuser) to obscure (e.g., the pattern in the floor tile, a dog barking outside the window) and because the patient may have limited ability to help decipher what is occurring.

The other sense of the term *traumatic transference* refers to the much more pervasive set of negative interpersonal expectations that the patient brings to the treatment situation—and whose elaboration, and successful transformation, is often the most important determinant of treatment outcome. These transferences range from frank conscious or unconscious fears of assault by the therapist to subtler expectations that the therapist will not care about her, or will condemn her or disbelieve her, or will put her needs second—the list of possibilities is long. Several years into a treatment with a patient who is improving steadily, with a seemingly trusting therapeutic relationship, the therapist may be taken aback to learn that the patient still comes to each session fearing that this will be the day when the clinician will finally make sexual advances. The patient's psyche is typically ruled by a host of negative cognitive schemas (e.g., "I am unlovable, in fact disgusting and loathsome"; "My fate is to have a horrible life, so any positive development is just a setup for a worse disappointment"), and in the therapeutic relationship these pre-existing schemas are transformed into transference, with the clinician perceived as holding these same negative views or as being the person through whom they will be enacted.

The exploration of these transferences, and the patient's eventual experience of disconfirming them in the treatment situation, usually serves as the clinician's most powerful ally in the patient's movement toward health. Confronted with the patient's seemingly unshakable negative convictions, the clinician's stance is crucial. Here we adapt Jay Greenberg's view on the evolution of the meaning of "neutrality" in post-Freudian metapsychologies, wherein the clinician adjusts his or her responses to achieve optimal relational positioning for the exploration of the material that is relevant at that moment. In our view, for instance, when the patient begins with a deep conviction that her sexual abuse was her fault, making her irreparably "dirty," strong pressure will have to be applied in the opposite direction, with the clinician stating clearly his or her belief that sexual abuse is never the child's responsibility and is not the patient's fault. This stance is necessary to provide a context in which the patient can begin to even *question* her long-held beliefs. When the clinician states his or her position as to the patient's blamelessness, the clinician does not imagine that the patient will thereby immediately change her view, and the clinician does not preclude detailed exploration of why the patient blames herself, but he or she is attempting to improve what begins as a severely unbalanced contest between the patient's entrenched negative belief and the possibility of her entertaining a less damaging view. We contend that the patient has a better chance of successfully examining her pathological self-blame if she knows that the therapist does not agree with it than she will if the therapist never states his or her position. Although at first seeming like a departure from classical neutrality, this leveling of the playing field best approximates a "neutral" frame for the necessary therapeutic work to occur.

The traumatic transference also emerges as the most formidable treatment resistance, with "resistance" here seen along the lines of Kohut's notion of resistance as fear of retraumatization. The patient's pervasive mistrust, her expectation that the therapist will be revealed eventually as just another exploiter, and her conviction that the therapist thinks as badly of her as she does of herself, all undermine her ability to reveal important information and to participate in the therapeutic relationship. These transference feelings will need to be explored repeatedly.

In addition to the overarching concept of traumatic transference, a few specific transference phenomena deserve mention here. A patient with DID by definition presents with multiple, subjectively separate personality states, so the patient's mix of, for instance, trusting and mistrusting feelings toward the clinician will usually emerge in a "split" fashion, with some parts of the patient that feel trusting, alternating in an all-or-nothing fashion with other parts that voice absolute determination never to trust the clinician. At such times, if the clinician were to ask, "Does this patient trust me?" the correct answer would be "somewhat"—the clinician keeping in mind that the opposing transference views, which the patient does not attempt to reconcile and experiences as coming from different people, are in fact all aspects of one person's fluid and evolving transference. However, on a practical basis and for a long time in the treatment, the clinician cannot avoid the complexity of processing multiple different transferences, as if he or she were treating multiple different people of different ages, genders, and attitudes, sometimes needing to switch between multiple transference configurations within one session.

Typically, there is another side to the negative transferences detailed above: although the patient fears and expects retraumatization, she also intensely desires the positive attachment of which she was so deprived. Freud noted, referring to libidinal cathexis, "the patient's need and longing should be allowed to persist in her in order that they may serve as forces impelling her to do the work and to make changes."

The DID patient's desire for a redoing of her childhood with a better parent (the clinician) serves as fuel for therapeutic work but also presents a powerful and potentially problematic transference. Patients often develop unrealistic wishes to be reparented by the clinician—especially when there are child alters, which is usually the case—and this often leads the patient to look to the therapist to fill an actual parenting role or to the patient's treatment becoming stuck as she enjoys the feeling of finally having a caring parental figure, and this starts to take precedence over moving ahead in therapy. This configuration has been described as "wanting to be loved into health." When this transference meets with understandable, caring maternal countertransference, parent/child caretaking enactments can derail treatment (this is discussed further under the topic of countertransference errors later in this chapter). However, if managed properly, the patient's strong desire for a relationship with a caring figure helps to motivate her to do the difficult work of therapy. This is especially relevant when the therapist is confronted with so-called persecutory alters, who may voice hatred of both the patient and the clinician. Invariably, this overt devaluing of the clinician covers an even stronger wish to be able to value the clinician and to be valued by the clinician.

Patients with DID are at high risk of revictimization, and after emerging from a childhood filled with trauma, they often find themselves victimized repeatedly in adulthood as well. Sexual victimization of patients with DID by their clinicians has been reported with such frequency that Richard Kluft labeled it the "sitting duck syndrome." Revictimization is a complex, multidetermined phenomenon with its own literature, with important determinants being the DID patient's lack of an appropriate frame of reference for what constitutes a violation and her difficulty finding an appropriate stance between blanket mistrust and unearned overtrust. It is also not uncommon for a sexualized alter to overtly propose a sexual involvement with the clinician. Often this occurs because her transference is that sexual accommodation is a necessary precondition for receiving any sort of caring; at other times, the dynamic is a passive-into-active approach, wherein the patient expects she will ultimately be victimized, so she initiates the activity in order to gain some sense of control. This becomes a test of the therapist's corruptibility, and when the therapist "passes" by refusing the sexual activity, it may offer an opportunity to challenge one of the patient's negative schemas. Of course, if the therapist fails this test, although this may initially be described as countertransference, it passes beyond that into the realm of therapist narcissistic pathology and egregious harm to the patient.

Countertransference

The transferences encountered in the treatment of a patient with DID are so multitudinous and shifting and the intensity of the feelings—angry, mistrustful, beseeching, sexual—so high that clinicians new to DID are certain to feel overwhelmed at times and will inevitably be drawn into a number of compelling countertransference enactments with the patient. Experienced clinicians are usually able to recognize these enactments earlier, engage in them less deeply, and extricate themselves more gracefully, hopefully able to utilize them as important opportunities for learning and growth. A review of some common countertransference errors follows.

Many errors are rooted in the most fundamental issue the clinician faces in the treatment of DID—namely, finding the optimal stance regarding the patient's multiplicity. The paradox, as discussed earlier, is the necessity to enter the patient's world of multiple self-states on its own terms as the only way to engage all dissociated aspects of the patient's memories, feelings, and impulses while providing a consistent counterforce in the direction of integration, steadily pushing the patient to acknowledge all parts of herself as parts of *herself.*

Clinicians experienced in the treatment of the patient with DID agree on the necessity of engaging alters directly, more or less on their own terms. For instance, a middle-aged female patient named Louise presents a male teenage alter named Louis. There will usually be points in the therapy at which it is important for the clinician to confront this alter explicitly with the fact that the patient is in fact female and not a teenager; however, in general the clinician will not choose this path of empathic failure, or possible iatrogenic treatment rupture, by routinely refusing to call her Louis or by repeatedly confronting her with the reality of her age and gender. It is easy to see, however, that this then becomes a delicate balancing act and that once the clinician is participating in the patient's reality, it would be easy to reify the experience of Louis to the point at which it feels as if one really is having a relationship with a separate person of that name. Maintaining this dialectic (the patient's deeply rooted experience of multiplicity vs. the reality of one-person-ness) in a state of dynamic tension is part of all DID treatment and does not have to be problematic. However, along the way there are various pitfalls related to the topic of separateness, including the potential for the clinician to take sides in disputes between different parts of the patient or to join the patient in evasion of responsibility for negative behaviors, such as self-harm, ostensibly committed by one part of the patient. Both of these errors are usually born out of the clinician's tendency to favor the more sympathetic, or overtly health-seeking, aspects of the patient's personality over the more destructive ones—which unfortunately then ends up reinforcing the splitting off of these aspects, which is already occurring.

> At a difficult juncture in treatment, Jane, the "host" personality state, reports that she feels helpless in the face of other personality states who are determined to take an overdose. The clinician allies with this beleaguered part of the patient, empathizing with her feeling that she is unable to control the dangerous behavior of the "others." Jane feels warmly

supported by her therapist but continues to feel helpless in the face of suicidal urges, which feel as if they belong to other people. The clinician, gravely concerned for the patient's safety, seeks supervision. The supervisor reminds the clinician that, in actuality, all personality states represent the attitudes and behaviors of one conflicted person. At the next session, the clinician points out that although the other parts may feel alien, they represent feelings and impulses that must be understood and claimed as belonging to the patient. The clinician now takes the position that the patient as a whole person, and thus by extension each part of the patient, is responsible for actions such as overdosing and must take part in the problem solving. When Jane says, "Yes, I'm depressed, but I don't want to kill myself. I'm just afraid that Amanda will overdose, and I can't control her," the clinician now responds, "I know you are saying that you don't want to overdose, but would it perhaps be more accurate to say that you are feeling ambivalence about it, and that the ambivalence is what opens the door for Amanda to self-harm? I believe if you decide 100% that you will not permit the self-harm to happen, it won't." The patient is thereby pushed to acknowledge significant overlap between her own emotional state and behaviors and those of parts that were being considered as "other," and that the behavior of one part is intertwined with the behavior of others. Once she does this, two things happen: the patient is challenged to take responsibility for safety and feels more power to do so; simultaneously, she begins, ever so slightly, to experience herself as not totally disconnected from other aspects of herself.

The countertransference error of treating parts as if they were separate people is most prevalent when dealing with child alters. These parts of the patient, self-describing as young children who carry feelings from the traumatic childhood (loneliness, terror, longing for love, often accompanied by preserved fragments of childlike trust and innocence), are often confused in an ongoing, flashback-like way about the distinction between past and present, so that in 2015 the patient may feel terrified each night of being raped by her father, who in fact passed away 10 years earlier and who committed the rapes in 1990. Who would not feel strong sympathy for such a child or would not want to rescue her from such an ongoing nightmare? The clinician may be even more inclined to a parental, doting response when the child alter's emergence in session provides a shift from the adult's grim and depressed perspective into a lighter one. It is easy for the clinician to begin to attend selectively to these child aspects, with both patient and clinician feeling gratified in the short term by the child's grateful response to adult caring.

Although it is in fact a necessary step in the therapy for the child aspects of the patient to express and analyze negative schemas, such as the expectation of an uncaring response, and eventually to rework them, thinking that this will occur by simply reparenting the internal children is a common countertransference error—the clinician's counterpart to the patient's desire to be "loved into health." This can be seen as a particular variant of a rescue fantasy that could occur in any treatment but whose pull is exponentially increased when the patient presents as a traumatized child in need of love. In a successful treatment, the clinician's empathetic responses are not an end in themselves but are used to help the patient reevaluate her schemas and eventually to mourn the loving childhood that she did not have and will never have, rather than attempting to give her that childhood in the present. Simultaneously, through positive empathic interactions with the therapist, the patient learns to respond compassionately to her own internal emotional needs, childlike and otherwise.

Just as the clinician can find himself or herself choosing gratifyingly warm interactions with a child part over other more difficult therapeutic work, the clinician is often tempted to retreat from the horrible realities of the patient's traumatic past. This retreat can take a number of forms and often resonates with the patient's own wish to avoid these realities. The therapist may gravitate toward spending time in session with more upbeat alters, may find himself or herself intending to focus on traumatic material and then realizing near the end of the session that other issues ended up taking precedence and the trauma work was never undertaken, or may find himself or herself uncomfortable with the level of emotional upset occurring during trauma discussions and step in prematurely with reassurance. Increased self-scrutiny or supervision may be indicated for this countertransference avoidance.

Kluft and others have pointed out that DID is a condition that results from broken boundaries in childhood, making the establishment of a secure treatment frame with consistent boundaries even more important than for other conditions. However, Kluft also suggests, "Take an active, warm, and flexible therapeutic stance." The activity and flexibility are necessary because of the high degree of negative interpersonal expectations carried by the patient with DID—so that traditional passive, less interpersonally responsive analytic stances are likely to be experienced by the patient with DID as critical or withholding or even as signaling abusive tendencies. However, achieving a balance between flexibility and firm boundaries is often a hard-won battle. The patient with DID can present such an array of clinical challenges, including self-harm and suicidality, sexual acting-out, and victimization situations, often disremembered, as well as disagreement or frank warfare between parts, that the clinician who attempts to stick to one strict set of unvarying rules will almost certainly find himself or herself backed into a corner of trying to enforce dictates that seem increasingly inadequate. On the other hand, the chaos of many DID patients' lives and their at times desperate clinical needs often lead to successively greater boundary bending, most commonly about frequency or types of outside-of-session contact, until the therapeutic frame has been distorted in ways that make the therapist uncomfortable and that are then difficult to undo.

> In the early phases of treatment, a patient alludes to terrible abuse that she is too ashamed to discuss. A child part, in particular, pleads movingly for a chance to discuss the abuse by telephone rather than in person, "so I won't see you looking at me." The therapist, who desires to help this child part and hopes to move past a therapeutic impasse, consents to extra phone time. Gradually, other parts make it known that they, too, would like to talk on the phone and hint that if they cannot, they would feel less cared about than the original child part. Over time, the therapist finds himself having daily phone contact in addition to in-person therapy; he comes to feel increasingly resentful, until one day he angrily confronts the patient with her "manipulations," causing a serious therapeutic rupture.

It is usually a struggle to achieve a safe, consistent frame that meets the needs of both parties, and countertransference needs for rigid control, or countertransference difficulties with setting adequate boundaries, each can result in poor outcomes. The potential for ever-increasing involvement, which begins in response to genuine clinical need but culminates in insupportable overinvolvement, often then followed by painful overcorrection, has been observed as far back as Anna O's treatment with Joseph Breuer.

A final note concerns countertransferences around the "special" quality that tends to adhere to the DID diagnosis, both negatively and positively. The dismissive and skeptical opinions about DID that are at times encountered within the mental health professions would of course constitute a profound negative countertransference—if the clinician's starting point is believing that the diagnosis does not exist, effective treatment of a patient with DID would seem impossible. At the other extreme, the disorder's dramatic media portrayals and at times colorful clinical presentation can lead to an overfascination with the phenomenology of the disorder (sometimes manifested in desires to write books about the treatment), which distorts the treatment frame in a different way. However, by the time the clinician is treating his or her third patient with DID, this fascination is replaced by a more straightforward recognition of the complicated, painstaking work that treating the disorder entails.

CONCLUSION

The treatment of the patient with DID is typically arduous and demanding for both clinician and patient, requiring facility with the issues commonly encountered in the treatment of both PTSD and BPD, as well as a skill set specific to approaching multiple personality states and amnesia. However, this can also be one of the most rewarding conditions to treat, because DID, when approached properly, is a condition in which one can achieve tremendous improvement with exploratory psycho therapy as the primary treatment modality.

CHAPTER 12

THE ANTISOCIAL PATIENT

The antisocial patient presents special problems for the interviewer. The patient's pervasive tendencies to manipulate, lie, cheat, act irresponsibly, steal, demand special attention, hurt others, and not feel guilt are disturbing to the clinician. The terms that have been applied to them in the past—*psychopath* and *sociopath*—have become pejoratives that reflect the countertransference and societal indignation that their character pathology arouses.

What is now called *antisocial personality disorder* was the first of the personality disorders to be described. This occurred in the nineteenth century, when psychiatric attention focused on defining the psychological attributes of the so-called criminal personality. At the beginning of the twentieth century, Kraepelin delineated a variety of psychopathic personalities, but the range of pathology in his descriptions was much broader than the current definition of antisocial personality disorder. During World War II, a frequent diagnosis given to servicemen who were discharged as unfit for duty because of their behavior was "chronic psychopathic inferiority." Cleckley's 1941 monograph *The Mask of Sanity* provided the first comprehensive clinical description of the antisocial patient. He used the term *psychopath* and described the lying, narcissism, poor object relations, irresponsibility, and lack of remorse for violent or cruel actions characteristic of the more extreme antisocial patient. He felt that these individuals were so out of touch with reality that they were fundamentally psychotic. His term *psychopath*, used through the 1950s, was replaced by *sociopath,* which in turn was replaced by *antisocial personality disorder*. Each of these name changes reflects an attempt to evade the stigma attached to the category, but because the accrued stigma is based on unchanging core features of these patients' behavior, it inevitably returns. Stone criticized the DSM-IV criteria for antisocial personality disorder as narrowly behavioral and posits that the more psychodynamic concept of psychopathy as defined by Hare has several advantages. Hare's definition of *psychopathy* includes superficial charm, glibness, grandiosity, pathological lying, shallow affect, lack of empathy, and superego deficits such as lack of remorse or guilt and failure to accept responsibility for actions. Stone feels that Hare's psychopathy can be viewed as a distinct, more malignant subset within the larger domain of antisocial personality disorder. This subset contains the dangerous and violent repeat criminals, the serial killers, the hit men, the arsonists, and so on. Not all individuals with antisocial personality disorder meet the core criteria for Hare's psychopathy. In Stone's view antisocial personality disorder is a broad concept, and not all such individuals lack remorse or compassion; hence, it is more heterogeneous than Hare's psychopathy.

Some would suggest that antisocial individuals should be regarded as criminals, not patients, and because of their behavior belong in the hands of the legal-justice system, not in the office of the mental health practitioner. Some patients with severe antisocial personality disorder may be "untreatable" by any current psychiatric methods and use the mental health setting as just another opportunity to exploit and manipulate to further their impulsive desires. However, "antisocial" is not one simple entity but represents a continuum of psychopathology. Some antisocial persons may be responsive to clinical intervention. One of the clinician's tasks in interviewing an antisocial patient is to make an evaluation of the utility of treatment versus nontreatment while self-monitoring the sense of moral outrage that the patient's behavior and attitudes often arouses and that can easily disrupt clinical objectivity.

Genetic and constitutional factors are probably important in the etiology of antisocial personality disorder (Box 12–1). Children who manifest attention-deficit/hyperactivity disorder (ADHD), which almost certainly has a neurobiological substrate, are at significantly higher risk to develop antisocial personality disorder in adulthood. ADHD children are also significantly more likely to develop substance abuse problems in adolescence and adulthood. Substance abuse disorders frequently accompany antisocial personality disorder and may come to dominate the patient's behavior because constant craving for the drug leads to robbery, stealing, and such in order to obtain money to buy drugs. This cycle tends to be repetitive, and antisocial patients with concomitant substance abuse are often incarcerated. They constitute a significant proportion of the prison population.

BOX 12–1. DSM-5 Criteria for Antisocial Personality Disorder

A. A pervasive pattern of disregard for and violation of the rights of others, occurring since age 15 years, as indicated by three (or more) of the following:

1. Failure to conform to social norms with respect to lawful behaviors, as
indicated by repeatedly performing acts that are grounds for arrest.
2. Deceitfulness, as indicated by repeated lying, use of aliases, or conning
others for personal profit or pleasure.
3. Impulsivity or failure to plan ahead.
4. Irritability and aggressiveness, as indicated by repeated physical fights
or assaults.
5. Reckless disregard for safety of self or others.
6. Consistent irresponsibility, as indicated by repeated failure to sustain
consistent work behavior or honor financial obligations.
7. Lack of remorse, as indicated by being indifferent to or rationalizing
having hurt, mistreated, or stolen from another.

B. The individual is at least age 18 years.
C. There is evidence of conduct disorder with onset before age 15 years.
D. The occurrence of antisocial behavior is not exclusively during the course
of schizophrenia or bipolar disorder.

Source. Reprinted from American Psychiatric Association: *Diagnostic and Statistical
Manual of Mental Disorders,* 5th Edition. Arlington, VA, American Psychiatric Association, 2013. Copyright 2013, American Psychiatric Association. Used with permission.

It is possible that the impulsivity, irritability, and low frustration tolerance of children with ADHD become the substrate around which
crystallizes the personality of the later antisocial patient. Most children
with ADHD, however, do not go on to develop antisocial personality
disorder. Conduct disorder (Box 12–2), seen in children before the age
of 15 years, is the anlage to antisocial personality disorder.

BOX 12–2. DSM-5 Criteria for Conduct Disorder

A. A repetitive and persistent pattern of behavior in which the basic rights of
others or major age-appropriate societal norms or rules are violated, as
manifested by the presence of at least three of the following 15 criteria in
the past 12 months from any of the categories below, with at least one criterion present in the past 6 months:

Aggression to People and Animals

1. Often bullies, threatens, or intimidates others.
2. Often initiates physical fights.

3. Has used a weapon that can cause serious physical harm to others (e.g., a bat, brick, broken bottle, knife, gun).
4. Has been physically cruel to people.
5. Has been physically cruel to animals.
6. Has stolen while confronting a victim (e.g., mugging, purse snatching, extortion, armed robbery).
7. Has forced someone into sexual activity.

Destruction of Property

8. Has deliberately engaged in fire setting with the intention of causing serious damage.
9. Has deliberately destroyed others' property (other than by fire setting).

Deceitfulness or Theft

10. Has broken into someone else's house, building, or car.
11. Often lies to obtain goods or favors or to avoid obligations (i.e., "cons" others).
12. Has stolen items of nontrivial value without confronting a victim (e.g., shoplifting, but without breaking and entering; forgery).

Serious Violations of Rules

13. Often stays out at night despite parental prohibitions, beginning before age 13 years.
14. Has run away from home overnight at least twice while living in the parental or parental surrogate home, or once without returning for a lengthy period.
15. Is often truant from school, beginning before age 13 years.

B. The disturbance in behavior causes clinically significant impairment in social, academic, or occupational functioning.
C. If the individual is age 18 years or older, criteria are not met for antisocial personality disorder.

Specify whether:

312.81 (F91.1) **Childhood-onset type:** Individuals show at least one symptom characteristic of conduct disorder prior to age 10 years.
312.82 (F91.2) **Adolescent-onset type:** Individuals show no symptom characteristic of conduct disorder prior to age 10 years.
312.89 (F91.9) **Unspecified onset:** Criteria for a diagnosis of conduct disorder are met, but there is not enough information available to determine whether the onset of the first symptom was before or after age 10 years.

Specify if:

With limited prosocial emotions: To qualify for this specifier, an individual must have displayed at least two of the following characteristics persistently over at least 12 months and in multiple relationships and settings.

These characteristics reflect the individual's typical pattern of interpersonal and emotional functioning over this period and not just occasional occurrences in some situations. Thus, to assess the criteria for the specifier, multiple information sources are necessary. In addition to the individual's self-report, it is necessary to consider reports by others who have known the individual for extended periods of time (e.g., parents, teachers, co-workers, extended family members, peers).

Lack of remorse or guilt: Does not feel bad or guilty when he or she does something wrong (exclude remorse when expressed only when caught and/or facing punishment). The individual shows a general lack of concern about the negative consequences of his or her actions. For example, the individual is not remorseful after hurting someone or does not care about the consequences of breaking rules.

Callous—lack of empathy: Disregards and is unconcerned about the feelings of others. The individual is described as cold and uncaring. The person appears more concerned about the effects of his or her actions on himself or herself, rather than their effects on others, even when they result in substantial harm to others.

Unconcerned about performance: Does not show concern about poor/problematic performance at school, at work, or in other important activities. The individual does not put forth the effort necessary to perform well, even when expectations are clear, and typically blames others for his or her poor performance.

Shallow or deficient affect: Does not express feelings or show emotions to others, except in ways that seem shallow, insincere, or superficial (e.g., actions contradict the emotion displayed; can turn emotions "on" or "off" quickly) or when emotional expressions are used for gain (e.g., emotions displayed to manipulate or intimidate others).

Specify current severity:

Mild: Few if any conduct problems in excess of those required to make the diagnosis are present, and conduct problems cause relatively minor harm to others (e.g., lying, truancy, staying out after dark without permission, other rule breaking).

Moderate: The number of conduct problems and the effect on others are intermediate between those specified in "mild" and those in "severe" (e.g., stealing without confronting a victim, vandalism).

Severe: Many conduct problems in excess of those required to make the diagnosis are present, or conduct problems cause considerable harm to others (e.g., forced sex, physical cruelty, use of a weapon, stealing while confronting a victim, breaking and entering).

Finally, it should be noted that antisocial mechanisms are found in everyone, even the most overtly conscience-ridden and morally scrupulous person. Their expression depends on context, opportunity, desire that overwhelms ego and superego controls, and so on. It is when such mechanisms become the dominant and, sometimes, only mode of behavior that we speak of antisocial personality disorder.

PSYCHOPATHOLOGY AND PSYCHODYNAMICS

Behavior is antisocial when the gratification of basic motives is of overriding importance. The controlling and regulating functions of the ego are defective, and the individual pursues immediate gratification with little regard for other aspects of psychic functioning, the wishes or feelings of others, moral codes or strictures, or the demands of external reality. The primary goals of antisocial behavior are to avoid the tension that results when impulses are not gratified, to avoid the anxiety that appears when frustration is imminent, and, furthermore, to protect the ego from feelings of inadequacy.

The traits of the antisocial personality are designed to ensure the gratification of impulses and to provide the security and tension relief that result. There is little regard for the demands of conscience, affectivity is shallow, and there is little capacity to tolerate anxiety. The antisocial patient's failure to develop adequate ego defenses makes it necessary for him to escape from frustration and anxiety, as compared with the neurotic person, who has mental mechanisms that control anxiety while providing partial gratification of feared impulses. The antisocial individual shuns responsibility and avoids situations that expose his affective deficit.

The antisocial individual is relatively indifferent to his important others apart from what they can do for him. He has little concern for the security, comfort, or pleasure of others. Inner drives are experienced as urgent and overwhelming; delay or substitution does not seem possible. The feeling that results from gratifying his drives has a quality of tension relief, or satiation, rather than the more complex happiness with tender feelings toward others and increased self-esteem that characterize the neurotic individual.

Although the formal diagnosis of antisocial personality involves overt social behavior, underlying psychodynamic issues are an essential and integral part of the syndrome. An antisocial patient does not conform to social standards and participates in activities that are illegal or immoral, but *antisocial* is not merely a technical term for social misbehavior. It implies that certain developmental experiences and psychodynamic patterns have led to fixed disturbances of behavior that are antithetic to the basic moral standards of the society in which the person was raised. However, there are times and situations in which apparently antisocial behavior may be psychodynamically normal. It is therefore important to take the patient's age and cultural background into account when evaluating his psychopathology. For example, normal adolescents will experiment with behavior that is superficially antisocial; in fact, the absence of such experimentation may be suggestive of psychopathology. Members of deprived and oppressed subcultures may be viewed by the dominant culture as exhibiting similar tendencies, because the lack of opportunity to resolve their conflicts more adaptively is associated with an increased utilization of seemingly antisocial mechanisms. Persons raised in families that are committed to lives of crime and antisocial behavior may identify with familial goals and values, with resulting patterns of criminal behavior without psychological abnormality—a pattern that was once called "dyssocial reaction." Such individuals experience loyalty and love and can control their impulses so that they conform with the requirements of their own subculture. In each of these situations, overtly antisocial behavior does not necessarily signify that the individual has antisocial personality disorder.

Clinical Features

The antisocial individual, failing to develop control over the expression of his basic needs, retains relatively primitive impulses as his primary motives. Painful affects are poorly tolerated, and the capacity for mature pleasure and positive affectivity is impaired. Failure to develop mature ego functions is associated with inadequate or pathological object relations early in life, and adult object relations are severely disturbed. Therefore, the patient with a preponderance of antisocial mechanisms is likely to show defects not only in his basic impulses and his mode of handling them but also in his affectivity, including anxiety, guilt, and the capacity to love. His object relations are shallow and uncaring, leading to disturbances in his patterns of behavior.

Impulses

Impulses are the mental representations of needs and motives that form the driving force behind all behavior. Some antisocial patients experience their impulses as ego-syntonic—that is, they feel that they want to act on them—but others have a subjective sense of an urgent and compelling external force. Combinations of these attitudes are common. For example, a substance abuser explains his desire for drugs by the pleasurable experiences that they offer, but he has neither the interest nor the capacity to defer the pleasure when he learns of the long-term dangers associated with it. If he is deprived of the drug, his need is experienced as more urgent. He is unable to postpone gratification because of the feeling that each opportunity may be his last and that he must take advantage of it. This philosophy of immediacy is associated with a lack of concern about the consequences of his behavior.

The antisocial individual is impatient and hedonistic, but the acts that are customarily associated with pleasure for others are more likely to bring him only a transient relief of tension. Those pleasures that he does experience have a primitive oral quality and are more related to physiological responses than to interpersonal relationships. The drink, the "hit," the opportunity for sexual gratification, or the acquisition of property offers a temporary diminution of his inner pressure for gratification. There is no long-lasting shift in his psychic economy, no change in his perception of himself or his relationship to others. The neurotic patient who engages in a pleasurable sexual relationship develops a new attitude toward his partner, enhances his own self-esteem, and enriches his personal life in a way that lasts far longer than the effects of the physical sexual act. The antisocial patient is more likely to experience the event as a relief of a bodily need.

The patient's inability to control or modulate his impulses leads to outbursts of aggression. These may be active or passive, and although they can be triggered by relatively minor slights, they usually involve a reaction to some frustration. The patient's deficit in empathy and concern for others may lead to extreme cruelty and sadism, although characteristically he will have little emotional reaction to his own behavior after it is over.

Affect

Anxiety. The antisocial patient is often described as having little or no anxiety. In fact, he has a very low tolerance for anxiety, and many antisocial mechanisms are designed to forestall, defend against, or allay even minimal anxiety. The slightest threat that his needs will not be gratified leads to unbearable discomfort. He will go to great lengths to guarantee his security, but of course frequent frustrations are inevitable, and constant diffuse tension is the result. A common defense is denial, with the appearance of external composure that leads to the erroneous claim that these patients do not experience anxiety. The patient is likely to deny not only his anxiety but also the urgent, compelling nature of his inner needs. However, this denial can be maintained only if constant gratification is available. When gratification is not available and the denial fails, anxiety, depression, rage, and impulsive behavior are common.

Guilt.   The role of guilt is another controversial issue in the discussion of antisocial patients. In one view, there is a diminished tolerance for guilt, but in the other there is a relative lack of guilt. In our opinion, either of these features may be present, and they are integrally related in the early development of the patient. The antisocial patient experiences the more primitive precursors of guilt. He may feel shame and fear public disapproval for his unacceptable behavior, or he may become depressed if his behavior is exposed. However, he has not developed an autonomous internalized system of behavioral controls that function without the threat of discovery and that provide for regulation of impulses before they lead to overt behavior.

Shallowness.   The affective responses of the antisocial patient have a superficial quality. This may not be apparent at first contact, and even when it is, the inexperienced interviewer may think that it is he, rather than the patient, who has failed to connect. The patient may go through all the motions, and even do so with a dramatic flair, but his feelings are unconvincing. When the patient's sham or façade affect is penetrated, one usually finds feelings that the patient may describe as depression but that seem more like free-floating anxiety mixed with emptiness and a lack of relatedness to other people. These patients seek stimulation from the outside to fill this inner void, and any experience is better than the tense, isolated feeling that they are trying to escape.

Object Relations

The emotional investments of the antisocial patient are narcissistically focused on himself. Other people are transient characters in his life; they come and go, or may be replaced by substitutes, with little feeling of loss. He is most concerned with how they supply his needs, so that his primary style in interpersonal relations is ingratiating, extractive, and exploitative.

A sadomasochistic relationship typically exists between the patient and one or both of his parents or their surrogates. When the patient marries, this attitude is displaced to the spouse, who becomes both the victim and the silent partner in the patient's antisocial behavior. As the victim, the parent or spouse is hurt directly or indirectly. An example is the wife of the embezzler who experiences economic hardships as a result of his behavior. A not-uncommon story is that of the wife who begins a relationship through letters or e-mail with a white-collar criminal while he was incarcerated. Upon his release from prison they marry, and she believes her love for him will prevent future transgressions. She gets her father to take her spouse into the family business when he leaves jail. He promptly begins to abuse his trust and embezzles funds from the firm. The antisocial patient's need to punish his loved ones is universal, and often the patient has little awareness of the amount of rage that is discharged in this pattern.

The patient prefers to avoid controversial issues, and if he senses the interviewer's feelings on some issue, he will simulate a similar position first. He has little sense of self and therefore no desire to take a stand that will leave him feeling isolated and alone.

The antisocial person fears passivity in his personal relationships. Much of his aggressive behavior is designed to avoid a feeling of submissiveness, and many episodes of criminal violence that occur in antisocial individuals are triggered by direct or symbolic threats that make the patient feel passive. Antisocial prisoners are often more disturbed by the enforced passivity of prison life than by the disruption of social relations.

Because he is interested only in what he can get from other people, the antisocial individual seeks out persons of power or status. He is not concerned with the weak or powerless unless he can earn favor from others by displaying this interest. He frequently becomes involved with members of the opposite sex, and his air of cool self-assurance may make him quite attractive sexually. His dashing and exciting exterior bears some resemblance to a romantic folk hero, and he is appealing to those who seek exciting or glamorous romantic involvement. Here again, however, his primary interest is extractive, and his lovers are doomed to disappointment.

At times, the patient appears to be playing a game, and the phrase "as if" has been used to describe this role-playing quality. This is exhibited in mild form by the man at a cocktail party who makes himself more attractive and interesting by assuming glamorous and exciting roles. One patient would pick up women in bars and relate elaborate descriptions of his job, social connections, and past life, varying the story to suit the interest of each new woman. The most extreme illustration occurs in the impostor syndromes in which the patient consciously acts out a false identity. Frequently these involve prestigious or romantic roles as a scientist, explorer, or entrepreneur. One of us saw an English professor who lived a double life, traveling to Europe each summer and convincing his acquaintances there that he was a nuclear scientist working on secret projects for the government.

The patient may sometimes simulate the role of psychological health. When an individual is interviewed in some depth and is seemingly without any emotional or psychological conflicts at all, not even the stresses and strains of normal life, one should suspect an underlying antisocial disorder. Closer scrutiny may reveal deficits in affectivity and object relations. Another role that the patient may assume in the interview is that of the psychiatric patient. This usually involves claims of subjective distress. However, these are not communications of inner pain but rather attempts to deflect the conversation from the more uncomfortable topic of the patient's interaction with his environment.

Behavioral Patterns

Antisocial behavior. Antisocial behavior includes a wide variety of disturbances, such as pathological lying, cheating, embezzling, stealing, and substance abuse. The motivational context of this behavior ranges from the apparently rational financial manipulations of the shady entrepreneur to the bizarre and highly sexualized fire setting of the pyromaniac.

The antisocial individual usually seeks to avoid punishment, but the threat of possible punishment often does not serve as an effective deterrent to his behavior. The patient's inability to postpone gratification, poor impulse control, lack of guilt, and intolerance of anxiety contribute to an inability to consider the consequences of his actions. At the same time the usual social restraints are less important to the antisocial person; the shallowness of his object relations and his lack of tender or warm emotionality render him indifferent to the loss of social ties.

The patient often feels that he is entitled to do what he does, although he may recognize that others will not agree. He thinks that he has been unjustly treated in the past and that his current behavior will help even the balance. For example, a heroin addict who had been apprehended by the police for stealing explained that his early life was so marked by pain and deprivation that he felt he should suffer no further discomfort. He explained that he had a right to take things from others who were more privileged and that the comfort he achieved by doing so was society's debt to him.

Assets. Antisocial mechanisms may also lead to useful character traits. The absence of neurotic anxiety can be associated with a calm self-control and daring behavior that superficially resemble courage and bravery. The antisocial individual may develop great skill at tasks that would cause considerable anxiety in most others. For example, antisocial traits are common in persons who pursue dangerous careers. These skills are most evident when a single episode of brilliance will suffice, and sustained goal-directed effort over a long period of time is not required. Lack of patience and susceptibility to impulsive distractions cause difficulty with long-term pursuits.

The antisocial person's social skill and smooth charm can make him successful in dealing with others, and he is master at the art of manipulating people. To the uninitiated, he does not seem to be antisocial. He has often cultivated social manners and graces to an extent that ranges from "slick" to sincerely charming. Although the antisocial individual might utilize antisocial behavior when he feels it is necessary to obtain personal gratification, ordinarily he uses his social skills in order to control the interviewer and to make the interview as friendly and comfortable as possible.

Defensive and Adaptive Techniques

In the antisocial patient, anxiety leads directly to action, in contrast to the neurotic patient, whose mental processes are designed to control and bind anxiety or to substitute symbolic action. However, there are certain psychological defenses that the antisocial individual does utilize. These involve attempts to deny anxiety and a variety of maneuvers, including isolation, displacement, projection, and rationalization, that minimize the guilt and social discomfort that he might otherwise experience.

Defenses against anxiety. The antisocial patient attempts to transfer his own anxiety to others. If he is successful, his own fear is diminished. Phobic patients also try to elicit anxiety in others, but if they are successful, they become quite anxious themselves and usually search for calmer partners whom they cannot disturb as easily. The antisocial patient, in contrast, prefers those who react most intensely, because he seems to gain some reassurance from the other person's discomfort. His provocation may begin with the opening words of the interview. One of us treated an antisocial patient who started the first interview by mentioning that he was acquainted with one of the clinician's medical school classmates and later dropped innuendoes regarding information he had concerning the clinician's earlier life. A favorite technique for evoking anxiety is to detect some weakness in the interviewer and then to focus on it. One patient asked about the clinician's fidgeting in his chair, inquiring whether he was nervous about something. This behavior also occurs outside the interview. A medical student would question his colleagues about obscure details before examinations, implying that he was familiar with this material and that they were in serious trouble if they were not.

In addition to making the clinician anxious, the patient will deny his own anxiety, with the resulting picture of detachment described earlier. Antisocial individuals are relatively skillful at concealing the overt expression of emotions, and the clinician may miss the clues to underlying anxiety.

Psychological control of guilt.   The antisocial individual copes with his discomfort about his impulsive behavior by a series of defensive maneuvers. The simplest is the patient who claims, "I didn't do it," denying his overt behavior. This is common, for example, in alcoholic patients, who frequently state that they drink very little and have no problem with alcohol.

Slightly more complex is the patient whose position is described by the statement "I think it was all right." He admits the behavior but denies awareness of its social significance. This attitude is common in adolescent delinquents.

A related defense is represented by the idea "Everyone else does it." This involves a projection of the patient's impulses onto others. The individual with antisocial trends often feels that everyone has a gimmick and that all people are extractive and exploitative, looking out only for their own advantage. He quickly extends this view to the interviewer and may more or less directly suggest that the clinician has a good deal going. This is done in a tone of grudging admiration, often coupled with an offer of conspiratorial assistance. The patient might suggest that he could pay the clinician in cash, with the implication that the clinician cheats on his taxes.

The next step in the sequence can be characterized by the feeling "No one cares anyway." The patient feels that others are indifferent to his behavior. This patient may claim that others expect it. For example, a college student who wanted a medical excuse from an examination even though he was not ill explained that his professor knew what was going on but wanted an official letter. Patients will frequently employ this mechanism in dealing with fees that are paid by or to third parties, such as insurance companies. They attempt to enlist the clinician's assistance in falsifying information in order to save money, insisting, "It's all part of the system."

The ultimate defense in this series can be represented by the narcissistic claim of "I'm special." The patient may include the clinician in his "special" category, saying, "You and I aren't like the rest." Various explanations for this privileged position can be offered: that he is more gifted or intelligent, that his needs are somehow different, that he is more sensitive than others, or that his earlier experiences entitle him to special consideration.

Defenses against failing self-esteem.   The antisocial patient finds that others disapprove of his behavior. Although he may attach relatively little significance to specific other people, some general sense of respect from the world is important to him, if only in the form of an outer display of social approval. An example is the powerful organized crime figure who is active in his church. If he not able to gain this respect from others, he feels increased loneliness and diminished self-esteem. These feelings lead to defensive and reparative operations.

One of the simplest defenses is to treat his vices as virtues. This patient presents his callousness, indifference, or ruthlessness as an admirable trait. Adolescent delinquents frequently demonstrate this mechanism. It appears in milder form in the individual who brags about his numerous brief sexual relationships. Emotional isolation also serves to protect the patient from the pain of depression. It is common for the patient to become visibly more depressed as a relationship with the clinician develops and this defense diminishes.

Alcoholism and substance abuse.   Environmental agents may become involved in antisocial patterns of behavior, and their secondary effects may strongly influence the resulting clinical picture. The most common examples are alcoholism and substance abuse.

The patient's life becomes organized around obtaining a drug for the resulting elevation of his mood and self-esteem. Because these effects are temporary, he experiences periodic cycles of need, consummation, satiation, and renewed need. He usually claims that the satiated state is the desirable one and that his behavior is designed to regain this experience after it has been lost. Contact with this individual suggests that the entire cycle is an integral part of his personality and that it is as necessary for him to crave and to seek gratification as it is to experience the state of satiation and euphoria that results.

Society frowns on the addict, and legal and social institutions are often harsh to the point of cruelty. By finding a magic chemical route to pleasure, the addict acts out universal unconscious fantasies of magical gratification for oral dependent needs. Anyone who openly acts out the secret and forbidden wishes of others becomes an outcast. These societal attitudes become issues in the interview, and it is common for the patient to cast the clinician in the role of policeman or judge rather than therapist.

Developmental Psychodynamics

The antisocial individual's mistrust of others begins early in life. The "normal" infant's feelings that his needs will be met is based on his early relationship with his mother or other primary caretaker and his repeated experience that frustration and delay, however stressful, is inevitably followed by gratification and security. Although the child may respond to each frustration with anxiety and protest, this occurs within the context of repeated gratification. Furthermore, the child learns not only that needs will be met but also that this will occur in spite of angry protests directed at the need-fulfilling objects, his parents. In fact, this protest behavior disappears if it is unsuccessful, and the child whose cries bring no aid eventually stops crying and lies quietly and passively.

There are several reasons that the future antisocial individual does not follow this pathway. Early experiences may lead to the feeling that no one can be trusted and that security must be derived from some source other than a close human relationship. There may be constitutional determinants that contribute to an increased pressure from basic drives or a decreased tolerance for frustration such as is seen in the child with ADHD.

When a child has been abandoned by his parents or has drifted through a series of foster homes and child-care institutions, syndromes that resemble adult antisocial behavior may appear very early in life. There is much overt display of affection but little real feeling, and the shyness and inhibition that most children experience with strangers are absent. The child is skillful at extracting love and attention from adults, but the relationship that is so quickly established is of little importance and will quickly be severed if a more rewarding parental figure can be found. These children can be seen in child-care institutions, where their immediate and appealing charm is quickly directed to every new adult who appears on the scene. It is clearly a highly adaptive pattern of behavior for such a life, both protecting the child from the pain of repeated separations and facilitating his immediate adaptation to new social situations.

The severe ego pathology arising in the earliest years of life is further complicated at the stage of the developing conscience or superego. The capacity of the ego to mature through identification with important objects fails to develop. Furthermore, the parental figures who were associated with the deprivations of the first years of life offer pathological models for identification. The same mother whose care never led to a sense of basic trust may have social and moral attitudes that, when incorporated by the child, will lead to a distorted sense of right and wrong. The child acts out the unconscious forbidden wishes of a parent who may also be antisocial.

These defects in conscience formation can also occur in the absence of serious primary ego pathology. The concept of "superego lacunae" has been offered to describe individuals who have isolated specific disturbances in their personalities. For example, one of us knew a man who was a pillar of his community and an elder in his church but whose business success depended on selling overpriced merchandise to poor people who did not understand time payment plans. His daughter was arrested for selling drugs to her high school classmates. Although the overt behavior of her parents met the highest moral standards of society, the child perceived hidden or unconscious parental attitudes and translated them into action. If the family of a delinquent adolescent is available for a careful interview, one can frequently obtain a history of behavior patterns in the parents' earlier years that are similar to the child's current difficulties and that were overtly concealed from the child but covertly manifest in the parents' attitudes and behavior.

The peculiar attitude of the antisocial individual toward tension and anxiety may also stem from early experiences with the caretaker. The child's needs are ignored on one occasion, but on another his protests are quickly silenced by overindulgence in an attempt to placate his anger and shut him up. He grows frightened of the tension associated with his needs, because gratification is erratic and not motivated by love. At the same time, the process of getting what he wants becomes equivalent to extracting a bribe, and he feels entitled to take everything he can possibly get because he feels deprived of that which is most important: love and security. When this pattern continues into adult life, we see the ego-syntonic and guiltless extractive qualities of the antisocial individual.

As the individual with prominent antisocial tendencies enters puberty and adolescence, he frequently has less difficulty than his peers. Shifts in identity and allegiance present no problem to him, and he is not troubled by guilt in response to his defiance. His acquaintances look up to him and envy his social and personal ease. He has no close friends but is an object of admiration for many. In later years, these same friends are surprised to learn that the former big man on campus ended up friendless and a failure.

Adult life, and particularly old age, presents great problems. Marriage is frequently unsuccessful, and when it lasts, it is usually in spite of a distant and impersonal relationship with the spouse. If there are children, they are seen as competitors or potential sources of gratification, attitudes that rarely lead to close family ties, or they too may become antisocial and partners in crime. Life is lonely and empty, and solace may be sought in drugs or alcohol.

Differential Diagnosis

Severe narcissistic personality disorder overlaps with antisocial personality disorder. Both are characterized by tendencies to be exploitative and unempathic to others. Kernberg has suggested that antisocial personality disorder is simply a very primitive variant of narcissistic personality disorder. Borderline personality disorder can also merge with antisocial personality disorder, although the former is usually more object-connected, albeit in a primitive manner.

Antisocial patients must be differentiated from paranoid individuals, who also have difficulty controlling their anger and may have poor reality testing. This combination can result in episodes of explosive violence. When the paranoid patient's delusional view of the world is taken into account, however, his behavior is understandable. The paranoid patient may feel guilt and remorse after an episode of rage, he may attempt to defend his behavior, or he may disown responsibility for it, but it usually takes him a long time to simmer down. In contrast, the angry outbursts of the antisocial person can disappear as suddenly as they began, and the patient may be tranquil, almost to the point of disinterest, after the episode. He cannot understand why others attribute such significance to his violence.

Histrionic patients are also manipulative and extractive in personal relationships and show great variations in values or behavior according to social cues. However, the histrionic patient establishes important relationships with other people and is distressed when these do not go well. The antisocial individual views others more as vehicles for gratification and is less concerned about the disruption of specific relationships. The histrionic patient also exhibits sham emotionality and role playing. However, the roles assumed by the histrionic patient are dramatizations of unconscious fantasies, and there are consistent themes that relate to the patient's inner conflicts. The role is a vehicle for expressing and resolving a conflict, not an end in itself. It may have manipulative or extractive functions within the immediate interpersonal context, but this is only a secondary issue. The histrionic patient tries to be someone else because he rejects certain facets of himself; the antisocial person tries to be someone else because he feels that otherwise he is no one at all.

The obsessive-compulsive individual often expects disapproval, whereas the antisocial person wants the respect and admiration of others. The obsessive-compulsive person is more likely to emphasize his defiance of authority, denying his fear and submissiveness. The antisocial individual will speak of his skill or agility in getting what he wants.

MANAGEMENT OF THE INTERVIEW

Although the interview behavior of the antisocial patient is not as consistent as that of the obsessive-compulsive or the histrionic patient, there are specific problems in interviewing that are associated with the patient's use of antisocial mechanisms. These occur both in antisocial characters and in others with antisocial traits.

Several major themes can be described. The patient may be charming, ingratiating, and superficially cooperative, although simultaneously evasive and dishonest. This is a common initial presentation. Later, often in response to direct confrontation by the interviewer, he can become uncooperative or overtly angry. This attitude might appear initially if the patient has been coerced to see the clinician. As the patient attempts varying methods of pursuing his goals, these established patterns may alternate.

The antisocial patient studies the interviewer from the very first moment of contact. He covertly searches for evidence that will help him to decide whether the clinician can be conned and, at the same time, mentally registers any sign of weakness or uncertainty. Although the clinician often feels on guard, he has difficulty identifying the source of the feeling. He may experience a negative reaction to the patient, or he may be overly enthusiastic and develop rescue fantasies, but he is uncertain about the reason for these responses.

Action is far more important than reflection or contemplation for the antisocial individual. A major problem in interview technique arises from the patient's tendency to act before, or instead of, talking. He does not see how talking to another person can be of any use, unless that person is a means to some concrete end.

The Opening Phase

Pre-Interview Behavior

The antisocial patient seizes the initiative at the very first contact. When the clinician greets him in the waiting room, he may inquire, "How are you today?" and will often chat while walking into the office.

He is sensitive to the clinician's interests and attitudes, but unlike the histrionic patient, he is more interested in establishing a general atmosphere of permission and receptivity than in eliciting a specific emotional response. He may comment appreciatively on a picture on the wall or the political views suggested by a book on the clinician's shelf, comments that are aimed at disclosing something about the clinician's status or position. "Nice setup you have here" or "Have you been in this office very long?" is a typical opening remark. One patient, noticing that a Harvard diploma was displayed on the wall, said, "I see you trained in Boston." The recognition of the clinician's status was slightly disguised but nonetheless obvious.

The First Minutes

As the interview continues, there is ongoing scrutiny of the clinician and a tendency to focus on any flaws that may appear. For example, one patient began his first interview by commenting, "I noticed an article in one of the magazines in your waiting room." He went on to indicate that he agreed with the article's political views and then added, "I guess you must be much too busy to really get involved in that sort of stuff." The message was clear: the clinician was not only successful but perhaps preoccupied with his success and inconsiderate of the needs of others. These comments provide important information for the interviewer, but any attempt to reply to them early in the interview will leave the patient feeling angry, uncomfortable, and defensive.

The patient appears to be composed, pleasant, and engaging; at times he may be smooth and charming. He speaks freely, but at a level of generality that sometimes leaves the interviewer feeling that he is lost and must have missed some key material. In spite of this, every sentence is clear and relevant, and there is no suggestion of a thought disturbance. He compliments the clinician on the insightful comments he makes or the penetrating question that he raises. The patient seems to say, "We'll get along just fine." The clinician may feel pleased and flattered, or he may sense that the praise is somewhat extreme and that something is not quite right. As a rule, however, any comment on this will be met with indignant denial, the patient insisting that he could not be more sincere. It is not wise to challenge or confront the patient at this point. He does not trust the interviewer anyway, and any indication that he is not trusted himself will only make things worse. The patient's false flattery is a product of his need to con the interviewer, which is based on his mistrust, a central theme in treatment. Mistrust can be interpreted most effectively after it has been brought into the open, and premature confrontation is likely to encourage the patient to conceal his negative feelings. It is preferable to ignore his attempts to con the clinician until the patient has more completely exposed his suspicions.

The Chief Complaint

The clinician must establish the antisocial patient's reason for seeking treatment, a process that is not the same as eliciting the neurotic patient's chief complaint. The antisocial patient's complaints sound quite similar to those of the neurotic, but they rarely explain why he has come for help now. He may describe conflict and anxiety but seldom displays these feelings directly. If he complains of depression, he quickly shifts to expressing his frustration and irritation over a lost love object. The patient experiences more anxiety than is apparent to the clinician, and it is preferable initially to accept the patient's description of his feelings rather than to confront him with the superficial quality of his affective response.

The antisocial patient often seeks some relatively concrete goal and hopes to elicit the clinician's assistance in achieving it. If he was referred by the courts, he hopes for an acquittal or a lighter sentence; if referred by a school, he hopes to be pardoned for delinquent behavior or excused from some responsibility. Perhaps the most common situation is the patient who wants an ally in a battle with a spouse or other family member. In all these situations, the patient also experiences painful inner feelings, but he rarely comes to the clinician with any hope of help for his inner pain; he only seeks assistance in his struggle with the outside world. The therapist is perceived as a real person who can be the patient's agent rather than only a transference figure.

Exploration of the Patient's Problem

Withholding and Secrecy

The antisocial individual is frequently referred by another person or institution, and thus the clinician often has some advance information about the patient. The patient frequently does not mention that he is in trouble, thereby presenting the interviewer with a problem. If the clinician allows the interview to unfold in the usual manner, important material will not be discussed. On the other hand, if he introduces the information himself, he will have difficulty learning its emotional meaning to the patient. Also, such action is likely to be perceived by the patient as a judgment or criticism. The problem is further complicated if the patient knows that the clinician has the information. The clinician often learns that the "confidential" correspondence he received from the referring agency has already been seen by the patient and that the question in the patient's mind is not what the clinician knows but whether he will be open about it. As with any other patient, it is essential that the clinician not keep secrets. Therefore, he refers to the information in a general way and asks the patient to discuss it. An example will best illustrate the problems that arise.

> An adolescent male high school student was referred by his school because he had been caught stealing books from the school bookstore. He came to the interview and discussed a variety of academic problems, not mentioning the stolen items. After listening for a while, the clinician said, "I understand you've had some difficulties with the bookstore." The patient quite characteristically replied, "What do you know about that?" At this point the clinician did not go into detail but replied, "I guess

you don't feel comfortable talking to me about it," thereby commenting on the patient's unwillingness to discuss the matter himself. The patient persisted in trying to find out what the clinician already knew, and the clinician then added, "I guess you don't fully trust me." This approach shifted the interview from an attempt to find out what happened in the bookstore—a fruitless and basically unimportant quest—to a discussion of the patient's mode of dealing with other people.

The antisocial patient frequently invites inquisition rather than a psychiatric interview. He seems to be withholding or frankly lying, he may become openly resistant or uncooperative, and the material that does emerge may suggest antisocial or criminal behavior. The clinician is tempted to try to piece together the truth by ingenious or coercive questioning. The interview is not furthered by getting the goods on the patient, and it is far more important to earn his trust and respect than to pin down the facts. It may be helpful to interpret this dilemma to the patient, suggesting, "I'm interested in your problem, but I see no point in my conducting an interrogation. You seem to cast me in the role of district attorney." The patient is establishing a pattern of relationship based on his past experiences with authority figures. He tries to get the interviewer to play the role of the suspicious and mistrustful parent, unjustly accusing and exploiting him. If the patient is successful, he feels justified in concealing his behavior and trying to manipulate the clinician so that he can achieve his own goals. This is the way the patient deals with others, and he feels that it is the way they deal with him.

With most other patients, the clinician will, in time, learn about the patient's inner mental life. This is not the case with the typical antisocial patient, who is unwilling or unable to share such material. In fact, he is not even likely to tell the clinician the daily events of his external life, let alone his fantasies. This prevents the therapist from obtaining the essential psychological information that he utilizes with other patients in understanding the psychodynamics of the treatment process. Some of these missing data may be offered by ancillary informants, such as a telephone call from one of the patient's relatives. The therapist accepts this information and tells the patient about each call. It is mandatory that the clinician not betray the patient's confidence in any way. However, it is not necessary for the clinician to tell the patient everything that he has learned about him if this would alienate the relative. The clinician can utilize these events to discuss the difficulties created by the patient's withholding.

Clarification and Confrontation

As the interview progresses, the clinician directs his attention to the patient's style of life and his mode of relating to people in general and to the interviewer in particular. The clinician must shift the discussion from those issues that the patient has volunteered to the painful feelings that he tries to avoid. This usually requires a more or less direct confrontation. Despite cautious phrasing and careful timing, a negative response frequently follows. A conflict of interest develops between the patient and the clinician. The patient wants to use the clinician to elicit an emotional reaction or to obtain some assistance in pursuing a concrete goal; the clinician wants to establish a relationship that will permit exploration of what the patient wants and how he goes about getting it.

The initial confrontation should aim at exploring the patient's behavior or elucidating his defenses but not attacking them. For example, a young man sought consultation because of depression and somatic symptoms that were accentuated each time he was abandoned by a sexual partner. He seemed somewhat depressed during the interview but emphasized his incapacitating anxiety while discussing the reasons for his consultation. The patient seemed more interested in what he could learn about the interviewer than in relating his own problems and started the conversation by commenting, "I understand that you're on the staff of the medical school. Do you spend a lot of time teaching up there?" These comments were made with considerable social charm, and it was easy to imagine the patient's success as a personnel manager, his chosen profession. After some minutes the interviewer interrupted, saying, "I guess you're more comfortable talking about me than discussing the difficulties you've been having in your personal life." This is a somewhat supportive confrontation. Any more direct statement this early in the interview will interfere with the patient's communication. For example, the question "If you're so upset about your own problems, why do you spend so much time talking about me?" would provoke an angry or withdrawn response.

The Patient's Anger

The antisocial patient's anger may be denied behind a façade of rationalization. He will offer elaborate explanations of why his behavior has a meaning other than the obvious one. This is intended to circumvent the meaning that the interviewer has attached to it while maintaining the appearance of goodwill in the interview.

> A student who was referred to the college psychiatrist after he had been caught cheating in a major examination insisted that he had only been making notes on a scrap of paper, which the proctor thought was a "crib sheet." He went on to elaborate on how the paper came from a book of lecture notes that contained material related to the course. The psychia-

trist commented, "I guess the dean didn't completely believe your explanation or he wouldn't have asked you to come here. What do you think he had in mind?" The student responded by further protesting his innocence and explaining why he thought that the administration might be discriminating against him. The interviewer then said, "Obviously you are the only one who knows what happened at the examination, but I'm not sure that that is really so important. Whatever actually went on, you are now in a jam. Have you thought about what to do?"

When the rationalization is both elaborate and transparent, the clinician is often tempted to reply by suggesting that so complex an explanation must be covering something. This is a fairly direct accusation of lying, and whether or not the patient is lying, it will seldom improve communication. When the clinician does want to confront the patient with an obvious lie, this can be done by comments such as "I find it hard to believe that what you say is true." This allows the possibility of discussing why the patient's statement is unbelievable, even if he continues to insist that it is true.

The patient may respond to the clinician's confrontation by sullen withdrawal. He controls his angry feelings, playing the role of the injured party and thereby appealing to the guilt or sympathy of the interviewer. This was seen in a patient who frequented different hospital emergency rooms, presenting multiple somatic complaints and obtaining analgesics. She would collect prescriptions by lying about her previous medical contacts. When an intern who had seen her on a previous occasion recognized her and rather sharply questioned her about her story, she refused to speak and sat staring at the floor, at first pouting and then beginning to cry. The intern, not certain of what was going on, immediately became warmer and more supportive, and the patient constructed still another story.

A different type of response to the interviewer's confrontation is acceptance followed by renegotiation. The patient adopts a new tack as he learns more about the clinician, often openly admitting that what came before was "a line" and suggesting that he is now serious and straightforward. The clinician may feel flattered as the patient praises his perspicacity and insight. It is this patient's manipulative style, his readiness to use and then to discard a line, rather than any specific tactic that is the essential point.

A physician learned that a recently hospitalized patient had become involved in an extensive net of gambling and bribery that involved several hospital employees. When confronted, the patient quickly sized up the situation and then said, "OK—you're smart and you're right. I got hooked into this by the attendants. The whole staff situation is really pretty rotten, but I can help you find out who's behind it." The patient offered to make a deal to protect himself and to placate the doctor.

The Patient's Relatives

The antisocial person's problems usually involve other people, and the clinician often has direct contact with the patient's family. This may take the form of letters, e-mails, telephone calls, or interviews that may or may not include the patient. Antisocial mechanisms that may be obvious in the patient are often mirrored, although in subtler form, in other members of the family. A case involving a patient treated by one of us illustrates some of these points:

> The patient, an adolescent male, entered treatment because of academic difficulties in school and conflict with his family over his use of marijuana. His parents, whom he described as "middle class and materialistic," were divorced and lived in another city. Shortly after treatment began, the clinician received a letter from the patient's father expressing his support for the treatment program and enclosing some insurance forms. The items that the father had already completed suggested that he was capitalizing on the similarity of his own name to that of his son to collect on a policy that did not actually cover his son. The problem became more complex when the patient started to miss sessions, insisting that whether he kept his appointments was privileged information that was not to be shared with his father. It was clear that the father would be enraged if he learned that he was paying for sessions that were not actually held. Thus the patient had enlisted the clinician in a conspiracy against the father by offering him full payment for an open hour, and the father had engaged the clinician's assistance in extracting money from the insurance company.
>   Finally the clinician told the patient, "I'm not here to get paid to read a magazine." The patient replied, "You said what happens here is confidential; you can't tell him about my not coming." The clinician answered, "That's true, but if I decide you're not motivated for treatment, we will stop. If that happens, I'll have to tell your father that I felt further treatment was not useful." At the same time, the clinician explored the patient's anger at what his father was doing with the insurance. Eventually the patient and his father were seen together, and the clinician discussed the family pattern that each member practiced himself while protesting similar behavior in the other.

It is particularly important to keep the patient informed of every contact that the clinician has with the patient's family, although the clinician may keep the details to himself. If the clinician receives a letter or an e-mail, he may show it to the patient; if he has a phone conversation, he should discuss it at the next session. If the relatives are to be seen by the clinician, it is usually advisable to have the patient present.

Relatives often use subtle devices to induce the clinician to betray the patient's confidence. For instance, a teenager's mother called the physician and said, "I guess Mike told you what happened with the car this weekend." Either "Yes" or "No" betrays the patient. Instead, the clinician might reply, "Anything Mike does or does not tell me is confidential. What was it that you wanted to say?"

Acting Out

The antisocial individual prefers action to language or thought. When he feels anxious, he is more likely to do something than to talk about it. If his relationship with another person gives rise to uncomfortable emotions, these will appear in his behavior rather than in his report of internal mental processes. For example, a young female patient with antisocial tendencies would indulge in promiscuous sexuality shortly before her therapist's vacations, although she persistently denied any emotional response to his leaving. It is this tendency to action that makes the standard techniques of psychotherapy difficult with this patient.

The term *acting out*, when used strictly, refers to behavior that is based on feelings that arise in the transference relationship and are then displaced onto persons in the patient's everyday life. The purpose and result are to keep the expression of these feelings away from the therapist. Such behavior is a common resistance in all patients, but it can be particularly troublesome in the patient with antisocial tendencies. A neurotic patient also may displace his transference feelings, but he is more likely to inhibit the accompanying activity. The antisocial patient has a lower threshold for action and less restraint on his impulses. The result is that feelings arising in the treatment situation may directly lead to inappropriate and maladaptive behavior in the outside world.

The acting out of transference feelings can also occur within the treatment without displacement to other figures. It is this acting out in the transference that produces some of the most difficult technical problems in the interview. The antisocial patient may not follow the rules of simply sitting in his chair and talking. He will frequently try to read the clinician's mail or peruse the papers on his desk or even open his computer if the clinician is called from the room. These acts are usually concealed in the initial interview, unless the patient's defenses are inadequate or are too quickly challenged.

In general, the role of the interviewer is to link acting-out behavior with the underlying feeling and to point out the displacements that have occurred. It is rarely useful to interdict the behavior early in treatment and almost never effective if these interpretations have not preceded the interdiction. The exception is when the behavior directly impinges on the rights or interest of the therapist. Here, as with the psychotic patient, it is not helpful to allow the patient to abuse his relationship with the doctor. The patient who cannot set his own limits requires others to assist him in this.

The Role of Interpretation

The limited value of intellectual insight into the psychodynamic mechanisms underlying pathological behavior is nowhere so clear as in the antisocial patient. This individual may be quick to understand the therapist's interpretations, and he will frequently repeat and extend them at appropriate points in therapy. The patient is often misperceived as an excellent treatment case by beginning students.

Although the antisocial individual may be skillful in manipulating abstractions, only concrete things have emotional significance to him. The simplest comment linked to an act or a thing is far more powerful than an insight into unconscious patterns that are not connected to an immediate person or behavior in the patient's life. The patient will make many concrete demands, asking for analgesic medication, money for a parking meter, recommendations for a restaurant in the neighborhood, or renewal of prescription for a medication written by another physician. Initially, the therapist responds to these directly, either accepting or rejecting them. At some point, when the patient has at least partially accepted the mode of treatment, the therapist will suggest that these requests have underlying psychological significance. The patient will either accept or deny this, but it will have little emotional impact. However, if the therapist links his interpretation to a change in his own behavior, no longer gratifying the demand that he has now interpreted, the patient will respond dramatically and at times violently.

The Closing Phase

As the interview draws to a close, the antisocial patient senses the clinician's intention of stopping. He may seize the opportunity to seek some favor or permission, avoiding the necessity of full discussion. For example, a patient with addictive tendencies visited the emergency department of a general hospital during the course of his evaluation in the psychiatric clinic. He told the emergency department doctor of his anxiety since the last clinic visit and discussed his family problems. The doctor reviewed the patient's difficulties and confirmed that he had a follow-up appointment in the clinic. Just as he rose to terminate the interview, the patient said, "Oh, one more thing, Doc. I've just run out of my Valium, and I need a new prescription." The waiting room was crowded and the doctor was hurried. The patient was counting on this pressure to coerce the doctor to grant his request. There is obviously no time for exploration or interpretation in this situation, but the doctor could have replied, "Why don't you call your regular doctor in the morning and discuss a new prescription with him? I'll let him know about our talk tonight." The patient is forced to explore his behavior with his primary doctor.

The end of the interview provides an opportunity for the clinician to counteract the patient's tendency to relate to him impersonally. With the antisocial patient, as with the borderline patient, it is helpful for the clinician to foster and maintain a real relationship. Brief social amenities at the end of the interview—plans for the weekend or comments about the weather—are usually seen as a form of resistance in neurotic patients. The antisocial patient has difficulty establishing interpersonal relationships, and the clinician is not only an object for transference but also a potential primary person with whom he can safely experience personal feelings that are intense and genuine. The patient often has developed social skills in an almost hypertrophied form, but these are not connected with appropriate subjective feelings. Although it rarely occurs early in treatment, the patient should be encouraged when he does make a sincere social gesture toward the clinician.

TRANSFERENCE AND COUNTERTRANSFERENCE

The patient's need for a sadomasochistic relationship soon appears in the transference. The most common manifestation is to stimulate the clinician's hopes that the therapy will succeed. This is partially due to the fact that the patient's deep mistrust is not verbalized early in therapy, and instead the patient will often feign trust by playing the role of a good patient. As treatment progresses, it becomes apparent that the problems do not magically disappear, and the clinician is disappointed. Although the clinician is fully aware that neurotic and psychotic symptoms do not vanish quickly, he seems to expect that they will in this patient. Such attitudes ensure his disappointment. It must be remembered that deceit is a way of life for this person, and then it can be viewed as any other character trait.

Narcissistic pathology is universal in antisocial patients. As a consequence the real person of the therapist is relatively unimportant to the patient. He may forget the clinician's name or have little concern about shifting to a new clinician. The antisocial patient will show defensive interest in the clinician and possibly curiosity about his status or his therapeutic technique, but he will be strangely devoid of curiosity about the clinician's more human attributes—his family or his personal life. When he does ask questions, they are designed to shift the spotlight to the clinician, either to charm him or to make him uncomfortable rather than to know him.

If, in spite of this, an important relationship with the therapist does develop, it is difficult (if not impossible) for the patient to replace him with a substitute. When the clinician finally does become a total object for this patient, he is a *real* object, and the patient may retain such a relationship, if only in fantasy, for the rest of his life. If the patient does begin to recognize the therapist as a person, his problems with trust will be manifested in a different fashion. For example, he might tell his friends some personal information that the clinician has offered about himself. Here the clinician can comment, "You don't seem to consider things that go on between us as private" or "You have betrayed my confidence." This response shows the patient that the clinician really is different from his parents.

> The patient's tendency to view the therapist as a nonperson is illustrated by the adolescent who was seeing a clinician because of chronic truancy. The patient perceived therapy as a route to increased privileges and the removal of restrictions on his freedom that his parents had imposed in an attempt to control his behavior. He came to the clinician but involved himself only at a superficial level. His interest never deviated from the issue of when he would again be allowed to use the family car or not be grounded. He would talk about his feelings or discuss the day's events, but always with his mind's eye trained on his goal. When he regained the lost privileges, he abruptly stopped treatment.

It is valuable to make the patients' concerns as explicit as possible early in the treatment. For example, when this patient said, "I feel anxious about being tied down in the house all of the time," the clinician could have replied, "You must be annoyed about not being allowed to use the car." This directs the interview to the issue that is most prominent in the patient's mind. Later, the clinician could add, "I imagine you have some idea of what your parents want to happen before they'll let you use the car again. What do you think that is?" As the discussion shifts to parental demands and the patient's response to these, the clinician can offer his services in helping him to understand the connection between his desire and his parents' behavior and to work out a relationship with them that will accommodate both the patient and his parents. It is necessary to explore the parental encouragement of the patient's behavior. Why did the father buy a fancy sports car? What traits does the mother admire in a man, and what avenues are available for the patient to emulate these? At the same time, the clinician must avoid taking sides. He must neither blame the parents, thereby relieving the patient of any sense of responsibility for his own behavior, nor scold the patient while ignoring the parents' implicit communications. If the clinician can resolve this dilemma, the relationship with the patient shifts from that of adversary or co-conspirator to a therapeutic framework.

The antisocial patient elicits major countertransference problems in the interviewer. The clinician is confronted with suspiciousness and distrust coupled with evasion and, at times, outright deception. The patient shows little guilt or anxiety about this behavior and angrily denies it if confronted directly. Furthermore, the clinician senses that the patient is trying to manipulate him. The most common patterns of countertransference are the clinician who makes himself oblivious to the patient's behavior; the clinician who assumes the role of the angry parent, threatening and admonishing the patient for behavior that is often linked to unacceptable impulses of the clinician himself; and the clinician who is more strongly motivated than the patient to continue treatment. If his own therapeutic success makes the patient a feather in his cap, this dream turns out to be short-lived, because the patient inevitably disappoints him. The clinician may then react to his disappointment much as the patient's parents have done. Paradoxically, the antisocial patient may stimulate unconscious admiration or even envy in the clinician. The patient is seen as getting away with behavior that is gratifying or pleasurable but that is conflictual or forbidden for others. The clinician's unconscious envy is often accompanied by some degree of identification with the patient, and exaggerated negative responses to these patients may represent the clinician's rejection of similar unacceptable impulses in himself.

The inexperienced clinician is particularly prone to accept the patient's self-presentation as valid and to ignore more covert antisocial dynamics. This clinician expects to believe his patients and is more comfortable relying on the clinical data that the patient provides rather than his own vague, subjective, and often contradictory responses.

> A resident was evaluating a man referred by the courts after a fourth arrest for passing bad checks. The clinician was moved by the patient's description of his early life deprivation, his desire for another chance, and his plans for schooling and vocational training. However, the clinic administrator would not support the clinician's recommendation that the court drop the charges and refer the patient for vocational rehabilitation. Before the disagreement could be resolved, the patient had jumped bail and disappeared. The resident angrily explained the pa-

tient's behavior as a result of the clinic's failure to provide support and assistance. This view was modified when it was learned that the patient had continued his check-writing habits throughout the initial evaluation, although claiming to the resident that he had "gone straight." When the patient returned, he indicated a preference for the senior clinician, whom he had met briefly during a conference and with whom he had developed good rapport. The patient was aware of the disagreement among the staff and felt more comfortable with a clinician who understood him than with one who was taken in by his subterfuges.

The antisocial patient has his own program for the interview and his own goals in mind. He presents an image of himself as he would like to appear, and he fears the humiliation that would result if this picture were challenged. He will go to great lengths and will often lie to prevent exposure and does not welcome distraction or interruption. His response to early confrontation is usually negative. This may take one of several forms, the simplest of which is angry denial. The patient insists that he does not know what the interviewer is talking about, that he is being misunderstood, and it is clear that he is quite hurt by the clinician's failure to understand him. The patient may be both insistent and convincing, and it is not uncommon for the beginning interviewer to retreat in confusion and guilt, apologizing for his comment and letting the patient continue to control the interview.

> A nurse was referred for consultation because of her extensive use of narcotics for vague abdominal pains. After she described her symptoms and her drug regimen, the clinician commented, "It sounds to me as if you have become addicted." The patient became enraged and said that several previous doctors had sympathized with her pain and had prescribed the narcotics. His labeling of the patient as an addict had reflected a pejorative view, and he quickly became anxious and did not know how to respond when she detected this feeling and reacted to it. Now uncertain, he apologized and shifted to a more detailed discussion of her physical symptoms. Had he been more comfortable, he could have interrupted her attack and said, "You're responding as if I just accused you of a crime. Perhaps it sounded that way, but I'm sure you know of the addiction that can develop to narcotics, and I guess I was wondering how you have been handling that."

The example illustrates several points: first, the importance of carefully obtaining the data before making an interpretation; second, the value of searching for a phrase that will "save face" for the patient and allow a comfortable response (e.g., he could have said, "With that much use of narcotics, you must be worried that you will become addicted"); and third, the problems created by the interviewer's countertransference.

The interviewer is often struck by the patient's callous indifference in personal relations or his apparent comfort in violating social and ethical norms. Such responses may be elicited by material that is peripheral to the explicit theme of the interview but reveals the patient's general attitude toward other people. A female patient revealed such a facet to her character when she was at first indifferent to and then annoyed by the friendly overtures of a small child who was in the waiting room of the clinician's office. The clinician's spontaneous reaction is to the lack of human feeling in the patient's behavior. For example, one clinician, consciously unaware of his hostility, asked a patient who was being evaluated after an arrest for sexually molesting children, "Have you ever had any normal sexual feelings?" Early in an interview with a heroin addict, another clinician asked, "Do you serve any useful role in society?" Such comments reveal the interviewer's feelings and prevent the establishment of a relationship with the patient.

The clinician who becomes inappropriately angry and judgmental, adopting a disciplinary rather than a therapeutic position, probably represents the most common countertransference response to these patients. This may follow the response just described, when the clinician who feels that he has been duped switches from blind acceptance to blind rejection. The patient is accustomed to similar responses in the outside world, and he will often work hard at provoking them in the therapist. If they occur, he knows where he stands, and his mistrust is justified. The patient who provokes countertransference rejection by placing the clinician in the role of inquisitor is a common example.

The last form of countertransference, the encouragement of acting out, also repeats a pattern common in the parents of antisocial patients. The clinician vicariously enjoys the patient's behavior, although he may loudly condemn it. His pleasure is often revealed by the delight he has in recounting his patient's exploits in discussions with other clinicians or his fascination with the mechanical or operational details of the patient's exploits. One clinician would entertain his professional friends with anecdotes of his patient's sexual conquests. Another would explore his patient's technique of income tax evasion in great detail; the patient, sensing what was going on, would spend long periods of time tutoring the clinician in sophisticated methods of accounting. Antisocial patients are quick to sense the conspiratorial potentialities of such a situation.

CONCLUSION

Antisocial behavior is only partially explained by psychodynamic concepts. It is an unfortunate corollary that many clinicians ignore psychodynamic principles when interviewing these patients and instead utilize a style that would be more appropriate for a law enforcement officer or an anthropologist trying to make sense of an exotic and unfamiliar culture. The interview with the antisocial patient affords an opportunity to explore aspects of behavior that are often concealed for many years in neurotics and that may be too fragmented or disorganized to be understood in psychotic patients. The core psychopathology is often difficult to treat, but some of these patients experience considerable gain from psychotherapy.

CHAPTER 13

THE PARANOID PATIENT

The paranoid patient suffers deeply from pervasive feelings of being mistreated and misunderstood, hypervigilance, and an acute sensitivity to real or imagined slights. He is suspicious of other people's motives and may distrust those he loves most or to whom he is most attached. This patient harbors simmering anger and grudges toward those he feels may have deceived him or taken unfair advantage. His persistent fear and conviction of not being liked, appreciated, or treated properly become a self-fulfilling prophecy as friends, acquaintances, and workmates become alienated by his hostility, suspiciousness, and constant indignation at the insults or psychological injuries to which he believes he has been subjected.

The paranoid patient is constantly on the alert for evidence of deliberate intent that he is being abused, ignored, or subjected to humiliation. He finds subtle clues to confirm this conviction of deliberate mistreatment. Inadvertent or minor social miscues by another person will convince him that he is being purposely ignored or insulted. He need not be delusional, but he misinterprets the significance of events or social interactions to confirm his conviction that he is an object of denigration. The narcissistic aspects of this type of preoccupation are apparent, and, indeed, paranoid thinking is frequently found in the more disturbed narcissistic patient who feels he does not receive the appropriate recognition that his grandiose self-image demands. To the paranoid patient, the world is a malevolent place that is intent on causing him injury. Ultimately, the patient suffers the rejections, aversion, and avoidance that he most fears because of his distortions of reality.

The DSM-5 criteria for paranoid personality disorder capture this crippling cognitive style in its more florid form (Box 13–1). Milder variations, however, occur in patients with many other personality types or diagnoses. This less disturbed individual will fixate on an insensitive or maladroit comment by a friend or acquaintance, even if it is innocent at heart, and feel intensely affronted. He will react with inner indignation and self-righteous feelings of having been deliberately demeaned by the other person. Simultaneously, he is often highly critical of other people but exempts himself from inner criticism through the mechanism of projection. It is always the other person who is obtuse or thoughtless or who says the hurtful thing. Unconsciously, he gains considerable satisfaction in possessing the moral high ground—the other person is the provocative or insensitive one, never him. These paranoid themes are often present in obsessive, masochistic, or narcissistic patients. More extreme paranoid themes are found in borderline patients with primitive fantasies of being controlled, manipulated, or used in some degrading fashion. The psychotic paranoid has developed a delusional belief that he is being deliberately persecuted because a plot has been engineered against him.

BOX 13–1. DSM-5 Diagnostic Criteria for Paranoid Personality Disorder

---

A. A pervasive distrust and suspiciousness of others such that their motives are interpreted as malevolent, beginning by early adulthood and present in a variety of contexts, as indicated by four (or more) of the following:
   1. Suspects, without sufficient basis, that others are exploiting, harming, or deceiving him or her.
   2. Is preoccupied with unjustified doubts about the loyalty or trustworthiness of friends or associates.
   3. Is reluctant to confide in others because of unwarranted fear that the information will be used maliciously against him or her.
   4. Reads hidden demeaning or threatening meanings into benign remarks or events.
   5. Persistently bears grudges (i.e., is unforgiving of insults, injuries, or slights).
   6. Perceives attacks on his or her character or reputation that are not apparent to others and is quick to react angrily or to counterattack.
   7. Has recurrent suspicions, without justification, regarding fidelity of spouse or sexual partner.
B. Does not occur exclusively during the course of schizophrenia, a bipolar disorder or depressive disorder with psychotic features, or another psychotic disorder and is not attributable to the physiological effects of another medical condition.

Note: If criteria are met prior to the onset of schizophrenia, add "premorbid," i.e., "paranoid personality disorder (premorbid)."

Source. Reprinted from American Psychiatric Association: *Diagnostic and Statistical Manual of Mental Disorders,* 5th Edition. Arlington, VA, American Psychiatric Association, 2013. Copyright 2013, American Psychiatric Association. Used with permission.

Paranoid mechanisms are found in everyone and can be clinically prominent in a wide variety of psychotic, organic, and neurotic disorders. Although the range of psychopathology is great, there are psychodynamic patterns and mechanisms of defense that are common to all of these patients. The greater the degree of paranoia, the more difficult the interview, because the paranoid patient resists the establishment of a therapeutic working relationship. The patient typically comes to complain about something other than his own psychological difficulties or is brought to the clinician by someone else against his will. The paranoid patient is not readily liked and accepted by other people, and the clinician may also respond negatively to him.

PSYCHOPATHOLOGY AND PSYCHODYNAMICS

Paranoid Character Traits

Suspiciousness

The paranoid person is tense, anxious, and basically unsure of himself. He is mistrustful of others and suspicious of their intentions and looks for hidden meanings and motives in their behavior. He has few close relationships, and although he may have contact with many others, he feels himself to be a loner. He may be impressive and even charming at first meeting; however, as people know him better, they like him less.

The paranoid person sees himself as the center of the universe and views events in terms of their bearing on himself. All actions, attitudes, and feelings of others are understood and reacted to in terms of their reference to him. The paranoid patient lacks awareness of his own aggressive impulses but instead fears that he will be attacked or treated unfairly by others, whom he views as unreliable and untrustworthy, thereby justifying his own secretive and seclusive behavior.

Chronic Resentment

This patient's difficulties relating to others realistically cause him to feel awkward and ill at ease in social situations. Every slight is interpreted as a personal rejection. He collects injustices, and his vivid memories of these experiences are never forgotten. He is argumentative and quarrelsome, manifesting impatience and angry emotional outbursts in situations in which others contain themselves. Inappropriate reactions of anger occur in heavy automobile traffic, while waiting in line, or in response to being pushed and bumped in a crowd. The paranoid person, like the narcissistic patient, expresses resentment over his feeling of being unloved and unappreciated by the world. The paranoid person, however, goes further, attributing malevolent motives to those who do not appreciate him. He frequently fixates these feelings on a specific individual or group whom he feels does not like him. The narcissistic patient says, "That is just the way people are," with an attitude of arrogant contempt. The paranoid person, however, says, "He has been out to get me," with angry resentment.

Justice and Rules

Justice and fairness are major preoccupations for the paranoid person. In his concern about safeguarding his rights, he may obtain instruction in the art of self-defense, such as boxing or karate, and he may possess firearms, knives, or other weapons. A compulsive concern with honesty and dedication is a thin disguise for concealed rage. The mistrust of the paranoid patient underlies his concern with the literal interpretation and rigid enforcement of rules and regulations. At the same time, he is unable to appreciate the spirit of rules, and he tends to interpret them mechanically without considering people's feelings.

He also uses the rules to control the direct expression of his own aggression. For example, one patient described how he had spent many hours scrutinizing the laws in anticipation of preparing his income tax return. He reported triumphantly that he could deduct the cost of the postage for mailing the forms. He was determined to get everything that was due him without breaking the law. At times the patient's own minor violations lead to exaggerated fears of detection, but at the same time he searches out loopholes that permit him to express some of his aggression while denying the significance of his behavior.

A similar rigidity concerning rules is found in obsessive patients, but the obsessive person is more likely to bend the regulations for his friends. The obsessive patient is concerned with the authority and status issues represented by rules—who has the power to make them and who has the power to violate them. Rules stimulate his obedience–defiance conflict. Because paranoid and obsessive traits frequently coexist, it is common to find both mechanisms in the same patient.

Grandiosity

The paranoid patient creates an impression of capability and independence, neither needing nor accepting assistance from others. He is opinionated and insists that he is right. His tactlessness and attitudes of superiority, arrogance, and grandiosity antagonize other people. These traits also make him an easy target for insincere flattery and praise, and such recognition quickly reestablishes his childhood feelings of grandiose omnipotence. The paranoid patient is resentful of others when appreciation is not immediately forthcoming. That person is then viewed as stupid, contemptible, and incompetent. This patient frequently reports receiving recognition before he has earned it through adequate achievement. He describes such experiences with a feeling of having been rescued and may relate that his performance actually improved after this unearned and unconditional acceptance.

Because the paranoid person is confident that his goals and ambitions are for the betterment of mankind, he sincerely believes that his ends justify his means. He frequently develops missionary zeal and expects to convert the world to a more perfect place, but he loses sight of how he treats other human beings while accomplishing his purpose. The paranoid personality is attracted to extremist groups, both political and religious; he is more concerned with the rigid application of a system of ideas than the principles contained in them. He is a revolutionary, but he is always disenchanted, even if his revolution succeeds.

Shame

It is common for the paranoid patient to report that he was treated sadistically in early childhood, with repeated experiences of shame and humiliation. Many of the patient's problems stem from his constant sense of humiliation over his failure to control and regulate himself and his environment properly. When he becomes aware of some deficiency, he reacts as though he had soiled himself publicly and everyone were ridiculing him.

He finds it difficult to apologize for a transgression and equally difficult to accept the apologies of others. The paranoid patient confuses forgiveness with the admission of having erred. One patient who had experienced a realistic slight from her therapist delineated this problem by saying, "If I forgive you, that means that I was wrong."

Envy and Jealousy

Envy is a prominent paranoid character trait. The paranoid person is more concerned with the privileges and gratification that others receive than with his own deprived and emotionally barren existence. His preoccupation is with fairness as defined by him. He does not have the narcissistic person's eternal quest for power and status. He is unable to trust, which precludes his ability to love others or to allow them to love him. He longs to trust others, but his preoccupation with betrayal blocks any love relationship. If he begins to trust another person, he imagines signs of betrayal and accuses his partner of cheating on him.

The paranoid person is extremely jealous because of his inability to love and his strong narcissistic needs. He has an intense longing to be loved and an equally intense fear of betrayal. This is discussed in greater detail later, under "Psychodynamic Theories of Paranoia."

Depression and Masochism

Paranoid patients can have an underlying depressive trend. Clinically, when a paranoid defense is no longer effective, depressive feelings may overwhelm the patient. Suicide is not uncommon in acutely paranoid patients. The paranoid person believes that he is not loved, has not been loved, and never will be loved. Feeling persecuted, he considers himself a loser, and his life is spent in suffering (according to his view) at the hands of others. Even the patient with grandiose delusions loses, because he is inevitably confronted by reality when these delusions do not come true. Many of these patients are now recognized as having a bipolar type II illness. The paranoid person is an eternal pessimist, always expecting the worst. He interprets his misfortunes, disappointments, and frustrations not as chance but as the result of personal malevolence from someone else. He is unable to ask for love directly and can only obtain it through pain, self-sacrifice, and humiliation. The intensity of his demands is exorbitant and ensures disappointment. Unable to accept real gratification of his need to be loved, he substitutes fantasies of revenge. Too much of his enjoyment comes from observing the misfortunes and failures of others rather than from his own success.

Success has its own difficulty for the paranoid person. He expects that others will react to his success with intense jealousy and that he will soon become the victim of their retaliatory rage. Therefore, his acceptance of success leads to fear and anticipation of punishment. He cannot enjoy being a winner any more than he can enjoy the role of loser. He disbelieves or depreciates his success to avoid feeling that he has outdone his competitors.

The grandiose paranoid patient is better able to accept success, particularly when it is associated with some idealistic cause. His success is always for the enhancement of "the cause" rather than for personal gains. In his private life, the masochistic aspect becomes more apparent, with asceticism a prominent feature.

The obsessive-phobic character also has fears of success, but the psychodynamic conflict is more clearly related to the patient's competitive relationship with the parent of the same sex for the love of the parent of the opposite sex. The conflict in the paranoid patient is at an earlier developmental level.

Differential Diagnosis

As with the other serious personality disorders, the major differential diagnoses include borderline personality disorder, obsessive-compulsive personality disorder, narcissistic personality disorder, masochistic personality disorder, antisocial personality disorder, and bipolar spectrum disorders. In certain ways both the paranoid patient and the masochistic patient are extensions of narcissistic personality disorder in their unconscious belief that they are the center of the universe, albeit a distorted universe. The thematic element that distinguishes the paranoid patient is that of misplaced trust, fear of betrayal, and explosive anger. The paranoid patient longs for a loving relationship, but his mistrust or trusting the wrong person precludes love and becomes a self-fulfilling prophecy of rejection. The future narcissistic patient, as a child, is made to feel special, whereas the future paranoid patient is mistreated during childhood in many subtle or overt ways and frequently goes on to mistreat others. This element of abusing others can overlap with the antisocial personality. The future paranoid patient as a child is not happy, is often angry, is frequently a loner, and may be either a victim or a bully. There is much more overt aggression in both the history and the presentation of the paranoid patient than one finds with the narcissistic patient. The paranoid patient is often sensitive to only his own dynamics, which are suffused with suspiciousness and hostility; thus he is remarkably insensitive to much that goes on around him, which is in contrast to the narcissistic patient. It is as if he is only resonating to one tune, that of potential mistreatment and betrayal. Paranoid rage has been described as a "red rage," one that is seething and has a potential for violent explosion. This stands in contrast to the "white rage" of the offended obsessive patient, whose self-control inhibits striking out but who is ragefully planning "cool" vengeances against those who have crossed him. Potential or real explosive aggression is the leitmotif of the paranoid patient and can be disturbing to the interviewer.

The grandiosity of the paranoid patient differs from that of the manic or narcissistic patient. The grandiosity of the paranoid patient revolves around his belief that he is the center of the universe and that malevolent forces are arraigned against him because of his specialness. He is on the alert for attack and betrayal. The manic patient is far more expansive and elated in contrast to the foreboding of the paranoid patient. The manic patient may see himself as a "genius" who should be recognized as such, although he can become paranoid if rebuked, crossed, or not acknowledged. The narcissistic patient merely feels that he is far more important than anyone else and can generously dispense his glory to those around him, all of whom should rightfully acknowledge his grandness. Again the differentiating factor lies in the quotient of intense aggression that imbues the paranoid patient in contrast to the narcissistic patient.

Psychodynamic Theories of Paranoia

Freud's conception of the nature of paranoia was based on his study of the memoir of the distinguished German jurist Schreber, who developed a late-onset psychosis replete with complex persecutory and grandiose delusions. Freud felt that the basic motivation at the core of the disturbance related to unconscious homosexuality. In the Schreber case, Freud postulated that unconscious homosexual tendencies were warded off by denial, reaction formation, and projection. The feeling that "I love him" was denied and through reaction formation became "I do not love him; I hate him," and then through projection was transformed into "It is not I who hate him; it is he who hates me." The patient once again experienced the feeling of hate, but now he rationalized, "I hate him because he hates me." In Freud's view, this series of defensive maneuvers was involved in delusions of persecution. In the formation of grandiose delusions, the denial of homosexual impulses occurred through the process: "I do not love him; I do not love anyone—I love only myself."

Freud thought that unconscious homosexuality was also the foundation for delusions of jealousy. The patient's preoccupation with jealous thoughts was the residue of his ego's attempt to ward off threatening impulses. Through the mechanism of projection, unconscious wishes of the patient were attributed to others. The patient asserted, "I do not love him; she loves him." The "other man" whom the paranoid patient suspects his wife of loving was actually a man to whom the patient felt attracted. This is often borne out clinically when the wife of the patient confides to the clinician, "I actually have been interested in other men, but it has never been anyone whom he suspects." The paranoid man often wishes to possess a beautiful female in order to attract the attention of other males. His self-esteem is elevated by other men's attraction to his "trophy woman," just as though it were his penis that was being admired. This phenomenon is also seen in narcissistic men. Heterosexual impulses to be unfaithful also may be projected onto the spouse, leading to pathological jealousy.

Freud felt that narcissistic regression had contributed to unconscious homosexual wishes in that the paranoid patient had withdrawn his interest from others and concentrated it upon himself. His ambivalent feelings of self-love and self-hate were expressed when he became enamored of another person who unconsciously represented himself. He inevitably turned against these love objects, attacking them for the same qualities that he hated in himself. This process was the same whether the love object was a real person or a delusional figure. The intense interest in persons of the same sex aroused unconscious erotic feelings and fears of homosexuality. The patient's narcissistic wish to meet his own body and parts thereof in the external world is reflected by certain clinical material. Patients may reveal that some parts of the body of persons in their delusional world remind them of parts of themselves. Often the buttocks are involved in such thoughts. The frequency of anal preoccupation in paranoid patients often reflects their obsessive conflicts and passive submissive longing for intimacy.

Although conflicts referring to homosexuality are clinically common in paranoid patients, Freud's view of the etiological centrality of unconscious homosexuality is no longer accepted. Some writers claim that a significant number of paranoid patients have no concern with this problem. It is difficult to test Freud's theory, since paranoid patients are typically secretive and often withhold material from the interviewer that pertains to homosexual conflicts. For example, one patient initially denied homosexual concerns in association with his delusions of being poisoned. Finally he admitted that the "poison" was "hormones," and then he acknowledged that it was "sex hormones." Ultimately he revealed his belief that he was receiving female sex hormones. Some paranoid patients are treated for years before disclosing such material. However, contemporary psychoanalysts have emphasized the paranoid patient's preoccupation with being inferior, demeaned, and viewed with contempt, with homosexuality a concrete symbol of that state in our culture, particularly for heterosexual men. For some female paranoid patients, accusations of being promiscuous or a prostitute play the same role.

Mechanisms of Defense

Primitive denial, reaction formation, and projection are the basic defenses in paranoid persons. They are most prominent in the overtly delusional patient. These defenses are first encountered early in the interview, when the patient indicates that he has no problem and does not need to be a patient or does not require hospitalization. The paranoid person utilizes reaction formation to defend himself from awareness of his aggression, his needs for dependency, and his warm or affectionate feelings. In this way he is protected from betrayal and rejection by others. One patient reported, "If I say I don't care about you, then you can't deflate me."

The paranoid person utilizes denial to avoid awareness of painful aspects of reality. Fantasy serves to bolster this denial. This mechanism underlies delusions of grandeur as well as other feelings of omnipotence. Although the paranoid patient sometimes reports his own experiences in great detail, he often completely disclaims any emotional response to a given event. Although the paranoid patient is hypersensitive to those traits in others that he denies in himself, he is a poor observer of others except in the narrow area of his own hypervigilance.

The paranoid person is consumed with anger and hostility. Unable to face or accept responsibility for his rage, he projects his resentment and anger onto others. He then relies on rules to protect himself from fantasied acts of attack or discrimination, which represent his own projected impulses. The patient denies the aggressive significance of his own behavior and is insensitive to its impact on others. If the patient with persecutory delusions is able to recognize some of his anger, he views it as an appropriate response to the persecution he receives in his delusional world. The patient with grandiose delusions is more apt to feel that others resent him because he is so great. He, of course, considers himself to be above feelings of anger. The mechanism of projection enables the patient to imagine that he is loved by someone to whom he is attracted, or he may use projection as a defense against unconscious impulses that he finds unacceptable in himself. The latter case is exemplified by the 75-year-old unmarried woman who imagines that men are breaking into her apartment with some sexual designs. Her delusion reveals not only her frustrated sexual wishes but also her projected hostility toward men.

Another aspect of projection is exemplified by the patient's own superego criticisms that are projected when denial and reaction formation fail to handle his guilt feelings. This is illustrated by the patient who believes that his persecutors are accusing him of dishonesty. Many delusions are critical or frightening, thereby implying a projection of superego processes. Furthermore, paranoid mechanisms are often triggered by intense feelings of guilt.

The defense of externalization as used by the paranoid person is similar to projection in its genesis. The patient accepts no responsibility in interpersonal situations because of extreme inner feelings of shame and worthlessness. Everything that goes wrong must be seen as someone else's fault. Obviously, the paranoid person alienates himself from others by constantly blaming them for his own misdeeds or failures.

Paranoid symptoms involve regression to earlier levels of functioning. This regression affects the entire personality, including ego and superego functions. Superego regression is revealed by a return to the early stages of conscience formation, when the patient was fearful of being watched by his parents.

The fundamental feeling that is projected by every paranoid patient is his self-image of inadequacy and worthlessness. In the male heterosexual patient, this may be symbolized by the self-accusation of homosexuality. The projected accusations in the delusions of female paranoid patients often involve prostitution or fears of heterosexual attack and exploitation rather than homosexuality. This difference can be traced to the girl's early relationship with her parents. When she turns to her father for the maternal love that she is unable to receive from her mother, she begins to develop heterosexual desires rather than homosexual wishes. These are later repudiated and projected in fears of rape or hallucinated accusations of prostitution. The common theme in both male and female patients is that of being a degraded and worthless sexual object.

The paranoid man's childhood power struggle with figures of authority may also contribute to his fear of homosexuality. The homosexual thoughts and feelings reflect the incomplete resolution of this power conflict, with the resulting development of inappropriate attitudes of submission and regression to dependent modes of adaptation, which are symbolically represented by homosexuality. Phrases such as "getting screwed" or "getting the shaft" illustrate the symbolic homosexual significance that our culture attributes to a situation in which one is forced to submit to unfair treatment. Because of intense ambivalence over such wishes, paranoid persons may resist normal cooperation on one occasion only to submit to some totally unreasonable demand on another.

A further understanding of the psychodynamics of the paranoid patient has been developed by Auchincloss and Weiss. They noted that anyone may become paranoid when his or her security or *connectedness* with important others is severely threatened. This can happen, for instance, to a soldier in a frightening combat situation and occurred frequently during the murderous trench warfare of the First World War. They suggested that the paranoid patient, in contrast to other people, regularly suffers from a failure of *object constancy*—that is, the psychological capacity to maintain a mental image of another person even in his or her absence—and thus his connectedness to others is always threatened, even when no obvious external threat exists. The paranoid person cannot maintain a constant loving attachment to the internal mental representation of another person. In the face of intense frustration or rage toward that person, often precipitated by separation, he resorts to thinking about him or her in magical, concrete ways. For instance, the paranoid patient is convinced he "knows" what the therapist is thinking and what the therapist is trying to do to control the patient's thoughts or actions. Through this pathological mechanism the paranoid patient maintains his connectedness, often feeling he is constantly being thought about by the therapist. Inwardly, when faced with this paranoid self-referentiality, the therapist may be tempted to say, "You're not that important; not everybody constantly is thinking about you." The paranoid person can only feel connected to another person by thinking about that person all the time, even if in a hostile way, thus maintaining a sense of connectedness. An intolerance to indifference—to not being thought about constantly—is one factor at the core of the paranoid patient's psychopathology, reflecting problems with object constancy. This inability to maintain a constant mental representation of another person, even in the face of separation or empathic failures, precipitates defensive fantasies in the paranoid person of being secretly controlled, manipulated, or otherwise used unfairly.

Paranoid Syndromes

Hypochondriasis

Hypochondriasis is not a disease entity but a symptom complex found in paranoid illnesses, schizophrenia, depression, anxiety disorders, organic psychoses, and some personality disorders. Paranoid patients may complain of insomnia, irritability, weakness, or fatigue as well as strange sensations in their eyes, ears, nose, mouth, skin, genitals, and ano-rectal area. These areas represent the chief routes through which the patient's body can be penetrated or invaded by others.

Paranoid hypochondriasis is often accompanied by withdrawal from emotional involvement with other people. The ego develops as the infant differentiates his own body from the external world. Direct observation of infants reveals that the initial discovery of one's own body is a pleasurable process. However, in hypochondriasis the rediscovery of the body is intensely painful. As the patient's interest fixates on his physical self, he experiences fears of damage and death. This may symbolize castration anxiety, or it may directly reflect an awareness of impending psychological disorganization. The threat of psychosis may be defended against as the patient symbolically attempts to localize or wall off the disintegrative process in one part of his body.

In the patient's view, his social withdrawal is caused by his physical suffering. He is relieved to find an organic basis for his suffering that further fixates his attention. If no organic basis for his complaint is found, he is likely to seek medical help elsewhere. In more severe cases, the interviewer will respond to the hypochondriacal symptoms as he would to a delusion; this is discussed later. Other variants of hypochondriacal reactions may be found in depressed, anxious, and narcissistic patients.

The negative or painful feelings associated with hypochondriasis reflect the patient's hostile, antagonistic feelings that have been withdrawn from others and turned against himself. Although these patients have always experienced some social isolation, the further withdrawal of interest from others is now accelerated. The patient may report that since the onset of his physical preoccupation, he has quit his job and stopped seeing his few friends, and he now devotes all of his time to matters related to his illness.

The specific symptom choice may represent the patient's ambivalent identification with a parent or parent surrogate. To illustrate, a patient who was preoccupied with his bowels revealed that his father had died of a carcinoma of the rectum. Exploration of the symptom revealed both the positive aspect of the identification and the hostile competitive feelings toward the father that were now turned inward. The interviewer can learn much about the patient's psychodynamics through a careful study of his hypochondriacal symptoms.

Paranoid Psychoses

Paranoid themes are common in psychoses, particularly schizophrenia but also delusional disorders, affective disorders (both manic and depressed), and organic brain syndromes. Although the etiology of these conditions is different, the problems in interviewing are essentially the same.

The paranoid schizophrenic psychosis usually has a gradual onset. The patient withdraws from emotional contact with the people in his life. A common sequence is hypochondriasis, persecutory delusions, and then grandiose delusions. Although there is some controversy over the nature of delusions, one psychodynamic view is that they serve a reparative function. The patient who has been preoccupied with himself shifts his interest from his own body and attempts to reestablish contact with those persons from whom he has withdrawn. He is unable to accomplish this, and the world appears to be chaotic and disturbing. He cannot make sense out of the behavior of others, and he desperately searches for the clue that will explain their actions. The delusional concepts that emerge represent the patient's effort to organize himself and to reestablish contact with the real world. Cameron coined the term *pseudo-community* to describe the group of real and imagined persons who are united (in the patient's mind) for the purpose of carrying out some actions against him. As the patient becomes a more active participant in his pseudo-community, he behaves in a more grossly psychotic manner. The fantasy world of the delusion is designed to protect the ego from the pain of reality.

A delusion is a fixed belief that is usually false but, more fundamentally, is impervious to evidence, reason, or persuasion by one's normal reference group. It is usually based on denial, reaction formation, and projection. It reflects a degree of confusion between the self and the outer world. The essence of delusional thinking is not just the lack of correspondence with external reality but the fixity of the patient's conviction and his inability to alter his ideas in response to evidence of their irrationality. The capacity for delusion formation rather than the specific type of delusion is the patient's basic pathology. In paranoid characters the same rigidity of persecutory thinking exists and is not responsive to evidence of irrationality, but this patient is not necessarily delusional.

Closely related to delusional thought is the paranoid person's fascination with extrasensory perception, mental telepathy, and similar occult phenomena. The paranoid patient's affinity for these strange modes of communication is consistent with his regression to the magical thinking of childhood. The process is defensive in that it validates the patient's reparative distortions and convinces him that he is right. It also reflects his basic social ataxia and lack of understanding of interpersonal relations. Because he has withdrawn his emotional investment from others and has fixated on himself, his ability to relate to others is impaired. These unusual means of communicating represent his attempt to restore contact with other humans by those primitive techniques that are still available.

The content of the patient's delusions is determined by his psychodynamic conflicts, by the general cultural values of the society in which he lives, and by the specific characteristics of the family in which he was raised. The clinician can learn the patient's psychodynamic conflicts most quickly through a careful study of the patient's delusions. The defense mechanisms and psychodynamics of delusions have already been discussed. Different types of delusions are delineated in the following sections.

Delusions of persecution. Delusions of persecution are the most common delusions found in paranoid patients. The persecutor represents not only the ambivalently loved object but also a projection of aspects of the patient. There usually is some realistic basis for paranoid projections, although it has been vastly exaggerated by the patient. The patient's tendency to distort reality is furthered by the patient's particular sensitivity to the unconscious motives and feelings of others. However, he cannot differentiate their unconscious feelings from his own.

Persecutory delusions usually reflect the social issues of concern to the culture in which the patient resides. Political conspiracies, modern science (e.g., computers, cyberspace, genetic engineering), racism, sexual attitudes, and organized crime are the most popular themes in paranoid American patients today, whereas the Japanese and Germans were more prominent in delusions 60 years ago, and until the collapse of the Soviet Union, communist conspiracies were common.

Delusions of grandeur.   Feelings of great artistic or inventive talent or of being a messiah provide the most common content of delusions of grandeur. They are, however, far more common in the delusions of the manic patient. From the viewpoint of differential diagnosis, such delusions in the manic patient are accompanied by an elevation of mood state, a euphoric grandiosity that is not present in the paranoid patient. The patient may or may not be aware that his fantasized abilities are unappreciated by the rest of the world. Sometimes grandiose delusions have been preceded by delusions of persecution. The patient may seek to avoid the painful feeling of persecution by telling himself that he must be a very important person to merit such treatment. Compensatory grandiosity assists projection in defending the ego from the full significance of the entry of unacceptable impulses into consciousness as well as warding off feelings of inadequacy.

Erotomania or delusions of being loved.   Erotomanic delusions most often occur in female patients. The basically grandiose delusional system becomes centered and fixated on one individual, usually an older male. The patient believes that this man has fallen in love with her and is communicating that love through various secret signs and signals.

Milder nonpsychotic forms of this problem are seen in the female student and the older male teacher—often an English or a French teacher. The student does extra academic work, stays after school to assist the teacher, and soon becomes his pet. The teacher is romanticized and endowed with magical omnipotence and omniscience. His attention and interest are misinterpreted by her as she attempts to compensate for feeling unattractive to boys her own age. This state blends imperceptibly into psychosis in the case of the girl who feels that her teacher's selections of poetry are chosen particularly with reference to her and that they contain covert messages of his devotion.

The erotomanic patient may develop intense rage toward the object of her delusion. Such reactions can occur independently of any real rejection on the part of this person, or they may occur as reactions to a trivial slight. Male patients may develop erotomanic delusions involving a female pop singer or actress. If he pursues her, he is usually jailed for harassment. He can become dangerous.

Somatic delusions. Patients with somatic delusions have a more severe form of pathology than those previously discussed as hypochondriacal. Their preoccupations have become focused on a particular part of their body and have reached delusional proportions. The parts of the body and the psychic mechanisms most commonly involved are the same as those discussed in the earlier section on "Hypochondriasis." The specific choice of symptoms always has psychodynamic significance.

Delusions of jealousy. Although all paranoid patients are extremely jealous, this can only be considered delusional when an organized system has been constructed by the patient. The patient's partner is the most frequent target for this delusional jealousy.

Drug-Induced Paranoid States

Cocaine, lysergic acid, marijuana, phencyclidine, and amphetamines readily induce acute paranoid states that are reversible when the drug use is stopped. The use of anabolic steroids by professional athletes, bodybuilders, and fitness enthusiasts can also lead to severe rage-filled paranoid conditions in some individuals. One articulate athlete described his condition thus:

> It was like I was always in a slow burn, prepared to jump out of my car at any time and confront anyone on the road who bothered me by driving too close, too slow, or weaving in front of me. I would explode at other people at the drop of a hat—in restaurants if the service was not fast enough, at my elevator man if the car was held at another floor, at my wife if she was 30 seconds late. My flashpoint was so low I could be set off by anything. Now that I've stopped using the drugs, it's hard to believe what I became when I was on them. I was some sort of monster ready to erupt at any minute.

Developmental Psychodynamics

Although genetic, constitutional, and cultural factors are also important in the development of paranoid disturbances, this section focuses on the role of psychological conflict. The focus is on clinical observations, without regard to their etiological significance. Nevertheless, we hope that these observations will provide the clinician with guidelines for investigation during interviews with such patients.

Melanie Klein postulated that everyone goes through a *paranoid–schizoid position* during early development. The infant, in her view, is terrified of the "bad"—that is, frustrating—mother and projects his own aggression aroused by this frustration back at the mother. This mechanism of projection is combined with introjection of the "good" or satisfying mother. The image of the mother is thus split, and this process of projection and introjection continues until, with further development, the images of "good" and "bad" mother are integrated into a single mental representation of the parent that combines both characteristics. These mechanisms are believed by object relations theorists to be central to the splitting found in borderline patients, in whom a person important to them may go from being idealized to denigrated in bewildering fashion, an experience often encountered by their therapist. The mechanism of projecting "badness" onto external figures, a residue of the paranoid-schizoid position, is felt by object relations theorists to be at the heart of the psychopathology of the paranoid patient. In the Kleinian view, the infant fears that malevolent objects from the outside will invade and destroy him. Whether or not this theory is correct, such unconscious fantasies can be found in the adult paranoid patient.

From the viewpoint of the ego-psychological conflict model of development, the paranoid person experiences difficulty in establishing a warm and trusting relationship with his mother. His feeling of rejection leads to difficulty in developing a sense of identity in this early symbiotic relationship. Feelings of worthlessness alternate with contradictory and compensatory feelings of grandiose omnipotence. Perceiving his mother as rejecting, the future paranoid patient turns to his father as a substitute. In the male, this leads to fears of passive homosexual wishes. These fears are accentuated by the parents' anxiety over their young son's turning primarily to his father for nurturing love and closeness. In the female, fears of sexual involvement arise as she turns to the father for the affection that she is unable to obtain from her mother, causing a regression to earlier homosexual attachments. These fears are later interpreted in oedipal terms, with the result that the girl's fear of attack from her mother is intensified. She develops a secondary fear of attack by men as her incestuous desires are warded off through projection.

This patient learns early in life that his parents are motivated by feelings other than love and closeness. Their behavior is inconsistent with their words; consequently, the future patient is forced to rely on his own observations and on what he is able to read between the lines. Sadistic parental attacks are common from either or both parents. The father may be rigid, distant, and sadistic; weak and ineffectual; or possibly totally absent. The obsessive patient typically receives parental love and approval as long as he is obedient. The paranoid patient, however, submits to authority only to escape attack and receives little and inconsistent nurturing love and warmth as a reward. The patient equates his parents' attacks as a form of rape, and this is later apparent in his fears of penetration. This fear is also a defense against his passive, submissive feelings toward his father, which stem from a longing for his love, as well as a defense against the rage felt toward him. Intense feelings of anger and hate develop and are dealt with by denial, reaction formation, and projection. Identification with the aggressor becomes a prominent mechanism of defense in his actual life behavior as well as in the structure of his delusions.

The mother in such families is often overly controlling and frequently seductive, exposing the child to sexual stimulation either directly herself or indirectly through siblings, with total denial of the significance of such stimulation. If the mother is the sadistic parental figure, she is likely to have prominent paranoid features. Her grandiosity leads her to feel that she is always right and the child is always wrong. Under these circumstances, the child develops little sense of worth or individuality but instead denies his ambivalence and attempts to ally himself with his all-knowing, all-powerful mother. The more the child is rebuffed in his attempt to identify with the aggressor, the more likely it is that persecutory attitudes will later develop. Because his self-esteem is achieved through identification with an omnipotent, aggressive parent, he feels that he should automatically and immediately be recognized without demonstrating his worth. The patient's mother often attempts to dominate and control her offspring through the threat of frustration and withdrawal. Therefore, intimacy and closeness become dangerous. The child's occasional intimate experiences with the mother typically lead to humiliation or rejection. The resultant fear of intimacy is prominent in the paranoid patient, and closeness is avoided at all cost. As a result, the future paranoid patient also learns to deny his warm, tender, and sexual feelings. The child expects that all close relationships require the abandonment of independence and the adoption of a passive, submissive attitude, reawakening his rage when others do not submit to him and thereby demonstrate their love. His defense is the identification with the aggressor.

Just as his parents have inadequate social skills, the paranoid person also is unable to acquire the coping mechanisms necessary for acceptance by others in his environment. His parents' lack of consideration for his rights as a human being leads him to lack appreciation either of his own rights or of the rights of others. He compensates for his isolation and loneliness with an increase in his grandiosity. This attitude in turn leads to renewed rejections from others and further entrenches his feelings of persecution.

Although obsessive, phobic, depressive, histrionic, and narcissistic symptoms are common in childhood and preadolescence, paranoid symptoms are unusual before middle adolescence. Paranoid psychotic patients tend to show less severe regression or deterioration than other schizophrenic patients, an observation that seems in part to be explained by the later age of development. Although this is not well understood, it may be related to the fact that full-fledged paranoid syndromes require experience with a rejecting environment other than that of the patient's family. Another factor is the highly developed capacity for logical thinking associated with the production of delusions.

Paranoid behavior is, in part, learned behavior and is based on the attitudes of the parents. This patient may develop a close peer relationship during the preadolescent years; however, his parents warn him not to trust his friends and not to reveal confidences about himself or his family. Puberty, with its intensification of sexual impulses, creates problems for the paranoid person. He is unable to make the transition from preadolescence to adolescence, with the consequent shift of emotional interest from members of the same sex to members of the opposite sex. His deflated sense of self-esteem and fear of sexual impulses cause him to remain distant and aloof from members of the opposite sex. The young boy is fearful of women and relates better to other males. His fears include both fear of domination and fear of rejection. His avoidance of women requires intensification of his defenses against homosexuality. Similar problems occur with a girl who fears either sadistic attack or rejection and disinterest such as she experienced from her father.

Precipitating Stress

There are two classes of stress that precipitate paranoid reactions. The first consists of situations similar to those that precipitate depressive episodes. These include the real, fantasied, or anticipated loss of love objects. Closely related are experiences of adaptive failure with consequent loss of self-esteem, such as occurs after losing a job or failing in school, with the associated expectation that significant other persons will reject the patient. Paradoxically, success as well as failure may precipitate paranoid episodes as a result of the patient's fantasy of retaliation from envious competitors. The third major category of situations that precipitate paranoid reactions includes those in which the patient has been forced to submit passively to real or fantasied assault or humiliation. These range from injury incurred through an accident or an assault to situations in which the patient is forced into a passive, submissive role in his occupation. In the latter case, the patient may project his wishes to submit passively, with the resulting fantasy of having been overpowered or assaulted. Competitive experiences may lead a paranoid person to feel that he must submit or they may stimulate intense feelings of aggression. Situations in which there is an intensified stimulation of homosexual feelings, such as confinement in a closed space with other males on a navy or merchant ship, can lead to acute paranoid reactions. In all of these instances, the paranoid response may be initiated by the intense guilt or feeling of shame that overwhelms the patient. He may experience this guilt over his failures, his successes, or his passive submissive wishes.

MANAGEMENT OF THE INTERVIEW

The paranoid patient's anger is a prominent feature in the initial interview. This may emerge as negativistic withdrawal, an angry filibuster, assaultiveness, or irrational demands. Once the interview is under way, the patient's profound mistrust presents additional problems. His hypersensitivity and fear of rejection make interpretation and confrontation extremely difficult. However, when psychotherapy progresses successfully and a trusting therapeutic relationship slowly develops, the therapist becomes the most important person in the patient's life.

The Opening Phase

Anger and Silence

The patient who has been brought for psychiatric care against his will frequently expresses his angry feelings by refusing to talk. However, unlike the catatonic or severely depressed patient, the angry psychotic paranoid person does not remain aloof from his human environment. His withdrawal is not only a defense against anger but also a means of expressing such feelings. The patient welcomes any opportunity to give vent to his anger and hate. The interviewer can establish initial rapport with the patient by recognizing this and commenting, "You seem to have been brought here against your will" or "I gather you felt coerced into coming here." The clinician has not agreed with the patient's interpretation but has shown an interest in learning more about it. Usually such remarks will start the patient on a long, angry diatribe that allows the interviewer to engage the patient. If the patient is already hospitalized and this approach does not induce him to talk, it is helpful to say, "I have to assume that you were admitted to the hospital for some reason, and at least until I have evidence that these reasons were not good, or are no longer valid, you will have to remain. Under the circumstances, talking with me can only improve your chances of being released." The interviewer must make it clear to the patient that although discussion may lead to his *eventual* release, there is no promise of immediate action. This honest approach will often enable the otherwise noncommunicative psychotic paranoid patient to be interviewed.

The clinician can sympathize with the patient's feeling of being mistreated. For example, a hospitalized psychotic paranoid woman who had been interviewed by several different clinicians earlier in the day began the interview by saying, "I have told my story to enough doctors, and I am tired and fed up and I am not going to talk to you!" When the interviewer sympathized with the patient's feeling of injustice in being utilized in this way, the patient angrily continued, "Yes, and furthermore, the male patients who have jobs are excused to go to work and do not have to be subjected to these interviews." This additional statement about the special treatment received by the male patients provided an opening for a sympathetic response, and within 2 or 3 minutes the patient was talking freely with the interviewer.

The more seriously ill psychotic paranoid patient who has frightening hallucinations and delusions is better motivated to communicate with the interviewer in order to obtain his protection; however, the pattern of the interview very quickly assumes the same characteristics as that with other paranoid persons.

The "Paranoid Stare"

The paranoid patient observes every detail of the interviewer's behavior and of the surrounding environment. His "paranoid stare" makes many interviewers feel uncomfortable, and they may react by averting their gaze from the patient's eyes. The patient is reassured if the interviewer watches him closely throughout the interview. Experiencing this as evidence of interest rather than mistrust, he is reassured that the interviewer is paying close attention and is not afraid of him.

The Filibuster

The interview with a paranoid patient is better described as a filibuster rather than an interaction between two participants. This filibuster is usually most pronounced in the opening and the closing phase of the interview. Since the paranoid person, like the obsessive person, experiences his greatest difficulty in establishing emotional contact and then in separating from another individual once contact has been made, it is easy to understand the adaptive value of this symptomatic behavior. By not allowing the other person to talk at the start of the interview, the patient controls the degree of his engagement in the relationship. Once he has developed emotional rapport, he must ward off the dangers of imminent rejection. He accomplishes this by rejecting the interviewer first, using words to keep him at a distance, but at the same time "hanging on" by continuing to speak.

A basic sense of worthlessness and inadequacy underlies the patient's attempt to dominate the therapist with his tirade of words. In order to permit engagement, the interviewer must allow the patient to tell his story. However, if this filibuster is permitted to continue throughout the interview, there will be no contact with the patient. Although one may occasionally confront this defense in the first interview with a comment such as "I have the feeling that I am being subjected to a filibuster," this technique will often alienate the patient. It is usually preferable to say, "I would like to hear the details of your story, and over the course of our sessions together I certainly will. However, there are issues that we must discuss now so that I may be able to help you." Another way to limit the patient's tirade without provoking him is to ask, "How can I be of help to you with these problems?" In this way the interviewer indicates that he will not be dominated by the patient, and he takes some control away from him. It may be necessary to repeat similar statements on more than one occasion during the interview if the patient attempts to reestablish the filibuster.

Denial

The paranoid person often refuses to accept the role of patient. This is a form of denial. For him the acceptance of this role implies a humiliating loss of dignity. If the interviewer attempts to force this person to admit that he is a patient, it will further threaten an already tenuous balance of self-esteem. On the other hand, if he does not insist, the patient will often respond by demonstrating further psychopathology, once again inviting the interviewer to force him into the role of the patient. The interviewer, even though he recognizes and understands this cycle, should not interpret it to the patient during the early stages of treatment.

The patient who denies problems of his own and wants to discuss his delusional complaints, but who has come to the hospital voluntarily, offers an easy opportunity for engagement. After listening to the patient for 10–15 minutes, the clinician can say, "Since you have come to a hospital to consult a psychiatrist rather than the police, you must have had something in mind about how a psychiatrist could be helpful to you." The patient's attention is thereby directed away from the content of his delusions. He may indicate that he had already consulted the police and that they laughed at him or told him that he was crazy. Emotional rapport is facilitated if the interviewer empathizes with the patient's predicament. For example, he might say to the patient, "It must have been terribly humiliating being treated in that way."

Mistrust

The management of the patient's mistrust and hostility becomes the crucial issue in conducting the interview. Beneath the patient's hostility are deep wishes for, and also fears of, a close, trusting relationship. However any attempt at closeness with the paranoid patient leads to fear and mistrust, with further hostility. This occurs because of the patient's fear of passivity and his conviction that only rejection can follow closeness, which is the reason that he wants to reject the clinician first. When the patient is not openly antagonistic and angry toward the interviewer, he will be distrustful and suspicious. The interviewer should refrain from assuring the patient that he is a friend, that he has come to help him, or that the patient can trust him as an ally. Instead, he can agree with the patient that he is a total stranger and that there is, indeed, no rational reason that the patient should immediately trust him or perceive him as an ally. The interviewer expresses his human compassion for the patient's suffering without becoming his intimate friend. His relationship with the patient is real and authentic, but professional rather than personal.

The paranoid person has great difficulty in determining whom he can trust and whom he cannot trust. The interviewer's recognition of the patient's mistrust shows understanding of the problems. If the patient accuses the interviewer of having wired the room, the patient could be given freedom to look about and check for himself. The interviewer might then pursue the patient's feeling that people are not trustworthy by asking him to relate experiences when he has been betrayed.

Nonpsychotic patients with paranoid personality traits express their mistrust of the clinician in more subtle ways. The psychodynamic issues involved are the same as those found in the more seriously disturbed patients. Some patients show their suspicion at the start of the interview. A patient may begin with a tone of firm conviction, "I was just curious, but did you leave that magazine on top of the pile so that I would see the cover story?" or "I think you left that picture crooked as a test!" The interviewer is advised to pursue these ideas further before providing an answer. He could reply, "What might I hope to learn from such a test?" One patient answered, "Oh, you could see if I am an aggressive type of woman who goes around straightening other people's pictures." Since the patient resisted her impulse, she felt that she had passed the test and therefore had no such problem. The interviewer did not challenge this view but mentally registered the incident in his evaluation of the patient.

Other patients evidence their suspicion and fear by attempting to keep "one up" on the interviewer. An example is the patient who says, "I'll bet I know why you asked me that question" or "I know what you're trying to do; you want to get me angry." If the interviewer explores the motives that the patient ascribes to him, he will uncover the power conflict and the patient's fear of being controlled. Persons with paranoid character traits tend to be secretive about revealing the names of former therapists or even friends whom they are discussing in the interview. The patient typically asks, "Why do you need to know that?" The interviewer can explore the patient's fear of damaging other persons as well as his fear of betrayal by the clinician. If the interviewer tries to pressure the patient into revealing such information, it only reinforces the patient's fear. It is more helpful if the interviewer interprets the patient's mistrust of him.

Demands for Action

On occasion, a paranoid psychotic patient may begin the interview not only with denial of any emotional problems but also with some bizarre demand based on his delusional thoughts. For example, a patient came to the emergency department complaining that he had been shot in the back. When the intern could find no evidence of a wound, he suggested psychiatric consultation. The patient, however, replied that he had been shot with an invisible bullet and demanded a magnetic resonance imaging (MRI) scan be done. Attempts to establish rapport with such a patient by acceding to his outlandish demands are doomed to failure. Some part of the patient's ego maintains awareness of the irrational aspect of his request, and the clinician who humors the patient subjects him to later feelings of humiliation. Instead, the interviewer can indicate that the patient's perception is valid but that his interpretation is impossible. On might say, for example, "You feel that you have been wounded in the back, which is frightening, but there are several possible explanations for that feeling. I would not consider giving you an MRI; there are no invisible bullets." The inexperienced interviewer often expects that the patient will angrily leave the emergency room at this point; however, if the clinician is able to express his genuine interest with his tone of voice and attitude, the interview will then proceed.

A similar situation occurred with a patient who came to an emergency department demanding an X ray of his skull, claiming, "There is a cell phone in my brain." The patient was hallucinating, and again the relationship was enhanced by the clinician's indication that he was sincerely interested in aiding the patient but that he did not accept the patient's interpretation of his experience.

The interviewer is advised to limit his early confrontations concerning delusions to situations in which a patient demands immediate unreasonable action on the part of the interviewer. These demands can also be managed by exploring how the patient would feel if the X ray failed to confirm his belief. This will sometimes provide an opportunity for discussion of the problem that the patient attempts to deny with his delusions. The patient may then be able to express his fear that the voice may be a hallucination and therefore a reflection of mental illness.

It is sometimes necessary to accede to some unrealistic request on the part of a paranoid patient in order to establish an initial therapeutic relationship. For example, a paranoid patient entered the clinician's office and at once complained that he could not discuss his problems unless the interviewer pulled the window shade because he was being watched from the next building. The interviewer granted his request, but it became readily apparent that even though the shade was pulled, he still was not discussing his problem. When this was pointed out, the patient first became angry but then proceeded to reveal his difficulties. In these situations, the patient's demand is not as bizarre as those described earlier, and the interviewer set the stage for challenging the patient's rationalization by yielding to his request. One paranoid patient refused to be interviewed in a room where the partition did not go to the ceiling, even though he was assured that there was no one in the adjacent room. The patient's request for greater privacy was granted by moving to a different room.

A difficult problem is presented by the patient who refuses to be interviewed unless the clinician will promise not to hospitalize him. Obviously, no such blanket promise can be given. The interviewer might reply, "I do not believe in forcing treatment on someone against his will. Nevertheless, people who have uncontrollable impulses to harm themselves or others are treated in a hospital until they regain their own self-control." Often this will reassure the patient at a deep level so that the interview can continue. If the patient has come voluntarily but further discussion convinces the interviewer that the patient would be best treated in a hospital, he should attempt to convince the patient to accept hospitalization, and if the patient still refuses, he can refuse to treat him unless he agrees. If the patient has been brought by someone else and these techniques fail, with the patient insisting on the promise before speaking, the interviewer could say, "If I do not hear the problem from you, I will have to base my decision exclusively on what your friends and relatives can tell me."

Establishment of the Therapeutic Alliance

Challenging the Delusion

Every beginning clinician is tempted to argue the psychotic patient out of his delusional system by the use of logic. The impossibility of this task soon becomes apparent. It is more helpful if the interviewer asks the patient what is responsible for this persecution—why people should be against him and what he could possibly have done that offended them. The interviewer neither agrees with the delusions nor challenges them. The patient, however, usually interprets the interviewer's interest as a sign of tacit agreement. It is essential for their later relationship that the interviewer makes no deceptive statements in order to gain the patient's trust and confidence momentarily.

If the patient directly inquires whether the clinician believes his story, the interviewer could reply, "I know that you feel just as you say and that you are telling me the truth as you see it; however, the meaning that you attribute to your feelings is a matter for further clarification." The interviewer might address himself to the patient's anxiety about convincing the interviewer of the accuracy of his views so quickly and indicate that time is required to evaluate these problems. In general, the more bizarre the delusional material, the more open the interviewer must be in directly questioning the patient's interpretation of his experiences. In doing so, it is helpful for the interviewer to state the logical foundation behind his own position but to avoid debating it with the patient. Frequently, this involves a challenge to the patient's grandiosity. For example, the clinician might say, "I have no doubt that the green car you described actually drove around the block; however I see no reason to believe that it contained foreign agents or that anyone in the car was interested in you more than anyone else. Nothing you have told me indicates why the foreign agents should consider you so important that they would bother to make your life difficult."

The interviewer can often point out that the patient's relatives disagree with his delusional system and that they believe their view just as strongly as the patient believes in his. He can then ask, "Why should I believe that you are right and that your relatives are crazy?" Any doubt or fluctuation in the patient's feelings provides a foothold for establishing a therapeutic relationship. Later in treatment, increased or renewed delusional material should be traced to specific precipitating stresses.

Differentiating Delusions From Reality

Paranoid delusions often contain some kernel of truth. When the delusion is somewhat plausible, beginning interviewers often attempt to determine how much of the patient's production is actually delusional and how much is real. This is an error, because it does not really matter exactly where reality begins and ends, and one can never actually make such a determination. It is far more important to establish rapport through the acknowledgment of the plausible elements of the delusion. The most important aspects of a delusion are the patient's preoccupation with it, his irrational certainty that it is true, and its use to explain his frustrations, disappointments, and failures. The interviewer should suggest to the patient that his preoccupation with the delusion interferes with a constructive and useful life. In this manner, he can avoid arguments concerning the degree of truth in the delusion.

The interviewer inquires whether the patient has ever taken action or contemplated action based on his delusional system. It is important not to ask these questions in a tone that suggests that the patient should have taken action. The nature of any action that the patient did take will enable the interviewer to evaluate the patient's judgment and impulse control.

Developing the Treatment Plan

It is important that the patient function as an active participant in the development of a treatment plan. Otherwise, he is likely to feel passive and submissive and then express his resentment by not following the clinician's advice. To avoid this problem, the interviewer must stimulate the patient's motivation to receive help. The patient who is delusional may not feel that he requires treatment for his delusion but may willingly accept help aimed at his irritability, insomnia, or inability to concentrate. He might acknowledge a problem in his social life or on his job that could be treated with psychotherapy. Once the patient has indicated that he recognizes problems for which he desires help, the clinician can offer a tentative recommendation for treatment. Statements such as "These are problems we could work on together" or "I believe I can help you to arrive at a solution to this difficulty" emphasize that the patient plays an active role in treatment and is not merely submitting to the clinician. If the therapist is overly enthusiastic in offering therapeutic recommendations, the patient is more likely to resist them.

When it is necessary to refer a paranoid patient to another therapist, the clinician can anticipate trouble. The patient will often question the qualifications of the therapist to whom he is referred. The interviewer can review these qualifications and then ask, "Did you think I would send you to someone not adequately qualified?" The patient will usually hasten to reassure the interviewer that he had no such thought. The interviewer could then comment, "Perhaps you feel hurt or angry that I do not have time to work with you myself." If the patient acknowledges such feelings and the interviewer is not defensive, the referral is more likely to proceed smoothly. If the patient denies such feelings, the interviewer can expect a call from the patient saying that he did not like the new clinician for a variety of reasons. In general, the interviewer should advise the patient to go back to the other clinician and discuss these feelings with him, rather than send the patient to still another therapist.

The psychotic paranoid patient is hypersensitive to restrictions of freedom or situations of enforced passivity. He does not readily accept medication or hospitalization. The interviewer should not bring up these subjects until he has established a trusting relationship with the patient. When hospital treatment is required, every attempt should be made to convince the patient to accept voluntary hospitalization, avoiding physical or social coercion. The psychotic paranoid patient's fear that others will exert influence over his behavior extends into the area of medication. The clinician who hands a prescription to the patient and says, "Take this according to the directions" will have little success. Instead, the clinician might advise the patient concerning the name of the medication as well as the therapeutic action and possible side effects to be expected. He can then ask the patient if there are any questions concerning the prescription. The patient is now a partner in planning the treatment and is more likely to work for its success.

Maintaining Openness and Consistency

The therapist works to establish a relationship with the remaining healthy portion of the patient's ego. It is not the patient's delusional system that requires treatment but the frightened, angry person who has created it. Firmness and steadiness characterize the secure therapist's attitude. The patient should be granted no special favors or privileges, and the clinician must maintain the most scrupulous honesty at all times. The punctuality, predictability, and consistency of the therapist's behavior are of great importance in enabling this patient to develop a trusting relationship. When a paranoid person is treated on an outpatient basis, a clear statement about the rules of treatment, the charges for missed sessions, and so on will help prevent misunderstandings that otherwise may threaten the therapy. For example, this patient can easily make the clinician angry by not respecting his personal rights or property.

The clinician does not help the patient by allowing him to intrude into his private life or to abuse the furniture in his office. The interviewer may sympathize directly with the patient's hate of hypocrisy, inconsistency, and unpredictability. Accurate perceptions should be reinforced, including perceptions about the interviewer, even though these may be negative. At all times, the interviewer must be forthright about areas of disagreement, making statements to the patient such as "We can agree to disagree." Such statements underline that the patient and interviewer each have their own identity. Whenever possible, the therapist can emphasize and support the patient's right and ability to make his own decisions.

Managing Anxiety in the Therapist

Some therapists have such strong dislike or fear of paranoid patients that they should not treat them until these problems are resolved. If the therapist is frightened of the patient's potential assaultiveness, he should conduct the interview only in the presence of an attendant or other adequate safeguard.

The paranoid patient tends to disrupt his relationship with the therapist as he has done with significant persons in the past, first by making him anxious and then by perceiving his reaction as a rejection. The therapist must understand that there is some validity in the patient's complaints. The paranoid patient requires a secure therapist whose self-esteem is not challenged by angry, and at times accurate, criticisms.

When the patient expresses hostile, critical feelings, the therapist who needs to be liked and appreciated will feel hurt and will respond with anger or withdrawal. When the patient expresses positive feelings, this therapist will accept the benevolent parental role that the patient ascribes to him, thereby inflating the clinician's ego and infantilizing the patient.

The interviewer may advise the paranoid patient that, in due time, he will grow suspicious of the therapist but that this does not justify terminating the relationship. Instead, it is an indication for exploration, improved communication, and a better mutual understanding of the clinician's and the patient's feelings. Because of the patient's extreme sensitivity to rejection, he must be prepared long in advance for any vacation or absence from treatment on the part of the therapist.

Infinite patience is required in order to tolerate the continuing mistrust and suspiciousness that are directed at the therapist. The patient's extreme sensitivity to criticism and his alternation between clinging submissive ingratiation and defensive aggression often stimulate anger in the therapist.

Avoiding Humor

The paranoid person thinks of himself as having a good sense of humor. In actuality, he lacks the ability to reflect on himself, to relax, and to accept the subtlety and ambiguity required for true humor. His sardonic laugh reflects his pleasure in the sadism or aggression in a situation, but more complex types of humor are beyond his grasp. The interviewer therefore should avoid witty or humorous remarks, particularly if they are directed at the patient, because this person has no sense of humor about anything applied to himself. He reacts to such attempts, no matter how skillfully conducted, as though the interviewer were making fun of him. Irony and metaphor are also dangerous, because the patient's concreteness makes him likely to miss the desired meaning.

The most frequent joke attempted by the therapist is an exaggeration of the paranoid patient's tendency to be suspicious or mistrustful. If the "clever" sarcastic remarks of the paranoid patient are returned in kind, the patient feels hurt and misunderstood. For example, a paranoid patient made sarcastic, humorous remarks about her therapist's scheduling her appointments during the lunch hour. The interviewer misperceived the meaning of the patient's "jokes" and quipped, "The next thing I know, you'll be accusing me of trying to starve you." Not long thereafter, the patient developed a delusion that the therapist was plotting her starvation. The inexperienced clinician displays his anxiety and unconscious hostility to the patient with such remarks.

Avoiding Inappropriate Reassurance

The interviewer sometimes offers inappropriate reassurance prior to understanding the patient's specific fears. For example, an obviously psychotic paranoid patient began an interview by asking a resident psychiatrist, "Do I seem 'crazy' to you?" The resident replied that he did not, thereby hoping to foster a supportive therapeutic relationship. Although some initial rapport was established by this method, the clinician soon learned that the patient had many crazy thoughts and feelings. By allowing himself to be manipulated, the clinician appeared naïve and foolish in the patient's eyes. It would have been better had he said, "What makes you ask if you are crazy?" or "Let's talk and see if there is anything crazy." The patient was testing the clinician to determine his willingness to admit uncertainty. The clinician's lack of hypocrisy, despite the coercive pressure for an insincere reply, would have been comforting.

Use of Interpretations

Understanding the Importance of Timing

Interpretations are intrusions in the patient's life, and paranoid persons are unable to tolerate intrusion. Clarification or explanations may be offered early in treatment, but interpretations must be delayed until a trusting relationship has developed.

Dynamic interpretations of grossly psychotic paranoid distortions must wait until the psychosis has improved. However, it is necessary to stimulate doubt and uncertainty in the patient's mind concerning his delusional systems. Teaching the patient to consider alternate explanations of his observations undermines his projective defenses. As an example, a patient reported that people in the apartment across the street were making videotapes of him. The therapist agreed that there might indeed be people across the street making videotapes but suggested that there might be other explanations of what was being filmed. When the patient argued that the purpose of the filming was to obtain evidence concerning his sexual practices, the clinician inquired whether the patient felt embarrassed and ashamed about his sex life. This was, in fact, the case, and it initiated a discussion of a major problem area.

Interpretations directed at the role the patient plays in bringing about his own misfortunes must be slow, gentle, and tentative. This topic can easily precipitate severe anxiety with total loss of self-esteem and overwhelming depression, a constant problem for the paranoid patient. When the patient does achieve some insight into this aspect of his behavior, he experiences a sense of acute panic and feels that the problem must be resolved magically, immediately, and permanently. For example, a therapist interpreted that the patient's fear of male figures of authority had caused him to behave provocatively with his boss. During the following session he reported, "Well, I have now solved that problem of being afraid of my father." Further exploration was thereby closed off. This makes any "uncovering" approach to psychotherapy difficult with a paranoid patient. The patient is unable to live up to his ego ideal and feels intense shame whenever the discrepancy is brought to his attention.

Early in treatment, the therapist can offer interpretive comments that are aimed at reducing the patient's guilt, even though the patient denies any feeling of guilt. The paranoid person is tortured by unconscious feelings of guilt, and such comments reduce his need to project his self-contempt onto others. Some early clarification of the patient's continuing search for closeness and his intense fear of it may be productive. Exploration of the patient's unconscious fears of homosexuality is best not pursued in the early or middle phases of therapy if they are not brought up by the patient and if the patient is able to deny the significance of such material.

Interpreting the Transference

When the patient produces fantasy material about the therapist in the early stages of treatment, it is helpful to provide appropriate realistic data and then to explore how the patient came to his own conclusions. An analysis of the paranoid patient's transference fantasies while the therapist remains anonymous is doomed to failure.

As a positive relationship evolves, the paranoid patient typically develops an unrealistic overestimation of his clinician as omniscient and omnipotent. The interviewer can diminish this projection of the patient's grandiosity by occasionally dropping specific data about himself that challenge the patient's idealized distortion. For instance, a paranoid man indicated that the clinician was always fair and reasonable. The therapist reminded the patient that he had once overheard the therapist speaking impatiently to the doorman. Another patient made a reference to a historical novel and the therapist indicated that he had not read that book. The patient immediately offered excuses for the clinician's ignorance, but the therapist remarked, "You have uncovered an area in which I am not well informed, and you seem reluctant to accept my deficiency." This technique can stimulate disturbing fantasies and must be utilized with caution and never early in treatment.

The interviewer can indicate to the paranoid patient that his recognition of slights may be quite accurate but that his interpretation of motives may be quite erroneous. The paranoid person views the world as though people had no unconscious motives and all acts were deliberate. The patient's accusations may pertain to the motivation of the interviewer. One of us had a patient who became justifiably angry when he found that the clinician had forgotten to leave the waiting room door unlocked and suggested that this was evidence of the therapist's wish to get rid of him. The therapist responded by admitting that he had left the waiting room door locked, thereby supporting the patient's right to be angry, but then added, "You are certainly entitled to analyze me if you wish to do so; however, isn't it only fair that you find out what I think happened and how I feel about it before jumping to conclusions concerning my motives?" In this way, the interviewer not only addressed himself to the patient's feeling of righteous indignation but also established a foundation for analyzing the patient's projective defenses. Every opportunity for the patient to expand his awareness of how he makes conclusions about the motives of others without adequate information has a therapeutic effect. It was later explained that the clinician was unlocking his front door when the telephone rang. He rushed to answer the phone, leaving the door ajar but still locked. A passerby closed the door, and soon thereafter the patient arrived. It is helpful to the paranoid patient for the clinician to show him that other factors in the interviewer's life not related to the patient may at times affect his mood and his treatment of the patient.

The therapist must be tolerant of the patient's overreactions to mistakes and shortcomings, an attitude that is the opposite of that expressed by the patient's parents. It is common for the patient to collect a series of minor grievances and temporarily withhold them from the therapist. He will often confront the clinician much later with something that the patient misinterpreted as a slight, quoting the therapist's exact words. While he keeps his injuries secret, the patient may feel superior to his therapist. The patient's tendency to withhold his resentments makes exploration and understanding impossible.

The paranoid patient attempts to maintain a one-up position by anticipating the clinician's behavior and interpretations, and he defends himself from their impact by analyzing the motivation behind the therapist's comments. The patient's eventual awareness of his underlying grandiosity and its role as a defense against feelings of worthlessness and inadequacy is only the beginning. It allows exploration of the developmental problems that led to the development of such defenses. The introduction of reality into the treatment process provides an important therapeutic lever. However, in discussing the patient's delusional system in terms of reality, the therapist must protect the patient from feeling humiliated.

The Dangerous Patient

The assessment of homicidal risk is in many ways quite similar to the assessment of suicidal risk. As with the suicidal patient, the interviewer inquires if the patient has formulated a specific plan as to how he would commit the murder and whether he has taken any action toward the implementation of this plan. The interviewer might ask if he has had similar feelings in the past and how he managed to overcome them on those occasions. A family history of murder or sadistic beating is of importance. Inquiry into past episodes in which the patient had lost control of aggressive impulses and the outcome of these episodes provides important data. A past history of vengeful, destructive behavior indicates that the patient may require external control. In this regard, the interviewer could inquire if the patient has ever caused anyone's death. A history of torturing and killing animals in childhood is pertinent to the assessment of homicidal risk. Such behavior is frequently found in the history of people who kill others. Precipitating stress is important in understanding the development of destructive impulses. When specific stresses can be uncovered, the clinician has a greater opportunity to recommend helpful manipulations of the patient's environment. Persons accompanying the patient, including police officers, should always be interviewed. Often the homicidal significance of the behavior is denied by the patient's relatives and professional personnel as well.

The interviewer should realize that it is possible to assassinate anyone. The patient who is unambivalent concerning his homicidal impulses is not likely to be interviewed by the clinician, or at least he will not mention these feelings. If the patient brings the subject up for discussion, this is already evidence that he has not completely decided to commit murder and may therefore be influenced away from this course of action. The interviewer can interpret that the patient is frightened and upset at the possibility of becoming a murderer and comment on the predicament in which the patient finds himself. The therapist offers to help the patient understand the reasons behind his desire to commit murder and to help the patient obtain additional control in restraining his impulses if needed. The latter may be in the form of medication or temporary hospitalization until the patient feels more capable of controlling himself. If the interviewer has evidence of homicidal intent, for example, if the patient states that he intends to kill someone for whatever reason, delusional or not, the confidentiality of the interview no longer applies. The clinician is legally bound to inform both the putative victim and the legal authorities of this declared intent. The patient should be informed that this action has to be taken because it is mandated by law.

> A 17-year-old adolescent was brought to the emergency department by his parents because he had become reclusive and refused to attend school. He had been seen obtaining information on firearms from the Internet and would sometimes lock himself in his room for hours. In the interview he was sullen and withdrawn, responding evasively when asked about violent or aggressive impulses. A history of fire setting and cruelty to animals was elicited from the parents. On one occasion he had almost choked another boy. He repeatedly denied any need for treat-

ment and asked to be allowed to return home. The interviewer told the patient, "I have the uneasy feeling that you may be planning to kill someone." The patient did not reply but looked away from the interviewer. The clinician continued, "Under the circumstances, I feel that you belong in a hospital until I am convinced that you are well enough to return home." On other occasions, the interviewer's admission of discomfort with the patient would facilitate the interview. He might say to the patient, "If you are trying to scare me, you are succeeding. I can't help you if you put me in this position, so let's try and find out why you need to do this!"

It is worthwhile to remember that the patient who threatens the life of a clinician often behaves in this fashion because he is afraid. The interviewer who realizes that the patient is more anxious than he is has a distinct advantage. For example, a frightening incident occurred when one of us, as a fourth-year medical student, had started to deliver a baby at the mother's home. The expectant father suddenly burst into the room, intoxicated and waving a pistol. He shouted, "The baby better be OK, Doc!" The student physician started to pack up his equipment and said, "If you don't put down that gun and leave immediately, I will leave your wife and not deliver the baby." The man put down the gun and left without further trouble.

Although a paranoid patient may be assaultive in initial interviews, it is rare for him to harbor specific homicidal impulses toward his therapist until treatment has progressed. It is easy to panic when a patient announces that he is formulating a plan to kill the therapist or some member of his family. It can be devastating for the patient if the interviewer panics and calls the police behind the patient's back, arranging for him to be hospitalized under force. The arrangements for hospitalization must be openly discussed, *with the patient under constant observation*, until they can be implemented. If the patient indicates that he is carrying a weapon, the clinician should ask him to relinquish it until the patient has reestablished confidence in his ability to control himself. The therapist might well remember that the patient fears he will be rejected because of his intense homicidal impulses. The therapist's ability to accept the patient in spite of these feelings will often lead to their prompt amelioration.

CONCLUSION

As this chapter has shown, the paranoid patient presents multiple challenges to the interviewer. Gradually, as psychotherapeutic treatment progresses, these patients can develop some understanding of how their attitudes and behavior affect others. As they learn to trust the support and affection of their therapist, they can then appreciate that life is not always black or white and that people are able to genuinely care about them without their becoming the center of their universe.

CHAPTER 14

THE PSYCHOTIC PATIENT

The psychotic patient poses special challenges for the interviewer. The patient with acute psychosis may be agitated, incoherent, and frightened, or he may be euphoric, aggressively overbearing, and delusional. For the interviewer who has had limited clinical exposure to patients with this degree of mental disturbance, considerable anxiety will be aroused, mirroring, to some extent, what the patient is also experiencing. While inwardly acknowledging this shared aspect of subjective state, the interviewer has to adopt a highly empathic response to the disorganization or heightened mood of the psychotic patient, one that is predicated on an attempt at understanding. What is the patient experiencing? How does he understand it? What does it mean for him? To some degree, the interviewer has to function as an external ego for the acutely psychotic patient, empathically connecting to and acknowledging the disruption of personality and the emotional storm that is sweeping through the patient.

The patient who has a chronic or insidious-onset psychosis poses a different set of problems. He may be suspicious, uncooperative, and withdrawn. Again the interviewer has to be highly empathic, patiently attempting to gain access to the patient's hidden world. The immediate countertransference danger for the interviewer dealing with either the acutely or chronically psychotic patient is that of objectifying him as "crazy" and "not-me." This is a defensive response in the interviewer engendered by an unconscious fear that "I, too, could become like this." As Sullivan aptly observed, the psychotic patient is "more human than otherwise." Being constantly cognizant of the validity of Sullivan's observation is crucial for establishing rapport with the psychotic patient and ensuring that the interview is therapeutic.

During the 1940s and on into the 1950s, Harry Stack Sullivan and his contemporaries at the Washington School of Psychiatry, William Alanson

White Institute, and Chestnut Lodge were particularly interested in the psychotic patient. Papers published by Frieda Fromm-Reichmann, Harold Searles, and others emphasized an empathic approach that they believed was helpful to these patients. They listened with great sensitivity in order to help the psychotic patient find understanding in the midst of internal chaos. Many psychotic patients responded to their clinician's attempts to understand them and bring some degree of order to their inner disorganization.

These patients were able to recognize the clinician's efforts to reach them, but this did not "cure" their psychosis. By the mid-1950s reserpine and chlorpromazine had been introduced as antipsychotic agents, and they often had a dramatic therapeutic impact, particularly with the acutely ill patient. Lithium carbonate became a standard treatment for bipolar illness in the late 1960s. Since that time, there has been a continuing development of newer and better antipsychotics. Unfortunately, this positive therapeutic development has led to a marked diminution in the attention given to understanding the subjective experience of the individual psychotic patient. Fewer clinicians have been interested in making sense out of the patient's strange behavior and peculiar communications except for the purpose of diagnostic classification and neurobiological research. In the clinical situation, psychosis has often been reduced to being simply a manifestation of disturbances in the patient's neurochemistry. Although we recognize the great value and potential therapeutic importance of neurobiological research and believe that psychotic disorders have an "organic" etiology, this chapter is dedicated to the psychological means of establishing a deep connection with the psychotic patient. We do not subscribe to a dualistic view that sees psychosis as simply a "brain disease" separate from the patient's psychological issues, neurotic conflicts, and problems in ordinary life. Psychosis is expressed through the personality of the individual patient; hence, that person's psychology, personal history, and particular character structure determine many aspects of the psychotic experience and should be recognized and addressed in both the interview and ongoing therapeutic work.

Like anyone else, the psychotic patient has neurotic conflicts. These may be obscured or exaggerated by the gross disruption of normal psychological function that the psychosis entails, but they should be recognized nonetheless because they will form the basis for psychotherapeutic work alongside appropriate psychopharmacological interventions. Psychodynamic insight into the personal meaning of the disorder and into the patient's capacity for attachment to others, especially the therapist, forms an essential foundation for therapeutic efforts. This makes the initial interview of critical importance. An interview with an empathic, connected, and unfrightened clinician who can accept the patient in the acute or chronic phase with all of his or her frightening or strange symptoms will often later be remembered by the patient as a positive, crucial healing experience. One sometimes encounters the mistaken notion that the acute, disorganized psychotic patient cannot be interviewed until he is medicated. A beginning psychiatric resident told his supervisor of a newly admitted psychotic patient: "I haven't interviewed the patient yet. We are waiting for the antipsychotics to work." They went to see the patient; the supervisor interviewed the patient, who calmed down and was responsive in the interview even though the medication had not yet taken effect.

Frequently the beginning clinician does not fully appreciate the patient's capacity to move into and out of psychotic mentation in a particular interview. In the days before the advent of modern antipsychotics, a recovering patient would often say, "Thank you for the hours that you sat with me. I felt that you cared despite the fact that I was so incapable of participating in the session." Although psychodynamic mechanisms are readily observable in psychotic patients, they do not cause the illness. Nevertheless they do reveal the patient's unconscious psychological conflicts.

In the absence of knowledge of specific biological markers, psychosis remains a phenomenological diagnosis. This is reflected in DSM-5. Psychosis represents a spectrum of disorders acute and chronic, and the reader is referred to DSM-5 for delineation of the diagnostic criteria that differentiate among them. The clinician's greatest contribution to both the initial interview and ongoing therapeutic work with the psychotic patient, alongside appropriate somatic interventions, is the maintenance of a thoughtful, sensitive, and, most important, highly empathic posture that can have a healing effect in its own right. This chapter focuses on the influence of psychosis on the interview.

PSYCHOPATHOLOGY AND PSYCHODYNAMICS

The Acutely Psychotic Patient

Positive and Negative Symptoms

The acutely psychotic patient usually presents with gross disturbances of thinking, affect, and behavior. The patient may appear profoundly mentally disorganized and behaviorally inappropriate. The interviewer should understand that he is encountering a massively altered state of consciousness causing, in the case of the schizophrenic patient, a frightening and phantasmagoric subjective experience or, in the case of the manic bipolar patient, often a wildly elated and euphoric experience. The acutely psychotic bipolar patient can, however, present with extreme dysphoria and agitation. The common thread in the acutely psychotic bipolar patient appears to be a radical *heightening* of mood states, whether euphoric, dysphoric, or mixed, accompanied by racing thoughts and increased psychomotor activity.

One conception of acute psychosis postulates three main sets of determinants. First, neurobiological disturbances lead to heightened awareness and intensification of normal sensory experience together with the invasion of perceptual and cognitive modalities. One patient described the onset of his illness in the following words: "I felt that the sun had filled my body and that light was emanating from me. I was radiant, a special enlightened being directly in touch with God." This initial ecstatic experience was transient and rapidly replaced by feelings of persecution and tormenting auditory hallucinations accusing him of evil. A second group of determinants are individual and reflect the patient's personality, history, and neurotic conflicts. These determine the particular content of the psychotic experience. "My father is the most dangerous person in the universe and must be destroyed," declared an acutely psychotic young man who was envious and in awe of his father's considerable financial power and influence. Finally, it is the psychosocial context of the patient's current life that determines the initial clinical presentation. A freshman college student who had been extremely homesick and anxious during his first two semesters became psychotic when he returned to college at the end of the spring vacation. Used to having his own private bedroom as a teenager, he had been particularly disturbed at having to share with a male roommate, a situation that had made him acutely self-conscious and uncomfortable. When he returned to the campus, he had the conviction that the whole university had been subjected to a nuclear holocaust and that everyone was dead. "I was walking through a huge cemetery covered in gray ash." This patient's illness responded well to a combination of medication and psychotherapy, and he went on to marry and have a productive career.

A useful clinical distinction has been made between the positive symptoms—hallucinations, delusions, thought disorder, and anxiety-driven agitation—found in both acutely schizophrenic and psychotic bipolar patients and the negative symptoms usually found in schizophrenia alone. Positive symptoms may reflect an exaggeration and elaboration of normal psychological processes. They commonly have "meaning" in terms of their content relevant to the psychodynamics of the individual patient.

Negative symptoms, which include blunted affect, impoverishment of thought, apathy, and the absence of pleasure in life (anhedonia), may be a reflection of the loss of ordinary psychological functions. This diminution of normal psychological experience is generally associated with chronic or insidious-onset forms of schizophrenia. Although less dramatic, and less "crazy" to a layman, the negative symptoms are associated with a more dire prognosis, are more resistant to treatment, and cause greater suffering over the course of the patient's lifetime.

Disturbances of Thought and Affect

The manic patient.   The acutely manic psychotic patient is often agitated or excited as if the psychic "thermostat" has been turned to high. The torrent of words, ideas, and tangential associations to external stimuli that pour out of the patient may elicit in the interviewer a sense of being overwhelmed. The affective state may be one of elation and wild expansiveness, a type of extreme grandiosity that can lead to spending sprees, promiscuity, and insistent claims by the patient for his genius and originality. The expansive mood state has an "enthusiastic" quality to it—everything within the patient's purview is "wonderful," "extraordinary," "marvelous," "original." The relentless energy and grandiose exuberance of the manic psychotic are exhausting to all around him, including the interviewer. Sleep disturbances are common, usually manifested in a radically decreased need for sleep. The manic individual will stay up all night telephoning friends, superficial acquaintances, and public agencies, barraging them with ideas, plans, and irrational schemes. Elation and euphoria may alternate with periods of intense irritability. When challenged or thwarted, he may become enraged and furious at the person who questions his extravagant claims and behaviors. The psychotic manic patient seems to have a type of psychic storm: tempestuous, wild, and wind-blown. It seems like a cerebral "discharge" phenomenon, overwhelming the surrounding psychological landscape with its fury. A bipolar patient described the ecstatic onset of his psychosis as follows: "From the very beginning, the experience seemed to be one of transcendence. The ordinary beauties of nature took on an extraordinary quality. I felt so close to God, so inspired by his spirit that in a sense I was God. I saw the future, organized the universe, and saved mankind. I was both male and female. The whole universe existed within me." This mystical elated state was transient and followed by a deep and dangerous depression wherein the urge to kill himself was incessantly forcing itself into consciousness.

One psychodynamic concept of the phenomenology of mania suggests that it can be compared to sleep. It is like the dream of a small child, with the wish fulfillments of the narcissistic pleasure ego. This view postulates that the ecstatic mood state of the manic patient relives the nonverbal experience of union at the mother's breast and is a defense against the painful frustrations and disappointments of life. One manic patient described her experience thus:

> At orgasm, I melt into the other person. It is hard to describe, but there is a certain oneness, a loss of my body in the other person, as if I were part of him without my individual identity, yet in him part of a larger whole. At other times, I am the dominant individual and he the lost one, so that I become the perfect whole—When he seemed to enter me, I gained his attributes, for example, his aesthetic taste, which was better than mine. It seemed as if I absorbed the beauty he made me aware of.

The first part of this description of sexual experience, the sense of oneness with the partner, is within the realm of normal ego regression that may occur in lovemaking. The psychotic element has to do with the second part, where ego boundaries are disturbed and personal identity is lost.

The acutely schizophrenic patient.   In contrast to the acutely psychotic patient with mania, whose secondary process is often still functioning, albeit in an accelerated and unrealistic form, the acutely schizophrenic patient may be sullen and withdrawn, mute or stuporous, or posturing bizarrely, or he may appear agitated and incoherent, beset by persecutory auditory hallucinations accusing him of evil and manifesting incoherent speech that makes it difficult for the interviewer to understand what he is attempting to say. In the more cognitively organized, acutely schizophrenic patient, apocalyptic end-of-the-world fantasies are common. This is often a projection of the internal mental catastrophe that has occurred within the patient. Delusional ideas may permeate his thinking. "Now I know what happened to me," related an acutely schizophrenic patient. "The CIA and the FBI have targeted me because I have special knowledge that will change the world." This fantasy had the narcissistic function of reassuring the patient that the intrapsychic chaos that had beset him had a purpose, that he was unique and was on a glorious mission. Such defensive fantasies are usually ineffective in calming the patient. They may become crystallized into a rigid and sustained delusional explanation for the subjective experience that has affected the patient. When this fades, the patient becomes more anxious and agitated. Fantasies such as these establish "meaning"—a universal human need—for that which is meaningless and overwhelming, in this case the experience of psychosis. "Why is this happening to me?" is replaced by "This is happening to me because I have a special calling."

Delusions and Hallucinations

As noted, delusions, which can occur in both manic and schizophrenic patients, may have a restorative function. They can represent an attempt at psychological repair and provide an explanation for the intrapsychic catastrophe that has occurred. A differentiating point between the delusions found in the manic patient versus the schizophrenic patient revolves around the *fixed*, crystallized, and unchanging form of delusion found in the schizophrenic patient. This contrasts with the *fluidity* of delusions in the manic patient, which keep shifting. It almost seems as though the manic patient is making up the delusions as he goes along, and they keep changing in content. One delusion will be dropped as another appears.

The ego defense mechanisms of projection and denial are central to a psychodynamic understanding of both delusions and hallucinations. Freud speculated that in hallucinations and delusions something that had been forgotten in childhood returns and forces itself into consciousness. For Freud, the essence was that there is not only *method in madness* but also a kernel of historical truth—that is, delusions contain, albeit in distorted form, an element of individual history. This formulation is relevant to the interviewer, who should not simply dismiss the delusional structure as "completely crazy" but rather be curious as to what its latent meaning might actually be and what aspect of reality and history relevant to the patient's life is contained in the psychotic elaboration. This may be helpful regarding areas to be explored after the patient is no longer psychotic.

Freud first drew attention to the utilization of the defense mechanisms of denial and projection in delusional formation. (For a more extensive account of Freud's conception of delusional formation, the reader is referred to Chapter 13, "The Paranoid Patient.") Later, Freud acknowledged the enormous role that aggression plays in delusional formation. Further developments in the psychodynamic understanding of both auditory hallucinations and delusional ideas emphasized the projection of the psychotic patient's superego. The persecutor observes and criticizes the patient—that is, the persecutor represents a projection of the patient's bad conscience. The patient may feel that he is being controlled, observed, and criticized for his sexual desires, which are depicted as dirty or forbidden. One psychotic patient lamented, "My thoughts are filthy and evil. I will be punished for them by God's retribution. I deserve to be persecuted in Hell for my sexual desires."

Delusions are not all simply persecutory, however. There are hypochondriacal delusions that the body is corrupted and diseased in some fashion, nihilistic delusions that the world has been or will soon be destroyed, grandiose delusions of being the new messiah or a Napoleonic individual who will change the world.

The Schizophrenic Patient Presenting in the Nonacute Phase

Schizophrenia is a chronic disease, and the majority of clinical contacts with schizophrenic patients will occur in the nonacute phase of the illness. Furthermore, many schizophrenic patients have an insidious and gradual onset to their illness. Such a patient does not generally present to the clinician in the acute agitated form described earlier. His withdrawal from the world and increasing social isolation, together with a tendency to conceal delusional ideas, may lead to the illness smoldering unaddressed by a clinician for months or years.

The family members of these patients sometimes collude in a form of denial, ascribing the patient's escalating withdrawn and odd behavior to "eccentricity." In such cases of family denial, help will only be sought when the patient's behavior reaches an intolerable crescendo.

Schizophrenic patients have the same problems and conflicts as neurotic or normal individuals—hopes and fears about family, work, sex, aging, illness, and so on. The schizophrenic person is an individual with an unusual way of thinking, feeling, and talking about the same subjects that all of us think, feel, and talk about. The interviewer can often serve his most valuable function by recognizing this and relating to the patient as a separate and important person.

Disturbances of Affect

The schizophrenic patient may show a disturbance in the regulation and expression of his affect or emotions. The interviewer normally relies on the patient's affective responses as a guide to how the patient is relating to him, and therefore he must adjust to the patient's mode of affective communication. With the schizophrenic patient, subjective emotional experience may be diminished, flattened, or blunted. In addition, the patient may have difficulty expressing and communicating the emotional responses of which he is aware. More subtle gradations of feeling tone are lost, and the emotionality that does emerge may seem exaggerated. Warm and positive feelings are sporadic and unreliable. The patient somehow fears them, as though his continued independent existence would be threatened if he felt tenderly toward another person. When affection does appear, it is often directed toward an unusual object. A schizophrenic patient may feel positively for his pet or someone with whom he has little real contact or whom others might consider far beneath him in social status. One young adult schizophrenic patient claimed to have no concern for her family but was intensely involved with her cat.

Some schizophrenic patients complain that they feel as though they are only playing a role or that other people seem to be actors. This phenomenon can also be seen in patients with personality disorders. The sensation of playacting results from the patient's defense of emotionally isolating himself in response to a disturbing situation. In this way he remains distant from both his own feelings and those of others. This is common in those with borderline personality. Those with histrionic or antisocial personality may also seem to be playing a role, but this is rarely described by the patient himself; rather, it is an observation of the interviewer, who perceives the patient's false self.

The physical and bodily components of affect may rise to central importance in the schizophrenic patient. These affective components, of course, are present in everyone, although they frequently occur without subjective awareness. The patient will often be fully aware of them but will deny their emotional significance and explain them as responses to physical stimuli. Thus an anxious schizophrenic patient may attribute the beads of sweat on his forehead to the warmth of the room, or a grieving patient will wipe away his tears as he explains that something got into his eye.

The interviewer may find it difficult to empathize or may not trust his own empathic responses to the patient. Affects that he expects to find in the patient do not appear, and the signs that normally help him to understand the patient's feelings are unreliable or denied. A successful psychiatric interview always involves emotionally significant communication, and if the patient appears to have minimal affect, the problem is to evoke and reach this affect while tolerating the patient's level of feeling and avoiding criticizing or challenging the patient's defensive capacity. Some therapists use dramatic or unusual methods to develop an affective interchange with relatively affectless patients. They realize that they must use their own feelings as stimuli before the patient will permit an emotional interaction to develop. This is preferable to a passive technique of emotional neutrality that allows the interview to unfold without emotion, but the interviewer must constantly monitor the difference between what is being avoided and what is not possible for the patient to acknowledge.

The beginning interviewer is reluctant to use his own feelings in so active a manner. He fears that he will create problems or disturb the patient and is concerned lest he inadvertently reveal too much about himself. He may indeed make mistakes, but if these help to generate an affective interchange where none was present, they may be preferable to a safer but emotionally bland approach.

The patient's feelings may seem inappropriate to the apparent content of his thought, to the interview situation, or to both. However, emotional responses are always appropriate to the patient's inner experience, although this may be hidden from the interviewer. After identifying the patient's emotions, the interviewer's task is to elicit and identify the thoughts that are linked to them. Often the patient has responded to something that seems trivial or unusual to the interviewer. The clinician will better understand the patient if he attempts to unravel the meaning of the patient's reactions as the patient experiences them. The interviewer should not expect customary emotional responses in a schizophrenic patient; the patient may sense this expectation and react by concealing his true emotions. For example, if a social acquaintance spoke of his mother's recent death, the spontaneous response would be sympathy and an indication of willingness to share the experience of grief. The interviewer's response to most patients would be similar. However, this might disturb a schizophrenic patient, because it would indicate that the clinician expected a response that differed from the patient's actual feelings. The patient would then react with evasion and withdrawal, unable to correct the interviewer's error. His true feelings would not emerge. An open-ended inquiry concerning his feelings allows the patient greater freedom in his response.

Disturbances of Thought

The schizophrenic patient often has difficulty organizing his thoughts by the usual rules of logic and reality. His ideas may emerge in a confused and bewildering sequence. Every conceivable aspect of organization is potentially defective, as exemplified by loosening of associations, tangentiality, circumstantiality, irrelevance, incoherence, and so forth.

The disorganization of thought and communication is not random. Although the etiology of such difficulties may ultimately be explained biologically, the process of disorganization can best be understood in a dynamic framework. Disorganization blurs and confuses, and it appears when the patient experiences emerging anxiety. The patient's confusion serves as a defense by obscuring an uncomfortable topic.

These cognitive defects have secondary interpersonal effects as well. Circumstantiality and tangentiality are likely to distance and annoy the listener and therefore may become a vehicle for expressing hostility. Gross incoherence and loosening of associations evoke sympathy, although at the cost of emphasizing the patient's difference from other people and promoting his social isolation. These effects may be exploited by the patient, usually unconsciously. In general, they should not be interpreted early in the treatment because they represent a minimal secondary gain that helps to compensate for a larger primary loss. Later they may become an important source of resistance that must be worked through.

The schizophrenic patient may also have difficulty with the symbolic aspect of language, manifested by his tendency toward inappropriately concrete or abstract thinking. Not only are the connections between words disturbed, but the words themselves may have a different range of meanings than is generally accepted by others and may become important in themselves rather than serve as symbols for underlying thoughts. The patient will frequently interpret the interviewer's words in a strangely literal way, such as when a patient was asked what had brought him to the hospital and he replied that he had taken the bus. At times the opposite will occur, as when a college student who was acutely psychotic complained of a fear that "My behavior has violated the categorical imperative." It was several hours before he revealed that he was worried about masturbatory impulses. He had transformed his guilty feelings into ruminations about abstract philosophical systems that deal with right and wrong. By the time he came to see the clinician, it was these philosophical systems, and not sexual thoughts, that consciously preoccupied him. Language functions that are normally autonomous may become involved with sexual or aggressive feelings. Seemingly everyday words are assigned special meaning. One young schizophrenic woman became embarrassed when the word "leg" was used in her presence because she felt that it had sexual significance.

In addition to difficulty in organizing his thinking and in maintaining an appropriate level of abstractness, the schizophrenic patient may accent obscure features while ignoring central issues. For example, a hospitalized man with paranoid delusions who had formerly worked as an attorney became involved in a campaign to get the United States out of the United Nations, writing letters to the president and members of Congress. At the same time, he was uninterested in resuming his regular employment or even in more traditional political activities. Another schizophrenic patient, a post office employee who had developed asthma, spent several years collecting affidavits attesting to the dust-ridden conditions to which he had been exposed during his employment. His realistic problems with his health, his family, and his occupation were ignored while he pursued a relatively small disability compensation. When his persistence was finally rewarded, he became even more disorganized.

The schizophrenic patient may spend much of his time preoccupied with fantasies that are unusual in content but have special meaning to the patient. If the patient trusts the interviewer enough to reveal them, they can provide valuable insights concerning his emotional life. However, the patient is often afraid to expose his fantasies to others. For the schizophrenic patient, as for any other person, fantasies represent a retreat from reality and an attempt to solve problems by constructing a private world. However, this universal function of fantasy may be less apparent because of the patient's personalized use of symbols and his peculiar style of thinking. Furthermore, he is not sure where fantasy stops. At times his overt behavior can only be understood in terms of his inner reality. The idiosyncratic nature of the fantasy may distract the interviewer from its dynamic significance. In general, the psychotherapeutic exploration of the dynamic origins of fantasies is best deferred until later in treatment, because prematurely focusing on his fantasy life may further impair his contact with reality. The psychological function of the patient's fantasy life is illustrated by the young man who spent many hours planning trips to other planets and developing methods for communication with alien beings. His life on Earth was lonely, and he had trouble mastering the more mundane art of communicating with friends and family.

The schizophrenic patient may develop more complex systems of ideas, entire worlds of his own, if his fantasies are elaborated. When reality testing is intact, these are confined to his mental life, but if the patient is unable to differentiate fantasy from reality, the fantasy becomes the basis of a delusion. Often these ideas are religious or philosophical in nature. As the patient struggles with the nature of his own existence, the struggles are generalized into questions about the meaning of the universe. Religiosity is a common symptom, and schizophrenic patients often turn to studies of religion or existential philosophy before seeking treatment more directly. Less sophisticated individuals may become deeply involved in their church, synagogue, or mosque, usually with the accent on fundamental questions of theology rather than the daily activities of the congregation. A preoccupation with the existence of God is a typical example. The more delusional patient may have the conviction that he receives messages from God or has a special relationship with Him.

Disturbances of Behavior

The chronically schizophrenic patient with prominent negative symptoms may lack initiative and motivation. He seems to not care what happens and is not interested in doing anything, fearing that any activity may reveal him as inadequate or incompetent. His obvious problems seem to distress his family or the interviewer far more than they do the patient himself. Like the apparent absence of affect, the seeming absence of purpose or motivation can provide the patient the secondary gain of avoiding discomfort. However, it often leads to frustration and hopelessness in others, further increasing the patient's isolation. At times the interviewer can overcome this defense by searching for those areas in which the patient remains capable of acknowledging involvement and, at the same time, exploring the fears that inhibit his interest in other aspects of his life.

Disturbances in Interpersonal Relations

The chronically schizophrenic patient may have difficulty relating to others. Dynamic psychotherapy utilizes the exploration of transference as a major tool in helping the neurotic patient to understand his conflicts and to modify his patterns of behavior. This assumes that the patient has a simultaneous nonneurotic relationship with the doctor that allows him to look at his transference feelings objectively. It was once thought that the schizophrenic patient did not establish a transference relationship and therefore could not be treated by psychodynamic psychotherapy. In fact, he often establishes an intense transference quickly, but the resulting feelings may threaten the basic alliance between patient and therapist. The greatest problem is thus to maintain the therapeutic alliance, and in view of this, interpretations of the neurotic origins of the transference must be focused on those that enhance the therapeutic alliance.

A close relative of the schizophrenic patient frequently seeks professional help for the purpose of better understanding a daughter, son, or spouse:

> A man in his early 60s had a chronically schizophrenic son, age 40. He complained to his consultant that he had invited his son to a fine restaurant. The son had attempted to be appropriate in order to please his father, who then scolded him severely for wearing a pair of dirty sneakers with his blue suit. The man added that he felt embarrassed and humiliated by his son's behavior. The consultant asked how he understood his son's behavior. He replied, "He did it to annoy me. I told him it was a dressy place and to wear a suit. Do you think I was too hard on him?" The interviewer replied, "Your son has no job or other connection to the world into which he was born except through you. He tried to please you, but he felt alienated from himself, disguised as a normal person. Those dirty sneakers are a reflection of his inner identity." The father appeared shaken and asked, "Is there something I can do to fix the pain that I caused him?" "Yes," the interviewer replied, "you can apologize to him and share your enlightened understanding of his dirty sneakers and ask him to dinner again." Two weeks later, he again invited his son to the restaurant, this time with no instructions. His son arrived in the same blue suit but wearing a brand-new pair of sneakers. The interaction led to a moving exchange between father and son.

Assertion, Aggression, and the Struggle for Power and Control

The schizophrenic patient sometimes harbors hostile and angry feelings that he experiences as overwhelming. The patient is anxious lest these hostile feelings emerge and he be allowed to destroy others. He usually suppresses his healthy assertive capacity along with his violent rage. His judgment is often poor in evaluating both his destructive potential and his ability to control it. Although excessive inhibition is the usual result, there are times when his fear seems well founded, and he may be capable of violence. Therapy attempts to develop his awareness and integration of both his inner hostility and his controls without forcing him into premature and frightening assertive behavior. One patient was unable to obtain a driver's license because he could not tolerate the frustration and resulting rage at having to wait in line, and he was fearful of his inability to control his responses. Months later he deliberately rammed his parents' car into a number of parked vehicles at a supermarket, creating a scene that resembled a demolition derby.

Suicide and Violence

Suicide is an ever-present danger with the psychotic patient. Suicide is the leading cause of premature death in both schizophrenic and psychotic bipolar patients. A careful inquiry into suicidal ideation is crucial in the interview, because the presence of suicidal ideation has been shown to be predictive. Most psychotic patients do not spontaneously report suicidal ideation, and the clinician must be active in the interview about inquiry into its presence and pervasiveness in the patient's mental life. This can be approached tactfully: "You have been so upset; I wonder if sometimes you think that life is not worth living?" If the patient responds by saying, "I do sometimes think it would be better if I weren't around" or some equivalent that may be euphemistically expressed—for example, "I'm such a burden" or "Life is such a torment"—this should precipitate more direct inquiry by the interviewer into how suicide would be effected. If the patient reveals a thought-out plan, this should alert the interviewer to the fact that suicide is an imminent danger. The concomitant presence of depressive symptomatology—"The world is empty"; "I'm such a failure"; "Nothing has any meaning"; "I have no pleasure in life"; "It all seems worthless"; or "My situation is hopeless"—is also a red flag to the interviewer that suicide is a real possibility.

Command hallucinations to kill themselves or harm others are critical indicators for potential suicide or violence in schizophrenic patients. Although only a small minority of schizophrenic patients are violent, schizophrenia is associated with an increased risk of aggressive behavior. Some schizophrenic patients may act on their paranoid delusions, and the interviewer should not only empathically explore the nature of the patient's delusions but also ask whether he is tempted to take action against those whom he feels are harmfully investigating him or whom he feels are persecuting him.

Comorbidities

The most common comorbidity in schizophrenia is substance abuse. Schizophrenic persons have six times the risk of developing a substance use disorder that the general population has. It is possible that the attraction to mind-altering substances is predicated on a desire to control and change the painful mental state that the schizophrenic patient often endures. However, the use of such substances can precipitate exacerbations of the disorder, and the interviewer should carefully investigate the patient's use of drugs and alcohol, which when regularly abused indicate specific treatment.

Both alcoholism and substance abuse are common comorbid conditions in bipolar illness. Substance abuse may exaggerate mood states or precipitate acute episodes, and careful inquiry should be made by the interviewer concerning the bipolar patient's use of these agents. The combination of alcohol or drug abuse with bipolar illness can be particularly deadly, and the clinician must monitor this issue with great care. When the bipolar patient slides into the depressed side of the disorder, the use of alcohol or sedatives as self-medication can easily lead to overdose and death.

MANAGEMENT OF THE INTERVIEW

It may be difficult to establish emotional rapport with a psychotic patient, but as with any other patient, this is the primary task of the interviewer. The patient's intense sensitivity to rejection may lead him to protect himself through the use of isolation and withdrawal. In most psychiatric interviews the patient is encouraged to reveal his conflicts and problems with as little intervention as possible from the interviewer. The clinician serves as a neutral empathic figure who recognizes the patient's needs but does not gratify them directly and who avoids becoming involved in the patient's life outside the sessions. The interview with a psychotic patient requires modification. The patient feels rejected if the interviewer merely recognizes his needs. It is necessary for the clinician to convey his understanding more actively by expressing his own emotional response or by providing symbolic or token gratification for the patient's needs.

Should the psychotic patient ask the interviewer to recommend a coffee shop near the office, the therapist should answer directly and provide the information without further interpretation. With a neurotic patient, on the other hand, the therapist might provide the information and also register and possibly interpret the unconscious wish incorporated in the patient's request, for example, a wish for dependency gratification or for the avoidance of more meaningful material. In the early phase of work with the psychotic patient, the clinician accepts whatever limited emotional contact is possible. The patient will accept gratification from the therapist only on his own terms. The therapist should accept these terms as the basis for the initial relationship as long as they are within the realm of reality.

Prior history of psychiatric hospitalization, medication, and other treatments are an important area of inquiry. This includes dates, duration of hospitalizations, and names and dosages of medications. A history of side effects is also crucial, because these are the major reasons that patients do not comply with a treatment plan. An encounter illustrating this occurred some years ago when a colleague consulted one of us regarding a patient with chronic schizophrenia who seemed to be re-experiencing psychotic symptoms:

> The author listened to the story and suggested that he was the wrong consultant and that it sounded like the patient should consult a psychopharmacologist. The colleague persisted: "You are the right person to see this patient." The author accepted the request only to learn after the first 15 minutes of the interview that the patient had secretly discontinued her medication because of unpleasant side effects. The consultant remarked to the patient in a warm tone, "You like Dr. A, don't you?" "Very much," the patient replied. The interviewer continued: "You wouldn't want to disappoint him, would you?" The patient appeared sad and outpoured her confession of discontinuing her medication. The interviewer asked her permission to report his findings to Dr. A in a manner that he was certain would not hurt Dr. A's feelings and told her that Dr. A would help her further with this problem. She had lied to her psychiatrist because "He is so nice, and I know he cares about me and wants to help me, but I didn't want to hurt his feelings by rejecting his medication." This revelation opened an important area for psychotherapeutic exploration and interpretation. In a jocular tone, the consultant showed his report to his colleague. "I told you that it sounded like your patient had a medication problem," he said. The treating doctor replied, "I told you that you were the right consultant." This is not a unique or even unusual experience working with bipolar or schizophrenic patients.

The Acutely Psychotic Patient

Although the acutely psychotic patient may sometimes present in the clinician's office after making a scheduled appointment, many are encountered in the emergency department, where they are often brought by family, friends, or social agencies.

The patient's agitation, fueled by his acute anxiety, is often the most prominent clinical feature and requires both somatic and psychological interventions. The interviewer's most important psychotherapeutic intervention during this acute phase is that of providing psychological support and a "container" for disruptive affects—what amounts to an external ego for the patient. The patient's reality testing is often fragmented, and the interviewer, by adopting a calm, measured, empathic approach, can provide an external psychological structure that helps to mitigate the patient's sense of internal chaos. The interviewer has to self-monitor the danger of being "infected" by the patient's rampant anxiety. He must soberly assess the patient's potential for violent or self-destructive behavior. In extreme cases, external restraints may be necessary to prevent the patient from violent outbursts, elopement, or attempts to commit suicide.

When the acute, agitated phase has subsided, the interviewer can begin an exploration of the precipitating event. What factors, intrapsychic or contextual, triggered the onset of the illness? A careful inquiry into drug use should be made, from the patient if possible or from family or friends, because many agents—such as cocaine, methamphetamine, and phencyclidine—can induce an acute psychosis. The interviewer must sort through the chaos of the patient's acute psychosis to discern the sequence and role of events, conflicts, and symbolic or real losses that may have led to the acute illness. The psychotic patient may possess a biological diathesis for the disease, but environmental precipitants are usually involved in onset or acute exacerbations. An example is the acutely psychotic young adult who stated wistfully, "I'm due to be married in 2 months. Maybe this is making me crazy. Marriage scares me, even though I love my fiancée." This patient was indeed terrified of this developmental step. Each developmental milestone involves losses as well as gains. In this patient's case, the loss was that of being an adored child with omnipotent parents who would always protect him. He was torn between the desire to be a child and his attraction to his fiancée and wish to be grown-up. This conflict, combined with genetic vulnerability, had indeed driven him "crazy."

Careful inquiry into the nature of the patient's delusions can be very productive in understanding both acutely and chronically schizophrenic patients. A delusion provides special access into getting to know the patient because it embodies his core wishes and concerns. The delusion is a special creation, much like the dream, which in Freud's words is "the royal road to the unconscious." For the patient, the delusion explains everything. It is not a false belief, a universal phenomenon in normal human psychology, but a defensively held, fixed belief system that is clung to in spite of evidence to the contrary. The interviewer should not argue with the patient about the irrationality of the delusion but be curious as to its content and larger meaning for the patient. It is a creation with significant individual meaning.

The bizarre behavior of a regressed, acutely psychotic patient has a disconcerting effect on most interviewers. The patient may sit on the floor in the corner of the room, holding his coat over his head, or constantly interrupt the interviewer to converse with a third, but nonexistent, person. The interviewer can help this patient to control such behavior and promote rapport by indicating that he expects something different. If the behavior does not annoy the clinician, he might say, "Are you telling me that someone considers you to be crazy?" Another interviewer might sit on the floor in the corner with the patient. This indicates that the interviewer is neither impressed nor intimidated by the patient's behavior. If the clinician is annoyed, it is best to first explore the hostile or provocative aspect of the patient's behavior. The impact of the mental health practitioner communicating his expectations is illustrated by the clinician who was called to the emergency department to see an acutely psychotic patient who was standing in a corner and shouting at the staff, "Repent of your sins…Jesus saves!" The clinician interrupted the patient and said, "You'll have to sit down here and stop screaming for a few minutes if we are going to talk." The patient responded promptly to the interviewer's expectation of normal social behavior.

The patient's behavior may include inappropriate demands upon the interviewer. A patient may enter the office and, without removing his overcoat and two sweaters, ask that the interviewer turn off the heat and open the window because he may become overheated and then catch a cold when going out-of-doors. The interviewer is well advised not to comply with such unrealistic demands. In exploring the content of a delusional system, the interviewer may ask questions concerning the details of the delusion as though the delusion were reality. In taking a genuine interest in the content of the patient's delusions, it is important that the interviewer not suggest that he believes them. In the case just mentioned, the interviewer could ask the patient if his mother used to caution him about catching cold when he went out-of-doors in an overheated state. If the inquiry is productive, the clinician could inquire about what feelings accompanied the experience.

If the patient exhibits destructive behavior, the interviewer should stop the patient from doing damage to the interviewer's or the hospital's property, because it is not helpful to allow a patient to infringe on the rights of others. The patient who is permitted to continue such behavior will often become ashamed and guilty when he is less psychotic and will justifiably be angry with the clinician who did not supply the needed controls.

Development of the Therapeutic Alliance

The most common problem encountered in the interview with the psychotic patient involves the consequence of his inner disorganization. Furthermore, the psychotic patient's difficulty in organizing his thinking can be used defensively to avoid communicating with others. For example, a psychotic patient may speak freely from the beginning of the interview, manifesting little anxiety or hesitation; however, the interviewer soon encounters difficulty in following the trend of the conversation. The patient starts to answer a question but then leaves the topic. The interviewer may respond with confusion, boredom, or irritation. Often he does not recognize that the patient has changed the subject until the patient is in the middle of a new topic. On other occasions, the patient may seem to adhere to the topic under discussion; his words and even his sentences make sense, but somehow they do not fit together. This disorganization tests the interviewer's interest and attention and serves to block effective communication. The interviewer must reveal his difficulty in understanding the patient rather than responding, as in most social situations, with feigned understanding and concealed boredom, eagerly anticipating the termination of the contact. He can support the patient by avoiding statements that tend to berate him or that suggest that he is responsible for the interviewer's lack of understanding. Rather than saying "You're not making yourself clear," the interviewer can say, "I'm having difficulty following what you are saying." Similarly, "I don't understand how we got on this subject" is preferable to "Why do you keep changing the subject?"

Although it may be possible to understand the content of the disorganized patient's communication, it is nevertheless important to deal with the process of disorganization and its effect upon the developing relationship between the interviewer and patient. The long-term goals of treatment include helping the patient to communicate more effectively with other figures in his life as well as with the therapist.

Disorganization is sometimes apparent within the first few moments of the interview. The patient may be unable to describe a chief complaint. He might say, "I haven't been feeling too well lately" or indicate that one of his close relatives thought that he should come to see the clinician. One young man came to a hospital emergency department late at night asking to see a psychiatrist but was unable to formulate any specific problem; he simply stated that he was upset. His waxlike face and vacant stare suggested a psychotic illness. When the clinician directly inquired about his current life, he revealed that he had just come back from a business trip and had discovered that his wife had taken their small child and left him. He felt panicky and helpless, but in his own mind he did not connect these feelings with the traumatic events that he had just experienced.

When a patient answers the interviewer's opening inquiry with a vague reply, it is helpful to inquire whether the patient himself decided to consult a clinician. If the patient indicates that it was not his own idea, the interviewer can explore why another person felt that such a consultation was indicated. Furthermore, the interviewer might inquire whether the patient felt he was "dragged against his will" or pressured to come. Sympathizing with the patient's resentment concerning such a process facilitates early rapport.

The interviewer might then inquire if this is the first time that the patient has consulted a clinician. If not, prior contacts are carefully explored. In discussing previous psychiatric contacts, explicit inquiry about past psychiatric hospitalization is important. Psychotic patients often indicate that there have been prior hospitalizations but seem unable to describe what led to them. The interviewer could ask about the circumstances of the hospitalization and inquire about the symptoms. It is appropriate to inquire about a previous history of secondary symptoms with every grossly psychotic patient. While making these inquiries, the interviewer communicates his interest in understanding the patient rather than his interest in establishing a diagnosis. For example, instead of merely asking the patient if he heard voices, the interviewer would go on to ask what they said, how the patient interpreted them, and what he felt had caused these experiences. If the patient does describe the symptoms of previous psychotic episodes, the interviewer can inquire about their recurrence in the present. With regard to delusions, the interviewer should inquire as to what the belief is, how systematized and elaborated the delusion is, how the patient feels other people view his convictions, and how certain he is of his delusional conviction.

The clinician actively assists the psychotic patient in defining problems and focusing on issues. This is true even for the patient who does not have a serious disorganization of thought processes. Despite such efforts, some patients remain unable to identify the problem that is the theme for the interview. The interviewer can help by pursuing specific precipitants of the request for consultation. Questions such as "What was the final straw?" or "Why did you come today rather than last week?" may be helpful. It is also valuable to inquire about the patient's expectations of the interview. For example, if he communicates that he has difficulty finding a job, the interviewer attempts to pinpoint the specific difficulty encountered. The interviewer can gradually shift the focus from the external environmental problem to the intrapsychic issues. Often this will involve interpretive comments concerning precipitating stresses in the patient's current life. As an illustration, the interviewer might say, "Your trouble at work seems to have started at the time that your wife became ill. Perhaps this upset you in some way?"

It is easy to overlook the adaptive skills of psychotic patients. In focusing the interview, the clinician should direct attention to the patient's assets and areas of healthy functioning as well as to his pathology. The emphasis of the interview thereby shifts from exposing the patient's deficiencies to supporting his attempts to cope with the stresses in his life and the conflicts within himself. This also involves an evaluation of the patient's living situation. With whom does he live? What is the nature of their relationship? Can the patient take care of himself, pay the rent, cook meals, take his medication? What has he done recently that he enjoyed? What are his interests?

The interview may seem to be rambling or aimless despite the interviewer's attempt to provide structure. In this situation, the interviewer looks for topics and themes that recur repeatedly, even though they may not occur sequentially in the interview. Thus, the interviewer might say, "You keep coming back to the trouble with your boss. I guess it is on your mind." Even if the interpretation is inaccurate, this comment indicates an interest in searching for the meaning of the patient's thoughts rather than treating them as incoherent productions. Accuracy is only one determinant of the effect of any interpretation. Timing, tact, and the transference meaning of the interpretive activity are all important factors that influence its impact on the patient. The patient can be helped by observing how the interviewer tries to determine what is happening regardless of whether the attempt is successful. In addition, the therapist tries to demonstrate that he is interested in understanding rather than judging or condemning. Accuracy becomes increasingly important as a patient learns to trust the therapist and to use the insights that he gains in therapy. This process is particularly slow with psychotic patients, and therefore it is an error for the therapist to refrain from interpretive activity early in the treatment because he is not sure what is happening. If he is open about his uncertainty and invites the patient to join him in a search for meaning, the development of a therapeutic alliance will be fostered even if he is wrong in his interpretation. Phrases such as "I'm not sure I fully understand what has been happening here, but it seemed to me…" or "I'm sure that this is only part of it, but could it be…" are helpful.

As the patient becomes better acquainted with the clinician, he may reveal a surprising degree of insight into the social significance of his disorganized thought processes. For example, one young woman explained that when another person would nod in agreement even though she knew that the person did not really understand her, her communication would become even more diffuse and incoherent.

Some patients express acute emotional turmoil in association with the disorganization of their thought processes. The interviewer first works with this patient's feelings. He utilizes any communication that seems related to the patient's overall feeling tone and links it to the emotion the patient displays. For example, an agitated, disturbed young woman appeared in the emergency department of the hospital muttering incoherently. The interviewer empathically inquired about what she was muttering, stating that if he could hear her words, perhaps he could understand what was happening to her. She became more coherent and revealed that her husband had just abandoned her and that she was laying a "curse" on him so that he would die a terrible death because of his cruel behavior toward her and their children. She calmed down considerably after she revealed this.

ROLE OF THE CLINICIAN

The patient's disturbance of affect leads to an extension of the clinician's traditional role. The patient may be better able to express his emotions in response to some similar expression on the part of the interviewer. Therefore the interviewer follows the patient's emotional cues and utilizes them to develop the affective tone of the interview. These cues may be difficult to detect, and the interviewer may have to be active in helping the patient both experience and express his own feelings. He may directly inquire if the patient is experiencing some particular feelings, asking, for example, "Are you angry right now?" The patient will often respond to such interventions with a total denial of any feeling similar to that suggested by the interviewer. After acknowledging that he may have been wrong, the interviewer can then discuss his difficulty in determining the patient's feelings. This will lead to an examination of the motivational aspects of the patient's defenses against feeling rather than to an argument about who knows more about the patient's inner mental state. If such an exploration is premature, the interviewer can let the subject rest. It is common for a psychotic patient to vigorously deny a response suggested by the interviewer and then, weeks or months later, refer to the episodes as though he had been in complete agreement.

There are occasions when the interviewer has no idea what the patient is feeling and the interview seems dull and flat. Flatness and the lack of interaction reinforce the patient's sense of loneliness, isolation, and alienation. The interviewer might utilize his own emotional response in such situations as a guide to the further conduct of the interview. To illustrate, the interviewer could say, "As I listen to your description of your life, a sense of boredom and loneliness comes through. Perhaps you have similar feelings?" or "It sounds as if your life feels purposeless and filled with meaningless detail. Was there ever a time when it was different?"

When the treatment has progressed sufficiently, the clinician may modify his role in other ways. For example, a patient might come into the office and comment, "It's a beautiful day outside." The clinician who has developed a stable positive relationship with the patient might agree and add, "Shall we go out for a walk?" The spontaneous suggestion of a change in routine may open up areas of rigidity in the patient, expose fears about obtaining forbidden pleasure, or initiate a discussion about his perception of the therapist as a real person. If the patient is able to accept such contact with the clinician, an opportunity is provided for sharing a new experience. The therapist must feel comfortable before making such a suggestion or the patient may perceive and interpret his discomfort as indicating that the therapist is ashamed to be seen with the patient in public. In the situation just described, the patient responded to the clinician's suggestion by stating, "You probably have colleagues in this neighborhood. Suppose one of them saw you walking with me?" The clinician responded, "So, then what?" "They would wonder what you were doing walking with this bag lady." This interchange led to a productive discussion while they walked.

Interpretations of the Defensive Pattern

With the ego's weakened capacity for repression, the psychotic patient may reveal unconscious material in the initial interview that would take months to uncover in a neurotic patient. The beginning interviewer is often intrigued by hearing the patient discuss conflicts that are normally unconscious in the same terms that appear in a textbook. However, the patient's intellectual insight into the unconscious is not to be encouraged, because it is a manifestation of basic psychopathology. The psychotic patient may sense that the clinician has become intrigued and might continue to produce such material in order to maintain his interest. The interviewer can best respond to such productions by asking the patient if he was helped by his attempt to understand his "Oedipus complex" or whatever other term the patient may have used. If the patient indicates that he was not, the interviewer can ask why the patient wishes to discuss the topic or suggest that they direct their attention to some other area that might be more helpful, while recognizing that the patient is trying to be cooperative with the therapy.

It is valuable to explore the minute details of day-to-day living with the psychotic patient, because it is his difficulty with these aspects of life that drives him to a defensive retreat and a world of his own. For example, a young psychotic woman came to the session after a shopping expedition that left her quite depressed. She was silent for the first 10 minutes, but with the clinician's encouragement, she related her conversation with the salesperson, and it became apparent that she had been coerced into buying something that she did not want because of her guilt about wasting the woman's time. She had been quite unaware of her response, or of her anger and withdrawal that followed it, and had felt only a sense of gloom. However, she was able to report the events in detail, and with the therapist's help, she reconstructed and reexperienced her emotional responses as well. Patterns such as this will require multiple new experiences of a similar nature before the patient can acquire the psychological template required to extinguish the old way.

On some occasions, the clinician's successful understanding of some aspect of a patient's private fantasy life may intensify the patient's fear of having his mind read and of losing his identity. The patient may retreat to a defensive posture, and his communication may become more obscure. It is important that the clinician then acknowledge his inability to understand, because this will reassure the patient that he is able to establish a separate identity and that he will not fuse into oneness with the interviewer.

> A seriously disturbed young woman had developed a strong positive tie to her therapist after several years of work. One day she presented a dream, an unusual event in the treatment, that concerned her anger at a grade-school teacher who had paid less attention to her than to her classmates. As was characteristic, she had no associations. The therapist intuitively understood the dream as soon as he heard it, recognizing its

transference implications and relating them to an attractive woman whom the patient had seen in his waiting room the preceding day. He told the patient his associations, and she was silent for some minutes. She then said that she thought that dreams were meaningless anyway and that was why she rarely discussed them. Over the next few months, she became increasingly guarded and evasive, until she finally quit treatment. Certainly this single episode was not the only cause, but it came to symbolize her fear that therapy represented a threat to her personal integrity and that as long as she was a patient, she could not maintain her personal boundaries.

The interviewer will be more successful if he attempts to see the world as it appears through the patient's eyes. In order to accomplish this, he must be prepared to share the patient's loneliness, isolation, and despair. The psychotic patient may evoke feelings of confusion and intense frustration in the clinician. It is often helpful if the therapist admits to the patient that he is experiencing such emotions and inquires whether the patient is experiencing similar feelings.

Ancillary and Ongoing Treatment

Although clinical research has dispelled pernicious notions of psychosis originating as a result of pathological parenting, there is considerable evidence that concurrent family interventions are useful. Psychoeducational family treatment efforts emphasizing emotional, empathic support for the patient while acknowledging the frustration, anger, and guilt that the family may experience in their dealing with him are directed at helping the psychotic patient's family deal with a debilitating illness. Simultaneously, the clinician has a crucial role in fostering and preserving a therapeutic alliance with the patient. Such an alliance helps to maintain medication compliance and makes the patient a partner in recognizing early exacerbations of the illness that require active psychopharmacological intervention. Helping patients develop insight into their illness, its reality, its meaning, and its value in understanding themselves and their conflicts can be highly therapeutic. For the patient with chronic psychosis, small gains in everyday functioning should be acknowledged and applauded by the clinician.

CONCLUSION

The clinician's psychotherapeutically supportive, consistent, and emotionally constant individual involvement with the psychotic patient—

an approach that is sensitive to both psychodynamics and the crippling impact on self-esteem that psychosis causes—can be of crucial healing benefit. This was eloquently expressed in a written account by a schizophrenic patient:

> Can I ever forget that I am schizophrenic? I am isolated and I am alone. I am never real. I playact my life, touching and feeling only shadows. My heart and soul are touched, but the feelings remain locked away, festering inside me because they cannot find expression…. One of the hardest issues for me to deal with has been trust. My mind has created so many reasons to fear the real world and the people in it that trusting a new person or moving to a new level of trust with a familiar person presents a terrifying conflict that must be hammered out over and over until I can find a way to overcome my fears or in a few cases give up the battle, even if just for the time being. The intensity of this conflict makes it hard to build relationships. It's hard for the family to help. It's difficult for them to understand the nature of the disease. Therapy with schizophrenics can go for years before a level of trust is built up sufficiently for the patient to use his therapist as a bridge between the two worlds he is confronted with. For me, each new experience of trust adds a new dimension to my life and brings me that much closer to living in reality.

CHAPTER 15

THE PSYCHOSOMATIC PATIENT

JOHN W. BARNHILL, M.D.

Everyone has psychosomatic aspects of their emotional lives. Reactions such as rage, guilt, fear, and love have physiological components mediated through the neuroendocrine system, and that same system can directly affect subjective aspects of emotion and cognition. These relationships among brain, mind, muscles, immune system, mood, cognition, and perception are dauntingly complex even before adding in variables such as age, licit and illicit drugs, motivation, and patterns of psychological conflict and defense.

Evaluating psychological components of a physical symptom is, therefore, complicated. Traditional questions to be answered in making this determination include the following:

1. Does the patient's symptomatology not fit into a known pattern of organic disease?
2. Can the physical symptoms be explained in terms of the patient's emotional conflicts?
3. Were emotional or interpersonal stresses prominent in the patient's life at the onset of the condition or clearly related to remissions and exacerbations?
4. Does the patient attach unusual psychological meaning to his symptoms?
5. Can a psychiatric condition be diagnosed, and are the physical symptoms consistent with this diagnosis?
6. Does the patient obtain secondary gain from his illness?

The exact degree to which such psychological factors contribute to physical complaints often remains uncertain. This uncertainty can frustrate everyone involved, including the psychiatrist, other physicians, and the patient. This chapter outlines an approach to the psychosomatic patient that emphasizes alliance building as well as techniques that can help determine the degree to which psychological factors are contributing to the physical complaints.

PSYCHOPATHOLOGY AND PSYCHODYNAMICS

Range of Psychopathology

There are multiple categories of psychosomatic illness. First, patients can have a psychological reaction to medical illness. The news of a serious illness may cause a previously healthy person, for example, to become sad or to have a catastrophic psychological response with prominent denial and distortion. Included in this category would be exacerbations of long-standing personality or Axis I disorders. Second, patients can have a medical illness that physiologically induces a psychiatric syndrome. For example, certain cancers evoke a cytokine cascade that can cause depression and irritability, which may in fact be the first sign of the malignant process. A third group of psychosomatic patients have definable medical illnesses that are worsened by psychological distress. Examples include irritable bowel syndrome, psoriasis, and asthma. This would also include a cluster of incompletely characterized disorders such as fibromyalgia, chronic fatigue syndrome, and multiple chemical sensitivities.

Two additional groups of psychosomatic patients tend to arouse particular physician concern. Somatoform patients have physical complaints that lack organic explanation and are presumed to have a psychological etiology. An example is conversion disorder, in which the complaints are neurological. A patient may present with seizures, but the movements do not appear typical and the electroencephalogram is negative. As with all somatoform disorders, the medical problem is not the result of intention but reflects unconscious conflict and anxiety. A final group of patients consciously fakes symptoms. The patient might be faking for obvious gain, as in malingering, or the patient might have factitious disorder in which he consciously feigns illness for reasons that are not clear to the patient but relate to being in the sick role. A severe variant of factitious disorder is Munchausen's syndrome, in which the pursuit of the sick role may lead patients to long hospitalizations, repeated surgeries, and even death.

In practice it is difficult to make these clinical distinctions. There are no definitive diagnostic tests for any psychosomatic illness. Some of the diagnostic distinctions rely on assumptions about unconscious processes, and it is unusual for the physician and patient to agree on a diagnosis of somatoform disorder, factitious disorder, or malingering. Finally, individual patients tend to straddle diagnostic boundaries. In any one patient, cancer might lead to a psychological response of sadness as well as a cytokine-mediated depressive response. The same patient's anxiety might lower his pain threshold and cause a dormant case of fibromyalgia to flare up, leading to multiple ill-defined pains that do not conform to the oncologist's expectations. That same patient might then seek pain medications by consciously dramatizing his pain symptoms while also seeking the sick role by exaggerating his level of disability. It is not surprising, then, that primary care physicians tend to view psychosomatic patents with trepidation.

Psychodynamic Issues

There are a broad range of psychodynamic issues that apply to the psychosomatic patient. For example, physical illness tends to induce regression. Depending on basic character structure, one patient may lapse into a helpless and dependent state, another may become sad and anxious, and yet another may appear to obtain significant gratification from his dependency. Disease can induce particular suffering in patients who unconsciously experience the illness as a punishment for prior misdeeds. Other patients use projection to convert this suffering into a punishment of loved ones while they appear to feel normal.

Denial is a common mechanism of defense in the psychosomatic patient. Even when the acknowledgment of emotional conflict is inescapable, the patient may deny any relationship of the conflict to his symptoms. For example, physical symptoms frequently have an overlay of neurotic complaints built upon a minimal degree of organic pathology. Physicians sometimes feel that these symptoms will disappear as soon as the minor physical ailment is clarified and treated. Instead, many of these patients end up feeling misunderstood by their physicians and cling even more tightly to their complaints.

Specific psychodynamic constellations have been proposed to explain the etiology of such medical disorders as asthma, peptic ulcers, hypertension, and inflammatory bowel disease. These attempts to predict symptoms from dynamic formulations have been largely unsuccessful. Not only are the psychological conflicts nonspecific, but their importance in the etiology of each condition is unknown and probably varies considerably.

Many people use their bodies as defenses. In somatization, painful emotional feelings are transferred to concern about body parts. This can make psychotherapy frustrating because such patients are unable to use words to describe feeling states. Conversion is characterized by the representation of intrapsychic conflict in physical and often symbolic terms. This can be seen in a young man whose urge to hit someone led to the psychogenic paralysis of his arm. In so doing, he converted his conflict over an unacceptable wish into motor symbolization and developed a conversion disorder.

Unconscious processes affect everyone, however, and they do so in ways that have more to do with the individual than with the particular medical complaint. The interview of the psychosomatic patient should, therefore, be aimed at understanding the person rather than applying preformed psychodynamic theories to a symptom cluster.

Differential Diagnosis

Many patients have physical complaints that are secondary to a primary Axis I disorder, and these, although "psychosomatic," are not discussed in this chapter. For example, many patients with major depression present with solely somatic complaints. Similarly, anxiety can increase the tendency to focus on physical sensations, and panic disorder often mimics a heart attack. Alcohol and substance abuse lead to insomnia, aches and pains, and a variety of withdrawal effects that can be misinterpreted or misreported by the patient. Some psychotic disorders present with somatic delusions. For example, parasitosis refers to belief of infestation. It is a delusion that can be neatly circumscribed, leaving the patient otherwise rational and functional. This is in contrast to the patient with schizophrenia who may have somatic delusions that are part of a more obviously bizarre cluster of symptoms. When interviewing patients with prominent somatic complaints, it is important to screen for these primary psychiatric diagnoses, because the interview and the treatment will be quite different.

MANAGEMENT OF THE INTERVIEW

The Opening Phase

The patient with a psychosomatic problem may be particularly uncomfortable coming to see a psychiatrist. Rather than perceiving the psychiatrist as a source of help, the patient fears that the referral means that his primary physician considers his complaints imaginary or that he may be crazy. Therefore, it is helpful if the interviewer spends time at the beginning of the interview putting the patient at ease. For example, ask the patient, "What did Dr. X tell you about the reasons for this referral?" This development of a therapeutic alliance is critical and is promoted by beginning with a series of medical-model questions. The particular questions should be individualized based not only on the patient's presentation but also on the information earlier gleaned from the referring physician and a careful consideration of available medical records. The nature of the physical complaint should be addressed early in the initial meeting, and premature psychologizing should be avoided. Instead, find out from the patient how he views the consultation and clarify misunderstandings.

Many of these patients will hesitate to begin the interview without some notion of how it might help. A typical response might be, "I'm not certain that it will help, and that's what you and I will determine. It sounds like your medical problems are difficult for you. Many people with similar difficulties have found talking about it helpful."

Patients with puzzling physical complaints are often leery of a psychiatric consultant, fearing that their physical problems will be ignored. This concern can be addressed in several ways, including by demonstrating an interest in the problems and an intention to help with those problems. For example, the following interchange took place with a woman with unusual neurological problems.

> Patient (*angrily*): My doctors haven't done anything to help me. They don't understand or care how I do.
> Interviewer: You feel that they have been uncaring, but you have also emphasized that they have been active in ordering tests and prescribing medications.
> Patient: They had been active. They are getting tired of me. I think I was an interesting diagnostic dilemma, but now even the medical students find me boring.
> Interviewer: Do you think that may be why they called me?
> Patient: Yes, because they don't care anymore.
> Interviewer: Maybe they see me as another type of test or treatment. Something that will give them some clue about how to help you.
> Patient (*pausing, and with a significant change in mood*): Do you think you can actually help?

Exploration of the Presenting Symptoms

The medical model is particularly helpful with a wary interviewee. Ask about the symptoms that are most bothersome: "What do they feel like? When did they start? Is there a pattern? How serious are they? How disabling? What helps and hurts?" Develop a medical history that focuses on both present concerns and previous treatments and hospitalizations. A brief family and personal history and a description of the patient's life situation are often obtained in the early phase of the interview. Most patients are accepting of such structural questions as long as they conform to their expectations of a medical interview. Long silences can increase patient discomfort and erode the budding alliance, so the interviewer should remain interpersonally active and supportive of the patient's characteristic defenses. It is ineffective to ask such a patient to "say what comes to mind."

In addition to a longitudinal medical history, it is useful to obtain a detailed parallel history of the patient's life at the onset of the illness. It is seldom effective to ask questions such as "What was going on in your life when the pains began?" Many of these patients do not spontaneously link conflict with symptoms. Furthermore, such an approach may inform the patient that the interviewer is relatively unconcerned about his patient's somatic concerns and intends, instead, to focus on a presumed psychological etiology.

It is often more useful to take parallel histories. The first covers the physical complaints using a medical model. The second is a survey of the patient's life, with particular attention paid to clues concerning psychosocial stresses that might be related to the patient's complaints. The interviewer may quickly detect links that have remained out of the patient's awareness. It is often reasonable to suggest that certain emotional responses may have been temporally related to the onset of the physical symptoms and then evaluate the patient's response. As in other interviews, if the patient becomes mistrustful and withholding, it is often useful to back up and discuss the patient's mistrust, along with the concerns that motivate it. The interviewer can explain (or reexplain) that a goal of the interview is to get to know the patient as a person, that such an effort has been useful in cases similar to his, and that it is important to understand how the disease affects the patient's life as well as the physiology of the symptoms.

Frequently, it is useful to ask the patient if he has known anyone with an illness similar to his own. The answer may reveal unconscious attitudes about his illness and clues concerning its origin. Although psychosomatic patients frequently resist attempts to correlate symptoms with specific psychological situations, they will often indicate that their symptoms occur when they are nervous. At this point the interviewer inquires, "What kind of situation makes you nervous?" Other questions include "What did you notice first?"; "How did it all begin?"; or "When do you last recall feeling well?" On some occasions, asking the patient to describe a typical day in detail, or to describe all of the events of the past week, will successfully circumvent the patient's defenses.

As the interview progresses, the physician may develop the sense that psychological factors play a significant role in the patient's complaints. Even so, many patients will remain reluctant to link somatic symptoms and emotion. Certain techniques can help the patient develop a greater awareness and heightened sensitivity to his feelings. The patient may deny the role of anxiety, fear, or anger in the production of his physical symptoms, for example, but may readily acknowledge psychological symptoms such as tension, depression, insomnia, anorexia, fatigue, nightmares, or sexual disturbances. He will often explain that his physical illness is making him nervous or upset. The interviewer is advised not to challenge this patient, nor the one who totally denies nervousness, too early in the interview. The goal is not to push the patient into agreeing to a connection but rather to intrigue the patient into a curiosity about himself. The interviewer might wait until the patient has displayed anxiety, blushing, or sweating during the interview, for example, and then inquire whether the patient links this behavior with nervousness.

A common psychosomatic consultation is for pain, a complex subjective phenomenon. All pain is "real." It is almost always ineffective and inaccurate to suggest that pain is being consciously faked or exaggerated. Instead, the interviewer can begin by obtaining a careful description of the pain, when it began, what seems to bring it on, and what seems to help it, as well as the patient's understanding of its cause and significance. Patients whose complaint of pain or preoccupation with physical symptoms is a manifestation of depression may initially deny awareness of depressed feelings. However, if the interviewer refers to the pain and other symptoms by saying to the patient, "It must be terribly depressing to suffer like this," the patient may readily acknowledge that depression is a reaction to his pain. It may be more difficult for the patient to accept that pain is intensified by depression. As with many psychodynamic possibilities, it is more useful to suggest the link and await the patient's response. Further insight may not even be necessary. If the pain can be treated with some combination of medication, supportive psychotherapy, yoga, and acupuncture, for example, then the patient's depressive complaints may diminish without regard to his level of insight. The management of these problems is further discussed in Chapter 7, "The Depressed Patient." The management of the patient with acute anxiety symptoms is discussed in Chapter 8, "The Anxiety Disorder Patient."

To better understand the psychodynamic significance and possible secondary gain of the symptoms, the psychiatrist might ask, "What does your illness keep you from doing?" or "What would you do if you were well that you are not able to do now?" It is also useful to ask how family members and doctors view the patient's complaints as well as how the patient views the doctors. This can open a window onto the patient's object relationships and his level of psychological sophistication and capacity for trust. It can also promote an alliance by allowing the interviewer to point out the patient's disappointment and unfulfilled expectations.

In exploring both the central meaning and the secondary gain of the symptoms, it is important to explore who within the family is affected by them. Disabling symptoms may have led to a family dynamic in which the patient has become gratifyingly central. That patient's unconscious reward may make treatment difficult. A different patient may say, "My husband doesn't realize how much I suffer with these terrible backaches." The interviewer could reply, "What does he think about them?" As the patient proceeds to discuss her husband's feelings about illness and his lack of sympathetic understanding, the connections between the meaning of her symptoms and his disapproving, rejecting attitude will gradually emerge.

The interviewer is often unable to discover any specific precipitating stress in the patient's life, but instead the illness seems to arise as a result of the cumulative effects of life stress. This is particularly true of the individual who lives under the constant pressure of an obsessive-compulsive personality. The interviewer should refrain from offering well-meaning advice such as "Stop worrying" or "Try to relax." Instead, he might explain that chronic stress seems to be worsening the physical symptoms. This can lead to discussions of chronic worries and tensions and ways in which such problems can be reduced or addressed.

Exploration of the Psychological Problems

Many psychosomatic patients are concretely literal. Repeated questions that begin with "why" may frustrate them and undermine the early alliance. The interviewer should allow the patient to describe his emotional reaction to the symptoms without suggesting a cause-and-effect relationship. Some patients with unexplained medical complaints are introspective and psychologically minded and may relish the opportunity to share their theories. At times, these theories may appear to be a psychoanalytic caricature, as in the patient who believed that her abdominal pain was secondary to unconscious identification with her pregnant mother when she had been in labor with the patient. The psychiatrist could ask, "Was your mother's delivery of you quite painful?" If the patient replies affirmatively, the interviewer could continue, "And has she ever implied that you continue to cause her pain?"

Regardless of the levels of apparent insight or pseudo-insight, it is useful to explore the patient's understanding and feelings about his illness. It is also helpful to assess the limitations the symptoms impose and the patient's theories about the cause of the symptoms and the prognosis. Patients may freely admit that their symptoms worsen under stress. This admission creates a natural segue to a discussion of situations that cause stress and anxiety.

The patient should be asked how he has helped himself; for instance, has he tried diet, meditation, exercise, or massage? By mentioning these types of treatments, the interviewer has not only stamped them with legitimacy but also demonstrated a belief that nonverbal efforts can be helpful. Similarly, it is useful to demonstrate knowledge of subsyndromal constellations. For example, the interviewer might ask a hypochondriacal patient if his concern is predominately focused on his body, a fear of disease, or a conviction of having a disease. Such spontaneous discussion of details helps not only with treatment strategies but also with development of the therapeutic alliance. Similarly, the interviewer might comment on the patient's strengths, such as the ability of the person with hypochondriasis to focus intently on small details or the ability of the severely abused woman with somatization disorder to maintain her household in the midst of much stress. The interviewer should try to avoid exacerbating the shame that regularly overwhelms psychosomatic patients.

Some of these people have suffered with various illnesses for many years, and their medical complaints and physical disabilities have gradually structured their self-concept, their social situation, and their interpersonal relationships. Few of these patients will want or be able to recognize their unconscious compromises. Although the interviewer may want to link such a patient's symptoms and life situation, the patient will likely respond defensively. Reassurance and supportive treatment based on the interviewer's psychodynamic understanding of the problems are more effective. If tactfully inducted into therapy, such a patient may eventually become curious about himself and develop a more psychological approach to conflict. Early confrontation is unlikely to accomplish anything other than undermining the alliance and reducing the likelihood that such a patient will become curious about his condition. If reassurance had worked, the patient would presumably not have been sent for a consultation.

Each of these patients warrants a biopsychosocial evaluation. In particular, efforts at defining intrapsychic etiology and psychological ramifications should be intermingled with an awareness of the patient's social milieu as well as an understanding of biological disease models and the patient's particular medical situation. In other words, attempts to use psychodynamic paradigms to fully explain somatic symptoms have been as unsuccessful as attempts to rely on physical examinations, laboratory tests, and computed tomography scans or to rely fully on an investigation into the accompanying secondary gain of the illness.

The Patient's Expectations of the Consultant

The psychosomatic patient expects to ask questions and to receive answers from the psychiatric consultant. Frequently the patient will ask the doctor, "How is talking going to help me?" The physician might explain that emotions have an important effect on the body and offer a brief explanation of how emotional factors can produce or intensify symptoms. Long and complicated explanations give the interview the quality of a lecture and are best avoided.

On some occasions the patient will ask, "Do you think I'm crazy, Doctor?" or "Is it all in my mind?" The physician could reassure the patient that his symptoms are real and that he is not going crazy. The psychiatrist may want to follow up such concerns by discussing the possibility that psychological issues could be intensifying the patient's medical complaints but that this does not mean the patient is insane.

In another situation the patient may surprise the interviewer by asking, "What's my diagnosis, Doctor?" or "What is really wrong with me?" This can be an excellent opportunity to explore the patient's fears and fantasies about his illness. Reassurance is more effective when it is specific to the patient's situation. For example, the patient may have vague abdominal pains that have yielded no diagnosis but that the patient believes are caused by AIDS. He may have, for example, developed vague fantasies of retribution for sexual behavior that he finds shameful. In the patient's mind, the abdominal pain indicates AIDS, which indicates painful death. This equation binds his free-form anxiety and allows him to focus on only one big problem: dying from AIDS. After noting his recurrently negative HIV tests and his shameful feelings about his sexual activity, the psychiatrist can tactfully point out this link. The doctor can then indicate to the patient that the anxiety will persist and that longer-term therapy can be useful to work on the bigger issues of free-floating anxiety and shame.

A different patient with vague abdominal pain may have developed intense anxiety after being diagnosed with colon cancer. After prolonged hesitation, he might ask the psychiatrist how long until he dies the same painful death that was suffered by his own mother, who had the same disease. Reassurance in this case could include clarifying the reality that treatments for cancer and pain have both significantly improved since his mother died. Tactful honesty remains the goal, but it is important to appreciate the specific situation. The patient who asks, "Doctor, do I have cancer?" and then adds, "If I do, I will kill myself" will likely need the truth deferred while his psychological state is explored.

Countertransference

As in other clinical situations, the psychiatrist's interview of the psychosomatic patient should combine tact, timing, honesty, and curiosity. Diagnosis and treatment can occur simultaneously. Awareness of both transference and countertransference helps to guide the interview. There are, however, important differences from the typical interview, not least because the nature of the presenting complaint can lead the interviewer to a disregard of each of the above principles. The disregard often stems from unanalyzed countertransference toward a difficult patient, but it can also stem from the interviewer's anxiety about stepping into medical waters that are unknown or long forgotten.

The interviewer may collude with the patient in avoiding painful feelings by conducting a dryly insensitive fact-finding mission. Alternatively, the interviewer may pursue affect-laden personal and psychodynamic information in an effort to uncover the hidden origins of the medical complaint while avoiding physical reality. The interviewer may think it unobjectionable to link symptoms to their psychological meaning, but this patient will likely recognize that such a perspective is not his own. This patient tends not to believe that psychology plays a role in his symptoms, and an initial interview that is focused only on feelings and intrapsychic conflicts will be experienced as intrusive, unempathic, and adversarial.

Psychosomatic symptoms have eluded complete characterization, and uncertainty tends to prompt medical skepticism. The patient is often a vague or unreliable historian, and if not, he tends to be scrupulously and obsessively focused on symptoms that appear exaggerated. As the clinician becomes frustrated, a somatoform disorder is often considered, which tends to lead to disinterest in the patient's actual experience and a focus on behavior management. As the patient feels increasingly misunderstood and criticized, he may become increasingly angry or hurt, which tends to confirm the doctor's diagnosis of psychological causation. When the patient abandons treatment for another round of "doctor shopping," the physician is both convinced of the diagnosis and relieved.

The psychiatrist may feel that both the patient and the referring physician possess expectations of magical relief. This pressure can lead to various types of errors, including the attempt to quickly wrap up the patient's psychological issues during the first session. It may be useful to recall that symptoms may have been developing over a lifetime and that useful biopsychosocial interventions may require a considerable effort by the consultant and the referring doctor as well as family and social services.

When confronting a situation in which the patient and the primary physician are at odds, the interviewer will find it useful to explore the situation rather than take sides in the battle. Early interpretations tend to be ineffective, whether addressed to the patient (e.g., "Your anger at your doctor is actually a projection of your own primitive rage") or to the referring physician (e.g., "Your premature diagnostic closure is a defense against anxiety"). Such comments are unlikely to have an impact except to focus hostility toward the psychiatric consultant.

The interviewer's underlying attitude should be of respectful, tactful skepticism toward all information. While maintaining an explicit interest in the patient's experience, for example, the interviewer should look for obvious secondary gain and precipitating psychological stressors. Similarly, the interviewer should be attentive to the fact that the difficult patient can lead to an uncharacteristically incomplete medical evaluation and that the interview is another opportunity to detect a treatable organic illness. If the psychiatrist concludes that psychological issues play an important role in the development of the medical complaint, he should help the medical treatment team develop a reliable safety net of good care while minimizing invasive procedures.

The Closing Phase

The murkiness of many psychosomatic complaints should not necessarily lead to parallel uncertainty in the interviewer. When possible, the psychiatrist should make diagnoses that fulfill criteria for Axis I disorders such as major depression and panic disorder. The interviewer may be able to develop conviction about the possibility of a somatoform disorder, factitious disorder, or malingering. Most other psychosomatic illnesses inspire a formulation rather than a diagnosis, but as much as possible, the interviewer should clarify the extent to which he believes that psychological factors are contributing to the somatic complaint.

As the interview draws to a close, it may be helpful for the physician to explain to the patient what he has learned. This should initially stick closely to the patient's report. It may be useful to reorder the information in such a way that implies a psychological formulation. In this way, the physician not only has an opportunity to clarify misunderstandings but also can obtain some measure of the patient's receptivity to psychological insights concerning his illness. For example, after interviewing a young adult with recurrent stomach pain without physical findings, the psychiatrist might say, "It seems that you get pain every morning during the week, and this pain keeps you from going to work, but you don't get the pain on weekends and holidays." The interviewer can then wait and see how the patient reacts before explicitly theorizing a more specific link between work and the stomachache.

In reviewing the situation, it can sometimes be useful to frame the patient's concerns in terms of being especially sensitive to physical sensations. The interviewer might say that the patient seems to have a particular ability to appreciate subtle physical sensations and then remind the patient that most people have physical pains every week without any demonstrable organic pathology. The patient's sensitivity may be making the patient unduly worried. By normalizing aches and pains and creating a framework to experience bodily sensations, the interviewer can help reduce the patient's tendency to "catastrophize."

Before ending the interview, the therapist should allow the patient sufficient time to ask questions. If the patient's questions and comments remain stuck on physical symptoms, the patient is unlikely to be amenable to suggestions of insight-oriented psychotherapy. If, on the other hand, the patient proceeds to inquire about matters related to his emotional life, he may be more responsive to an uncovering psychotherapy.

People who are especially sensitive to discomfort are often quite sensitive to the side effects of all medications, including, for example, antidepressants. Adequate time should be allowed to explain the rationale for the medication, the dosage regimen, the expected benefits, and the expected side effects. Similarly, many of these patients are sensitive to the suggestion of psychotherapeutic treatments. Explanation and reassurance are often needed before a psychosomatic patient is likely to be intrigued by the possibility of therapy.

CONCLUSION

The psychosomatic patient is often difficult to interview, and it is useful to recall that most difficult patients are making an unconscious effort to hold themselves together. The misuse of others, the denial and projection of harsh emotions, and the rapid fluctuations between idealization and denigration may be uncomfortable for the interviewer but have become an important coping strategy for the patient. For many of these patients, symptoms have a useful purpose. Part of the responsibility of the interviewer is to model a sense of curiosity and compassionate interest. The interviewer should try to understand the patient individually rather than create a unified theory of either causation or response. The patient with psychosomatic complaints has intrigued and frustrated the greatest clinicians for centuries, offering an opportunity to balance the traditional medical effort to understand each patient with the central Hippocratic adage to do no harm.

CHAPTER 16

THE COGNITIVELY IMPAIRED PATIENT

JOHN W. BARNHILL, M.D.

Cognitive impairment affects millions of people, and this number continues to rise as people live longer and survive increasingly severe illnesses. Sophisticated imaging and laboratory evaluations have allowed for a deeper understanding of such syndromes as dementia and delirium, but these remain clinical diagnoses that are made on the basis of the interview. Although the diagnosis may be obvious, many cases are subtle enough to be missed by the family and clinician. Furthermore, few patients spontaneously complain about either the gradual cognitive decline of dementia or the acute confusion of delirium. These factors contribute to a 3-year diagnostic delay in the typical patient with Alzheimer's disease and to the reality that most cases of hospital-based delirium are never recognized by the treating staff.

Cognitive impairment strikes at the core of how we define ourselves. Memory loss, inattention, disorientation, environmental misperceptions, behavioral dyscontrol, and mood lability tend to accompany cognitive impairment, and this constellation of symptoms induces powerful feelings of being overwhelmed. These same symptoms undermine the patient's ability to participate effectively in social and health-related situations, leading to a psychological and financial drain on all who care for the patient. Effective interventions with the cognitively impaired patient require not only the ability to diagnose and treat but also facility with interview techniques that differ from those used with most other patients. Such interventions can be singularly useful not only to the patient but also to the family and medical staff. In this chapter, two prominent types of cognitive impairment are explored: delirium and dementia.

PSYCHOPATHOLOGY AND PSYCHODYNAMICS

Delirium

Delirium is an acute confusional state that can present with any level of activity, from severely agitated to quietly mute. Careful assessment of the delirious patient will detect problems with arousal, attention, orientation, perception, cognitive function, and mood, but most cases of delirium will be suspected by a confused look in the patient's eyes or by speech that is uncharacteristically garbled. Clouding of consciousness tends to fluctuate throughout the day, frequently worsening at night. Although uncommon in a typical outpatient psychiatric practice, delirium is found in 15% of hospitalized adults.

Some delirious patients present with increased activity. Such activity is often related to substance withdrawal or intoxication, and these hyperactive patients tend to be quickly recognized. Many others present with either a hypoactive delirium or a mixed state in which the activity level fluctuates over the course of the delirium. Quiet confusion is often seen in patients who have recently had surgery or who are in the intensive care unit, have a terminal illness, or are battling illnesses of any severity within the context of a dementia. Under these circumstances, hypoactive delirium is usually unrecognized. When the medical staff and relatives do notice that the patient appears "out of it," there is a tendency to "psychologize" this neurological dysfunction as a response to a serious biopsychosocial stressor. In such cases, the patient often receives diagnoses such as depression, apathy, or a catastrophic reaction to bad news. At other times, the patient receives no formal diagnosis but instead prompts the casual use of euphemisms. For example, the term *sundowning* stems from the frequent finding that the behavioral dyscontrol of delirium and dementia tends to worsen at night. Similarly, the term *ICU psychosis* is used because delirium occurs frequently among the very ill in intensive care units. By normalizing delirium, both terms diminish the motivation to search for etiology.

The search for etiology is important because the onset of delirium is frequently the first sign of a serious medical condition. Delirium can be precipitated, for example, by infection, medications, cancer, trauma, or metabolic abnormalities. Drug and alcohol intoxication and withdrawal frequently cause delirium. In the patient with dementia, a superimposed delirium can be induced by something as simple as a fever, anemia, or prolonged confinement to bed. Within a psychiatric population, antipsychotic medications can cause a delirium called neuroleptic malignant syndrome, whereas selective serotonin reuptake inhibitor antidepressants can cause a serotonin syndrome. The single best treatment for these iatrogenic disorders is prompt discontinuation of the offending psychiatric medication. Although delirium is generally considered to be acute and self-limited, all such confusional states are likely to continue as long as the underlying cause remains untreated. Underdiagnosis can lead to complications such as aspiration pneumonia, falls, and bedsores and can also exacerbate emotional distress in the patient and his family.

There are a number of difficulties in the diagnosis of delirium. Although classically of acute onset, the history may be difficult to elicit, especially if the patient is not accompanied by an observant caretaker. Delirium is generally time limited, but it can last indefinitely, especially in terminal illness, coexisting dementia, and complicated drug and alcohol withdrawal. Because fluctuating symptomatology is a core aspect of delirium, and symptoms tend to worsen at night, the daytime interviewer may underestimate the patient's problems. The underdiagnosis of delirium frequently stems from the reality that quiet confusion does not generally warrant a thorough interview until either the family becomes worried or the patient is unable to sign an informed consent form.

Although it has a medical cause, delirium is also a psychological disorder. Social isolation and sensory deprivation increase the risk for delirium in at-risk patients, and hospital-based psychosocial interventions have been shown to reduce the incidence of delirium in the elderly. Interventions can, therefore, reduce diagnostic and treatment delays, medical complications, and hospitalization lengths of stay.

Equally as important, the experience of delirium is upsetting to the patient and everyone involved in his care, including relatives and medical staff. When the delirium is recalled weeks later, the patient is often haunted by memories. In addition to possible medical interventions, the identification and explanation of delirium can significantly reduce the anxiety surrounding the experience.

Clinical Presentation

A delirium prodrome is often recognized first by the nurse or family member who appreciates subtle personality change and sleep problems well before the development of overt cognitive deficits. For example, it is common for family members to notice that their loved one "just doesn't look right" a day or two before the patient becomes more obviously delirious. Similarly, family members will often notice that even though the patient has improved enough to be discharged from the hospital, it may take several weeks or months before he fully recovers.

Once the delirium has developed, the patient may appear quite normal for periods of time only to relapse recurrently to states of agitation, confusion, or stupor. This is not necessarily accompanied by drowsiness, and in fact the delirious patient is frequently hypersensitive to environmental stimuli. The speed with which he recognizes others may be slowed, and he tends to appear perplexed or confused. When the interviewer looks at a delirious patient, it often appears that "no one is at home." Affective changes are often prominent, and irritable dysphoria is common. These personality changes often elicit the greatest concern in the family.

The loss of cognitive powers is reflected by the heightened effort required to perform routine intellectual chores. The patient has particular difficulty with abstract thought, performing better with concrete problems. Mild degrees of perseveration are reflected in slowness and an inability to shift easily from one topic to another. Inattentive and disoriented, the patient first loses awareness of the date and may also fail to recognize the place or the situation. It is fairly common to meet with a quietly delirious patient who appears bewildered and who, despite the presence of white-coated doctors and beeping ventilators, believes he is at home and that it is 1996.

Many delirious patients have perceptual abnormalities. These may begin with the complaint that noises seem too loud or that other sensory stimuli are annoying. Many delirious patients prefer to speak with their eyes shut or in a darkened room. This reflects their difficulty with editing out extraneous environmental cues, as though the world is too much with them. This leads to misperceptions of noise, conversations, or shadows. It is common for delirious patients to see bugs crawling on their turned-off television and to wonder about the people who are hanging from the hospital drapes. At times, this can have a distinctly paranoid flavor, but many delirious patients will calmly describe events that would generally be perceived as scary. For example, one patient described being kidnapped by neighbors after having been restrained by nursing staff, but he did so with equanimity. Some clinicians offer the distinction that the delirious patient usually misperceives by making the unfamiliar more familiar, whereas schizophrenic hallucinations worsen the feeling of alienation. The delirious patient often sees hospital personnel as relatives, for example, whereas the schizophrenic patient is more likely to see them as terrorists. Again in contrast to the schizophrenic person, the delirious patient is much more likely to experience visual and tactile hallucinations. Auditory hallucinations can occur and may be accompanied by poorly organized delusions. It is often difficult to tease apart a hallucination in a confused, medically ill patient from an illusory misperception of a real experience. Such a distinction is far less important, however, than the recognition that the patient is delirious in the first place.

Dementia

As the population has aged, dementia has become increasingly important to the family members and health care professionals who care for dementia patients every day.

Dementia is a chronic syndrome of global intellectual deterioration, often accompanied by affective and personality changes. Dementia interferes with activities of daily living and is accompanied by a clear consciousness. There are dozens of underlying etiologies for dementia, and almost all of these are brain disorders that are irreversible and progressive. This chapter focuses on the most common dementia, that due to Alzheimer's disease, although the underlying principles are broadly applicable.

The brain has a remarkable ability to develop compensatory mechanisms, and the typical early Alzheimer's patient functions well enough to avoid a dementia diagnosis for several years. Instead, the patient and his loved ones assume that the deficits are consistent with the mild cognitive impairment of normal aging. Despite months or years of warning signals, many families feel the dementia diagnosis as a sudden, severe blow. Most patients with dementia, meanwhile, bear the diagnosis with equanimity or even apathy.

Dementia is usually defined in contrast to other conditions. For example, in delirium, consciousness is clouded, whereas dementia patients are usually alert. The cognitive deficits in both intellectual disability and traumatic brain injury tend to be stable, whereas dementia tends to progress inexorably. In practice, these contrasts are often obscure. Cognitive and behavioral problems may abruptly worsen during periods of stress and at night so that the dementia may not appear "stable" to caretakers. Furthermore, dementia patients are highly vulnerable to the metabolic and psychological stressors that can induce a delirium. When the delirium clears, the dementia patient may return to his previous level of functioning or may fall to a lower baseline level of functioning. These speak to the frequent confusion in differentiating acute from chronic brain syndromes.

Clinical Presentation

Cognitive impairments in dementia are wide-ranging and include the learning of new information, the naming of objects, and the ability to do calculations. Abstraction, calculation, and visuospatial construction progressively decline and interfere with the patient's ability to function independently.

The patient with dementia often attempts to compensate for memory deficits by using descriptive phrases as substitutes for forgotten names. This might lead to circumstantiality in which the patient describes the hospital rather than naming it. A different patient might look around the hospital room and confabulate that he is in a hotel. It is not uncommon for patients to insist that staff members are relatives or that relatives are staff members. Patients often try to shut down the interview by claiming fatigue. They may truly be tired, but such insistence is often an attempt to dodge the embarrassment of having one's declining abilities exposed.

Although cognitive decline is central to the diagnosis of dementia, other neuropsychiatric symptoms often pose a greater threat to the dementia patient's autonomy and well-being. Poor insight and apathy are frequent, as is a passive disregard for himself and his loved ones. Although some dementia patients may become transiently hypersexual, most lose interest in sex as well as in sleep and food. Speech becomes impoverished, and the patient tends to rely on stereotyped phrases rather than spontaneous interchange. It may appear that all unique vitality has drained out of the person. This apathy should be differentiated from depression, which is also common in the dementia patient. The depression may seem to result from awareness of decline—especially early in the course—but most dementia patients are strikingly unworried about their situation. Instead, many dementia-related depressions seem related to neurological changes that are part of the underlying disease process.

Up to half of patients with dementia become delusional, focusing on such things as theft, persecution, and spousal infidelity. Hypochondriasis is frequent. Wandering, restlessness, hoarding, and even assaultiveness are not uncommon. Visual hallucinations and illusions occur, although auditory hallucinations are unusual. Many dementia patients become disinhibited and resistive. Dementia may appear to change personality so that a previously pleasant and refined elderly person may become verbally coarse, unreasonable, and labile. At other times, normal personality traits may become exaggerated. In one case, a mildly obsessive woman became relentlessly rigid and orderly as her dementia progressed. In another, an outgoing man became embarrassingly exhibitionistic and rude. Cognitive decline is painful for families, but it is these emotional and behavioral problems that tend to lead to family exhaustion and residential placement.

MANAGEMENT OF THE INTERVIEW

Cognitive decline affects the interview significantly. For example, few people with dementia or delirium complain of intellectual problems. They will rarely have requested to see a psychiatrist. They tend to lack cognitive and emotional flexibility. In the midst of one of life's tragedies, the cognitively impaired patient tends to discuss not existential loss but the mundane. Although the interviewer should strive to create a predictable and quiet interview setting so as to calm the easily distractible patient, hospital settings can be unpredictably chaotic and public. Although the initial interview is generally intended to be diagnostic, optimal clarity is not achieved unless an alliance is created, and this alliance can be undermined if the interviewer too quickly seeks to formally evaluate cognition. As with other types of interviews, words remain important, but some observation of the patient is required to put the words into perspective.

The effective interview must take into account these inherent obstacles while also making use of this population's strengths. Usually the patient and his relatives will not have a preexisting psychiatric diagnosis, for example, and so the treatment effort can be applied to the debilitating neurological process as well as to often mild neurotic issues. Conflicts and self-defeating behavior—found in both the patient and relatives—can often be readily and successfully addressed by the alert interviewer.

Finally, the interviewer should remain attentive to the reason for the interview. If another physician would like help with the management of acute agitation and confusion, it would be a mistake to gather only information related to family dynamics. Conversely, if two siblings have brought in a parent known to have dementia-related dyscontrol, it would be unwise to focus only on the exact extent of the patient's decline. For these reasons, the patient with cognitive impairment warrants a flexible, supportive interview that is modified based on the extent and type of impairment.

The Opening Phase

The initial moments of the interview should be devoted to several overlapping tasks. A friendly attitude is important. Patients and relatives appreciate warm handshakes and brief introductions. While saying hello, the interviewer observes the patient and the surroundings, looking for signs of health and disturbance. Grooming and posture are important keys not only to the patient's degree of cognitive impairment but also to the availability and attentiveness of family. In addition, the psychiatrist should look for any signs of personal history that can later be used to gain an alliance or to better understand the patient. Tactful appreciation of photographs of grandchildren or a well-worn baseball cap can be the starting point for an alliance. During these opening moments, the interviewer must make some important decisions that are based on immediately available information. A well-dressed patient with a reportedly mild cognitive decline might want to talk about aging and loss and can best do so in private. The psychiatrist will generally ask relatives or attendants to step outside. A moderately impaired patient with dementia or delirium may profit most from reassurance and explanation that are delivered in front of loved ones. Severely affected people are often unable to communicate verbally with the interviewer, and so the interview is primarily conducted with caretakers. In many cases, the decision about the presence or absence of family members will be made by the family and patient. The risk of compromised confidentiality is often outweighed by the reassurance and clarification that can be provided by a well-meaning friend or relative. Furthermore, it is often useful for family members to witness effective styles of interaction and then to have their own concerns directly answered by the interviewer.

Most interviews with delirious patients occur in hospitals at the request of other physicians (see Chapter 18, "The Hospitalized Patient"). After deciding whether the family should be present and while observing the patient and situation, the interviewer identifies himself, carefully sounding out his own name. After reducing distraction and enhancing privacy by drawing curtains and turning off the television, the psychiatrist should try to position himself at eye level with the patient and explore the patient's understanding of the reason for the consultation. "I am Dr. X. Did your doctor explain that I would be coming?" The physician guides his next response by the patient's reply to this introduction. If the patient understands that he is being interviewed by a psychiatrist, the interviewer may proceed. If not, the interviewer should tactfully explain why he was consulted. For example, he might say, "I understand that you have been upset" or "Dr. Jones tells me that you have had some periods of confusion" or "Your doctor thought I could help with your nightmares." The mildly impaired patient will then begin to discuss his problems, and the interviewer will follow the patient's lead. If physical discomfort is the matter of greatest concern to the patient, the interviewer should spend some time discussing the chief complaint. The severely delirious patient is likely to be diagnosed as soon as the interviewer enters the room. In addition to the pursuit of diagnosis, the interview with such patients can be therapeutic from the outset by providing structure and a tone of reassurance.

The interview with the dementia patient begins in a similar fashion, except that the patient is not as likely to be seriously medically ill. Again, someone other than the patient has usually requested help. Most often the patient is elderly and has been accompanied by a relative or friend.

Relationship With the Patient

Attitude of the Interviewer

Some interviewers may doubt the therapeutic value of a psychodynamic interview for patients with delirium or dementia. In talking to patients who are "out of it," the interviewer may want to concentrate on formal assessment of cognitive functioning. Even a patient who has significant confusion or dementia can, however, detect the interviewer's level of personal interest and respond to the doctor's respect, as does anyone else, by feeling reassured and becoming more cooperative. Patients with dementia and delirious patients need considerable support and will not react favorably to a physician who is aloof, distant, or overly neutral. Although a generally warm, interested, and friendly attitude is desirable, the interviewer may sometimes need to guide the patient firmly toward more socially acceptable or safe behavior.

Transference

Patients with mild organic impairment develop a transference that is primarily determined by their basic personality type. Patients with more severe disorders may relate to the doctor in ways that have more to do with their neuropsychiatric illness than with their lifelong character traits. The transference attitudes of these patients are not interpreted or worked through in their treatment. Nevertheless, recognition of the patient's attitudes can allow the interviewer to ally himself with the positive aspects of the transference. It might be useful, for example, for an interviewer to act parentally with a patient who is acting dependently, although it may be a challenge for a young interviewer to act parentally toward an elderly patient without sounding uncertain or patronizing. A common example is referring to an elderly patient using his first name. Other delirious patients and patients with dementia are mistrustful and frightened. It is useful to remember that such attitudes are often fed by confusion and that the interviewer should be straightforward, reassuring, and sober-minded.

Specific Techniques

Using Brief Interviews

A shorter interview is helpful if the patient fatigues easily. It may be better to see a patient several times in one day or on several successive days for 15-minute interviews.

Recognizing the Patient as a Person

After the patient's initial spontaneous remarks, the clinician determines the chief complaint and a brief history of the present illness and then may direct attention to the patient's personal background and current life situation. The patient with dementia is particularly dependent on recollections of past achievements and capabilities in order to maintain his self-esteem. Therefore, a review of the patient's earlier life is not only informative for the interviewer but also therapeutic for the patient.

Allowing the Patient Time

Memory loss, circumstantiality, perseveration, and a lack of spontaneity can frustrate the interviewer. The patient should be given the chance to tell his story in his own way. If the patient is too disorganized to provide structure, the interviewer can help by asking direct, concrete questions. Impatience and overly rapid questioning can increase the patient's disorganization.

Stimulating Memory Chains

The interviewer may be able to improve the patient's recall by stimulating associative patterns. It is often useful, for example, for the interviewer to concisely summarize what the patient has said and to help him maintain continuity when the patient loses his place. When the patient stops in the middle of a thought and asks, "What was I just talking about?" the interviewer should repeat the patient's words, thereby helping his concentration and focus. An empathic comment regarding how frustrating it must be to keep losing his place will be appreciated.

Speaking Clearly

The patient's recollections will be enhanced by simple declarative sentences that focus on one topic at a time. Humor is generally inappropriate as a therapeutic maneuver, although it can help as a diagnostic measure: both delirious patients and dementia patients are likely to respond blankly to any sort of wordplay.

Aiding Reality Testing

Frequently, when a physician discovers that a patient is disoriented or confused, he permits the patient to give wrong answers without any attempt to provide the correct information. Instead, it is helpful to tactfully reorient the patient by providing the date and place and the name of the interviewer.

Taking Interest in Physical Complaints

Alliance is enhanced when the interviewer takes an interest in what most troubles the patient. After discussing these chief complaints, many patients will be more amenable to discussing psychological and cognitive issues.

Assessing for Self-Destructiveness

Delirious patients and dementia patients hurt themselves in several different ways. They are at greatly increased risk for falls and other types of inadvertent injury. Since their ability to perform activities of daily living is impaired, they may become malnourished, dehydrated, and noncompliant with medications. The evaluation for depression and suicidality is complicated by several factors. Depressions in geriatric patients are frequently atypical, and these patients may present primarily with, for example, a disorder of executive functioning or with somatic preoccupation rather than with sadness, diurnal variation, or self-criticism. Furthermore, delirious patients sometimes kill themselves impulsively and without ever having mentioned suicidality or depression.

The Mental Status Examination

The mental status examination is an important tool in the diagnosis of cognitive decline. The write-up of the mental status exam can loom so large to the interviewer that the entire assessment is transformed into a simplistic cognitive exam. Such an examination may yield much data but little information. For example, one interviewer spent the bulk of his interview administering the Mini-Mental State Exam. The 80-year-old patient performed quite well, missing only occasional questions. Since the patient was completely oriented and scored 26 out of 30 on the examination, the interviewer concluded that neither delirium nor dementia was present. In looking down at his form and not looking at the patient, however, the interviewer failed to notice the glazed, perplexed look in the eyes of the patient or the prolonged pauses and the exertion required to answer the questions. In this case, the patient's very high baseline cognitive functioning allowed for a reasonably good examination score despite the fact that she had significant delirium. In addition to missing the diagnosis, the interviewer did not recognize that the relentless questioning had led the patient to feel alienated, threatened, bored, and annoyed.

Observation of the patient lies at the core of the mental status examination, and such observation begins immediately upon entering the room. Is the patient awake, sleepy, alert, hostile, stuporous, depressed? The patient's appearance, effort, and level of interaction help to make sense of the rest of the mental status exam. Speech is a particularly revealing window into the patient's cognitive and emotional worlds. Does the patient lack fluency, pace, spontaneity? Are there errors of syntax or word choice? These may be clues to a smoldering delirium or subtle dementia and can be readily assessed during the course of the interview.

The patient with cognitive decline tends to have poor insight into emotional states. Observation of affect is critical, as is acquisition of collateral information from relatives and loved ones. When sadness is accompanied by significant guilt, hopelessness, or suicidality, the patient should be carefully evaluated for a treatable major depression. Hallucinations and delusions may be denied if the patient is asked directly. Instead, the interviewer should pay attention to clues that the patient is experiencing these phenomena during the interview. Is the patient picking at his skin or reaching into the air? Is the patient looking oddly at the television or the curtains? Is the patient unduly wary of the interviewer or of the interviewer's request to contact members of the patient's family? Some patients may respond freely when asked if they are suicidal, and all patients should be asked. The yield is greater, however, when the patient is also asked if life has become not worth living or if he ever gets so frustrated or scared that he feels like he might just have to end it all. Similarly, many patients who deny the desire to hurt someone will admit that there is someone from whom they have to protect themselves. Such questions are intended not simply to identify suicidality and homicidality but to tactfully elicit paranoia and depression.

The most commonly administered "test" within the mental status examination is orientation to time, person, and place. This is often best begun by asking about the situation, the fourth axis in the evaluation of orientation. For example, the interviewer can ask the patient what brought him to the hospital or to the psychiatrist's office. If the patient seems puzzled by that or any other relatively straightforward question, the interviewer might say, "It seems that you might be having trouble remembering things." If the patient responds, "Why do you say that?" the interviewer might say, "Whenever I ask a question that taxes your memory, you change the subject. It seems that you might be having problems with your memory." Such a comment demonstrates that the interviewer understands the patient's situation, which can both increase the alliance and allow for an assessment of the patient's insight. The interviewer can then say he would like to ask a few questions about memory. Time is a sensitive measure of orientation and can be assessed by asking the date. One patient did not know the date or month, and when asked the season, she looked out the window to look for clues from the weather. The interviewer recognized that the patient was seeking clues from the weather and further clarified the extent of her confusion. The patient may try to deflect the question by saying that he had not been paying attention to such things, but tactful persistence will likely help the interviewer decide whether the patient lacks the knowledge because of cognitive decline or as a result of depression or oppositionalism. Orientation is, however, of limited usefulness. Many people with cognitive decline are fully oriented. Furthermore, disorientation can be caused by a range of difficulties related to inattention, memory, thought content, and language.

Bedside neuropsychiatric testing often focuses on memory, attention span, and concentration. Recall and short-term memory can be efficiently tested by asking the patient to repeat three objects immediately and then after a few minutes. Tests for attention and concentration are heavily affected by levels of education. For example, serial sevens are difficult for many medically ill and elderly people, so the interviewer should be quick to shift to a request for serial threes or repetition of the months backward. The Folstein Mini-Mental State Exam is useful in eliciting a host of such cognitive deficits, whereas the Clock-Drawing Test can provide a rapid estimate of executive functioning and constructional apraxia. If done as part of the routine assessment of at-risk patients, these tests are fairly quick and much more useful than simply inquiring into the level of orientation. They may also be useful in anticipating the potential for recovery and for following the patient's clinical course. The interview and collateral history, especially concerning home functioning, help put these tests into perspective.

Cognitive testing can have psychological significance. For example, when asked to spell "world" backwards, one elderly woman quickly recited "rawdlrow." This particular patient had become paranoid and noncompliant upon entering the hospital, and the medical team had been concerned about delirium or dementia. After hearing this repeated, the interviewer realized that the patient was spelling "World War" backward, which led to an extensive discussion of the patient's

Holocaust experience. The patient was not at all cognitively impaired but was, instead, frightened by the institutional setting and her own medical illness and loss of control.

Much of the mental status examination can be performed with a patient who says almost nothing. For example, an interviewer approached the hospital bed of an elderly man who was hospitalized for pneumonia. She found him lying at a 45° angle with a sheet over his head. The interviewer began by saying, "It looks like you're having a hard time. Would you like to tell me about it?" The patient lowered the sheet but remained quiet and fearful and kept his eyes squeezed shut. The interviewer continued by saying, "It looks to me like you may not be feeling safe." The patient responded, "I'm OK." The interviewer then said that it seemed like he might be feeling confused. The patient did not move. The interviewer then hypothesized that he was keeping his eyes shut because it was too hard to concentrate with all the lights and movement. The patient nodded. The interviewer asked what he was doing there, and the patient said he did not know. When asked where he thought he was, the patient said at home. The interviewer made a tentative diagnosis of delirium as soon as she saw the elderly patient lying diagonally in bed. This diagnosis was substantiated by the patient's disorientation, fearfulness, inability to edit external stimuli, and apparent clouding of consciousness. The interviewer concluded the interview by telling the patient that it seemed that he had become confused because of the infection and that the team would work to get him back to his usual self. She continued by saying that she would prescribe medications to help him get to sleep that night and help him get his thoughts straight. These words appeared to comfort the patient. This brief interaction would be incomplete without corroborating personal and medical history, a review of the chart, and a discussion with the primary medical team, but a reasonable working diagnosis can often be rapidly acquired through observation of the patient.

The Physical Evaluation

The diagnosis of either delirium or dementia warrants a thorough medical evaluation that includes a physical and neurological examination, laboratory tests, and neuroimaging. More than perhaps any other psychiatric diagnoses, these syndromes require a search for the underlying etiology.

The Therapeutic Plan

Efforts to gain trust and cooperation may seem futile with patients who may forget you before your next appointment. Nevertheless, patients and their families do recognize warmth, respect, and attention. Simple explanations and efforts at connection and reassurance can often be immensely therapeutic.

Successful resolution of delirium requires the maintenance of safety and treatment of the underlying medical problem. Low-dose antipsychotic medications are often warranted, especially as a means to ensure nighttime sleep. Clarification is important, both for the patient and for the family. For example, loved ones are often reassured by knowing that delirium has a generally favorable prognosis once the underlying medical problem is corrected. At the same time, delirium is often found in the terminally ill, and the job of the interviewer then includes counseling of both the patient and loved ones. The physician who realizes that his job is to improve, not necessarily cure, the patient's condition will be less likely to feel overwhelmed by the limitations created by the patient's disability or life situation.

People with mild dementia often profit from having a role in the family, such as chores and responsibilities in the home. Creative talents, avocational interests, and hobbies should be explored. The interviewer can demonstrate his interest by asking to see examples of work the patient has produced. Patients may want to discuss feelings of helplessness and vulnerability. Recognition and respect for the patient's premorbid accomplishments can have a substantial therapeutic effect. By carefully reflecting on the patient's life story, the therapist offers himself as a substitute or supplement for the patient's internalized lost love objects. This can yield significant benefits to the patient.

> An 80-year-old man, who had retired 15 years earlier, moved in with his daughter and son-in-law after his wife died. The daughter noticed periods of confusion, irritability, and memory loss and brought her father in for an evaluation. After a medical workup and a psychiatric evaluation, the patient was diagnosed as having age-related cognitive decline. In addition, it appeared that the patient's main source of self-esteem during his retirement had come from dominating his wife. He attempted this same technique in his new home, but he met constant rebuff and failure. In one session he reported that his daughter had said to him, "Dad, would you please stop telling us what to do all the time?" The interviewer asked, "How did you feel?" The patient replied, "I was only trying to be helpful." The interviewer continued, "But how did it make you feel?" The patient answered, "A little rejected, I guess. Maybe I'm a burden."
>
> The interviewer reviewed several incidents with the patient in which he was trying to be helpful. It emerged that the patient was reminding his family of chores that needed to be done. The interviewer asked, "Were these chores that were done by your wife when she was alive?"

The patient nodded, "Yes, now that you mention it." The interviewer added, "Perhaps they feel that you are being critical or nagging." The patient looked pensive. The clinician asked, "Would you be willing to try an experiment for 2 weeks?" The patient agreed, and the interviewer continued, "Tell your daughter and son-in-law that you would like to make a bigger contribution around the house and do some of the household chores." The patient said that he would think about it and then went on to talk about how much he missed his wife. The therapist asked, "Do you discuss your feelings with your family?" The patient said that he did not. The clinician responded, "You are depriving them of the opportunity to comfort you."

The clinician's intervention stemmed from his view that the patient had regressed in the context of his mild cognitive decline and the loss of his wife. Instead of pitching in, the patient had sat idly by, expecting to be taken care of as he had been by his wife. Although his wife had been willing to accept his irritable domination, his daughter and son-in-law were uninterested in re-creating that particular dynamic. Instead, the three of them had recognized tension but had known no way to identify and address the problem. At the patient's request, the therapist relayed these ideas to the daughter, who picked him up from his weekly sessions. During the ensuing weeks, the patient and the daughter reported significant improvement both in the patient's mood and in the family's level of relaxed intimacy.

The Patient's Family

Cognitively impaired patients prompt more involvement with relatives than is typical for a psychiatrist. Not only is there much greater communication, but family members may end up making significant decisions about the patient, sometimes in conflict with the patient's expressed wishes. It is useful for the interviewer to have contact with these relatives early in the evaluation. Some relatives have difficulty recognizing and accepting the degree of impairment in their loved one and feel guilty about and fearful of institutional care. This guilt is sometimes openly discussed. At other times it is expressed in the form of hostility toward the medical staff. Other families resent the patient and look for any opportunity to get him out of the home. A large percentage of caregivers of Alzheimer's patients become depressed. One psychiatrist found that his most useful intervention with family members was to remind them that they needed to get out and enjoy themselves on a regular basis. In order to allow for such freedom, the psychiatrist may have to focus not just on family guilt but on the many behavioral interventions that can be used with people with dementia.

COUNTERTRANSFERENCE

Patients with cognitive impairment can evoke avoidant, pessimistic attitudes in the interviewer. These stem from several related issues. First, delirium and dementia affect insight, cognition, and memory, qualities that tend to be highly valued by interviewers. Therapists tend to want their patients to improve, and many of these patients will never recover. Whether subtle or dramatic, personality changes are generally found, and they may bear little relation to historical events or current stressors. This can be disconcerting to interviewers who have been trained to assume that personality is relatively enduring over time and that personality and mood changes tend to have some connection to internal or external events. Finally, the interview with the cognitively impaired patient may require expertise in neurology that is beyond that of the typical clinician. When evaluating a patient with cognitive impairment, the interviewer may experience dread when trying to recall the dozens of dementing illnesses and the hundreds of underlying causes for delirium. This potential complexity may lead many interviewers to avoid this increasingly sizable portion of the population. The attendant anxiety from being confronted by such a patient can de-skill even an experienced interviewer.

Other interviewers react very differently to this population. Often reacting to concerns about the aging of their own parents or of themselves, they may become intensely involved with their patients. This can lead to both professional satisfaction and anxious fatigue.

CONCLUSION

It may be difficult for the young, healthy physician to empathize with the delirious or demented person whose cognition is impaired and who may face a bleak, lonely future. The interviewer's own uncertainty about treating this patient may be paralleled by that of the patient's friends and family, who should be encouraged to visit, call, and surround the patient with newspapers, pictures, and other things that remind him that there is continuity to his life. In addition to family involvement, it is often very useful for such a patient to feel that the doctor is paying attention and lending a sympathetic ear. A clear formulation of the patient's problem and life trajectory can help the patient feel loved and protected, thereby providing gratification for his dependent needs while also providing structure and perspective for his loved ones.

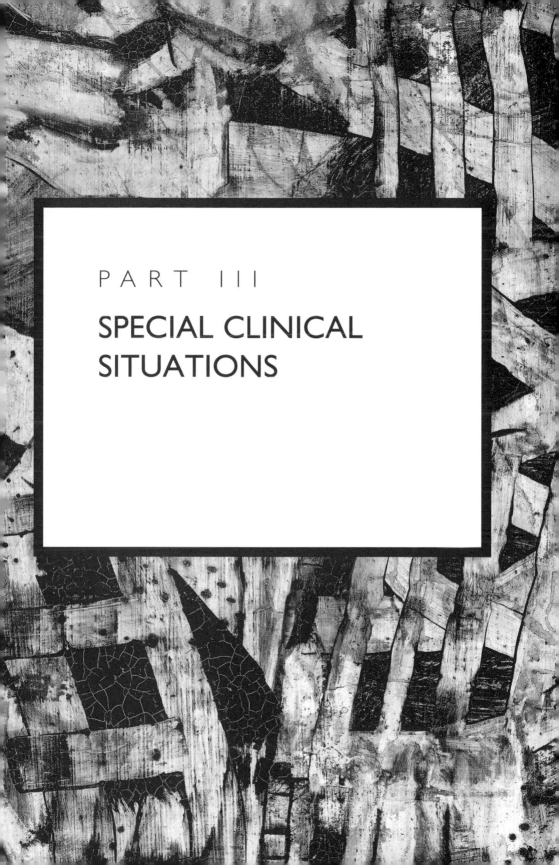

PART III

SPECIAL CLINICAL SITUATIONS

CHAPTER 17

THE EMERGENCY PATIENT

A psychiatric problem becomes an emergency when a person's anxiety has increased to the point that immediate aid is requested. The phrase "psychiatric emergency" does not define a single clinical situation, because many different types of patients may be interviewed under emergency conditions. A person may experience anxiety himself and seek help, or he may elicit anxiety in a partner who labels the situation an emergency and seeks assistance for the patient.

Previous chapters have emphasized the artificiality of boundaries between the initial diagnostic and later treatment interviews. This is particularly true in emergency situations in which therapy begins with the patient's awareness of the availability of treatment.

In all emergency situations—psychiatric, civil, military, and others—people do not know what to do. The clinician's most important functions are to project the feeling that he knows what *he* can do and to assist the patient and those who accompany him in developing a clear notion of what *they* can do. These role definitions convert the emergency into a problem and allow the individuals involved to employ their own adaptive skills in mobilizing the resources of their environment. The patient is not always an ally in this endeavor. If he is convinced that he is helpless and unable to cope with his problems, he may actually conceal his own resources in an attempt to make the clinician take care of him. After the emergency has subsided, it is not uncommon to find that the patient failed to mention a close relative, a supply of funds, or a contingency plan that would have been invoked if the clinician had failed him.

The sense of urgency that permeates every emergency is analogous to pathological anxiety in other situations: It impairs effective adaptive behavior and efficient utilization of resources. The clinician's task is to avoid being overwhelmed by this urgency, thereby reducing its impact upon his patient. His most important tool is the aura of competent self-assurance that he maintains throughout the interview. The clinician should convey the feeling that he is interested and is capable of assisting the patient with his problem. This professional approach, together with the early definition of roles, reduces the disorganizing effects of the crisis and establishes a firm basis for treatment.

PSYCHOPATHOLOGY AND PSYCHODYNAMICS

Psychiatric emergencies can best be understood by first classifying them according to three basic categories of presenting symptoms: intrapsychic, somatic, and interpersonal. A classification based on these three modes of presentation is initially more useful than the traditional diagnostic categories, since emergencies frequently require decisions and action before a diagnostic evaluation can be completed.

A central question in the psychodynamic evaluation of any crisis is Why did it occur now? or What has disrupted the patient's previous functioning? An understanding of the stress that altered the patient's psychological equilibrium and led to the presenting symptom is critical in managing the emergency. The precipitating stress may activate psychological conflicts directly, or it may operate at a physiological level, impairing the autonomous and executive functions of the ego. In either case, the individual will respond with characteristic patterns determined by his basic personality structure. Some individuals are crisis prone and frequently respond to stress with an emergency syndrome; others bind their anxiety more effectively and rarely experience crises.

The patient arrives not only with a presenting symptom and a precipitating stress but also with certain expectations concerning the treatment he will receive. These three factors determine the clinician's approach to the emergency interview.

Intrapsychic Problems

The most common intrapsychic problems are depression, anxiety, and confusion.

Depression

The patient's depression may stimulate anxiety either in himself or in a friend or loved one. The psychodynamics of depression have been discussed in Chapter 7, "The Depressed Patient." It commonly results from the real or imagined loss of love and the lowering of self-confidence and self-esteem. The emergency aspects of depression frequently develop from the possibility of suicide. This danger must be explored with every depressed individual, whether or not the patient introduces the subject himself. The discussion of suicidal thoughts and feelings is a route to increased understanding of the depressed person and again is dealt with in Chapter 7.

An acute grief reaction, the normal response to the death of a loved one, may present a picture that is quite similar to depression. The sadness and pain of grief, together with crying spells and insomnia, may bring individuals to seek emergency psychiatric help. The grief-stricken patient should be supported and given an opportunity to vent his feelings. He should be encouraged to accept help from others, to take medication if he has difficulty sleeping, and to rely upon friends and loved ones. Above all, the interviewer should make it clear that the patient's response is normal and healthy, that it will end in a short time, and that the patient will then be able to resume his normal role. Regressive desires and dependent needs should be supported and gratified during the acute stress, and the patient should be helped to work through the grieving process by being allowed to discuss his loss and express his sadness.

Anxiety

Anxiety, the emotional response to danger, is a cardinal feature of any psychiatric emergency. When it occurs in the patient, it may be the major presenting complaint. In emergency situations, this usually occurs when 1) an event in the patient's current life reawakens fears that have lain dormant in his unconscious or 2) the patient feels that his ability to control sexual or aggressive impulses is threatened, and he fears the consequences. He is rarely aware of the specific fear that has been aroused; instead, the patient feels an overwhelming sense of dread or panic. A common clinical example is the adolescent male who leaves home for college and is asked to share a room with another male for the first time in his life. Homosexual feelings become increasingly difficult to repress, and when he is under the influence of alcohol, his defenses are further weakened, and he begins to panic. Another typical emergency-department problem is the woman who becomes increasingly resentful of the burden of caring for her newborn infant. She becomes terrified that she will accidentally injure the baby, stick him with a pin, or drown him in the bath. Some patients will become aware of the feared impulses, but more often these impulses are denied, as in the postpartum woman, or projected, as in the male college student who responds to unconscious homosexual feelings by fearing that his roommate will attack him. In each of these situations, the balance between the patient's drives and his ego defenses has been disturbed, resulting in an acute increase in anxiety, which may be accompanied by new defenses.

Anxiety over the possible loss of control may disturb either the patient or significant figures in his environment, depending upon 1) whether the impulses involved are primarily transgressions against the patient's inner standards or against social mores and 2) whether it is the patient himself or others who feel that it is likely he will act upon them. Both of the examples given earlier are of patients who fear that they will act on impulses that they themselves consider repugnant. The parents of the adolescent female who bring her to the hospital because she has threatened to run away with her boyfriend and the woman who brings her alcoholic husband because she fears that he may injure their children in one of his drunken rages are examples of emerging impulses that disturb the patient's parents or partner rather than the patient himself.

Surgical procedures and other physical threats to the body are a common precipitant of anxiety because they symbolically reactivate primitive fears of bodily damage. Academic examinations may represent more abstract symbols of the same type of danger. The therapist must understand the relationship of the anxiety to the unconscious imagined danger, since the patient will focus on the realistic threat to his safety, although simple reassurances directed to this end will have little effect.

Anxiety can lead to neurotic symptom formation. Patients may present with acute panic attacks, social phobia, conversion reactions, or hyperventilation syndrome. These patients usually request help themselves, although others may be involved before they reach the clinician. The psychotic individual may respond to anxiety by fears of ego disintegration and gross disorganization. This patient is often unable to seek aid himself, and he may provoke others to define the situation as a psychiatric emergency.

Confusion

The confused patient may not know where he is or how he got there. He has difficulty communicating intelligibly, and his thought processes are fragmented and disorganized. He feels that his senses are unreliable and may misinterpret sights and sounds in strange ways. Anxiety and depression usually result from stresses that threaten the psychological defenses of the ego. They indicate difficulty in resolving conflicts, controlling impulses, and maintaining dependency gratification. Confusion, on the other hand, relates to those areas of ego functioning that are usually immune from psychological conflicts. These autonomous or conflict-free functions of the ego include memory, perception, and learning. They are impaired in brain syndromes and some acute functional psychoses. The patient is confused and bewildered. He is either frightened or so helpless that others are concerned about him, and often he passes through these two stages sequentially. For a more complete discussion see Chapter 16, "The Cognitively Impaired Patient."

The acute precipitant of the emergency may be an event that did not directly impair autonomous ego functioning but that instead placed new or increased demands upon an already damaged ego. The move to a new apartment, with the many adaptive tasks it entails, can precipitate an acute psychiatric crisis in an elderly and slightly brain-damaged person. He is unable to find the bathroom, forgets the location of the telephone, misses his familiar neighbors, and becomes agitated and frightened. His poor memory and impaired spatial thinking were adequate for a familiar environment but are not so for a new one. The interviewer must seek information pertaining to practical aspects of the patient's current life in order to evaluate what skills he retains and what type of assistance would allow him to utilize his remaining abilities most effectively. It may be quite unimportant whether an elderly man living alone knows the month and year or the name of the president, but it is crucial whether he remembers to turn off the gas or is able to find the grocery store.

This patient will usually be brought to the clinician by another person who is anxious to prevent the patient from acting irrationally or harming himself. Although the psychopathology is intrapsychic, the definition of the emergency and the plans for treatment involve interpersonal dynamics. A common error is to diagnose the underlying illness accurately (usually dementia) and to make appropriate recommendations, only to have the treatment plan fail because the needs and expectations of the emergency partner have been ignored.

Somatic Problems

Somatic symptoms that are based on psychological causes are easier to treat when the patient is aware of this relationship, or at least is aware of the existence of concomitant psychological problems. Unfortunately, in emergency situations this is seldom the case. The interviewer may quickly determine that the somatic complaint is only a symptomatic manifestation of a panic attack and thus focus the interview on the patient's emotional conflicts. However, at the end of what he thought was a successful interview, the patient may surprise him by asking, "But what about the pain in my chest?" Such experiences demonstrate that somatic symptoms must be treated as seriously and explored as thoroughly as any other psychological symptoms. Generally, the patient's medical examination and diagnostic studies have already indicated that he has not had a somatic crisis by the time the psychiatrist is summoned.

It is the patient whose symptoms include the somatic manifestations of anxiety or depression who is most likely to acknowledge the existence of emotional problems. Other psychiatric patients who complain of somatic problems will resist the suggestion of psychological conflict. Hypochondriasis, somatic delusions, conversion reactions, histrionic elaborations of physical symptoms, and psychosomatic reactions are usually not perceived by the patient himself as stemming from psychological conflicts. They are only seen as psychiatric emergencies when some other person feels that the problem is urgent and defines it as psychiatric (see Chapter 4, "The Histrionic Patient"; Chapter 14, "The Psychotic Patient"; and Chapter 15, "The Psychosomatic Patient").

Somatic symptoms are often associated with extensive denial of emotional problems, and therefore the patient is resistant to seeing a psychiatrist. He fears that the clinician will tell him that the problem is in his mind and will ignore his serious physical symptom. This is further complicated if the referring individual or emergency partner is a physician or member of the health profession. Again, the symptom must be taken seriously, discussed in detail, and explored with the patient. It is not sufficient to ascertain from a hospital chart that the referring physician performed a complete physical examination. Usually, if such an examination reassures the patient, he is not referred to the psychiatrist. Furthermore, the precise details of the physical symptoms and their course are an important source of information about the psychological problems.

Interpersonal Problems

Interpersonal problems frequently involve one individual complaining about the behavior of another—the wife whose husband is alcoholic, the adolescent male who threatens to leave home, or the psychotically agitated man who is brought by the police. These situations are furthest removed from the traditional medical doctor–patient model and therefore are often difficult for beginning clinicians. It is important to search for appropriate psychodynamic points of intervention rather than to become a judge or referee. When the patient is psychotic this may be easier, but when the major pathology is a character disorder, it may take some time to identify what the psychiatric problem is and which person (or persons) is best considered the patient.

A patient may be brought to the clinician by someone else because he is unable to recognize his own problems. The most obvious examples would be the very young or the very old—the child with uncontrolled aggressive outbursts whose parents frantically seek guidance or the elderly confused man brought by his family because he has been wandering aimlessly in the streets.

Whenever one person brings another—that is, whenever an emergency partner is involved—there is an interpersonal problem in the emergency situation, even if the basic psychopathology is intrapsychic.

Focus on the Present

Psychodynamic formulations rely heavily on developmental material, understanding the patient's conflicts by tracing them to his early experiences and his habitual modes of coping and relating. In an emergency, the patient's attention is directed to his current crisis, and time is usually limited. Therefore, it is necessary to focus on his means of coping with *this* stress, on his feelings and conflicts *now*. One must construct a formulation of the acute crisis rather than of the lifelong personality pattern. After the emergency has subsided, more developmental material can be obtained and a more complete psychodynamic explanation attempted. It is an error to concentrate on obtaining childhood historical material from a person with panic disorder—the focus of inquiry must always be on that which is immediately emotionally meaningful to the patient.

It is important to determine early in the interview which symptoms are acute and which have been present for a considerable time. More recent symptoms are more easily understood and provide clues to the problems and conflicts involved in converting a chronic problem or lifestyle into an acute crisis.

MANAGEMENT OF THE INTERVIEW

Emergencies seldom occur at convenient times or in convenient places. In spite of this, the traditional amenities of the interview should be maintained as far as possible. These include a quiet, comfortable place to sit and talk without a sense of hurry and a minimal number of interruptions.

The emergency interview invariably requires more time than the beginner anticipates. He should realize that even the most experienced clinician often devotes several hours to such problems. Otherwise, he will become dissatisfied with his own performance and annoyed with the patient. Furthermore, these patients are often unable to express appreciation for the clinician's efforts, and the clinician must obtain satisfaction independent of the patient's gratitude.

The exploration of the patient's problems follows the major outlines that have been discussed for nonemergency situations. A special characteristic is the increased emphasis on the precipitating stress and on the expectations of all persons concerned. In addition, the interviewer must structure the interview to include areas that are crucial for immediate therapeutic decisions.

Determination of Who Will Be Interviewed and When

If someone has accompanied the patient, the interviewer must decide who will be taken into the consultation room first. The customary procedure is to begin an interview by speaking to the patient alone. There are situations in which it is preferable to begin by jointly interviewing both the patient and the person accompanying him. The decision to include the partner in the interview is made when both the patient and the partner either verbally or nonverbally indicate their desire for a joint interview. If the patient seems reluctant to leave the partner, then both should be invited into the consultation room. This usually indicates that the person accompanying the patient is emotionally involved in the emergency and therefore must be considered in its management. If the initial portion of the joint interview reveals that the companion inhibits the patient's communication, he can then be excused. If, on the other hand, the patient leaves his partner in the waiting room and then seems unable to describe his problem, the partner could be invited to join the group.

Sometimes the person accompanying the patient will ask to speak with the clinician first, alone. Usually, it is a mistake to allow this, because the patient may no longer perceive the clinician as his ally. The interviewer can indicate that he is interested in what the companion has to say, but that he first wants to see both the patient and companion together. If the patient objects to this, the interviewer should see the patient alone. If the companion insists on a private interview, the interviewer should still see the patient first. Later in the interview, the patient usually agrees to a separate interview with his companion.

In a family or group crisis, there are actually multiple patients, and the entire family may be interviewed and given emergency treatment. One individual often becomes the focus of pathological interactions in a family, the scapegoat for family conflict. It is important to broaden this family's notion of who is in trouble, so that appropriate help may be made available to others.

The selection of the initial interview group is important, but it does not limit the clinician's freedom to change the membership of this group as the interview progresses. It is customary to ask the partner to wait outside after he has related his views of the problem. It may be useful to ask the various persons concerned to enter or leave the consultation room during the interview. This enables the clinician to obtain new information while mobilizing the interest and involvement of others. The establishment of direct relations with anxious family members is vital for the effectiveness of the treatment plan.

If the patient's companion is not included in the initial consultation, he should be asked to remain nearby in case the clinician should wish to speak to him later. This will also facilitate the patient's transportation home or, if necessary, to a hospital. The failure to make this request explicit may result in the clinician spending an hour or two attempting to reach the patient's husband, who has returned to his night job at a hard-to-locate factory, or otherwise struggling to make practical arrangements that the companion could have handled with little difficulty.

The Opening Phase

The more formal portion of the interview begins, as always, with a discussion of the issue of greatest concern to the patient—his chief complaint. While exploring this presenting problem, the clinician attempts to determine the following: 1) Who felt the need for help? 2) How was the problem identified as psychiatric? and 3) What was the precipitating stress? The first two questions are of crucial significance in assessing the patient's awareness that his problem is psychiatric; unless he has at least partially accepted this idea, it is unlikely that he will follow the interviewer's treatment plan.

Who Felt the Need for Help?

The need for help may have been felt by the patient, his family, friends, a social worker, a physician, or some other person. Mental health clinicians tend to be more accepting of self-referred patients, since they are more likely to have intrapsychic symptoms and to express emotional suffering in psychological terms. Beginners find them easier to engage psychotherapeutically and generally prefer them. Patients with somatic symptoms may be preferred by the general physician, but he becomes discouraged if their symptoms have no organic basis and the patient's complaints are not relieved by his therapeutic efforts. Such patients often antagonize the referring clinician with their clinging dependence, and a psychiatric referral may be as much an attempt to dispose of a problem as to solve it. Patients with interpersonal complaints may be self-referred but are more often accompanied by a family member or referred by a social services agency. Such patients may quickly sense that the clinician prefers patients who are self-referred and who seek psychotherapy. In order to please the clinician, the patient may alter his history. It then becomes necessary to explore the details of the search for help carefully in order to identify the actual referring source.

On occasion the clinician is called to see a patient when there is no valid indication for a psychiatric referral. For example, a surgeon requests a consultation after repairing the lacerations of a young man who was involved in a barroom brawl. The patient greets the clinician with protests that he was "only having a fight" and that he has no need to see a psychiatrist. If the clinician persists, asking if such incidents have occurred previously, the patient may answer, "Yes, so what?" The inexperienced clinician attempts to convince the patient that he must have emotional problems. However, the problem really concerns the interviewer, who is unsure of himself, reluctant to discharge the patient without completing a formal examination, and also reluctant to tell his surgical colleague that no consultation is indicated, because the patient has no awareness of a psychiatric problem and will not profit from the interview. This patient should be told, "You don't have to talk with me if you don't want to," and then should be given an opportunity to respond to this statement. The clinician's willingness to terminate the interview may stimulate the patient's desire to continue. If not, the therapist merely advises the patient of the availability of future psychiatric help if he changes his mind. For further discussion of this issue, see Chapter 18, "The Hospitalized Patient."

How Was the Problem Identified as Psychiatric?

The patient may be certain that his problem is psychiatric, he may tentatively consider the possibility, or he may be certain that it is not psychiatric. Often he has made some effort to obtain help prior to the interview, consulting a doctor, psychologist, minister, teacher, or social worker. He may have studied books on psychology or turned to prayer. His description of these attempts and their meaning to him will reveal his initial view of his problem and the way in which it came to be defined as psychiatric.

If the patient himself did not define the problem as psychiatric, he may have been referred to a psychiatrist for varying reasons. The referring physician may not have been able to fit the somatic complaints into a classical clinical syndrome, or he may have sensed underlying emotional problems. Occasionally, factors extraneous to the immediate emergency, such as past history of emotional illness, will determine the psychiatric referral. Understanding the reason for the referral and the patient's feeling about it will help in evaluating his attitude toward psychiatry and toward treatment.

A college student was referred to a psychiatrist by a family physician, who was also a close personal friend of his parents. The parents were devoutly religious and were greatly disturbed by their son's rejection of the church and its teaching. They were unable to see this as other than a symptom of illness and had enlisted the aid of the family doctor, a member of the same church, in reviving their son's faith. The young man was well aware of their feelings and saw the psychiatrist as just another agent of parental control. In fact, he was acutely troubled, but not over religion. His girlfriend had recently told him that she was pregnant, and he had become panicky and depressed and had contemplated suicide. He felt unable to discuss this with his family, and the religious issue kept them at an emotional distance. He was able to tell the story only after the clinician had clarified his role, explaining that he had no preconceived idea of what the problem was or of how it could be resolved but was willing to discuss whatever the patient thought was disturbing him and see if he could help.

What Was the Precipitating Stress?

The "Why now?" question considers what has happened in the patient's life that has disrupted his previously operating system of defenses. The changes may be in the intrapsychic, physiological, interpersonal, or external environment. Such information is usually not volunteered, and often not even conscious, but it is essential that it be elicited and understood early in the initial interview.

A direct question of "What brought you here today?" is often met with "Things just got to be too much for me" or "I couldn't take it any more." The interviewer should pursue the matter further. He might ask, "How did you select this hospital?"; "Have you sought help from anyone else?"; or "Did something happen that was the last straw?"

A detailed description of the events of the past week and particularly the past 24 hours is often illuminating. Important events in the patient's life or changes in his role are considered. Anniversaries and holidays lead to emotional reactions based on their symbolic meaning—for example, depressions can regularly recur on the anniversary of the loss of a loved one, and major holidays are common times for acute depressive reactions.

The clinician asks questions based on knowledge of the psychodynamics involved in specific symptom complexes. For example, if a depressed patient does not spontaneously report a loss, the interviewer inquires in this area. Similarly, if a patient is anxious about becoming psychotic, one can investigate recent experiences in which he feared losing control. One of us has had several emergency consultations with college students fearing impending psychosis without apparent cause. In response to specific inquiry, they revealed that the recent use of Ecstasy or marijuana had triggered their panic attacks. Such an episode will lead a patient to seek help, but his shame or fear of its significance may make him reluctant to reveal the crucial features of the history. He seeks reassurance but wants to avoid exposure. The clinician's direct questions not only elicit the specific information but also reduce the patient's anxiety by assuring him that the interviewer is familiar with this kind of problem and knows how to deal with it.

Specific Syndromes

In this chapter, only the emergency aspects of the specific syndromes are considered. For a discussion of these interviews in greater depth, the reader is referred to the appropriate chapters.

Depression and Suicide

When interviewing depressed patients in emergency situations, the most obvious area of structured inquiry is the exploration of suicidal risk. The patient should be asked about this directly. If the clinician is anxious about the topic or employs euphemisms such as "doing something to yourself," the patient feels inhibited. The interviewer determines the patient's thoughts and impulses, his attitude toward them, and the actions that have resulted. For example, if the clinician asks, "Have you had thoughts of suicide?" or "Have you wished to be dead?" the patient may reply, "Yes, I've felt that I should just end it all." An appropriate response from the clinician would be, "Did you go so far as to plan how you would do it?" If the patient replies, "No, the thought was too upsetting," and further inquiry reveals that he had not acted on impulses in the past, the risk would seem small. Another patient might reply to the initial question, "I had some thoughts of suicide last week, but not today." The alert clinician inquires further, "Did you think of how you would do it?" The reply "I wondered about shooting myself; in fact, I bought a gun and some ammunition a few days ago" would suggest a serious risk. If the clinician then asks, "Were you frightened?" and the patient replies, "Oh, I don't know; I think everyone would be better off if I were dead," immediate protective measures would be indicated.

Communications relating to suicidal impulses are frequently nonverbal or indirect. If a depressed patient arrives in the emergency department with his bag packed, he is asking to be hospitalized; if he has left the door of his home unlocked, spent his last few dollars on a good meal or a phone call to a distant friend, or is unconcerned about the time or place of the next visit, he may not expect to be alive very long. These messages indicate his ambivalence about living or dying. If someone cares enough about him, that person may succeed in tilting this ambivalence in the direction of life.

Persons who have had a close relative or friend who committed suicide present a greater risk, as do patients with a personal history of previous attempts at suicide. If the patient has recently made a will or straightened out his financial affairs, he may plan to die. A belief in life after death or the fantasy of reunion with a dead person that he loved is another important piece of information. A variety of demographic, ethnic, and social factors have a demonstrable relation to suicide risk.

The interviewer inquires who would remain behind if the patient killed himself. He may save the patient's life by convincing him that suicide would inflict great pain and suffering upon someone the patient loves. In the case of the suicidal patient who is physically ill, is elderly, and has no loved ones and no money, the clinician could say, "I can understand how badly you feel and how little you have to live for, but I have seen others who felt just as you do, who were then helped by treatment and recovered. You have nothing to lose by giving yourself a chance to get well." Beginning clinicians often attempt to reassure the patient with statements such as, "Don't worry—we won't let you kill yourself." This invites the patient to relinquish his own controls and to rely upon the clinician to arrest his self-destructive drive, and it is a promise that the clinician can rarely keep. The clinician may instead ask the suicidal patient if he would like to come into the hospital, where he may feel greater ability to resist his suicidal urge, until he is better. If hospitalization is not indicated, the clinician should let the patient know exactly where he can be reached, day or night, and whom the patient might call if the clinician is unavailable. Obviously, the person whom the patient can call must be told about the patient in advance.

Anxiety Attacks

The patient with acute panic attacks and hyperventilation syndrome may respond dramatically to direct explanation of his symptoms. This must, of course, be geared to his capacity to understand. An unsophisticated patient can be told, "When someone is frightened, he breathes very rapidly without knowing it. Fast breathing can cause many of your symptoms." The patient might be further convinced by asking him to hyperventilate deliberately and then showing him how to control his symptoms by regulating his respiratory rate.

Clinical Situations

The Anxious Patient

Patients with overwhelming anxiety have already been told by others to relax. If this had been helpful, the patient would not be seeking further assistance. The clinician should avoid repeating such advice and should instead reassure the patient that his problem will at last be understood rather than simply suppressed.

Simple reassurance is of little value to the patient who is afraid of going crazy. Rather than telling him that he is not going crazy, the clinician finds out what the word "crazy" means to him. This reveals the significance of his fears and allows exploration of the sources of his anxiety. The clinician can inquire, "What do you mean by 'crazy'?" or "What do you think it would be like to go crazy?" The patient can then be asked if he has ever seen anyone who was considered crazy, and what he observed at that time. Finally, the clinician finds out how the patient thinks people will respond to his craziness. Frequently the patient with an acute panic attack expresses fears concerning aggressive or sexual impulses. Once the specific fears are uncovered, the clinician's reassurance will have much greater impact.

The Confused Patient

The clinician is sometimes asked to see a patient who at first appears to be completely out of contact with his surroundings. The scene is the emergency department of a general hospital; the patient is lying on a stretcher, difficult to arouse, and disheveled. He does not respond to questions or mumbles incoherently without looking at the examiner. The first impression suggests the aftermath of a major neurological catastrophe. Patients with confusional syndromes need a constant input of sensory stimuli and orienting information in order to maintain their attention and contact with the outside world. The clinician should introduce himself and briefly assess the situation. He may then encourage the patient to sit up and, if possible, conduct the interview with the patient in a chair. The interviewer can initially structure the discussion by focusing the patient's attention on his immediate life situation. The response may be dramatic; on occasion it is possible to obtain a history and make a detailed evaluation of the patient's problem.

The Intoxicated Patient

One of the most difficult of the brain syndromes is seen in the alcoholic who is acutely intoxicated. This condition has many potential complications, some with a significant mortality. In addition to the medical complications of delirium tremens, hallucinosis, or pathological intoxication, the patient's emotional controls are weakened, and he is often depressed. Suicide or other impulsive behavior is a problem. The clinician must determine why the patient is drinking and whether this episode is different from previous ones. The interviewer will have little success in attempting to conduct an interview while the patient is acutely intoxicated, because the alcohol provides a chemical barrier that impairs effective communication. The patient has usually lost his emotional controls and is either belligerent and uncooperative or morose and depressed. If he can be observed for a few hours, a bewildering clinical picture often clears considerably, and a more careful evaluation is possible.

The Patient With a "Pseudo-Coronary"

The patient who is convinced that he is having a heart attack is a common emergency department problem. As with any patient with somatic symptoms, a careful medical history is indicated. The interviewer uses his questions in order to demonstrate the connection between symptoms and emotions. Someone who would be annoyed at a question like "Did you think the chest pain might have been because you were frightened?" will respond quite comfortably to "You must have worried a great deal about your chest pain." It is often useful to perform the physical examination personally; it provides an air of authenticity for later assurances about physical illness. Certainly if this patient proffers the affected portion of his body for examination, an examination should be performed. He wants to show his problem, and if this doctor appears disinterested he will seek another.

When the somatic symptom is pain, the interviewer never challenges its being real. Pain is a subjective sensation, and only the person experiencing it can tell whether it is present. This does not mean, however, that the clinician must accept the patient's explanation of its cause, because that is a medical matter. The clinician can say, "What you describe is certainly painful, but we need more information to determine the cause of the problem."

The Substance-Abusing Patient

One of the most difficult differential diagnostic problems in emergency psychiatry involves the patient suspected of malingering pain in order to obtain narcotic drugs. Although most patients with pain want medical treatment for their underlying condition, the patient with severe pain may initially seek only relief from his symptom. He will rarely specify how this is to be given, whereas the substance abuser who is malingering may have a specific drug and dosage in mind.

The Patient With an Interpersonal Crisis

The patient with an interpersonal crisis will initially tend to blame someone else for his difficulties and may indicate that he wants only environmental manipulation. As the clinician would not tell the patient with psychogenic pain that it is all in his mind, he similarly would not make massive assaults on this pattern of defenses. The interviewer who asks, "Why do you continually get into such messy situations?" may feel that he is searching for the origins of a psychological problem, but the patient will experience it as an accusation. Consider the adolescent female who is brought to the emergency department by her distraught parents after she has ingested 10 aspirins in a dramatic suicidal gesture. She has been fighting with her mother about her late hours and her current boyfriend. The mother is obviously controlling her rage as she asks whether her daughter is all right. She then adds, "We have tried to bring her up right, but we can't do anything with her."

The clinician finds himself torn between the patient's plea for sympathy and independence and the parents' frustrated helplessness. He is tempted to interpret either her manipulative coercion or their overcontrolling domination, thereby taking one side or the other. Instead, he can explore the events that precipitated the emergency. The process of discussion will provide the family with an alternative to the pattern of dramatic scenes and uproar that has been their characteristic mode of interaction.

The Assaultive Patient

The management of an interview with an assaultive patient is always a problem. If the scene is a hospital emergency department, by the time the clinician arrives he may find the patient lying on the floor, forcibly restrained by several attendants. Usually this demonstration of force will suffice to help the patient regain control over his aggressive impulses. The clinician can kneel beside the patient and ask him, "What is all the commotion about?" As the restrainers relax their grip, the clinician can quickly ascertain whether the patient plans to renew the struggle. If not (and this is usually the case), the clinician can ask, "Wouldn't you rather sit in a chair and talk with me?" and then help the patient to rise while the other personnel are dismissed. The interview continues with an immediate inquiry of "What happened?" and a discussion of the patient's loss of control. On some occasions, usually with organic psychoses, the patient must be kept in restraint while the clinician administers tranquilizers parenterally. When the medication becomes effective, the interview continues as it would under other circumstances.

Beginning interviewers are concerned that if they ask the wrong thing the patient will again become violent. Usually the patient is even more concerned about this than the clinician, and he should be asked to tell the interviewer if he feels his assaultive impulses recurring.

Some patients have not actually assaulted anyone, but they are on the verge. They may seem to be unaffected by the clinician's calm manner and continue to pace the floor in a state of great agitation. These patients are offered medication before continuing the interview. The therapist can remain with the patient while the medication takes effect and should not increase the patient's fear of being trapped by placing himself between the patient and the door. Such fears may provoke either aggression or flight.

If the clinician arrives to see the severely agitated patient just a few minutes too late he may find himself trying to interview someone who is heading out the front door. He should firmly but gently say, "Just a minute," and, if the patient stops, continue the interview wherever they are located, even if it is outdoors on the sidewalk. Rapport can be best established by exploring the patient's great haste to get away. Once this step is accomplished, the clinician suggests that the interview be continued in a more comfortable setting and proceeds as with other cases.

The assaultive patient is reassured by the confidence that the experienced clinician feels and exhibits. The same patient is quick to detect simulated confidence concealing fear, and he may react to the clinician's fear with assaultive behavior. If an inexperienced clinician continues to fear the patient, he should administer medication or utilize auxiliary personnel to control the patient so that he can conduct the interview more comfortably.

The Patient's Expectations

The patient comes to the clinician with expectations about the outcome of his visit. Such expectations are both conscious and unconscious, both positive and negative. They must be considered by the clinician early in the interview and reevaluated at its termination. Frequently, it is possible to help a patient modify his expectations during the course of the interview, after he has first gained an awareness of them. The clinician can demonstrate the inappropriateness of certain expectations while strengthening and supporting others that he can reasonably hope to satisfy. If the patient has not been able to formulate any realistic expectations, the clinician must do this for him. If the clinician fails to do so, the patient will be dissatisfied by the interview and will seek help elsewhere.

The patient should not be asked what kind of help he hopes to receive too early in the interview. He may interpret this as the interviewer's refusal to accept responsibility for ascertaining his difficulties or as a hostile rebuff. Nevertheless, once rapport has been established, this question can reveal a great deal. Inquiry regarding previous attempts at finding help is also useful. A patient who has sought the police before arriving at the emergency department often expects controls to be imposed. With patients who have sought help from religious advisors, one should inquire into the specific kind of help requested. The patient who sought the name of a psychiatrist has different expectations from the one who sought help through prayer. A difference even exists between the patient who prayed for strength in coping with a situation and the one who prayed for a solution through omnipotent intervention.

When there is an individual in the patient's life who would have been an obvious source of help but whom the patient avoided, questions concerning the avoidance may reveal some of the fearful expectations he has brought to the interview. The interviewer might also inquire directly concerning negative expectations. Such inquiry is not always successful, but the patient's feelings may be revealed indirectly through stories of his family's and friends' experiences with mental health practitioners, anecdotes about the hospital, jokes, and so on. If a patient starts the interview by joking, "Where are the men in the little white coats that cart you off to the insane asylum?" this reveals not only some ability to maintain a sense of humor but also fear of being seen as crazy, with all of the many possible unconscious implications.

The emergency partner will also have expectations, and these may be similar to or different from those of the patient. When the partner has initiated the request for help, his expectations must also be considered; otherwise the search will continue, regardless of the effectiveness of the interview with the patient.

Unconscious Expectations

The unconscious expectations of the patient are closely related to the psychodynamics of the precipitating stress. The most common unconscious expectation is that the clinician will directly resolve the patient's conflict. For example, the depressed patient wants his loss replaced, and an important early task is to shift this desire to a hope that his pain will be comforted and his diminished self-esteem restored. In the case of a man who is depressed following the loss of his job, the clinician inquires why the patient blames himself. By pointing out the discrepancy between the patient's critical attitude toward himself and his successful functioning in other areas of his life, the clinician focuses on his current adaptive skills and his desire to find a new job rather than his lost hopes and his fantasy that the clinician will somehow get his old position back for him.

Another situation is illustrated by the depressed woman who is angry with her husband but is fearful that he will leave her if she ventilates her rage. She feels that she is a martyr but is afraid to rebel. When she asks, "Do you think it is fair that I have to live like this?" she is seeking permission to act. This patient may become depressed if the clinician does not grant this permission, but she may be even more threatened if he does. It is important first to establish a trusting alliance and then to search for alternate patterns of behavior that may allow some gratification of her impulses without dire consequences.

Conscious Expectations

The conscious expectations of emergency patients include hospitalization, medical treatment, medication, environmental manipulation, psychotherapy, reassurance, no effect at all, and actual physical or psychological harm.

Hospitalization may be seen as a protection from the threat of inner impulses or as a means of influencing the environment. For example, a woman sought help a few weeks after giving birth to a child because of obsessive fears that she would drop or otherwise harm the infant. When the clinician inquired further, she said, "I hoped you would put me in the hospital or take my baby away before I kill him." She was seeking control. The very act of seeking control implied that some inner controls were working, and these had to be found and strengthened. The patient herself was the best ally.

If the patient views treatment as a means of controlling others, he may first insist that he be hospitalized and then be equally insistent that he be discharged 1 or 2 days later. A patient who loudly protests against hospitalization, while at the same time acting crazy, may actually be requesting hospitalization but refusing to accept responsibility for it. His expectation is that he will be forced into a hospital against his will, and he may become more upset if his expectation is not met.

A patient may fear that the clinician will select the wrong alternative in treating an impulse problem. Thus a religious patient who is concerned about sexual feelings may wish to remove or suppress them and may fear that the clinician will encourage sexuality. If his hopes and fears are made explicit, the patient can be helped. The clinician might say, "I have the feeling that you'd like to eliminate your sexual feelings and that you fear I may only make things worse by encouraging them."

Patients with little psychological sophistication and those with somatic symptoms will want medication. These patients may request medication early in the interview, and beginning therapists often comply much too quickly. The problem may appear different at the end of the interview, and advice concerning medication can wait until that time, even when the clinician feels confident that drugs will be necessary. If the patient feels that all the clinician can do is to prescribe medication, he loses interest in the interview once he receives his prescription, and what follows is anticlimactic. In an emergency situation, the prescription should be for only enough medication to last until the next visit. If the clinician reassures the patient that things will soon be better and then provides a 3-month supply of medicine, the patient may not trust the clinician's words. A beginning dose of medicine, supplied directly by the clinician and perhaps taken in his presence, has special value. It carries the magical power of the clinician's personal tool of therapy. A patient with whom the clinician is not thoroughly familiar should never be given a potentially dangerous quantity of medication. Even if the patient is not suicidal, he may feel that the clinician is either careless or unconcerned about his welfare.

The clinician often makes recommendations that involve manipulating the patient's environment. He may recommend a home helper or a leave of absence from school or a job. In doing this, he distinguishes between the patient who must be encouraged to relinquish his pathological sense of obligation and the patient whose tenuously maintained self-esteem is dependent upon his continued functioning. For example, the suggestion of a home helper could upset a mother who, despite her depression, takes pride in her continuing ability to care for her children. In this situation, the clinician recognizes the patient's devotion to her family, treats her depression, and asks the patient, "Is there a family member who can assist you in your responsibilities while we treat your depression?" If the patient has no helpful relative or friend but is open to the concept of accepting temporary assistance, a "personal helper" could be suggested.

The patient with interpersonal problems will often want the clinician to alter the environment and therefore remove the problem. Thus a woman might complain that her husband beats her and want the clinician to remove him from the home. The clinician might reply, "Only the police can do that, and you have told me that you have been to them many times. However, I might be able to help with the troubles that lead to his drinking, or your uncertainty about leaving him, if you are also bothered by those problems." The patient may already have some awareness of these considerations, and this can sometimes be elicited by comments such as, "If you only wanted someone to straighten out your husband, you would not have come to a psychiatrist." In this way the clinician is reinforcing the patient's more realistic expectations.

Psychotherapy is more likely to be expected by patients who are better educated or are from a higher social class and whose symptoms are psychological in nature. However, a patient's awareness of psychological problems does not mean that he will not need medication, direct guidance, or hospitalization. This patient's distress, like that of the patient with somatic symptoms, may be an indication for medication. Indeed, an acutely heightened awareness of inner conflicts is often indicative of the too rapid breakdown of defenses.

Negative Expectations and the Unwilling Patient

The patient with negative expectations anticipates no help and may expect further injury and humiliation. When depressed, he is likely to be suicidal; when paranoid, he will probably be belligerent and combative. He does not accept psychiatric intervention. These negative expectations must be openly discussed if there is to be any hope of engaging the patient's cooperation in a treatment plan. When discussing this patient's unconscious expectations, it is crucial that the clinician ally himself with the patient's unconscious hope rather than his unconscious fear.

It may be necessary to force treatment against a patient's will in order to protect him or others around him. This must be done openly. It is better to tell a patient, "I will have to send you to the hospital even if you don't agree to go," than to conceal this by saying, "We'll have to arrange for another consultation in the building across the street." The patient will ultimately appreciate the clinician's honesty and directness, and his attitude toward other clinicians will be favorably influenced.

Before involuntarily hospitalizing a patient, the interviewer should exhaust every possible means of convincing him to go voluntarily. This process begins by explaining the therapeutic rationale behind hospitalization at this time—usually the need to supply the patient with external assistance in controlling suicidal or assaultive impulses. If the patient did not wish to have these impulses curbed, he would not have allowed himself to be interviewed and would have kept their existence a secret until he was free to act upon them. This should be explicitly pointed out to the patient.

Few judges will force a commitment against the wishes of the patient's relatives unless he has committed a crime. Patients have been hospitalized repeatedly only to be signed out, against medical advice, by a relative on the following day. Therefore, it is necessary to gain the relatives' support when the clinician is recommending hospitalization. Frequently a relative, friend, priest, or someone else whom the patient trusts can exercise greater influence in helping the patient to accept hospitalization than can the clinician.

A careful discussion of the patient's fears of hospitalization is essential. He may think that he cannot obtain his own release when he no longer feels the need for hospitalization, or there may have been previous unpleasant experiences with psychiatric hospitals. Alternate plans that would provide assistance in controlling his impulses should be discussed. Sometimes this may convince the clinician that hospitalization is not the only way to cope with the emergency. The clinician should then feel free to alter his recommendation. Finally, when a patient indicates reluctance about accepting hospitalization, he should not be left unsupervised after the subject has been mentioned and especially not after a positive decision has been made.

The Treatment Plan

As the interview draws to a close, the clinician begins to formulate his suggestions and plans for further treatment. These must be conveyed to the patient in a way that will help him to accept them. The patient's own treatment plans are to be explored first. How has he handled similar problems in the past, and what were the results? If his plan differs radically from the clinician's, has he considered alternatives? If he indicates that he has already rejected the clinician's plan, one can point out that he thought of it himself, and at least considered it as a possibility. The interviewer finds the patient's own reasons for and against it, and deals with his arguments rather than with those of the clinician. If he has not considered the specific alternative that the doctor has in mind, it is suggested to him and he is asked to consider it during the interview. If he reaches the same plan as the clinician, he is far more likely to follow it than if he is simply informed of the clinician's thoughts.

> For example, an acutely depressed college student sought help in the week of his final examinations. He had never had a similar episode in the past. He described his problems, and the clinician inquired as to his plans. He replied that he expected to take his exams, but that, in his current state, he was sure that he would fail. The clinician asked, "Have you considered any alternatives?" The patient said, "Yes, I thought of asking to be excused from the exam, but the professor would probably say no, and anyway, it wouldn't be fair." The clinician asked, "Could you tell the professor that you weren't feeling well, and ask if you could make up the exam when you were better?" The patient had not considered this because, like most depressed people, he did not feel that he would get better. He replied, "Well, I don't know, I don't want the professor to know I've seen a psychiatrist. He would never understand." The clinician was then able to explore his reaction and to demonstrate that the patient's fear had no foundation in reality but was instead based upon his

diminished self-esteem and consequent assumption that others would be intolerant of him. This sort of discussion will help the patient to employ the clinician's recommendation, although initially he was quite resistant to it.

If the emergency partner has initiated the consultation, he too must be considered in the treatment plan. If the clinician does not reduce his anxiety, he will continue to pursue other avenues of help. It is not sufficient to merely acquaint him with the treatment plan if he was not present during its formulation. His expectations must also be made explicit, and any discrepancies between these and the actual plan must be discussed.

Closing the Interview

Because the emergency patient does not know the length of the appointment, the clinician should always indicate that time is drawing to a close when there are still a few minutes of the interview remaining. He can say, "We will have stop in a few minutes" or "Our time is almost up now." This provides the patient an opportunity to add more material or, more important, to ask questions. The clinician can ask, "Is there anything we have not talked about?" or "Is there something else you would like to tell me, or something you would like to ask me?" The patient's choice will reveal what he considers to be a crucial problem or major anxiety. Occasionally he will reply, "There is nothing." This reply does not necessarily mean that the patient is satisfied. The interviewer does not stop at this point but pursues discussion of an area that was not fully explored earlier. The topic can be one that, although affectively charged, was not developed because it was tangential to the emergency. The patient who has no questions to ask is provided an opportunity to reveal additional material through his trend of associations.

In closing the interview, it is preferable to give the emergency patient a specific appointment rather than suggesting vaguely that he come back later. If the problem was severe enough to precipitate an emergency, it should be reevaluated in a second interview. If he does not have a specific appointment, the patient may have to create another emergency in order to return.

CONCLUSION

The psychodynamics of emergency behavior encompass all of the specific clinical syndromes, but there are special considerations added by the emergency situation. An understanding of these additional dynamic issues will enable the clinician to utilize his existing knowledge most effectively. His systematic approach to the problem will allay his own anxiety by protecting him from the crisis atmosphere produced by the patient and partner. This allows the clinician to reduce the patient's anxiety, and as a result, the patient can mobilize his own adaptive skills to cope with his problems.

CHAPTER 18

THE HOSPITALIZED PATIENT

JOHN W. BARNHILL, M.D.

The patient in a medical hospital presents a unique opportunity for the psychodynamically informed clinician. Physiological and psychological stressors threaten the patient's customary way of being, leading even the most psychologically healthy of patients to feel discomforted. The hospital-based interviewer will work with many people who have never seen a psychiatrist or received a psychiatric diagnosis. Some of them will have symptoms that stem from psychological reactions to illness, whereas others will have symptoms that are secondary to physiological alterations. People with preexisting psychiatric illnesses may be especially vulnerable to subjective distress and may have coping styles that interfere with medical treatment. One group of these patients has long been in psychiatric care and welcomes the psychiatric interviewer as a potential ally in a strange environment. Another group has avoided psychiatric contact for decades, and the hospital-based interview may be their first and only opportunity to be evaluated, perhaps for a schizotypal personality or severe agoraphobia.

Psychiatric interviews within the hospital are generally conducted at the request of the patient's primary physician. Although the patient's psychological responses may be paramount to the interviewer, the primary physician often has specific practical concerns and is not interested in psychodynamic understanding of the patient or in the account of the process of the psychiatrist's data acquisition. Consultation requests often involve problems that have reduced compliance or have contributed to the medical complaints. The hospital-based interviewer should remain attentive to the diagnostic and treatment goals of the medical staff while at the same time maximizing the potential therapeutic experience for the patient. The interviewer of the hospitalized patient must be attentive to a host of neuropsychiatric and psychiatric syndromes, to the needs of the consulting physician, and to creation of an alliance with a patient who is sick, tired, and distracted.

The hospital-based interviewer does not act with the same independence as the outpatient clinician. As a consultant, the interviewer becomes a participating observer in a social network that includes the patient, the referring physician, other physician consultants, social workers, nurses, other staff, other patients, and the patient's family and friends. Each of these may have different—and conflicting—interests in the outcome. Amid this complexity is the reality that although many hospitalized patients are too acutely ill to profit from interpretations of their unconscious wishes or fears, the catastrophic nature of their illnesses may render them able to profit from brief focused psychodynamically based interventions.

PSYCHODYNAMICS

Psychodynamic Factors in the Patient

Patients exhibit an array of subjective and behavioral responses to illness and hospitalization. For most, hospitalization induces a regressive but trusting dependency that allows them to accept and participate in their medical care. Moderate amounts of sadness and anxiety are usual and can generally be attributed to the narcissistic injury secondary to the loss of their sense of invulnerability along with the loss of the ego-enhancing activities of everyday life. Furthermore, most illnesses sap energy, concentration, and enthusiasm. As they recover, most patients quickly revert to their prehospital personalities and regain their usual sense of autonomy. However, some experience a more severe amalgam of regression, sadness, confusion, sleep deprivation, and illness-induced fatigue. The extent of psychological disability may relate to premorbid psychological functioning, to the severity or chronicity of illness, or both, and it is usually impossible to predict a given person's response to illness and hospitalization.

Many typical features can be seen in the case of a 55-year-old businessman who had developed complications after a myocardial infarction and cardiac bypass surgery:

A psychiatric consultation was requested during his second week of hospitalization. The cardiology team felt that he was depressed, and they were concerned because he was refusing important procedures. The physical therapists reported that his poor motivation was impeding his recovery; the nursing staff noted that he was frequently demeaning and dismissive. The patient frequently threatened to sign out against medical advice. As he went to meet the patient, the psychiatrist suspected that the precipitating reason for the consultation was probably these behaviors rather than depression.

Although he had never before seen a psychiatrist, the patient was eager to speak, explaining that he felt that he was about to go crazy. He described himself as an institutional bond salesman, "a big earner who could outwork anyone on Wall Street," twice divorced with one adult child. He immediately launched into a series of complaints about the hospital, the staff, his friends, and his family. The nurses were slow to respond, the food was awful, his best friend had left on a golfing trip, and there were days when his daughter did not even call. The psychiatrist said, "Being a patient in the hospital is a humbling experience. It is especially difficult for a man as successful as you have been. Here you have been stripped of your dignity and authority and are dependent on your caretakers." These comments resonated with the patient. The patient said that he was not some "sad-sack loser" and went on to describe how he was accustomed to filling his evenings with client dinners and his weekends with buddies, women, and sports; then he spontaneously added that he had not realized how alone he really was. He had felt chest pain for months before going to a cardiologist, but throughout his life his ability to "suck it up" had proved valuable. He was worried that he might lose his job, and although he had some savings, his entire life would change. He felt a sense of irritable dysphoria that he had never experienced before.

When the psychiatrist asked if he had ever been in a hospital before, the patient said that he had always been as healthy as a horse. He then recounted that when he was 20, his father had died from heart failure. When asked to say more, the patient described how he had despised his father for being a failure at business. He said that his mother had died after his parents had divorced when he was 11 years old. He always thought that she had died of a broken heart and believed that both of his parents were weak. He felt that his own personal toughness had made him "a player on the Street," but now he feared that he was going to lose it all. He was angry at everyone, but especially at his own weakness.

This brief consultation illustrates many issues that are frequently seen in the hospitalized patient. The patient had a long-standing tendency toward denial of his emotions and a hypomanic defense against sadness. Although costly to his family life, these defenses had led to financial success and a degree of personal satisfaction. Denial of emotions and of his own physical symptoms had also led to the original delay in seeking treatment that had complicated his recovery. Many patients respond to the stress of illness—or fantasized illness—with denial, which can be adaptive when it allows the patient to function in the face of adversity but can be maladaptive when it leads to an impaired personal life, refusal of necessary procedures, or threatened premature discharge.

This patient also described significant self-criticism, dysphoria, hopelessness, and helplessness, which might suggest depression. The diagnosis of major depression in a medically ill patient is complicated by the many symptoms of depression that overlap with the physical symptoms of medical illness. In addition, many physical illnesses—including cardiac disease—can physiologically predispose an individual to depressive syndromes. Nevertheless, the patient's depressive symptoms seemed predominately a psychological reaction to his medical illness. Like many patients, his illness led to conscious fears that he would become an invalid, never to work again, as well as to fears that the least exertion might lead to sudden death, which might explain his poor effort in physical therapy. His illness had aroused long-standing conflicts concerning dependency in a man who had experienced multiple losses and deprivations following his mother's death. The patient's "hatred" for his father seemed to have been an unconscious defense against his painful feelings of loss and need. His self-loathing mirrored his loathing his father's weakness.

> The consultant told the patient, "The hospital is making you depressed. You can't do the things that made you feel good, like work, sports, and sex. You have spent your whole life as a successful, tough, and independent man, and now you can't even walk down the stairs by yourself. Furthermore, this is particularly scary for a guy whose own father died of heart failure and whose mother died of a broken heart." The patient laughed and said, "I don't know which is worse, having heart surgery or getting psychoanalyzed." The interviewer smiled and the patient went on, "Don't stop now, remember, I'm the tough guy." The interviewer continued, "Well, I was thinking about why they wanted you to see me, that you weren't going with the program. You're feeling weak and taking it out on everyone around you. The ironic thing is that the more you refuse physical therapy, the longer you'll be stuck in the hospital." The patient was intrigued, and more important, his behavior subsequently improved.

Psychodynamic Factors in the Staff

It is not the consultant's role to be therapist to the staff, but it is often useful to understand the person requesting the consultation. The complexity of medical science is less a challenge for many physicians than the stress of working with chronic illness, suffering, and death. These daily problems often elicit requests for psychiatric consultations, although the official excuse may be the patient's depression or anxiety. By recognizing that consultations often have multiple precipitants, the interviewer can function more effectively.

Consultations often stem from issues that have as much to do with the primary team as with the patient. For example, if the psychiatrist is asked to "hurry and get a note in the chart" a few hours before a scheduled discharge, it is likely that the consultation relates to administrative or medico-legal issues rather than to a desire for clinical guidance. This situation is in marked contrast to that in which the internist asks the psychiatrist to assess the possibility of panic disorder in a patient who is admitted with chest pain. Although this latter patient also may be admitted for only a few hours, it is far more likely that the referring physician in this case is interested in clinical recommendations.

The referring physician may ask how a patient can best be prepared for the psychiatric consultation. This concern may be related to the patient's irritability or perceived vulnerability and is one reason that many patients are never told about a request for a psychiatric consultation. If the patient has psychological concerns, it is useful to suggest that the referring physician describe the consultation as an attempt to help with those concerns, which can range from depression to placement issues to conflicts with staff.

Some patients provoke intense conflicts within the hospital staff. Such conflicts may reflect character pathology in the patient. For example, one patient idealized her primary physician while denigrating the house staff. This led the house staff to dislike her while her primary physician enjoyed her flattery. The psychiatric consultation was called by the house staff because they felt that the patient was irritable and difficult. The consultation revealed a lifelong pattern of unstable relationships, fear of abandonment, and mood instability, all of which worsened under stress. The psychiatrist theorized that the patient was splitting the staff into wholly positive and wholly negative. Staff members transiently and unconsciously accepted these roles, leading to some feeling benevolent while others felt misunderstood and angry. While the staff argued among themselves, the patient would lie back and "watch the action." *Splitting* is discussed in Chapter 9, "The Borderline Patient." In the hospital setting, the consultant's focus might be to address the patient's anxiety while bringing together members of the "split staff" and pointing out the patterns. In so doing, the staff can recognize that the disruption of their customary collegiality is actually diagnostic of particular psychopathology of the patient.

The staff may be divided over a request for psychiatric consultation in other situations. On occasion, paradoxically, staff bias can benefit disliked patients and adversely affect favored ones. For example, a consultation was requested to hasten discharge for a loud, argumentative patient. The consultant diagnosed alcohol withdrawal, and discharge was delayed in order to treat the impending withdrawal delirium. In another case an internist objected to a psychiatric consultation for a pleasant, elderly woman who had carcinoma of the breast and was moderately depressed. The physician later admitted that he did not want to pathologize a woman who reminded him of his own mother, who also had recently been diagnosed with cancer. Similar countertransference issues can lead a physician to hesitate in obtaining psychiatric consultation even for a patient who has made a serious suicide attempt. It is common for treating physicians to deny psychopathology by saying that delirium is normal in the intensive care unit and that suicidality is normal in the dying patient. In both cases, the consultant should remind his physician colleague that delirium and suicidality may be the response to severe illness but that they can be treated and warrant psychiatric intervention. Tactful, straightforward discussions with medical peers can lead to more appropriate and more timely consultations as well as more effective interventions.

Medical and nursing teams are relieved to find psychiatrists who use minimal psychiatric jargon and whose outward personal and professional characteristics resemble those of other physicians. For example, many hospital-based interviewers wear a white coat in order to "fit in" with the medical team.

MANAGEMENT OF THE INTERVIEW

The primary goal of the hospital consultation is the enhancement of the patient's overall medical care. There are related goals, including the diagnosis and treatment of psychiatric disorders and the development of a reassuring alliance, but the hospital-based psychiatrist has a mandate to answer the questions and concerns posed by the primary medical team. The interviewer's suggestions should reflect responsibility for the psychiatric aspects of the case without intrusion into areas that are best handled by medical and surgical colleagues. The consultant will be expected to suggest an approach to the psychiatric aspects of the case at the time of the interview, and the value of the suggestions will quickly be assessed by the primary medical team, the patient, and the patient's family.

Flexibility is essential in hospital interviews. Every variable—the patient, the consultation question, the frame of the interview, the medical team—can vary in ways that the interviewer cannot control. This combination of uncertainty and the need to respond to externally mandated demands can frustrate the psychiatric interviewer if he is not creative and pragmatic.

Before Meeting the Patient

Preparation dramatically increases the effectiveness of hospital consultations. The interviewer should clarify the reason for the consultation request and obtain as much information as possible through careful reading of the chart. Nurses' notes are often especially useful, since they tend to focus on psychosocial and behavioral issues. A brief discussion with a member of the primary medical team may be crucial. Tapping these sources of information increases the likelihood of a successful intervention instead of an aimless shuffle around a complex situation. A significant percentage of referral questions will prove to be incomplete or misleading, but these "errors" allow the consultant to be of particular use to colleagues whose focus and expertise are outside of psychiatry. For example, "depression" in the elderly is often delirium, and irritable noncompliance is often the reflection of a mood or personality disorder. The psychiatric consultant should remain attentive to diagnostic clues as well as to the referring physician, both explicitly and implicitly. For example, a patient who seemed to be overusing pain medications was referred for a psychiatric consultation. While talking to the medical resident, the psychiatrist realized that the real problem was not opiate abuse but rather a terminal illness that was upsetting to everyone involved. This had led to the underprescription of pain medications and to feelings of desperation in both the patient and his treatment team. This tentative formulation was possible before even meeting the patient.

Meeting the Patient

After talking with the primary team and reviewing the chart, the interviewer introduces himself to the patient. Many issues arise at that moment. Often, privacy is suboptimal. It may be necessary to ask relatives to leave the room. A hospital roommate may be present. In that case, it may be possible to move the interview into a private area or to ask the roommate to leave, but often the interview must be done within earshot of an awake and curious stranger. In that case, the curtains should be pulled around the bed to allow at least visual privacy. The interviewer should sit close to the patient, preferably at eye level, and speak as softly as possible. It may be useful to turn off the television, although conversely the television or radio may be left on in order to distract a roommate. If the patient seems reluctant to speak, the interviewer might comment on the lack of privacy and indicate that personal topics can be postponed for a more opportune time. In many cases, however, it is the interviewer who is most uncomfortable with the lack of privacy.

Although the hospital-based consultation requires the acquisition of much data, alliance building is also crucial. To a greater extent than in other psychiatric situations, the interviewer should be prepared to be active, personally revealing, and accessible to both the patient and the primary treating team. The judicious disclosure of personal life experiences, humor, and countertransference hunches can help ally the interviewer with the patient.

Countertransference

The hospital consultation is both especially challenging and especially rewarding to the clinician. Many problems stem from the structure of the interview. For example, privacy is thwarted because interviews frequently take place within earshot of other patients. Sessions can be interrupted at any time. Patients are often too ill to participate in lengthy discussions. Loved ones may intrude both in the interview and in the treatment plan, whereas in other cases relatives may avoid involvement although they are desperately needed. Missing charts and absent patients thwart efficiency. It is often imperative to read through medical charts and nursing notes, create an alliance with the primary treatment team, and interact meaningfully with the patient's relatives, all of which requires considerable effort and flexibility.

In addition, hospitalized patients are sick. The complexity of their medical problems may require significant medical knowledge outside of psychiatry. For trainees, the need to consider areas outside of their new specialty may challenge their developing professional identity, while the temptation to play medical consultant may distract from their psychiatric role. Beginning psychiatrists may be upset by very ill patients who are their own age as well as by older patients whose transferential expectations place the interviewer in the role of parent.

The hospital psychiatrist may be acutely aware of his limitations. Many patients face limited futures. This can induce feelings of inadequacy in interviewers who link their self-worth to patient outcome. Psychiatrists are often looked on by other medical staff with skepticism, denigration, and fear. For psychiatrists who desire a certain type of respect, the hospital consultation is difficult.

Finally, psychodynamic interpretations are often inappropriate in work with hospitalized patients. Hospitalization and serious illness interfere with customary life trajectories. Some psychiatrists may be dissatisfied working with patients who do not profit from "deep" interpretations but need a different sort of interview. The medical staff is even less interested in interpretation, perhaps especially when their unconscious issues may have precipitated an incompletely thought-out consultation or a patient–staff conflict. The result is that the psychodynamic understanding of the clinician is crucial, but it is often used to guide his treatment plan rather than as the theme of psychotherapeutic discussion.

Engagement and Alliance

After introducing himself and arranging to maximize privacy, the psychiatrist can ask whether the patient was expecting a psychiatrist and what the patient understood to be the reason for the consultation. If the patient has been adequately and accurately informed of the reasons for the consultation, the interviewer continues with the interview. If not, the psychiatrist informs the patient of the reason and awaits a response.

The interviewer then focuses on the patient's present illness. If the patient appears uninterested or hostile to such a discussion, the interviewer might shift to a topic about which the patient has some particular enthusiasm or interest. This shift of focus is intended to enhance the patient's self-esteem and make it easier for the patient to later explore less comfortable thoughts and feelings. For example, it may be useful to comment on bedside photographs, flowers, or cards. The clinician can ask about the ages of the grandchildren or the length of the marriage and then naturally ask about such issues as work or retirement.

> A psychiatrist was called to assess a frail, elderly woman who had refused the recommended home services. She had broken her arm in a recent fall, and the staff was concerned that she would injure herself further when she returned to her disorganized apartment. She was being evaluated for an involuntary nursing home placement. The internist had noted that the patient was isolated, stubborn, and quick to yell at the staff.
>
> When the interviewer entered the room, he noticed that the patient was remarkably well groomed and that the only personal item in the room was an old photograph of a young man. The interviewer introduced himself, and the patient immediately asked if she could have some ice water. After a trip to the ice machine, the psychiatrist handed her the glass of water and said, "I hear that there is some sort of confusion about your discharge." The patient responded, "Haven't they told you? We all hate each other." The psychiatrist smiled and said, "They told me about some conflicts, but they didn't mention you were from the South." The patient smiled and asked, "How'd you know I was from

the South?" to which he replied, "Well, you have a drawl." The interviewer continued by asking, "What are you doing in New York?" The patient smiled back and said that she had moved north when she got married. The psychiatrist pointed at the photograph and asked if that was her husband. She nodded and said that he had died the year before and quickly added, "No one has recognized my accent in years. Where are you from?" The interviewer told her, and the patient explained that she was from a neighboring state. The interviewer asked, "How did your husband die?" This led to a discussion of her husband and how his illness had led his relatives to "circle like vultures and try to grab anything that wasn't nailed down. They're as bad as the doctors and nurses around here, who are just trying to make a buck off of Medicare." The interviewer said that it sounded like she missed her husband very much, and the patient nodded. He then pointed out that it sounded like she was trying to keep her apartment and her husband's memories safe, which might be why she would not accept home services. "But," he continued, "if you don't let someone in to clean up, you might not be allowed to go back home." The patient bristled and changed the subject, but their conversation continued. Later in the interview, the patient asked, "What would you do?" The psychiatrist paused and asked her what she thought her husband would suggest. She smiled and said that her husband would tell her to quit being so paranoid. They smiled, and she later accepted home services after discharge.

The hospital interviewer had been able to develop a connection by offering water, sidestepping the patient–staff conflict by not blaming anyone, and recognizing the patient's accent. He revealed something about himself—his home state—that he might not reveal to a typical outpatient and was then able to deepen the interview by discussing how the husband's illness and death had affected the patient and led her to her current dilemma. This sort of interchange can strengthen the patient's hopefulness and improve ego functioning. Humor and anecdotes can also be effective in deepening the alliance. The psychiatrist did not challenge the patient's likely paranoia and projection but instead emphasized her feelings of loss. The enhanced alliance allowed the patient to develop the flexibility to imagine her husband's point of view and to even poke some fun at herself.

Exploration of Typical Defenses

Although most people weather the stress of illness and hospitalization remarkably well, a certain degree of regression is common and often embodied by the conflict of integrity versus disintegration and despair that Erikson used to characterize the final stage of life. Patients who feel that they are falling apart may present with a withdrawn blank stare, emotional numbing, behavioral constriction, and the inability to discuss ideas. This cluster can make the medically ill patient feel miserable and unable to participate in his medical care. In such cases, the active, attentive interviewer may be able to connect by asking the patient to talk about his life. "As you look back, what are the things of which you are especially proud? What are your disappointments and regrets?" The interviewer can encourage the patient to tell stories and make use of photographs or letters. Afterward the interviewer may attempt to construct an ego-syntonic life narrative. A typical one was given to a 40-year-old woman who had recently been diagnosed with breast cancer: "I think that you are refusing chemotherapy for a variety of reasons, but I think the biggest may relate to your sense of responsibility. You want to be as healthy as possible for as long as possible so that you can be there for your children, and you have seen how debilitating the chemo can be. And what's so terrible is that you promised yourself that you would never abandon your kids the way that your own mother abandoned you when she divorced your father. You're scared of being so sick that you can't take care of your kids, but the best chance you have of being there for your kids may be to get the chemo, deal with the side effects, and try to fight the illness."

In addition to regression, medically ill patients often become demoralized. Some may express their discouragement indirectly, such as by expressing sympathy for the doctor who works so hard with such poor results. Such patients often protect themselves from the psychological impact of illness through the use of denial. The primary physician may feel overwhelmed by the helplessness and futility of the patient's disease and the threat of death. Rather than participating in their shared hopelessness, the psychiatric consultant should try to empathize with the patient's situation and identify treatable family conflicts or primary psychiatric conditions. Even when there is no hope for the patient's long-term survival, the psychiatric consultant may be uniquely placed to have a profound impact on the dying patient, his surviving loved ones, and the hospital staff. For example, one consultant was asked to assess a man with metastatic pancreatic cancer for depression. The internist described the patient as fragile and possibly wanting to kill himself if he knew the true prognosis of his illness. Before the interviewer could enter the room, the patient's wife insisted that the patient not be told that his condition was terminal. After meeting twice with the patient and developing a friendly alliance, the consultant asked the patient if he had any ideas about his prognosis. He said that he was under the impression that he had a few months to live but asked the clinician not to tell his wife and children because he wanted to break the news to them gently. The psychiatrist asked, "What if your wife already knows your prognosis?" This caused the patient to become tearful for the first time since he had become ill. He explained that he suddenly recognized that he and his wife had been colluding by not talking about his death and that they now had to face it together.

The psychiatric interviewer should find ways to inject hope into a situation that has bogged down both the patient and the primary treating team. It is sometimes difficult for beginning psychiatrists to appreciate the potential power of a brief intervention in such situations.

Two types of resistance are particularly common in hospitalized patients. A patient may greet the psychiatrist with anger or sarcasm, beginning the interview with a statement such as "I suppose Dr. Jones thinks the problem is all in my mind" or "I guess Dr. Jones thinks I'm just imagining these headaches." These comments indicate that the patient has not accepted the consultation, which does not necessarily mean that the referring doctor neglected to prepare him. There are patients who are so fearful of psychiatry that even extraordinary efforts at preparation may be unsuccessful. In this case, prominent paranoid character traits led the patient to anticipate criticism and rejection. To the patient, the referral meant that his doctor was disapproving of and had given up on him. Reassurances that are directed to these issues are most effective. The consultant could reply, "Actually, when Dr. Jones called me, I had the feeling that he is quite concerned about you, and that he hoped that I might be another way for him to help you."

A second type of resistant patient is superficially agreeable but minimally motivated. This patient's passive superficiality is generally accompanied by defensive denial and lack of insight, features that tend to frustrate the consultant. If the psychiatrist appreciates that such attitudes are common with hospital patients, he is less likely to feel annoyed or impatient.

The hospital psychiatrist is often asked by the patient or family to answer questions about the medical illness. Although the interviewer might provide general information, most questions concerning more specific issues should be referred to the primary physician. In these ways, the interviewer indicates curiosity in what most interests the patient without straying too far either from the purpose of the interview or from the interviewer's expertise. The interviewer can be useful to both the patient and the medical team by facilitating communication between them.

A different situation is illustrated by the psychiatrist who was called to see a nurse-patient who had a bizarre hemorrhagic illness secondary to deliberate ingestion of anticoagulant medication. When the psychiatrist introduced himself, the patient promptly focused on her physical illness and resentfully protested that her internist had implied that she might be causing the condition herself. In fact, the laboratory evidence was conclusive that this was so. The psychiatrist replied, "It sounds like you and Dr. Jones are having a conflict, and he asked me to help out with the situation. My understanding is that the lab is saying that your condition must have come from ingesting an anticoagulant." Avoiding both the conflict and criticism of the patient, who appeared to have a factitious disorder, the interviewer continued by saying, "The fact that you treat yourself in this way means that there must be some serious difficulty in your life, and rather than getting into a discussion about the details, let us try to understand what might be troubling you." The psychiatrist emphasized the patient's right to be sick but indicated that the illness was designed to solve a problem in the patient's life. These assertions should be made in a straightforward, nonaccusatory tone, with the intention that the psychiatrist and patient together dispassionately observe the dysfunctional behavior. As is described in the next chapter, however, such patients do not easily agree to examine underlying psychological stressors, regardless of the interviewer's skill and tact.

Some consultations are called because the patient has a history of previous psychiatric illness. If the patient has long been stable and is cooperating with the treatment plan, the psychiatrist should reassure both the patient and the hospital staff without suggesting additional treatment. Some patients have a concurrent psychiatric disorder that remains active but does not interfere with treatment of the medical illness. In that case, treatment possibilities can be discussed with the patient. A subset of these patients will be relieved to gain a referral for their long-standing depression or anxiety disorder. Patients with personality disorders are generally less interested in treatment. A medical hospitalization is not the time to push forcefully for treatment of such conditions. Not only is the effort likely to be fruitless, it can lead to medical noncompliance and a premature discharge.

Special Situations

The Capacity Evaluation

In assessing a patient's capacity to consent or refuse, the interview includes a straightforward evaluation of the patient's cognitive ability to understand the procedure or placement option, the risk/benefit ratio, and its applicability to the patient. If the patient fulfills these criteria and is able to make a clear decision, then he is said to have capacity. The psychiatric interviewer, however, often goes beyond this basic structure. By exploring the illness and its meaning, the patient's life, the goals of the hospitalization, and the importance or unimportance of family, the "capacity consult" can become therapeutic. A patient may be refusing an important procedure because of anxiety or an exacerbation of a personality disorder. It is useful to uncover the personal meaning of the suggested procedure without being judgmental. One patient refused a magnetic resonance imaging scan because she was frightened by the noise. The offer of a preparatory sedative and allowing her husband to be in attendance led her to accept the procedure. Another patient refused a biopsy because her mother had died of cancer and she was frightened of having a similar cancer. The noncompliant and cognitively intact patient is more likely to accept a suggested intervention if he feels listened to and understood and if his worries are addressed.

Mixed Allegiances

Interviews within a hospital setting often involve *dual agency,* in which the psychiatrist has loyalties both to the patient and to another person or institution. For example, in interviewing a patient who is a potential organ recipient, the interviewer may decide that the patient's substance abuse or likely noncompliance makes him a poor risk. Although transplant might still be of value to that particular patient, the interviewer's role within the system might contribute to a judgment in favor of another potential recipient. The psychiatric interviewer who is an employee of the hospital may feel pressured to reduce length of stay, malpractice risk, or hospitalization of the uninsured. In each case, the interviewer should make clear to himself and, when necessary, to the patient whether he is acting as an advocate of the hospital or as a therapist. A slightly different dilemma occurs when the psychiatric interview for capacity leads to nursing home placement. In this case, the patient's wishes may conflict with his personal safety. The consulting interviewer may fully appreciate the inevitable philosophical conflicts between beneficence and autonomy, but clinically it is difficult to participate in the removal of an elderly person from his home of many years.

Substance Abuse

A significant number of hospitalized patients use mood-altering substances, often without informing the medical staff. The interviewer should ask about medication prescribed before the patient was admitted, alcohol and illicit drugs, tobacco, caffeine, and herbal and alternative medications. It is often useful to ask patients what is in their medicine cabinets and what they might have taken to improve their health or reduce their pain.

Unlike the more typical psychiatric interview in which people deceive for neurotic reasons, substance abusers often deceive to get drugs. As a rule, psychiatrists are not particularly adept at uncovering such deceit. Because of the high risk both for intoxication and life-threatening withdrawal, hospital-based interviews should often be accompanied by drug screenings.

Because substance abusers often have mood disorders and are perceived by hospital staff as manipulative and noncompliant, these patients receive frequent psychiatric consultations. The interview provides an opportunity for the patient to reflect upon his illness. What role does the substance play in his life? What does it provide? What are the pros and cons of using? What are the triggers for use? What efforts have been made to stop? What are the patient's views toward 12-Step programs? These questions help determine feasible treatment recommendations. A straightforward, friendly approach allows the clinician to avoid destructive moralizing and encourages the patient to observe his own behavior more objectively. Such an approach also encourages honesty, which is the first step toward recovery.

Other Common Diagnoses Within Hospitals

The focus of this chapter has been on patients who are dealing with the stress of medical hospitalization. In addition, many such patients have complaints that appear to have a prominent psychological component. Such patients are discussed in Chapter 15, "The Psychosomatic Patient." All hospital-based psychiatric interviews should screen for cognitive decline and mental status change. For a more in-depth discussion of dementia and delirium, see Chapter 16, "The Cognitively Impaired Patient." Finally, hospitalized patients can have any psychiatric diagnosis. The reader is referred to the appropriate chapters for such patients.

Closing the Interview

Ambitious personality reconstruction is not appropriate in a hospital consultation, but a psychodynamically informed interview can not only facilitate medical management but also provide significant relief for the patient. By the end of the initial interview, the psychiatrist should usually communicate to the patient in general terms what he has learned. He might schedule additional interviews, especially if the consultation was abbreviated because of the patient's illness or fatigue. He might plan outpatient follow-up. If indicated, he should obtain the patient's permission to speak with a relative or loved one in order to gain collateral information.

The hospitalized patient is generally pleased to find someone with whom he can discuss personal matters. This eagerness to talk is sometimes confused with motivation to pursue psychotherapy following discharge from the hospital. The neophyte is surprised to learn that his "well-motivated" patient no longer wishes to see a psychiatrist after he has recovered.

At times, hospital-based psychiatric interviews lead to involuntary psychiatric hospitalization or institutional placement. Nursing homes, rehabilitation centers, and psychiatric hospitals can arouse feelings of anxiety, especially in people whose lives are being significantly changed. The same psychiatrist who makes the decision about capacity or dangerousness can also help make the commitment less traumatic by spending some extra time and showing sensitivity to the fears of the patient and his family.

The consultation is not complete until the psychiatrist has written a note and discussed his findings with the referring physician. The same chart note is written for the primary team, insurance companies, and attorneys; the reality of multiple audiences makes a good note deceptively difficult to write. Referring physicians focus on the assessment and suggestions that conclude the note, and they prefer concise, jargon-free, and specifically helpful suggestions. Social workers and nurses read the note for help with patient management and discharge. Insurance companies value notes that cover a series of specific bases. In case of an untoward event, malpractice attorneys look for discrepancies, errors, and indications that risks were not considered by the medical team. Detailed psychodynamic formulations do not generally belong in such a chart note but, depending on the level of interest, can be relayed verbally to members of the primary team.

CONCLUSION

The goals of the hospital-based interview are generally limited by the patient's psychological and physical states and by the brevity of most hospitalizations. These same structural issues can cause the hospital consultation to be extremely important to the patient and his loved ones. After helping the patient safely complete such a dangerous journey, it is often useful for the psychiatrist to say goodbye to the patient prior to discharge and wish him well during the next phase of his life.

CHAPTER 19

THE PATIENT OF DIFFERENT BACKGROUND

The character structure of the patient, his psychopathology, and the setting and purpose of the interview are three major determinants of its course. The social and cultural context of the interview—and particularly social-cultural differences between the interviewer and the patient—is a fourth determinant. Issues such as language, ethnicity, social class, subculture, education, psychological sophistication, age, disability, sexual orientation, and hospitalization have a powerful influence on the interview. The interviewer's recognition and understanding of these issues, and particularly his use of that understanding, will determine the success or failure of the experience.

The underlying issue for the clinician is to acquire the necessary background, familiarity, and comfort for understanding a patient who is socially or culturally different. A fundamental purpose of the interview is for the interviewer to experience rapport with the patient and to determine how he views himself and how he is experienced by those around him. Everyone is unique in many ways, and everyone is vulnerable to feeling uncomfortable with people whose background is different from their own. The skilled interviewer makes contact with the patient in a way that allows the patient to share his anxiety about his "difference," not merely to reexperience it in the interview. The social meaning of a psychiatric interview often makes this more difficult, as does the stigma associated with psychiatry. This chapter elucidates factors that may increase this difficulty, along with strategies for minimizing them and even at times using them in an affirmative manner.

Cultural anthropology takes as its subject matter the investigation of different cultures and offers some insights into the challenging task of interviewing and understanding the patient of different background. Typically the anthropologist engages in fieldwork that involves a literal immersion in another culture, which is observed and studied at length. Unlike the clinical interviewer, however, the fieldworker lives among those being studied, partaking of their lives and customs in the role of a participating observer. The ethnographer Evans-Pritchard suggested that the anthropologist must develop the capacity "to abandon himself without reserve" and to attempt to think and feel like the subjects of his investigation.

Kracke, a psychoanalytically sophisticated anthropologist, recounted his personal psychological experience conducting fieldwork among the Kagwahiv Indians of Brazil. Early on, he noted that he experienced a feeling of exhilaration: "The excitement of discovery, as I quickly learned basic and important facts about Kagwahiv social culture." Gradually, he became aware of increasing irritability at not being fully understood by the Kagwahiv, which called to mind a pattern of interaction he had had with a younger sister, strongly tinged with sibling rivalry. His dreams became filled with memories from home and peopled by his family members. Kracke postulated a regressive trend in himself induced by the frustration and disorientation that had been aroused by attempting to understand a different culture. Most important he recognized the reawakening of his dependent experiences of childhood in response to the situation of having to learn another culture.

In an analogous way, the clinical interviewer faces some of the same psychological issues when trying to understand the patient of different background. Kracke noted a regressive pull from the attempt to understand someone whose culture, mores, and attitudes were radically different or even incomprehensible. He reexperienced aspects of childhood when elements of the grown-up world could not be understood or were mysterious. For the child this can lead to conscious feelings of frustration, helplessness, and inadequacy. Unconsciously, the same constellation of feelings may be aroused in the interviewer who cannot at first comprehend the world of a patient of different background. An open-minded and intellectually curious attitude on the part of the interviewer, combined with a self-monitoring awareness of the difficulty, frustration, and regression that may occur in attempting to comprehend such a patient, is crucial.

ETHNICITY, CULTURE, AND RACE

Everyone belongs to one or several ethnic groups. In the United States and in many other countries, an increasing portion of the population belongs to a minority ethnic group. One result is that the patient and the interviewer are frequently from different ethnic groups. Many customs or behaviors that are common and "go without saying" in one group may seem deviant and worthy of exploration in another, and differences between clinician and patient may lead to misunderstanding on this basis. For example, a serious young Jewish clinician persisted in questioning a woman of old English background as to why her 10-year-old son was about to go off to boarding school, a normal decision in the patient's family. Another clinician from a Northern European background questioned why a single woman patient in her late 20s still lived with her Greek immigrant parents—the usual arrangement in the patient's culture. The problem in both of these scenarios was the clinician's assumption that his particular segment of the world was the standard, or norm, and that variations were inherently deviant, rather than his maintaining an attitude of neutrality and curiosity toward his patient's life arrangements. It is often helpful if the interviewer knows something about the patient's culture, but it is even more important that he inquires respectfully, using the patient as a teacher and guide rather than imposing prejudicial assumptions.

It is important to differentiate culture, race, and ethnicity from one another because they are often erroneously used interchangeably. *Culture* constitutes a group of conceptual structures that determine the person's experience of life and includes sets of meanings, institutions, everyday practices, socially transmitted behavior patterns, arts, and beliefs. Usually *race* is the term applied to a more or less distinct group connected by common descent or origin and sometimes similar physical features. *Ethnicity* refers to a sense of belonging to a group with distinctive identity characterized by common national, religious, linguistic, or cultural heritage. Hence it includes aspects of both culture and race.

Culture

Culture is intrinsically complex. For instance, there are many different and culturally distinct Hispanic communities, and the Asian cultures of China, Japan, Korea, and Vietnam are quite different from one another. Black communities in Africa, the Caribbean, and the United States have disparate cultural experiences. A patient who identifies himself as "Puerto Rican" will respond positively if the interviewer expresses curiosity as to when the patient came to the mainland, where he lived in Puerto Rico, whether it was urban or rural, and what the local culture was like. This discussion not only gathers useful information but also transforms Puerto Rico from "elsewhere" into a unique and interesting alternative to "here."

It is also important to recognize that all differences are not explained by culture. One of us learned while working at a university health service that the staff frequently "explained away" unusual behavior in international students from other cultures, only to learn when mental health professionals from the students' own cultures were consulted that the students were seriously disturbed.

Cultures have distinctive ways of expressing and responding to psychological and emotional problems, and awareness of this is helpful in the interview. For example, the dominant culture in the United States is more psychologically and medically oriented than most of the world. In the United States, depression is widely recognized as a psychological disorder; in other parts of the world depression is experienced as physical rather than psychological. In the United States one might seek out a mental health professional to discuss feelings of hopelessness or despair. In other countries one would be more likely to see a religious or spiritual helper whose assistance might also be sought for hallucinations or disturbances of consciousness.

Interviewers should always assume that patients have previously sought help elsewhere. The way in which they have done so frequently reflects cultural attitudes toward their problems and the responses that are believed to be useful. Exploring one patient's visits to primary care physicians may be analogous to exploring the visits of a patient from a different culture to spiritualists or shamans, and the involvement of such healers in the second patient's treatment program might be as helpful as the involvement of a primary care physician in the treatment of the first. This recognition requires open-mindedness, flexibility, and adaptability on the part of the clinician, attitudes that are essential in bridging the gap between cultures.

Racism

Racial prejudice is common. The psychological impact of deliberate, conscious racism upon the victim is destructive. Unconscious racism is also common and is often reflected in the practice of professionals and on patterns of care in the health delivery system. As an example, studies have shown that African Americans are less likely than Caucasians to receive psychotherapy and more likely to receive only pharmacotherapy in mental health clinics.

The interviewer strives to examine his own prejudices and feelings of the superiority of his own subculture and achieve a neutral perspective with which to enter the world of a patient of different background. Everyone has prejudices, both positive and negative. Positive prejudices are based on overidentification with someone of a similar cultural and ethnic background and a consequent tendency to overlook their psychopathology. Such prejudices present their own problem for the interviewer and lead to a loss of clinical neutrality. Simultaneously, it is necessary to realize that most members of disadvantaged minority groups have experienced prejudice in one form or another from childhood through adulthood and have developed their own counter-prejudice. The interviewer who is a member of the dominant culture may feel embarrassed at exploring this issue in a manner similar to the discomfort that exists about finding out about the sexual life and fantasies of a patient. However, just as it is crucial to examine a patient's sexual life sensitively, it is important to understand the patient's experience of racial or ethnic prejudice. When did it occur? How did he react? How did he deal with it? What are its residual effects? Empathically connecting with this aspect of the minority patient's life experience will facilitate the development of an alliance and enhance the therapeutic impact of the interview. Conversely, the interviewer who is a member of a disadvantaged minority culture should be alert to indications of the patient's prejudices or discomfort and discuss them without defense or retaliation.

LANGUAGE AND INTERPRETERS

Language

The interview is a verbal interchange, and inevitable problems occur when the interviewer and patient do not share the same language. This is, of course, not the patient's problem alone but rather a problem between the patient and the interviewer, particularly if the clinician tends to react negatively to the patient in response. It is helpful to convey a desire to communicate as fully as possible and to enlist the patient's collaboration in searching for the best means to do so. This might entail finding alternate languages (perhaps written, or a shared second language, or pantomime or drawing) or using an interpreter when one is available.

Use of an Interpreter

Selecting the Interpreter

The ideal interpreter would be a unique communication machine that could convert one language into another, capturing the meaning of the words and sentences and translating them instantly, including the nuances and the feelings of both interviewer and patient. This, of course, is impossible. Often the translation of subtleties involves the loss of finer emotional tones or humor. The interpreter must have an intimate knowledge of both cultures in order to make even approximate translations in such situations. This is an exceedingly difficult task to perform rapidly and smoothly. The best example of this type of interpreting would be found at the United Nations, where a speech is translated line by line as it is being delivered.

Ideally, the interviewer would select a professional interpreter. In practice, this is usually not possible, and an attempt must be made to obtain the services of bilingual coworkers. There are many times when such personnel are not available, and the interviewer is obliged to utilize a family member or friend who accompanied the patient. If there is a choice, permit the patient to select the family member or friend with whom he feels most comfortable. Be sure that the person selected has a good command of English and seems capable of following instructions. Usually the patient will select an adult of the same sex. If he asks to utilize a child or a person of the opposite sex as an interpreter, he may be attempting to protect himself from certain aspects of the interview. On occasion he may suggest having more than one interpreter, but this is not a good plan because the two interpreters will often disrupt the interview with disagreements about the precise meaning of a certain phrase.

Giving Instructions to the Interpreter

The interpreter will be more helpful if the clinician instructs him concerning his role before starting the interview. It is preferable that he translate the patient's and clinician's statements rather than explain his understanding of their meaning. He should neither amplify remarks nor explore ideas of his own. The clinician can maintain better rapport with a sentence-by-sentence interpretation than with a summary that paraphrases the general content of the conversation. It is not desirable that the interpreter merely translate words without their accompanying feeling. His expression and voice should reflect the affective tone of each interchange. If the patient converses directly with the interpreter during the interview, it is likely that the interpreter has become involved in a defensive maneuver of the patient. A patient may seek out the interpreter after the interview in order to continue the discussion. This behavior reflects the patient's feeling that he needs direct, practical assistance that can be better provided by a member of his own culture. It might also mean that he feels closer to or better understood by the interpreter than by the clinician. The interviewer can support the patient's attempt to improve his social and adaptive skills. However, the patient's relationship to the interpreter can also be used as a resistance to involvement with the clinician. The clinician attempts to learn about and supervise these extrasession contacts so that the interpreter can become an auxiliary therapist.

When the interpreter is a close relative, it may be particularly difficult for him to adhere to his role. In fact, the interviewer may find himself conducting a family interview. This is not necessarily undesirable; however, it should be remembered that family members, particularly in an initial group interview, usually tend to protect each other and keep certain pertinent information away from the interviewer.

Transference and Countertransference

The interviewer should face the patient with the interpreter at the patient's side. He should speak as though the patient could understand his words, rather than saying to the interpreter, "Ask him if he does thus and such." If the interviewer addresses the interpreter in that manner, it encourages the patient to reply, "Tell him that...." The interviewer becomes anxious if he cannot "get to the patient," and his role as clinician is threatened. He responds by relating to the interpreter in a dependent way rather than utilizing the interpreter as his assistant. The patient's perception of a greater social closeness to the interpreter than to the clinician may further draw him to the interpreter. A third person in the room will inhibit both patient and interviewer; however, as the interview progresses, this effect tends to diminish. The extra time required by translation and the presence of the interpreter may make the clinician impatient.

When an individual is attempting to converse with someone who does not speak the same language, there is a tendency to speak louder, as though that would enable the person to understand. The interviewer should resist this tendency and speak in a normal tone of voice rather than behaving as though conversing with a deaf person. By speaking slowly, he allows himself to express feelings with his tone of voice, gestures, and facial expressions. This facilitates the development of rapport even though the patient does not directly understand the interviewer's words. If at some point in the discussion the patient inexplicably becomes upset or does not react as the clinician expects, one should go back in the conversation and determine whether something was translated incorrectly or if the clinician's lack of understanding of the patient's culture led him to a tactless comment or question.

Under most circumstances the patient will develop a transference to the clinician just as if the interpreter were not present. On some occasions the patient may utilize the interpreter in a defensive manner to avoid relating to the clinician. The therapist must guard against feeling rejected, angry, or depressed. Competitive attitudes toward the interpreter also may interfere with the therapist's functioning.

Modifications of the Interview

In an attempt to suppress any prejudice, the interviewer frequently ignores all references to the patient's race and ethnic background. The patient, however, correctly perceives these omissions as direct evidence of prejudice on the part of the interviewer. It is therefore important early in the interview to make inquiry into the patient's family background, length of stay in this country, present living conditions, and experiences in the new culture. In the case of a disadvantaged patient, the interviewer may be uncomfortable hearing data about how badly the patient has been treated by the majority group. However, a discussion of the patient's living conditions, economic circumstances, and happy and unhappy experiences in the new culture will give the interviewer a more intimate understanding of the problems and give the patient a feeling that someone is concerned.

If it seems that the interpreter is deviating from the instructions and is not translating every comment made by the patient, merely remind him of the nature of his task. Do not attempt to interpret his behavior. By concentrating his attention on the patient, the interviewer will enable the interpreter to feel more comfortable. This will minimize the likelihood of the interpreter's experiencing untoward emotional responses during the interview.

The patient will expect to concentrate less on past developmental material and direct attention more toward the present. It is always helpful to determine how the patient was referred for psychiatric care and who considered the problem to be psychiatric. When the interpreter is a family member or a friend, the interviewer should touch lightly on subjects that the patient may not wish to discuss in front of this person, such as sex, money, religion, and politics. However, each case should be evaluated individually. On some occasions the patient may come from a culture in which these subjects are less taboo.

Whenever the interviewer has difficulty understanding the data provided by the patient in terms of its cultural significance, he can be very open in admitting his ignorance of the patient's culture. He may then ask the patient directly if such behavior is considered normal, unusual, or significant in terms of the patient's own background. In this manner he can greatly reduce the obvious handicap of his limited knowledge and can give the patient confidence in the interviewer's genuine interest. If the interviewer has accumulated some knowledge of the patient's culture, he can facilitate more rapid development of a trusting relationship by demonstrating this understanding.

The interviewer often learns that the patient is able to speak more English than he initially revealed. This disclosure is evidence of the patient's greater trust, and no interpretation or comment from the interviewer is required because it will only make the patient feel criticized for his earlier behavior.

The patient needs time at the end of the interview to ask questions. Arrangements must be made for an interpreter to be present when the second interview is scheduled. As with all new experiences, the interviewer's comfort and proficiency will increase substantially as he acquires more experience in conducting his interviews with the assistance of an interpreter.

SOCIAL CLASS AND SUBCULTURE

Social Class

Socioeconomic status is correlated with ethnicity but is different from it. Mental health professionals are generally of middle class. Their education, career orientation, income, and family background determine this. Patients can be of any social class, although more severe psychiatric disorders tend to be correlated with lower social class. Social class is revealed through language, dress, manners, occupation, habits, expectations, and concerns as well as the class of one's parents. The interviewer wants to get to know the patient and at the same time to avoid offending or humiliating him in the process. Some aspects of the social asymmetry of the interview situation mimic social class asymmetries, and interviewers must be aware of this or they may unintentionally cause narcissistic injury and in the process sabotage their basic goals.

Although there is no way to avoid class differences, the interviewer strives to avoid even appearing to equate those differences with attitudes regarding personal worth or value. For example, one is always interested in the personal psychological meaning to the patient of the arrangements of everyday life. The sensitive interviewer is as interested in how the blue-collar worker spends free time hunting and fishing as in the wealthy patient's involvement in riding, sailing, or sponsoring charitable events. Watching television has become a leisure activity that transcends social class. Much can be learned about another person by inquiring about favorite programs and channels, how much time each week is devoted to watching television, and whether it is a shared experience. The goal is to learn how the patient views and organizes his free time and to demonstrate that the clinician is interested in the decisions that he makes in structuring the resources he has in life rather than only in the resources themselves. It is also to convey that the interviewer is not burdened by either envy or contempt, although he is sensitive to the patient's anticipation that he might experience either.

Subculture

The patient belongs to a culture and may live in the midst of a different dominant culture, such as the immigrant Asian family living in a large American city. However, he is frequently also a member of specific subcultures, such as a college campus community, an ultra-religious community, or an urban gang. Interviewing a patient who has an important identity as a member of such a subculture requires learning something about that group and the patient's place in it. It is usually more fruitful to make clear that one is ignorant and wants to learn than to exaggerate what little knowledge one might have. It is also important to be respectful.

A male clinician was startled when an ultra-orthodox Hassidic woman recoiled at his offer to shake hands on their meeting, unaware that to her this was forbidden. He then asked her help in arranging the seating for their interview, hoping to avoid another *faux pas*, and as the interview progressed was again surprised when she revealed her worldliness, autonomy, and competence in trying to cope with a difficult marriage and an abusive husband. She explained to him that both abortion and divorce were options in her community, although shaking hands with a strange man was not. He went on to demonstrate that although mental health practitioners may not be helpful in telling one what to do, they can help to identify and help the patient select among options, a task that she had been raised to avoid.

A young male counterculture patient arrived for an interview with his hair long and unkempt and his beard scraggly, and he was wearing a tie-dyed tee shirt, earrings, and a bracelet. He first seemed to have difficulty focusing on the conversation, as though "high" on drugs, but "settled down" as the interview progressed. The interviewer, groomed and dressed as the conservative professional woman that she was, invited him to tell her about his life. When he used terms about which she was uncertain—"crank," "dope," "old lady," and others—she asked what each meant. The message was that she was an interested tourist in the world in which he lived and that she welcomed his guidance. When he spoke of his anger at the police and his contempt for the establishment, she neither agreed nor disagreed and explored not only his own feelings but also his understanding of what other people thought. He grew increasingly comfortable telling her not only of his subculture but also of his personal problems and ultimately of his loneliness, because he trusted those within his subculture no more than outsiders and felt as estranged from them as he did from the larger society. He revealed that, in fact, his girlfriend was not much of an "old lady," just as his "old lady" mother had not been much of a mother, and he eventually was able to recognize that he had come seeking a therapist who might play this role for him.

PSYCHOLOGICAL SOPHISTICATION

Certain patients seem to be psychologically constricted and uninterested in themselves. Many interviewers prefer patients who think introspectively, describe themselves and others in terms of motives and feelings, and display insight. Constricted patients think concretely and may have nothing at all to say or, if they do, talk in terms of actions or events. When they describe a person, it is chiefly in terms of physical or occupational characteristics. Denial, projection, externalization, and inhibition of assertion and curiosity are major defenses.

In some patients, a genuine constriction of personality is a manifestation of individual psychopathology. These patients are inhibited even if viewed in the framework of their social and cultural background. In others, an apparent constriction of the personality is the product of social distance between the clinician and the patient. Such persons would not be viewed as constricted by the standards of those from their own environment.

Description of the Problem

It is important that the interviewer differentiate between the patient who is really constricted and the patient whose cultural background makes it difficult to relate in the manner to which the clinician is accustomed. The truly constricted patient will have difficulty relating and expressing himself on any topic, including those with which he has the greatest familiarity. He has few interests and generates little enthusiasm. Diagnostically, this patient may be depressed or have chronic psychosis or other syndromes such as Asperger's disorder.

The culturally constricted patient will seem less constricted when he is discussing subjects with which he is familiar and comfortable. He will express enthusiasm in his areas of individual interest, although these may be foreign to the interviewer. This difference in background creates the illusion of constriction. The patient of lower socioeconomic class may be constricted on the basis of both his deprived cultural background and his individual psychodynamics.

The interviewer often reacts to the unsophisticated patient with boredom or disinterest. This response in an individual who is interested in people and who has an opportunity to study someone different from himself stems from a defensive withdrawal secondary to the social distance between the clinician and the patient. The response changes with an increased knowledge of psychodynamics and interviewing skill. The patient's lack of familiarity with introspection often provides a unique opportunity for testing psychodynamic hypotheses without the contamination produced by educational exposure to psychological information. Dramatic responses to specific interpretations with accompanying relief of symptoms may occur. The psychodynamic derivatives of normal development—for example, dependency conflicts, sibling rivalry, castration anxiety, and oedipal conflicts—are often revealed with great clarity during the interview.

The observation has been made that the patient of lower socioeconomic class often drops out of psychodynamic psychotherapy after one or perhaps two sessions. This is sometimes a response to his dissatisfaction with the traditionally conducted psychiatric interview. Not only is the model of the traditional psychiatric interview poorly suited to this patient, but the inexperienced interviewer is frequently unfamiliar with the vastly different background of his patient. Another patient may feel that his difficulties have been alleviated after one or two interviews although the clinician considered them to be primarily diagnostic. The opportunity to ventilate his feelings provided dramatic relief.

Common forms of psychopathology leading to a request for psychiatric intervention include psychotic disturbance, psychophysiological disorders, substance abuse, and sexual disturbances. Although psychoneurotic reactions are common, they seldom motivate this patient to seek psychiatric help. For the person who is poor, unhappiness seems to stem from hardship directly related to his poverty. Often it is only after a person becomes more affluent that he discovers the existence of problems within himself that are not solved by the acquisition of more material goods.

Aspects of this patient's experience may differ from those of the middle-class patient. This leads to the development of styles of thinking. Less value is placed on intellectualization and intellectual achievement, which may lead the interviewer to grossly misjudge the patient's intelligence. Such patients may not be introspective and do not consider the subtleties of their emotional lives to be important. They do not think that talk can be helpful in the solution of their problems but are more concerned with action and therefore desire direct advice as to what they should do. They avoid philosophical discussions and are interested in ideas only for their practical value. They are not accustomed to describing their feelings about others, particularly to strangers, nor are they inclined to reveal highly personal material about themselves.

The patient of this type tends to blame the outside world rather than himself for his misfortunes and unhappiness. The tendency to externalize responsibility frequently influences the interviewer to consider this patient a poor candidate for insight-oriented psychotherapy.

Management of the Interview

The psychologically unsophisticated patient is not a single clinical entity. The methods of interviewing discussed here will be applicable to many, but not all, of these patients. If the interviewer develops a stereotyped approach to patients of lower socioeconomic status, he will grossly mismanage interviews with those who are educated and have developed middle-class values and attitudes. Conversely, a college-educated patient of higher socioeconomic class may be unable to discuss his subjective experience. The patient from a middle or upper socioeconomic class may present with the clinical problems of the psychologically unsophisticated patient, and the suggestions offered here would apply to this patient as well.

The Opening Phase

As with most other patients, the interview begins with an exploration of the patient's chief complaint; however, this patient will often say that he has no complaint or that he came to see the clinician because someone sent him. The interviewer can respond by asking who sent the patient and why this person felt that psychiatric help was indicated. The interview should proceed with a discussion of whatever material the patient offers, whether or not it seems immediately relevant to the patient's major problem. For example, the patient may refer to previous episodes of emotional difficulty or may indicate that he has recently quit his job, dropped out of school, separated from his spouse, or made some other change in his pattern of living. At an appropriate point, the interviewer can ask if such experiences have made the patient nervous. The term "nervous" is particularly useful because it circumvents the patient's denial of emotional problems.

The interview may be characterized by its sparseness. The patient volunteers little, and his answers to the clinician's questions are very brief. The interviewer feels that he is doing all the work and soon resents the patient for his inability to open up feelings. The clinician expresses his resentment by becoming less interested in the patient as the interview progresses, and he is inclined to dismiss the patient early. On the other hand, too great a show of warmth or too much personal interest may cause the patient to discontinue treatment.

The patient is not accustomed to discussing his feelings about friends and relatives with anyone, and particularly not with a stranger. Therefore, in the initial portion of the interview, concrete questions will usually produce more material than open-ended ones. For example, the interviewer should not say, "Describe your parents," but should instead ask, "What kind of work does your father do?" The interviewer might then inquire whether the patient's mother works outside the home. He could ask practical questions concerning their interests and hobbies and what they do for recreation rather than asking, "What are they like?" When the interviewer develops rapport with the patient he can inquire in a more open-ended fashion.

Early in the interview some approximate determination should be made concerning the patient's knowledge and education. The interviewer should be careful that he neither talks down to the patient nor talks above his capacity to understand. Any comments offered by the patient that emphasize the social distance between the patient and the interviewer should immediately be explored in an open manner.

Countertransference

The inexperienced interviewer mistakenly assumes that his interview is going badly when this patient fails to produce material containing psychological insights. He becomes frustrated and annoyed with the patient, as though the patient were deliberately interfering with the conduct of the interview. This response is less probable if the clinician realizes that he is working with a constricted patient who is unable to participate in an introspective discussion. Prolonged silences tend to become awkward, increasing the distance between patient and interviewer. Such silences are to be avoided, particularly in the initial interview, although brief pauses are to be expected while the patient or interviewer collects his thoughts.

The clinician asks this patient what he was thinking during a brief silence, and the patient replies, "I was just waiting for your next question." If the interviewer waits for the patient to volunteer something, the patient will typically respond, "Can you ask me some more questions?" A classic example of this patient recently consulted one of us:

"What brings you to see me?" the interviewer inquired. The patient replied, "You really ought to talk to my wife, she is the one with the complaints." The interviewer asked, "What are her complaints?" The patient dutifully listed her complaints that he did not listen to her, that he finished her sentences, that he never took her out, and that he did not love her. Asked how he felt about these complaints, he replied, "I do love her, but she does have a point about the rest. I try not to do those things but I just can't help myself." This was said in a bland tone with no evidence that the patient was distressed. He denied feeling angry with his wife. When asked about his childhood he responded, "I had a normal childhood. My parents loved me. I was an only child. I recall being happy." The interviewer asked for a biographical sketch of the patient's parents, and he answered, "Gee that's a tough one, they were nice people. They had friends. I'm not very good at this." The interviewer soon felt that he had to drag information from the patient. The patient was treating the clinician the same way he treated his wife—appearing to listen and adopting a cooperative tone of voice but not producing anything. All questions pertaining to childhood were answered with a sincere tone of voice, but the words were "Gee! I don't remember!" Trying to get into this patient's mind was like trying to find an entry into a house with no doors and no windows.

This patient was labeled in the clinician's mind as "the man with no history." In order to open up such a patient, the interview requires considerable modification. This was a striking case because the patient was an educated and worldly man. When he revealed that he had seen several psychiatrists in the past but felt that no good had come of it, the interviewer asked, "Are you really here to get your wife off your back?" "I guess that's it," the patient responded. "Have you ever told her that?" the interviewer continued. "Not really," the patient responded, and the beginning of a working alliance was established.

Modification of the Interview

Mutuality of the expectations of patient and therapist is a crucial factor determining the success or failure of an interview. When the interviewer directs the discussion toward the patient's expectations, the patient often responds by discussing the basis for his suffering in terms of external reality. For example, he may inform the clinician that he has come to the clinic to enlist professional help so that he might obtain a larger apartment through a social service agency. Because the patient's expectations of therapy are incongruous with those of the clinician, it is essential that the interviewer adopt a flexible and active approach in conducting the initial interview.

Treatment must be modified in order to address the patient's expectations. Direct answers to the patient's questions, practical help with environmental problems, and medication all facilitate the development of a trusting relationship. The clinician can gradually explain the manner in which the patient is expected to participate and at the same time define his own role. He should point out that the patient can be helped but that this will require time and that he, the clinician, has no magical cures. He can introduce the concept that talk constitutes work in psychotherapy, particularly talk accompanied by an expression of the patient's emotions, which in time leads to change in the patient's behavior. The patient needs help with guilt about critical feelings toward his family. As the therapy progresses, the patient will be able to accept a less structured interview.

If the therapist adjusts his conceptual framework to that of his patient he will avoid the use of analogies or metaphors that would be foreign to the patient's experience. The clinician will be more responsive to the patient's needs if he does not concentrate on past developmental material in the first interview but instead aims for simple insights related to the patient's current life situation.

The therapist may feel uncomfortable in an interview with a person who initially indicates no desire to be a patient. However, this individual may have a great desire to receive help. Because therapists tend to avoid constricted patients, the interviewer may be only too eager to accede to a verbal denial of motivation. It is only natural for someone unfamiliar with introspective thinking, unaccustomed to close interpersonal relations, and burdened with many reality problems to resist psychotherapy. The patient's initial demand may concern medication or environmental manipulation. The clinician can offer a considerable degree of help in these areas, and by so doing can make a substantial contribution. He will have to assume a directive role and may have to give practical advice. Early in treatment, intellectual interpretations based upon psychodynamic reconstructions of the past offer little help; they generally lead to frustration in the therapist and alienation of the patient.

The Closing Phase

Before terminating the interview, the therapist should establish definite arrangements for a second appointment rather than asking the patient when he wants to return or saying that he will contact him. By now the patient has revealed his conscious doubts and reservations concerning treatment; he has discussed his expectations, his own view of his problem, and the help he is hoping to receive. A few minutes should be allowed for the patient to raise additional questions. Finally, the clinician can make a brief statement to the patient, formulating the problems in simple terms as the clinician understands them and, at the same time, outlining a practical approach to treatment.

The therapist assumes an active role in reaching out to the unsophisticated patient so that understanding may be achieved at whatever level the patient's capabilities permit. This does not mean that the clinician limits his interventions to advising, reassuring, cajoling, lecturing, and so on. The therapist uses his knowledge of the role of unconscious processes in the formation of symptoms just as much with this patient as with any other. Ultimately, in a dynamic psychotherapy, the same unconscious conflicts must be worked through in order to resolve the patient's symptoms. The preliminary active interventions strengthen the patient's ego and coping mechanisms and enable him to accept interpretations of inner conflicts.

CONFLICT OF LOYALTY

The interviewer is establishing a relationship with the patient, but inevitably he has other relationships and other loyalties that are potentially in conflict. Mental health professionals are frequently called upon to interview the institutionalized patient, such as a hospital inpatient, a member of the armed forces, a student in school or college, or an incarcerated prisoner. Inevitably the patient's perceptions of the interviewer's relationship to the institution, as well as the reality of that relationship, become powerful determinants of the interview.

For whom is the interviewer really working? Is there confidentiality, and what are its limits? What is the potential impact of the interview on the institution's attitude toward the patient? The interview is most likely to be successful if the patient's interests are aligned with those of the interviewer. For example, the student health psychiatrist who is evaluating a college freshman after a suicide attempt is, at the same time, a vital member of a health care network and a potential threat to the student's continued career at the school. Usually it is best that, early in the interview, the interviewer inquire about the patient's understanding of the arrangements and then clarify the reality. The patient is more comfortable with the interviewer who is straightforward concerning any institutional limitations on traditional clinical boundaries, such as reporting, limits to confidentiality, or possibly adverse consequences of the interview, and perhaps even emphasizes these limitations, rather than with the interviewer who attempts to minimize, deny, or evade such issues.

DISABILITY

Disability is another important aspect of identity, and the disabled patient may be a member of a distinctive subculture. Deafness influences language and communication; wheelchair use may influence the physical setting of the interview or the availability of toilet facilities. It is important that the interviewer recognize and attend to these practical issues, or the patient will feel that his interests are not considered relevant or significant. It is also desirable that the interviewer recognize that the disabled individual resents the assumption that his disability is his primary identity. He is a person who happens to be blind or deaf or in a wheelchair rather than one of "the blind," "the deaf," or "the disabled." Incidentally, terms that underscore his differences, such as "handicapped," are often resented, whereas a description that emphasizes adaptation is preferred. He "uses a wheelchair for mobility" rather than being "confined to a wheelchair," and he is "differently abled" rather than "disabled." Similarly, the interviewer should explore how the patient adapts to his disability rather than how the disability interferes with his life. For example, one should ask, "What arrangements have you made for travel?" rather than stating, "That must interfere with your getting around." The emphasis is on the patient's identity as one who copes with adversity rather than as one whose life has been defined by it. A man who had had a successful academic career became severely disabled—quadriplegic—in late life. He described how his colleagues had reached out to him, including him in their social events. However, he was painfully aware that each time someone came over to talk to him at a cocktail party he or she became "trapped," unable to escape until replaced by someone else. Hating experiencing himself as a "trapper," he would dismiss his colleague in a manner experienced by others as arrogant. The interviewer recognized that this was a problem of character as much as disability and suggested that the patient bring along a graduate student who would be honored to be included and could serve as a social buffer, thereby reducing the pressure on colleagues, who would no longer be "trapped."

AGE

Patients may be either significantly younger or older than the interviewer. Although this often presents no special problem, it may lead to difficulty, particularly at either end of the age spectrum. The adolescent usually feels that he belongs to a generational subculture, one that is in conflict with the dominant adult culture to which the interviewer belongs. The interviewer should recognize the difference and show interest in it without trying to "pass" as a pseudo-adolescent or suggesting disapproval by assuming values and attitudes the adolescent associates with the adult world. If an adolescent patient mentions a current rock star whom he admires, it is useful to learn from the patient the reasons he finds his music so compelling, how it relates to his view of himself, whether his friends share this passion, and so on.

The problem is different at the other end of the age spectrum. The elderly patient has experiences and concerns that the interviewer has not lived through. Retirement, infirmity, becoming dependent on one's children, and the deaths of spouses or friends who formed one's cohort replace concerns with ambitions, raising children, and adapting to increasing power and responsibility. Once again the interviewer is interested in the life that the patient constructs from the raw material at his disposal and the role that the patient's character plays in shaping his destiny.

The elderly patient may arouse countertransference fears in the interviewer of his own aging and death and induce a reluctance to explore the patient's feelings about these issues, which are usually never far from the surface. Another common countertransference problem with the elderly patient is that of seeing him as a parental figure and unconsciously ascribing to him psychological attributes of the interviewer's parents, particularly those that may have aroused conflict in the clinician during development.

Many of the points made about labeling in discussing the patient with a disability apply to the elderly, who do not like being so classified. Being "old" is a challenge to most people, but in quite different ways and during quite a broad period of the life span. For a teenager "old" may be anyone as old or older than his parents. We all have our personal definitions of the *elderly*. As we ourselves age the term is more likely to connote frailty or those who are no longer able to care for themselves.

One of the most common countertransference problems is the failure of the interviewer to appreciate and acknowledge the continuing sexual needs of healthy elderly people. The elderly patient does have a sexual life. Sexual performance may sometimes be impaired, and this can be troubling to the elderly patient, who is often reluctant to discuss such issues even though they preoccupy him. Sensitive exploration of the elderly patient's sexual life should be a central part of the interview. Many elderly individuals have active sexual lives that remain a continuing source of satisfaction to them. A common countertransference problem is the interviewer's erroneous belief that sex is no longer important to the elderly patient. Sexual desires, fantasies, and activities are continuous throughout the life cycle.

As with the patient from another culture, social class, or educational experience, it is not essential for the interviewer to know the elderly patient's life circumstances in advance but rather to know how to help the patient to talk about them and to do so in ways that support the patient's pride in his identity. This is particularly true concerning retirement.

Retirement presents complex social, medical, and psychological issues that are a challenge for the interviewer. There is an old wives' joke that "Marriage is for better or for worse but not for lunch." The following is a prime example:

> The patient was the wife of a recent retiree from a prestigious firm where he was the senior managing partner. Their marriage, on the whole, had been successful; they had grown children and grandchildren whom they enjoyed. The husband had been inclined toward micromanagement at work, and in his retirement he drew a bead on the family dishwasher, which he previously had totally ignored. The patient promptly advised him that the kitchen was her domain and that he should "keep out." This quickly led to a power struggle because he had no one to boss around anymore.
>
> After a couple of history-taking sessions, the interviewer explained that it was sad that a man who had been so successful had found himself in a position in which he could find nowhere that he could be in charge. She replied, "I hadn't looked at it that way. I hope you aren't suggesting that now he should be in charge of me." "Not at all," the therapist replied, "All you need to do is to turn that job over to him; then you won't feel he is criticizing you by reloading the dishwasher." The patient decided that this could serve as a situational template by which she could allow her husband to feel useful and give him positive reinforcement. He had turned to her to fill some of the void created by his retirement, and the interviewer suggested that she could collaborate with him on finding pleasurable ways to fill the void in his life.

Another patient consulted one of us because he was being forced into an early retirement because of a rapidly failing memory. The psychiatrist took a careful medical history, including a list of all medications that the patient used. The patient stated that he had started a cardiac drug named Tenormin 6 months earlier. In the patient's presence, the psychiatrist consulted the *Physicians' Desk Reference* and learned that the drug can cause a dementia-like state. He read the piece to the patient and requested his permission to telephone the patient's wife and explain the situation to her, including the risks of stopping the drug abruptly and the importance of an immediate appointment with his cardiologist. Fortunately for all parties the diagnosis was correct and the story ended well.

The best predictors of a successful retirement include loved ones with whom the time can be shared, good physical health, adequate financial security, and the existence of rewarding hobbies and extra career interests prior to retirement. The interviewer can explore each of these areas, asking for examples to document the accuracy of the patient's general claims that everything is "fine" or "OK" in the retirement area. Such inquiries are most productive if the interviewer's questions arise from a genuine interest in the patient's new life and its connection to his past. Questions such as "What do you do with your additional free time?"; "Please describe a typical week"; "Do you miss the old job and do you maintain contact with former colleagues?"; "Do you ever feel depressed or bored?"; "How much television do you watch?"; and "What do you do for exercise?" are helpful. Inquiries about children, grandchildren, the patient's spouse, and additional family members are also productive.

A few questions concerning the patient's degree of satisfaction with his past life can be revealing. "If you could live your life over, what major decisions would you change?" or "What are the aspects of your life about which you feel the greatest pride and satisfaction?" are questions that provide useful entries into the patient's emotional life. If the patient replies that there is nothing that he ever reflected about or would have done differently, the interviewer can wait quietly and see what the patient brings up next, because it will probably relate to unconscious feelings elicited by the clinician's question.

Finally, the elderly patient is frequently responsive to psychotherapy and is often able to use the insights he gains productively.

SEXUAL ORIENTATION

The psychiatric profession officially removed the psychopathology label from homosexuality in 1980 in response to the recognition that such labeling was nothing more nor less than another manifestation of social prejudice. The harmful psychological effect of this prejudice on countless individuals has been grave. The prejudice results from homophobia and a belief in the moral superiority of heterosexuality, which has been termed *heterosexism*. Many of these negative beliefs are parallel to other prejudices, such as racism. For many years the result was that the gay or lesbian individual hid his or her sexual orientation and felt shame or guilt concerning it. In addition, many gay or lesbian patients have had painful childhoods because of their core sexual orientation. Just as with minority patients who have experienced racism, the interviewer should be sensitive to the impact of this overt or covert prejudice against gay or lesbian patients and gently explore this issue in the interview.

Transference and Countertransference

Years of discrimination, persisting into the present, and the prominent role of the mental health community in fostering that discrimination have made many gay and lesbian patients wary of psychiatric interviews. This pathologizing attitude toward homosexuality on the part of many psychiatrists and other mental health workers in the past is well known within the gay community. As a consequence, clinicians of any sexual orientation are advised to be aware of the uneasy feelings of many homosexual patients in an initial interview. Questions by gay patients such as "What is your professional background and orientation?" often signal the patient's underlying worries about the clinician's attitude toward homosexuality. The interviewer can respond empathically by saying, "You want to know if you would be comfortable working with me on your problems. As part of that I wonder if you don't also have some concerns about my attitude toward homosexuality?" The gay patient will usually confirm that he is fearful of putting himself in the hands of a clinician who believes homosexuality to be inherently pathological.

It is important in the initial interview with the gay or lesbian patient to establish whether the patient's problems directly involve his or her homosexuality. Being gay or lesbian may be conflict-free for many patients, who present with problems with relationships; conflicts regarding marriage, children, and establishing a family; or problems at work, but not with concerns about their sexual orientation. Some homosexual patients, however, may initially seek help wishing to change their sexual orientation or hoping to move a bisexual orientation in a heterosexual direction. A female patient who had had a number of intense love affairs with women and never with men professed confusion over her sexual identity in an initial interview: "I really don't know if I am gay. And, if I am, I don't know if I want to be." It quickly emerged that she was terrified of her parents' response if she came out. "They would never speak to me. I couldn't bear that." The clinician made clear to this patient that their task together was to understand the nature of the conflict concerning her homosexuality so that she would have more psychological freedom, but that the clinician would not push her in one direction or another. Some homosexual patients have internalized anti-homosexual societal biases and direct them against themselves, intensifying their conflict about their sexual orientation. Revealing and addressing this internal "homophobia" is often liberating for gay patients.

The interviewing problems with the gay and lesbian patient are similar to those with members of other social or cultural groups. The patient is expert about his personal world; the clinician's interest, curiosity, and lack of prejudice facilitate the exploration of how the patient fits into that world and what specific challenges he experiences. Developmental crises over attitudes of parents and siblings toward the patient's sexuality, conflicts about "coming out," and experiences of prejudice and discrimination are likely to be important. Homosexual sex is at least as complex and varied as heterosexual sex, and a history of sexual experiences comprises far more than the gender of the partner, including who does what to whom, with what fantasies, what anxieties about performance, what pleasure, what regard for the partner, what concern about consequences, and what precautions. Unfortunately, the gay community has had a special vulnerability in the AIDS epidemic, and interviews with most gay patients will include discussing how their lives have been affected by this plague.

The Gay Clinician and the Gay Patient

The homosexual clinician meeting with a gay or lesbian patient for the first time may encounter any of several situations. First, the patient may have been told directly by the referring clinician or other referral source that the practitioner is homosexual. Second, the patient may have requested referral to a homosexual clinician but may be unsure whether the clinician fits that bill. Third, the referring clinician may have referred the homosexual patient to a gay or lesbian clinician without ever revealing the sexual orientation of the clinician. Finally, the referral source may or may not have conveyed to the consulting clinician what he or she actually told the patient. Thus, as in other clinical situations, the clinical meeting with a gay or lesbian patient for the first time should explore how the patient came to seek a consultation in the first place, what qualities they requested in a clinician, what they were told about the clinician upon referral, and why they chose one clinician over another if they were given more than one name.

If the patient has been told that the consulting clinician is gay, asking the question "How did you imagine it might be helpful to have a gay clinician?" may prove instructive in delineating the patient's concerns and immediately highlights the fantasy elements of the meaning of a gay clinician to the patient. Answers such as "I thought I'd have an easier time talking about my sex life" or "I thought I wouldn't have to explain as much about the gay subculture" or "I thought you wouldn't be judgmental about me" should be carefully noted by the clinician because they are likely to be useful later in treatment as initial expressions of areas of concern or difficulty for the patient or indications of early transference tendencies.

For example, the patient who says he or she would not have to explain as much or would have more in common with the clinician is probably correct in certain concrete ways, because the gay clinician may have firsthand knowledge of places or people important in the gay subculture. However, the patient is also often making the erroneous, although understandable, assumption that the homosexual clinician is more like or has more inherently in common with him or her than would a heterosexual therapist. Assumptions that the clinician knows about or does similar things within the gay or lesbian community are common and are not necessarily accurate on the part of the patient. For example, the 20-year-old lesbian patient of a 40-year-old lesbian clinician was disappointed to realize that her clinician did not know of a particular new lesbian bar in town, whereas the clinician was bemused by the patient's image of her as a flirtatious, bar-hopping lesbian at a time when she was more preoccupied with raising her children and paying her mortgage. The fact that both were lesbian seemed less relevant than the generational gap between patient and clinician.

Another common assumption of similarity on the part of the patient is that the gay clinician will have shared common developmental difficulties or life experiences. One slight gay male patient who considered himself effeminate was disappointed to meet his burly, weightlifting gay male clinician because he suddenly realized that in requesting a gay man he had imagined that the clinician would share his childhood history of being bullied and teased as a sissy. Ironically, the clinician did share this developmental history, which in part accounted for his interest in bodybuilding as an adult, but the patient assumed based on his appearance that he did not. Highlighting and opening up such assumptions early in the therapeutic process can be a useful way to begin to engage a patient in an exploration of his or her inner world.

Even when a patient has requested a homosexual clinician, he or she may be ambivalent about actually getting one. Internalized homophobia on the part of the patient can make her worry that her lesbian clinician is somehow damaged or less than psychologically healthy. One early way of approaching this possibility with the patient who is aware that the clinician is gay is to include the question "Did you imagine there were things I might actually be less good at helping you with because I'm also gay?" along with questions about ways in which the therapist's homosexual orientation might be thought to be desirable. This tactic highlights more generally the evenhanded way with which complicated and conflict-laden material will be handled within the treatment. In addition, it highlights the very real possibility that the therapist may have blind spots in areas where his or her conflicts overlap with those of the patient.

As with most clinical situations in which the patient becomes aware of some important personal aspect of the clinician, knowing the clinician's sexual orientation often leads to additional questions on the part of the patient, such as whether the clinician is in a relationship, whether he or she has children, whether he or she experienced a difficult "coming out" process, and so on. As with any other personal information, the meaning of these questions should be analyzed, and the clinician must always be judicious in disclosing personal information about his or her life outside the office.

The fact that the patient begins therapy knowing that the clinician is homosexual does not rule out the possibility that the patient will fantasize about or even believe the clinician to be heterosexual at some point later in treatment. A gay male patient decided that his lesbian therapist had been "cured" in her own treatment and had a relationship with a man. He came to this conclusion when his therapist began wearing a wedding ring and became pregnant a short while later. He simultaneously felt that her walk had become less heavy footed and that she seemed less masculine. These feelings coincided with an altered sense of himself as less effeminate as well as the fact that the therapist's pregnancy stirred up issues related to having children as well. These issues ranged from envy of her capacity to have children to lingering internalized homophobic feelings that made him feel uneasy about whether it was fair for her to "force" her children to grow up in a gay household.

When the patient does not arrive at the consultation knowing of the clinician's sexual orientation, he or she may ask directly, "Are you gay?" Exploring what each answer would mean to the patient should ideally precede answering the question, but fostering and maintaining the therapeutic alliance as well as avoiding power struggles in the initial interview may lead the interviewer to choose to simply answer "yes" or "no." An intermediate position is for the clinician to say, "I'm not opposed to answering that question, but it may be useful to explore what it means to you first." Other patients may be curious but may not feel comfortable asking a direct question and may try instead to deduce the answer. One gay man referenced a popular club in a predominantly gay resort town in his initial consultation as a way of testing whether the clinician was familiar with it and thus presumably gay. This may provide an opportunity to elicit details about what the patient imagines a stereotypical homosexual is like. Finding out what the patient is looking for that would help him or her decide whether the clinician is gay can serve as a beginning for elucidating important aspects of a patient's representation of him- or herself as a homosexual person. Once again, using the patient's early behavior to attempt to engage him or her in the process of self-inquiry should be a cornerstone of the therapist's approach.

Still another patient may need to begin treatment and work in it for quite some time before he or she is ready to entertain the possibility that the therapist may also be homosexual. Sometimes this is an attempt on the part of the patient to keep erotic feelings at bay as well as the wish and fear that they might be acted upon by the therapist. At other times, a patient's own internalized antihomosexual bias may be so strong early in treatment that knowing the therapist is gay would cause him or her to devalue the therapist in a way that would render the therapy unworkable. In this case, it may be only after some of these issues have been explored and their intensity lessened that the patient becomes able to contemplate whether the therapist is gay. These situations and others like them, in which active forces in the patient prevent the patient from wondering about or wanting to know the therapist's sexual orientation, can be difficult for the inexperienced homosexual therapist, who may be tempted out of his or her own anxiety or interests to inform the patient of his or her sexual orientation or to aggressively question why the patient is not bringing it up. For many gay and lesbian therapists, being anonymous and an unknown entity to the patient seems to re-create the early life experience of being closeted, unseen and unknown by those around him or her. However, tolerating and understanding the nature of what can become an intense desire to tell the patient about his or her sexual orientation is a key aspect of countertransference management and self-analysis for the gay clinician.

Gays and lesbians, like members of many other minority groups in the United States, are living in the midst of a social revolution. They may be active participants or totally avoid involvement, but they cannot avoid awareness and choice. The interviewer's skill is reflected in his ability to explore these issues without conveying judgment, approval, condemnation, or persuasion but rather interest in how the patient approaches and selects among life's alternatives.

CONCLUSION

The experience of being "different" is universal, and clinical interviews are enriched by recognizing and exploring it, validating its existence and its universality, and understanding how the patient copes with it. The interviewer has to avoid several common pitfalls in doing so: first, pretending that it does not exist—that there is no prejudice, discrimination, or sociocultural tension in the world, and that the patient's experience of it is pathological; second, ignoring it—interviewing someone without inquiring of his experience of "difference"; and third, focusing on it exclusively, regarding the patient as a prototype or stereotype of a minority group rather than a unique individual who is a member of one of these groups. If the interviewer is successful, he can not only facilitate a successful interview but also have the added reward of learning about an aspect of the world he might not otherwise experience.

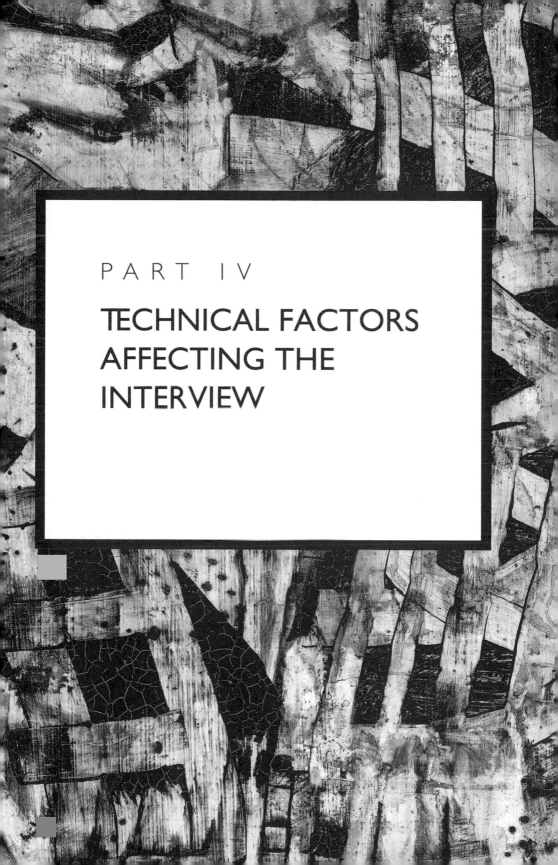

PART IV

TECHNICAL FACTORS AFFECTING THE INTERVIEW

CHAPTER 20

NOTE TAKING AND THE PSYCHIATRIC INTERVIEW

This chapter discusses the written record of the initial psychiatric evaluation and of subsequent therapeutic sessions. This written record is extremely useful for supervision and teaching because, unlike the prepared history that is organized around a more or less standard format, these notes reveal the process of the clinician–patient relationship as it unfolds.

The student is often distressed to learn that experienced psychiatrists vary considerably in their opinions concerning the optimal quantity and method of recording notes. The diversity of advice given the beginner is extreme. Notes are often suggested by a supervisor, thereby representing the intrusion of a third party into the interview situation. This may disturb either the patient or the interviewer. Therefore, a discussion of note taking requires consideration of the supervisory relationship. One supervisor may advise a student to make no notes whatsoever and instead to concentrate fully on what the patient is saying, relying on memory to reproduce the material. At the other extreme is the supervisor who recommends taking "verbatim notes." The student is always confused as to the definition of "verbatim," but in the spirit of cooperation, he writes frantically, trying to include everything said by both himself and the patient. The same supervisor may seem inconsistent, having a different approach for different students or for the same student with different patients or at different times in training. In order to understand this complex problem, it is necessary to establish some fundamental principles.

All interviewers make mental notes as they listen to the patient. One of the basic tasks in improving one's interviewing skill is learning to listen to and register the implied message and not only the explicit content. Simultaneously, the interviewer must observe the patient's behavior and affective reactions and his own responses to the patient. Furthermore, he is expected to note the correlation of specific topics with particular affective responses or body movements. Supervisors suggest that he learn to identify the "red thread," or the unconscious continuity that exists among the patient's associations. The interviewer is also expected to consider every remark that he will make to the patient and be able to recall his own comments, questions, interpretations, suggestions, advice, tone of voice, and so forth when reporting the interview. Since this is impossible, the result will be a compromise.

The pressure felt by the interviewer may be lessened by concentrating on one or more of the above-mentioned areas. Some emphasize historical data concerning the patient, whereas others direct attention to the interpersonal process that is taking place between interviewer and patient. Supervisors who emphasize historical data tend to be more demanding about note taking during the interview and usually want a precise record of the data concerning the patient in the order in which it was obtained. Those who emphasize the interpersonal process more often encourage a report of the interviewer's statements, regardless of whether the notes are recorded during or after the interview. Note taking is thus part of a much broader question: Which aspect of the interview will occupy the attention of the interviewer and his supervisor?

This chapter concentrates on the more narrow issue of what kind of record is to be made and when it is to be done in relation to the interview. The need for keeping written records about patients is ubiquitous in health care. There is a legal and moral responsibility to maintain an accurate record of each patient's diagnosis and treatment. Such requirements are quite broad; however, clinicians are subject to the policies of their particular institution. Although such policies undoubtedly influence attitudes, the precise manner in which the material is to be recorded is usually left to the discretion of the individual clinician. Another important purpose of record keeping is to aid one's own memory concerning each patient. Therefore, each individual has to decide what type of information he has the most difficulty remembering and use this knowledge as a guideline in his own system of record keeping. Basic identifying data such as the patient's name and address, the names of other family members, the ages of children, spouse, siblings, parents, and so forth should be written, because this information is not easily recalled. A concise description of the patient and his behavior during the initial interview along with initial diagnostic impressions often prove to be helpful later in treatment. Studies have suggested that therapists who prepare a written case formulation are consistently more successful than are those who only organize the material in their minds.

The chief problem in making notes during the interview is the potential distraction from attending to the patient. With experience, it becomes progressively easier to make notes with a minimum of distraction, giving almost full attention to the patient. Furthermore, one may be more distracted by attempting to remember information and more free to listen and attend to the patient if one knows that the critical data are written and preserved for future reference. Many therapists make fairly complete notes during the first few sessions while eliciting historical data. After that, most record new historical information, important events in the patient's life, medications prescribed, transference or countertransference trends, dreams, and general comments about the patient's progress.

The anxious or uncomfortable interviewer may find note taking a convenient refuge from emotional contact with the patient. It allows him to avert his eyes and occupy his thoughts with other matters. His note taking may fall a sentence or two behind the conversation. The interview fades into the background and whatever was making him anxious becomes less disturbing. When this occurs it is an indication that the notes should be put aside and the countertransference problems explored. As an example, a psychiatry resident told one of us that he had been particularly impressed by an article he had read that likened the maneuvers between beginning male therapists and female patients to the dating or courtship interaction. The resident felt that note taking helped him establish the feeling of having a professional identity and that he was relating to the patient in the proper and appropriate manner. Here, note taking functioned to reinforce a professional identity and to help provide a distraction so that the therapist could be more involved with the notes than with his feelings of attraction toward the patient.

There is a business-like quality to any note taking, and this can be used therapeutically. The clinician can establish a sense of heightened intimacy by putting his pen and paper aside. This is customary in discussing material about which the patient is expected to be reticent—his sexual life, his transference comments, or his negative feelings about a previous clinician.

In presenting material to a supervisor, the obsessive supervisee takes comfort in bringing copious notes. He is uncertain about what material is most important and is concerned that, if left to his own judgment, he is liable to bring the wrong data. He compensates for his inability to discriminate by attempting to bring everything. Invariably, he leaves out the most important things, those that took place on the way into the office or at the end of the interview when he had already put the notepad away. Since it is more difficult to write while talking than it is to write while listening, there is a tendency for the notes to be more complete and accurate concerning the remarks made by the patient than those made by the interviewer. Often when a supervisor suggests that the student might have said such-and-such or asked the patient about so-and-so at a certain point during the interview, the student quickly assures the supervisor that he did, in fact, say that, only he did not have a chance to write it down.

"Verbatim" notes are not actually verbatim. In fact, there is no such thing as a complete record of a session. Even a videotape is not a total report of all that transpired during the interview, as it contains only the externally observable behavior. Furthermore, many of the subtle verbal innuendos may be obscured by the recording equipment or completely missed if they are separated from the nonverbal cues that accompanied them. The crucial data of the interviewer's subjective feelings and responses cannot be directly recorded by any means. The quality of the relationship between the supervisor and the supervisee determines how much of the important material of the session is reproduced during a supervisory hour. If the supervisee respects and trusts his supervisor and does not perceive him as someone out to damage or weaken the trainee, more will be communicated. If the supervisee is frightened, the supervisor is not likely to learn many of the important things that transpired during the session, even though there are copious notes.

Audio- or videotapes are a kind of note taking that modern technology has made increasingly popular. When these methods are employed, one must consider the effect they have on both the patient and the clinician. The clinician's concern about the patient's rights and privileges is revealed by the manner in which he introduces these procedures to the patient. In the author's experience, it is uncommon for a patient to object to a recording, but every patient should have the procedure explained in advance and permission requested. The equipment should be started only after the patient knows about it, has given his permission, and understands who has access to the material and for what purpose. The patient is far more concerned with the clinician's attitude about invading his privacy than with the content of what might be revealed.

The interviewer, on the other hand, is often quite concerned about scrutiny by his colleagues and supervisors. This will stifle spontaneity and lead him to conduct a "safer," more stereotyped and more cognitive interview. In addition, his responses to the recording equipment are often projected onto the patient, and he may pursue the patient's anxiety about recording even though the patient is, in fact, relatively indifferent to it. One of the authors began his first interview on videotape with, "I imagine you're wondering about the television equipment," only to hear in reply, "Oh, don't you always do that?" On some occasions the doctor's exhibitionism will take over, and he will attempt dramatic maneuvers. In any event, he is responding to an unseen audience rather than to his patient.

Thus far, we have considered note taking largely from the point of view of the therapist and its effects upon him. Note taking also has effects on patients.

The paranoid patient is likely to be upset by note taking, and particularly by audio or video recording. He feels that the records represent damaging evidence that may later be used against him. In working with such patients, it is generally wise to confine note taking in the patient's presence to basic historical information. The interviewer should answer suspicious patients' questions about who has access to the notes. It is important to explore such patients' concerns and assure them that the interviewer will be discreet in his recording. Making notes at the end of the session will minimize some of these problems, but is often impractical.

The obsessive-compulsive patient may feel that the interviewer is getting the goods on him, but he is more prone to view the note taking as a cue to the significance of what he has said. The patient may also indicate his awareness of the importance of the notes by pausing periodically to facilitate the recording. The patient is usually unwilling to acknowledge that this behavior is motivated by his resentment that the interviewer shows more interest in the notes than in him.

Patients who are being treated by trainee therapists in academic training centers often have some awareness of the teaching role of the particular institution to which they have gone for help. They often do not ask directly about supervisors or supervision, but they will very frequently couch such curiosity in questions about the note taking. A common question is, "What do you use those notes for?" The trainee often senses that the inquiry is really directed at the supervisory process and represents a potential exposé of his inexperienced status. Therefore, he may be tempted to reply with a mild degree of dishonesty, offering such answers as "The notes are an important part of your treatment record" or "The clinic requires that treatment records are kept." Prominently concealed in such inquiries is the patient's fear that the clinician will breach his confidence. The evasiveness of the beginning therapist may also stem from guilt or discomfort at the idea of revealing his patient's confidences to a supervisor or at a conference. It is helpful to answer such inquiries by asking the patient if he has some specific idea concerning the purpose of the notes. The interviewer may uncover thoughts that the patient has concealed. Pursuing this point may lead to direct questions about the therapist's supervision. Such questions may be threatening to the novice, but he is surprised to learn how frequently the patient is reassured at the idea that his inexperienced therapist is being aided by a more experienced supervisor. At other times the patient already knows the answer to these questions and is relieved and impressed that his therapist is open and honest about his status.

On occasion a patient may ask, "What did you just write down?" or "Why did you write down what I just said?" Such questions indicate either the patient's search for some magical answer to his problem or his fear and mistrust of the clinician. The interviewer will gain more understanding of the underlying process if he does not answer the question directly but rather replies, "What do you think I wrote?" or "What is it that you are concerned about?" Uncovering the covert meaning of the question will shift the focus of the patient's interest from the notes to his own anxiety. Other variations of this situation occur when the patient tries to read the notes upside down while they are being written. This behavior may be accompanied by comments from the patient indicating that he has just read something. The interviewer might put down his pen at this point and explore the meaning of the patient's interest as suggested earlier.

Obsessive-compulsive and schizophrenic patients will frequently become concerned about the ownership of the notes. A common statement is "Those notes are about me so they must be mine." The clinician inquires about the patient's concern and may point out that the notes are really about their work together. Patients sometimes ask if they can read the notes or if they can have a copy of them. They may feel that the notes contain the magic answer that will immediately provide a solution to their problems, if only the clinician would share it with them. The interviewer should determine to which aspect of the note taking the patient is responding, rather than providing the notes to the patient. Once the interviewer has explored the basis of the patient's interest, the concern with the notes will be forgotten.

Ownership of the notes may also become a problem with patients who have a disturbance of impulse control. A typical patient might ask, "What would you do if I were to run over and grab those notes?" Interpretations about the patient's concern over loss of control are important. Such comments may be unsuccessful with very literal-minded patients, making it necessary for the interviewer to tell the patient that the notes belong to him, not to the patient, that the patient may not look at them, and that he will not allow the patient to take the notes away from him.

Histrionic and depressed patients tend to resent note taking. These individuals want the undivided attention of the therapist, and any interference provokes their anger and makes them feel deprived. Often their resentment about the notes is revealed in dreams long before they openly complain during the session. As with other patients who are disturbed by note taking, one can avoid the problem by making notes after the session. However, there may be a diminution in the quality of the notes. As with other transference cravings of such patients, the important issue is not whether the therapist accedes to the patient's desire but whether the desire is articulated and explored and whether this exploration contributes to the patient's self-understanding.

Like any other phenomenon that changes the frame of the interview situation, note taking will reflect transference and countertransference issues. When its impact is examined, note taking can usefully illuminate both the clinical and supervisory situations.

The supervisor's management of the student's note taking, including the exploration of the supervisee's transference to the supervisor that is reflected by these notes, often becomes an important educational experience in which supervision provides a "parallel process" to that of the therapy being supervised.

CHAPTER 21

TELEPHONES, E-MAIL, OTHER DIGITAL MEDIA, AND THE PSYCHIATRIC INTERVIEW

Electronic communication, starting with the telephone and, in recent years, e-mail, plays a significant role in contemporary clinical practice. At first glance the topic seems too simple or straightforward to warrant close attention. However, it involves an important area of clinical work with patients and therefore should be subject to study. Since it is not usually discussed in the training of mental health professionals, it is an area in which the personal style of each interviewer emerges with less self-scrutiny, and countertransference problems frequently develop and can be recognized.

Most patients make their initial contact with a clinician via the telephone, and many have subsequent occasions to call. Telephone calls can interrupt an interview and therefore present problems. Some professionals usually accept calls while interviewing a patient, whereas others never do, and still others occasionally accept telephone interruptions, with varying criteria for the decision. In addition, the telephone can be used to conduct clinical interviews both in emergencies and on an ongoing basis. Patients also contact their therapists via e-mail. Although in many ways this seems similar to leaving a message on a telephone answering machine, it often elicits an e-mail response with little possibility of a direct interaction with the recipient.

Other digital media, such as Facebook, pose complex issues for both clinician and patient. If the clinician is posted on Facebook, and depending on how much personal information is thereby available, the patient who has accessed this will enter the initial interview with knowledge about the clinician that has much preformed transference and voyeuristic valence. However, like any other "real" aspect of the clinician that the patient observes directly, such as appearance, office furnishings, and so forth, the impact of this indirect knowledge and its meaning for the patient need to be explored. The dangers of the reverse—the clinician who investigates the patient via the patient's Facebook posting—is captured in the following vignette:

> The clinician became aware in the early interviews with a patient that he was having considerable trouble obtaining a coherent history and narrative of the patient's past. He looked the patient up on a social media site and discovered that he had been a champion chess player as a teenager. Thinking to enhance the therapeutic alliance and that the patient would thus feel more understood and hence comfortable in revealing himself, the clinician shared this discovery with the patient. "I will never see you again," the patient responded and then stormed out. This did at least establish the diagnosis—a paranoid person who felt—correctly—that he had been spied on.

THE PATIENT TELEPHONES THE CLINICIAN

The Initial Telephone Call

Each clinician has his own way of handling an initial call from a prospective patient. Most expect some information concerning the patient before making the first appointment. Sometimes this has previously been provided by the referring person, but not infrequently the clinician does not know the individual who is telephoning to make an appointment.

It is expected that a caller will ask for the professional by name, will identify himself, and will make some explanatory comment pertaining to the purpose of the call. The prospective patient who telephones a clinician does not always follow these customary social expectations and thereby may provide clues concerning his personality pattern and the severity of his illness.

Even if the clinician answers his telephone by saying, "Hello," rather than by stating his name, a psychotic patient may immediately launch into a discussion of his problem. The interviewer can interrupt this with the inquiry, "To whom am I speaking?" The patient will usually respond by identifying himself and indicating that he wishes to make an appointment. If he only identifies himself and then continues with a discussion of his problems, the interviewer can interrupt him and ask, "Did you call in order to make an appointment?" Before actually making the appointment, it is useful to inquire, "Might I ask how you obtained my name?" If the patient obtained the clinician's name from an appropriate referral source, such as a colleague or social services agency, one may then ask the prospective patient if the problem he wishes to discuss pertains to himself. The caller may reply, "No, actually the patient is my wife" or "In fact, I want you to evaluate my son." In the example just given, the clinician responded, "How old is your son?" "He is 37," the patient replied. The patient continued, "He has this girlfriend we don't approve of, and he doesn't have a job and he still lives at home." Such situations require further telephone discussion before making the appointment, thus avoiding an inappropriate visit and a possible waste of time and money. The vignette just quoted reveals that the caller himself has difficulty coping with the person about whom he is calling, and that it would be more appropriate to arrange an appointment with the caller. However if, for example, the caller wants a physician to come to his home, posing as a guest, to arrange for commitment of a psychotic relative, some clarification of a psychiatrist's role is required. A brief telephone discussion will also help avoid unwanted appointments with salesmen, insurance agents, and others. If the patient indicates that he obtained the clinician's name from the classified telephone directory, one should determine whether he wants a general medical practitioner or a mental health professional, thus avoiding a misunderstanding.

Obsessive-compulsive or paranoid patients may take particular care that they are speaking to the clinician himself before disclosing anything about themselves. These patients are frequently insensitive to customary social expectations and may launch into a lengthy discussion of their problem over the phone. When this occurs, the clinician might say, "We can discuss this in more detail when you come to see me." The obsessive-compulsive patient often attempts to control the interviewer while making his first appointment by suggesting a list of times when he would be available. Rather than interpreting this behavior on the telephone, the clinician might indicate an hour that is convenient for him. The obsessive-compulsive patient will often inquire about the fee before scheduling an appointment. Such questions are best answered directly by telling the patient the fee. The patient may ask, "Is that subject to negotiation?" When the patient raises this issue during the initial telephone call, it often indicates ambivalence concerning treatment. Since an immediate exploration is not practical, the therapist must confront the ambivalence directly rather than accede to it. This is often done by replying that the fee for the initial consultation is not negotiable. The patient may then vacillate indecisively about scheduling the appointment. The clinician could then suggest that if the fee is too high the patient could be referred to another professional who might have a lower fee or to a clinic if appropriate.

A patient calling for a first appointment may ask for directions to the clinician's office or for information concerning parking in the neighborhood. It is appropriate to offer brief, factual answers to such questions. The patient may ask for permission to bring someone else with him to the office. If this person is involved in the problem or is a close relative of the patient, the clinician can agree without hesitation. If the relationship seems unclear, it is preferable to inquire about the patient's motives before indicating agreement.

Between the time of the initial call and the first appointment, the patient may telephone a second time. This might be to indicate that he will be late for the appointment or, if he is already late, he might ask, "Since only a few minutes of the hour are left, should I still come?" If the patient will have 15 minutes in the office, it is worthwhile to suggest that he come for the brief period; otherwise a new appointment should be scheduled. Another patient may telephone the morning of his session to say, "I have a cold, and my temperature is about 99°; should I come this afternoon?" The clinician could ask, "Do you have any reason for hesitation about the appointment other than the cold?" or "If you are leaving the decision up to me, does that mean you feel well enough to come?" Such comments indicate that one expects to see the patient at the scheduled hour and the conversation may be promptly terminated. After the first few interviews, when the clinician is familiar with the specific dynamic issues involved, other techniques may be more appropriate. A full discussion of these problems goes beyond the scope of this chapter.

Calls Following the First Interview

Different issues are involved when the patient telephones after the first visit. Something discussed during the interview may have upset the patient, and if this is not explored, the patient might be frightened away from further contact. On other occasions the patient telephones because he feels that he "left out" something important during the session. He might say, "Oh, I forgot to tell you" or "I made a mistake in telling you thus and such" or "I would like to add the following to what I reported." Such comments indicate that the patient was dissatisfied with the way that he felt he had expressed himself or with what he believes to be the interviewer's impression, or that he may have felt that the interviewer did not understand him or did not accept the patient's view of himself. The clinician might comment to that effect and then suggest that the issue could be explored further during the next appointment. Another patient may use the telephone to "confess" some embarrassing or humiliating information that he was unable to disclose during the face-to-face interview.

Phobic patients frequently telephone after the first hour, complaining of their symptoms and expressing a desire for reassurance. The interviewer could remark to such a patient, "Something during the visit may have upset you; this is not unusual, and we can discuss it at our next visit." It is essential to offer this type of reassurance to the phobic patient in the initial phase of treatment in order to help establish a working therapeutic relationship.

One example of covert hostile reactions to the therapist would be the patient who calls after the first session to say, "This is Elizabeth Smith, the patient you saw on Thursday morning at 10 A.M." The implication is that so little emotional contact was made that the interviewer might not remember the patient or that the patient's self-esteem is so low that she believes that no one would remember her. The interviewer may choose not to respond to this aspect of the comment until the next interview. However, on occasion, he may answer, "Yes, of course; I remember you."

At the end of the first interview, an anxious patient may ask the interviewer for his home telephone number. The patient might be asked if he is anticipating an emergency, because that is usually the reason for such a request. The clinician could explore what type of emergency the patient fears and how he has coped with such situations in the past. It was pointed out in Chapter 8, "The Anxiety Disorder Patient," that the phobic patient often requires the therapist to enter into various neurotic bargains before he will establish a therapeutic relationship. It is essential that the therapist tell this patient how he can be reached in an emergency.

We subscribe to the minority view that favors allowing most patients to obtain the clinician's home telephone number. This implies to the patient that the therapist is not afraid of the patient's dependent needs, nor will he feel unduly troubled or bothered if the patient has an emergency. Our experience has been that patients rarely abuse the clinician's privacy at home. The ability to contact the clinician quickly may relieve the patient's anxiety and actually decrease the frequency of his calls.

Severely depressed or suicidal patients are often so fearful of being a burden that they need permission to ask for the clinician's help. The clinician may provide this permission symbolically by giving his home telephone number directly to the patient rather than indicating that it can be obtained from the answering service. However, if the patient believes that the clinician is giving his home telephone number because of his own insecurity and anxiety, it may actually precipitate a crisis.

Occasionally the clinician telephones the patient following the first hour to change the time of the next appointment. Such requests do not require an explanation to the patient. The patient might ask, "Why is this necessary?" or say, "I hope nothing is wrong." It is sufficient to reply,

"Something has come up that makes it necessary to change the time." During the next session, the interviewer can explore the patient's reaction to the change in time as well as the meaning of his curiosity, if this seems indicated.

On occasion, a patient may intentionally try to interrupt the clinician with telephone calls, demonstrating the entitled, hostile, or inconsiderate themes in his personality. One should not become angry or abrupt with this patient; it is better to show him consideration, even though he may not be able to reciprocate. This helps the patient to adopt the therapist as a new ego ideal. One can say in a polite and friendly tone, "I'm busy just now. Could I call you back in a little while?"

In another situation, a message from a new patient leaves some confusion as to whether to return the patient's call. Messages are frequently garbled, and the clinician does not know his patient well enough after the first few interviews that he can be certain what is happening with the patient. Therefore, until the clinician is thoroughly acquainted with his patient, all telephone calls should be returned. This will forestall a number of potentially serious misunderstandings. A patient who is forced to cancel an appointment will appreciate the therapist calling to inquire about his problem.

At times the therapist must decide whether to telephone a patient who has missed an appointment without notification. During the initial interviews it is a good idea to telephone the patient under such circumstances. Such behavior on the patient's part often indicates a problem in the transference that requires immediate therapeutic intervention. If the patient has not called to reschedule at the earliest possible opportunity, a transference problem is usually at work.

When a patient has telephoned between sessions, it is usually helpful to refer to the call in the next session. The patient is then afforded the opportunity for discussion of his reactions to the telephone conversation and exploration of its deeper meaning to him when appropriate. The therapist will gear his analysis of the unconscious meanings of the call to the patient's capacity to develop insight. With more seriously ill patients, such an attempt at uncovering should be deferred until later in treatment.

TELEPHONE CALLS FROM OTHERS

Telephone Interruptions During the Interview

The clinician sometimes responds to telephone calls during a session with a patient. The resident who is "on call" would be an example. Other examples would include the clinician who has been playing "telephone tag" with someone who is difficult to reach and the need to speak with that person is urgent. The clinician could be a parent with a sick child who is expecting a return phone call from the child's physician. When the interviewer expects such a potential interruption, it is best to advise the patient, "I may receive a phone call that I must answer." Patients usually accept this and may inquire, "Would you prefer that I step outside if the call comes?" The clinician assesses the reality of the situation and uses his best judgment to answer "Yes, please" or "That won't be necessary." Whether or not the patient remains, the clinician must be alert to the patient's reaction to the interruption. If the patient hears the actual conversation, the likelihood of specific reactions increases as he is exposed to new data about the clinician as a person.

Telephone interruptions can be considered in terms of their effect on the ongoing interview as well as on the relationship between the clinician and the person who is calling. Many try to circumvent this problem by never accepting telephone calls when they are with a patient. This has both advantages and disadvantages. Their interviews are never interrupted; the patient and therapist are never distracted by an irrelevant conversation. However, not accepting phone calls during an interview reinforces the infantile omnipotence of the patient, encouraging his fantasy that he is the only person of concern to the therapist. Some clinicians who follow such a system permit the patient to hear their telephone ring before it is answered by a secretary or an answering service. Furthermore, they may continue with the interview, ignoring the ring as though it had not intruded. The patient is less likely to comment on the distracting influence of the telephone if the interviewer attempts to ignore it, but the patient will notice it nevertheless.

Others have an arrangement whereby they may turn off the ringer, allowing a light to flash instead. The usual practice is for the light to be placed where it is visible to the interviewer but not to the patient. It is then possible for the clinician to accept or not accept telephone calls depending on the patient, the situation, and his own mood. If he is not accepting calls during an interview, it is preferable that the patient be unaware that the telephone is ringing. In practice, we do not accept more than one telephone call during any given session.

In treatment of more seriously disturbed patients, the clinician's telephone conversations may help the patient to improve his reality testing and his recognition of emotions. For example, a psychotic patient may grossly misinterpret the nature of the call. The telephone interruption is useful if the therapist reconstructs the conversation and attempts to determine how the patient came to his conclusions. The therapist can point out gross distortions and at times disclose the true nature of the call. This helps the patient to cope with reality by improving his ability to communicate and to interpret the communications of others. As the patient demonstrates improvement, his speculations become more perceptive and accurate. Situations in which the patient continues to misinterpret are indications for further therapeutic work. The principles are similar to those used in working with the patient's reactions to the other members of a therapeutic group.

During the first few sessions of treatment, the patient often displays no reaction to telephone interruptions. In more advanced stages of therapy, reactions to a telephone call become obvious. These responses are manifestations of the transference and accordingly are subject to analytic study and interpretation. Hearing the therapist talk with another person on the telephone gives the patient an opportunity to experience a facet of the clinician's personality different from that elicited by the patient's personality. This may lead to a discovery that the therapist is capable of expressing tenderness, warmth, anger, and so forth, and in the later stages of treatment may help the patient achieve a more realistic image of his therapist. For example, one patient had abandoned his career as a teacher because of his feeling that it was a passive, feminine, and hence demeaning profession. He overheard his therapist's brief telephone conversation one day, and deduced that he was also a teacher and that he was able to function effectively as a man in this capacity. This helped the patient to work through his neurotic conflicts.

The effects of a telephone interruption on any given interview depend upon the problems of the patient, the personality of the clinician, and the specific events at the time of the interruption. The therapist who has a thorough knowledge of all of the factors can predict his patient's reactions to a given telephone interruption. When he feels that an interruption would have an unfavorable effect upon the therapy, he can turn off the telephone.

The Patient's Reaction to the Interruption

Patients may have a variety of reactions to their interviews being interrupted by telephone calls.

Relief

Patients may experience relief after telephone interruptions for several reasons. The discovery that other people have problems just as they do may be relieving. The clinician's willingness to accept urgent phone calls from others gives permission for this patient to call the clinician in a time of need. A third basis for relief is one that the patient describes as "saved by the bell." This typically occurs when the patient is just about to discuss difficult material.

In the first instance, the interviewer might explore the feelings underlying the patient's surprise at recognizing that others also have problems. Likewise, exploration would be indicated when the patient is relieved to learn that it is permissible to call the clinician in time of need. However, the patient who feels "saved by the bell" requires a different approach. He is using the interruption to support his resistance. Sometimes the interviewer can simply wait for the patient to return to the comments he was making when the telephone rang. On other occasions, it is more useful to explore the patient's feelings of relief at the interruption as a way of making the patient more aware of his resistance. If the patient continues to react in this manner, the clinician can turn off the telephone, particularly when the patient is discussing difficult material. The phobic patient will typically react with this type of response.

Distraction

The typical distracted response is characterized by the question "Where was I when the phone rang?" or "What was I saying?" Such a reaction also indicates resistance, although at a more unconscious level, and therefore this patient is less likely to accept an interpretation. An interruption may bring disturbing thoughts to the patient's awareness. After the call, the patient attempts to reconstitute his defenses by resuming his previous resistant discussion. Rather than exploring the resistant behavior directly, it may be useful to ask the patient what he was thinking while the telephone conversation was in progress. Often illuminating material will be revealed in response to such an inquiry.

Frequently it is appropriate for the clinician to say nothing after an interruption, thereby giving the patient the opportunity to pursue his own associations. During the initial interviews the clinician might completely ignore an interruption and merely help the patient to continue with what he had been saying. The therapist must exercise care in following the latter course, because it frequently serves to facilitate the avoidance of concealed responses of anger or curiosity about the telephone conversation. Once this is recognized by the clinician, he may work with the deeper feelings.

Anger

Angry responses to a telephone interruption include direct angry statements and indirect sarcastic remarks such as, "Can't you afford a secretary?" or "You owe me 3 minutes." It is important that the interviewer not respond with anger or defensive behavior. Explanatory remarks deflect the treatment from the important issue. The clinician either listens while the patient ventilates his rage and then continues with the interview, or interprets the patient's feeling that he is being cheated or deprived of the interviewer's complete attention. Such comments are supportive of the patient's anger and will help him feel that the interviewer really does understand him. If the call lasts more than a minute, the interviewer might ask the patient if he could stay a few minutes at the end of the session. Obsessive-compulsive or paranoid patients are most likely to feel overtly angry in response to interruptions.

Denial

The characteristic example of denial is the patient who ignores the call, seeming to remain in a state of suspended animation until the interviewer concludes his conversation. The patient will then finish his sentence as though there had been no interruption. This response can conceal the patient's anger or his intense interest in every detail of the telephone conversation and fantasies concerning the call, or it may reflect his struggle to retain his thoughts in spite of the interruption. Some patients will use fantasy formation to avoid overhearing the conversation. Such denial is a defense against expression of forbidden impulses. The denying patient also manifests a striking lack of distraction, and it is useful for the interviewer to comment, "You seem not to have been distracted by the telephone call." If the patient denies having distracting thoughts, the interviewer could let the matter drop. This type of response may occur in the histrionic patient who was interrupted in the middle of a rehearsed drama or with the obsessive-compulsive patient who was busily following his mental notes. If the interviewer successfully uncovers the patient's resentment, the focus of the interview is shifted to this issue.

Guilt or Feelings of Inadequacy

Responses of guilt or feelings of inadequacy reveal that the patient has carefully listened to the conversation. His typical remark will be "You have such important responsibilities" or "Why do you bother with me when there are other people who need you so much more than I do?" The patient may even offer to step outside while the clinician is in the middle of the telephone call. These responses basically stem from unconscious anger, which the patient turns inward against himself. The patient's self-esteem is low, and he does not feel entitled to ask for much in life. Underneath, he resents the necessity that he share the clinician with other people, whom he believes to have problems that are considered more important than his own. Because of his profound sense of inadequacy, he feels that he has no right to complain. Therapists are often tempted to interpret the patient's underlying resentment and usually make the patient feel worse. Instead, it is more helpful to comment to the patient that even in his illness he seems to feel that he is a failure—that his symptoms are less interesting or that his story is less engaging than that of someone else.

The patient who reacts in this manner also has hidden feelings of intense competitiveness. His response to the telephone interruption provides a ready opening for discussion of such feelings. Initially, the patient may only accept the idea that he is constantly making unfavorable comparisons between himself and others. Later he may acknowledge a feeling of resentment that he is always in the losing position. The patient may be more willing to accept this if the clinician does not immediately attempt to focus the feeling of resentment upon himself. Hostile feelings are easier to accept when they are directed toward someone not physically present. The interviewer's position as a figure of authority and a potential source of supportive care also inhibits the experience of hostile feelings by such a patient. The response of guilt or inadequacy is characteristic of the depressed patient or the patient with a masochistic character.

Envy or Competition

The openly envious or competitive response is a variation of the overtly angry reaction. After listening to the telephone conversation, the patient may ask, "Why can't you be that way with me?" The interviewer's warmth or friendliness to the caller has aroused feelings of competition and jealousy in the patient. The patient feels that the clinician does not care enough about him. Such feelings may be more subtly expressed with the comment, "That must not have been a patient!" When the patient is asked why or how he made such a determination, he replies that the interviewer sounded "so friendly." As in responding to openly angry reactions, the interviewer should not offer a defense or attempt to convince the patient that he is not being deprived. Instead, he might encourage the patient to further express his feelings of deprivation.

Paranoid Responses

A typical paranoid response would be "Were you talking about me?" or "Was the call for me?" If the patient is not too disturbed, the interviewer will learn more if he does not hasten to correct the patient's misinterpretation. First, he might explore the patient's fantasy and then determine the process through which the patient came to his decision. This avoids provoking the patient into an angry defense of his interpretation. Exploring the content of the fantasy will elucidate important transference feelings, and pinpointing the distortions in the thought process may be useful in helping the patient improve his reality testing. The paranoid patient does not know whom to trust. He compensates for this inability either by indiscriminately trusting everyone or by trusting no one. The clinician might inquire, "Whom did you think I was talking to?" and "What did you think we were discussing?" The fantasy revealed by the patient provides useful information concerning the psychodynamics of the patient's emotional disorder. After the interviewer has fully explored the patient's ideas, it is useful to tell him the reality, and together with him trace the process that led to his misinterpretation.

On occasion, a call may really be about the patient in the office. In this situation, it is wise for the interviewer to indicate to the patient the identity of the caller as soon as the interviewer has determined who it is. This can be done by addressing the caller by name and then proceeding with the conversation. This gesture helps the patient to recognize that the clinician is not holding secret discussions about him.

Curiosity

Curiosity, like denial, is a type of response in which the patient often has no awareness of any conscious emotional reaction. He has become involved in the conversation, but he is only aware of an interest in what is going on between the interviewer and the caller. Typical remarks would include "Was that your wife who called?"; "Is everything all right at home?"; or "I hope that wasn't bad news." The curiosity is usually a defense against a deeper emotional reaction, such as residual childhood curiosity concerning parental activities. Remarks displaying curiosity offer the interviewer an opportunity to comment, "Let's take a look at your curiosity." Rather than answering such questions, it is helpful to establish with the patient that he does have curiosity concerning such material. Another approach would be to explore the meaning of the patient's curiosity and to trace it back to his childhood.

Sympathy

The sympathetic response is elicited when it becomes apparent that the caller is in distress. The patient in the office may comment, "I hope that person will be all right," or he might volunteer to relinquish his appointment to enable the clinician to see the other person. Such reactions are frequently defenses against experiencing angry, envious, or guilty feelings. Interpreting the underlying emotion is difficult; the therapist can do very little at that time except continue the interview. Perhaps he may thank the patient for his good intentions. Responses of sympathy are more common in depressed or masochistic patients.

Fright

At times, when it is appropriate for the interviewer to express anger to the caller, the patient in the office may react with fear. An illustration of this occurred when an insurance agent interrupted a clinician for the third time and seemed unwilling to accept the clinician's statement that he was not free to speak. Instead, he insisted on completing his rehearsed speech. When the clinician became angry and abruptly terminated the call, the patient appeared shocked and said, "You certainly weren't very nice to that person!" The patient feared that he also might evoke an angry response from the clinician. Patients who inhibit their own aggression often fear that as a result of therapy they might lose control of their impounded rage and cause injury to others. Any indication that the clinician can get angry will increase this fear.

A variation of such a reaction might be characterized by the patient's disappointment in the clinician. This could happen when some unattractive aspect of the clinician's personality is demonstrated before the patient for the first time. The interviewer might cope with such reactions in different ways, for example, interpreting the patient's disappointment that the clinician is not perfect or helping the patient to recall previous experiences of disappointment in persons he admired.

Pleasure

The patient is sometimes pleased with the way in which the clinician conducts himself on the telephone. He may, for example, experience vicarious pleasure by hearing him express his anger in a way the patient has been unable to emulate. In this situation, the clinician could direct the interview toward the patient's characteristic ways of expressing anger and attempt to uncover the fears that prevent him from a more open type of emotional expression.

Another situation in which the patient might be pleased would be when the interviewer has obviously received good news. This reaction would require further discussion only if it seemed appropriate to explore an admixture of unconscious envy or competitiveness.

The Interviewer's Reaction to the Interruption

It is important that the interviewer be aware of his own emotional reactions to telephone interruptions. He may experience relief from boredom if the patient has been expressing hostility. He might be distracted and then experience guilt feelings for having lost the continuity of the interview. He could react by feeling happy or sad in response to good or bad news. He may become angry for several reasons: as a result of the interchange with the caller, merely because of the interruption, or because of the particular time at which the interruption occurred. He can recognize countertransference in some reactions, such as when he has used a telephone call in order to enhance his status in the eyes of the patient in his office.

Customarily, when answering the telephone, the interviewer indicates that he is not free to converse. However, if a brief conversation is unavoidable, the clinician can find useful therapeutic opportunities if he unobtrusively observes the patient's behavior during the call.

On rare occasions, the interviewer may ask the patient to leave the consultation room when he receives a telephone call. An example would be a call involving a serious emergency in the personal life of the interviewer. Under such circumstances, the clinician would place an undue burden upon the patient by the unnecessary disclosure of his personal problem.

At times, someone seeking to reach the patient may call the clinician's office. If the patient is in the office at the time, the clinician can simply hand the telephone to the patient. Should the patient not be there, he may take the message and convey it to the patient. If the matter was not sufficiently urgent to warrant the interruption, the clinician could analyze the patient's motivation for encouraging such behavior from friends or relatives.

Since most people possess a cellular phone, it is a rare occasion that the patient may ask to use the clinician's telephone. If the request is made at the end of the session and would cause the clinician inconvenience, it could be suggested that the patient make the call elsewhere. If the request is made at the beginning of the session, the clinician might permit the call but then direct the patient's attention to his reasons for not locating a telephone before his appointment. The patient's use of the clinician's telephone, however, can be therapeutically valuable. In one case, a patient asked to use the telephone and proceeded to phone her stockbroker, placing several "buy and sell" orders in an arrogant manner. Before the interviewer could comment on this unusual behavior, she volunteered, "You have just observed a portion of my personality of which I am very ashamed—I hope you will be able to help me."

TELEPHONE CALLS FROM PATIENTS' RELATIVES

Relatives of the patient may telephone the interviewer and ask either for an appointment or for information concerning the patient. The relative could be told, "I will tell John that you called and expressed an interest in his problem," without divulging any information. At times the relative may ask the clinician not to reveal the call. If the clinician agrees to such requests, he is placed in an untenable position and the therapy is inevitably damaged.

The therapist may accurately suspect that the caller wishes to interfere in the therapy. We believe that it is often an error to refuse to speak to such a caller if he is close to the patient. Frequently he exercises important influence over the patient's life, or the patient is dependent upon him. Alienating such persons can injure the patient. If the patient gives his consent, an interview with the relative could be arranged with or without the patient present.

Reciprocally, the clinician may need to contact a patient's relative or an institution such as a school or college. Another situation is the patient who has expressed suicidal or homicidal wishes or intentions. If a patient has expressed an intent to harm himself or another person, the clinician is concerned with both the safety of the threatened individual and the possible impact on the patient. The clinician has ethical and legal responsibilities to protect both the patient and others, and the patient should be informed of these. In the case of a serious suicidal intent, relatives may have to be contacted in order to effect the patient's hospitalization.

CONDUCTING SESSIONS BY TELEPHONE

Telephone Emergencies

A patient may telephone the clinician in a state of serious depression or acute anxiety that constitutes an emergency. It is apparent that the therapist is at a disadvantage in treating a patient over the telephone. His examination is limited to auditory material and he is unable to utilize other sensory impressions of the patient. Rather than work under such a handicap, some therapists insist that the patient come for a personal examination and otherwise refuse to aid the patient. Other therapists rely on their knowledge of the patient and the subtle communications that are more meaningful than verbal content. Tone of voice, pace of speech, and response time to the therapist's comments all convey a wealth of information.

A clinician's rigidity seriously limits his usefulness. Surely the patient is also aware that a personal interview is preferable to a telephone call. In an emergency, however, even a brief positive contact may be life-saving for the patient. It is essential, therefore, that one respond to such a patient with the same degree of respect and dignity as is shown in a personal interview. Therapists may react to a request for a telephone interview with annoyance and resentment, which are quickly communicated to the patient. Frequently, the telephone call is the patient's test to determine whether the therapist is an accepting or rejecting individual. It is a prejudice of some therapists that requests for telephone interviews are always manifestations of resistance. We disagree.

The clinician might begin by obtaining the patient's name, address, and telephone number, if the patient has not already identified himself. The patient may be reluctant to provide some of this information. In this situation, the patient can be asked why he feels that it is necessary to conceal such information. That patient has usually taken steps to circumvent the interviewer's caller-ID.

It has been our experience that the telephone patient has often had prior contact with a mental health clinician. It is therefore useful to make inquiry about such contacts early in the interview. This is particularly true of the patient who refuses to disclose his identity.

After a brief description of the presenting problem is obtained, it is useful to ask the patient if he has considered arranging for a personal interview. If it becomes apparent that the patient is psychotic, the clinician can ask if the patient fears that a personal visit might lead to hospitalization. If the patient does fear that, the therapist might then investigate specific symptoms that the patient feels might require hospital treatment. After such a discussion, it is frequently possible to reassure the patient that these symptoms do not require hospitalization. Such a patient can be told that treatment, in order to be successful, requires the cooperation of the patient, and that treatment forced upon the patient probably will not help. The clinician may further reassure the patient that he does indeed seem to have some motivation to receive help, as evidenced by his calling.

Telephone Interviews

Patients resort to telephone interviews for various reasons. The problem of physical distance prevents some patients from coming in person.

Other frequent motivations for telephone interviews are the fear of inordinate expense associated with psychiatric help or fear of humiliation as the result of discussing embarrassing material face-to-face. Some patients experience such intense desires to commit suicide that they fear that they may not live long enough to be interviewed in person and therefore are using the telephone contact as a measure of true desperation.

On rare occasion, at the conclusion of a consultation on the telephone, the clinician realizes that a patient who still refuses to come for a personal appointment is seriously in need of help. It may then be useful to make an appointment for a second telephone interview. After several such interviews, the patient usually will be willing to come for an appointment in person.

If someone other than the patient is calling, it is necessary to determine the relationship between the patient and the person on the telephone. In a recent example of this, one of us was telephoned by a very distraught colleague. Fifteen minutes of clinical presentation of what appeared to be a consultation had transpired before it became apparent that the patient was the colleague's wife and not a case from his practice. This was not a simple misunderstanding. It arose out of the colleague's strong need to detach himself from his own personal relationship, describing his wife merely as another patient about whom he was concerned.

It is important that the interviewer ask the age of the person to whom he is speaking early in a telephone contact. Meeting the patient in person provides visual clues about his age. Errors of many years can easily be made if estimates of the patient's age are based on the sound of his voice. Other basic identifying data that the clinician routinely obtains when speaking to the patient in person are also frequently overlooked during the telephone interview.

An obvious but often neglected technique for reducing the handicaps inherent in a telephone situation is to ask the patient to describe himself physically. Although no one answers such a question objectively, certain patients tend to distort more than others. This tendency is based on how they feel about themselves. It is possible for the clinician to reduce such distortion by asking the patient if the answer he has given is more a reflection of how he appears to others or how he feels about himself.

A clinician may decide to summon the police in response to a telephone call from a severely suicidal or homicidal patient who is on the brink of losing control of his impulses and cannot come to the hospital. This should be done openly, with the patient informed of the action. If the patient objects, the clinician can increase the patient's responsibility for this decision, pointing out that he just made such action necessary through the description of his problem.

For example, a patient may telephone a clinician and announce that he has just ingested a full bottle of sleeping pills. Obviously, the clinician asks the patient his name, address, and telephone number at once and then asks the name of the medication and the approximate number of pills. If he has taken a dangerous dose, the clinician can advise him that the police will be sent immediately, that the patient should open his door to facilitate their entry, and that he will call back as soon as he has summoned the police. He can also inquire about the name and phone number of the closest neighbor in the event that the police are not immediately available.

If the patient refuses to disclose his name and address, the clinician might comment, "You must have some uncertainty concerning your wish to die or you would not have called me. There are only a few minutes remaining in which you can change your mind. You have taken a fatal dose, and it may already be too late to save your life, but we can still try." Realizing that the outcome is already uncertain, the patient may allow "fate" to intervene and may provide the identifying data. An analogous situation could occur with the patient who is on the verge of homicide. In this situation of a specific victim at risk, the clinician should take immediate steps to protect that individual by calling him, the police, or appropriate third parties to facilitate the patient's hospitalization. In the later portion of the telephone interview, the clinician may inquire if there is anyone else with whom he can converse; by obtaining another person's view of the patient's problems the interviewer may gain information that would help him to assess the clinical situation.

A special problem of the telephone interview is silences, which occur as they do in conventional interviews. It often is difficult for the telephone interviewer to allow these silences to develop during the conversation and still remain focused on the patient. This is a reflection of the interviewer's discomfort, dissatisfaction, or impatience. Only through experience can a therapist relax and be professionally at ease while conducting a telephone interview.

Telephone Treatment Sessions

Not infrequently, treatment sessions may be conducted by telephone. For instance, a patient might be forced to interrupt an ongoing therapy because of a move, or might relocate to some part of the country where psychotherapy is unavailable. Business travel, out-of-town essential meetings, and so on may lead to missing a significant number of face-to-face sessions. Under these circumstances, treatment sessions may appropriately be conducted by telephone.

Three brief vignettes illustrate some major points. In the first case, a middle-aged depressed woman who had had several years of therapy went to another state for 6 weeks to obtain a divorce. Her marriage had contributed to her depression, but she was unable to face the prospect of the divorce without the emotional support of her therapy. Her treatment was successfully conducted twice a week for 6 weeks on the telephone.

The second case is that of a 30-year-old depressed woman with anxiety and hypochondriacal trends. After 1 year of treatment, she became pregnant and seemed likely to miscarry. Her obstetrician insisted that she remain in bed for 3 months. Her home situation was intolerable, and she lived too far away for the therapist to visit her at home. He treated her twice weekly by telephone during this period.

The third case involves a situation that was in some respects more unusual. The patient was a 30-year-old phobic housewife who moved to the suburbs after several years of treatment. One day, a severe snowstorm forced a cancellation. The patient waited until her appointed hour to telephone, because she had hoped to find some means of transportation. The therapist sensed that she was eager to terminate the call and commented to that effect. The patient revealed disturbing thoughts about the clinician that she had successfully suppressed while she was in the office. Because the patient would have isolated her feelings if the matter had been left until the next appointment, it was discussed at that time. Subsequently, the patient deliberately sought another telephone session the next time more difficult material emerged. That time the clinician refused, because it was clear that the patient's request was a form of resistance.

Admittedly, these are all special situations, but nonetheless they are scarcely unique. The arrangement to continue a patient's treatment by telephone implies that the patient's dependence upon the therapist is realistic. In situations in which this would be undesirable, telephone sessions are not indicated.

As the reader may surmise, the telephone consultation presents many challenging and difficult problems. The clinician who has developed skill and flexibility in this situation will be able to work more effectively with a wider variety of patients.

The Cellular Phone

Cellular phones, including smart phones, are ubiquitous, and many patients bring them into the consultation room. The patient may be talking on the phone, texting, or surfing the Web as the interviewer appears to greet him and escort him to the office. He may turn the phone off or leave it on during the interview. If the latter, it may ring or make a text notification sound and interrupt the interview. Once again, he may turn it off, take the call, or look at the text and then decide. In rare circumstances, a patient may even make a call during the session.

The most basic principle is that all of these behaviors are part of the interview—communications and enactments that have meaning can be explored, understood, and when appropriate discussed with the patient. Like all such enactments there is no simple relationship between a specific type of act and a specific meaning. It depends upon the context, the patient's personality, the dominant transference and countertransference themes, and the meaning that has been attributed (or not attributed) to similar enactments in the past.

Perhaps the simplest situation is the patient who is talking on a cell phone or texting when the clinician comes to the waiting room. Most often this calls for no comment, but the way in which the patient responds and the way in which he ends the call or the sending of an e-mail or text embodies a message about the relationship, just as with the patient who is continuing to read a magazine or begins taking off his overcoat when the interviewer approaches. "I'm sorry to keep you waiting," "This is more important than an extra few seconds with you," "You're not as important as my other business," or "See how busy I am" are all possibilities. The interviewer registers such behavior but is unlikely to comment on it early in a relationship.

The patient's decision to leave the cell phone on during the session or to answer a call or respond to a text is more likely to elicit a comment. The basic principle here is that the clinician is interested in understanding the behavior and in inviting the patient to participate in that understanding, not in ending or forbidding it. Comments such as "You have decided to leave your cell phone on," "Tell me about your taking that call," or "You looked to see who was calling. What was your thought?" may be helpful. The patient who replies, "My children are home alone," "My husband gets angry if he can't contact me," or "My girlfriend is always changing our plans for the evening" is opening an area for discussion.

Some patients may be less concerned about a specific call but know that they become anxious if their cell phone link to the outside world is interrupted. Often this patient provides a rationalization, but this serves to conceal phobic anxiety—the professional who explains that he is "on call" knows that the call can wait; the parent who is concerned about her children is aware that the concern is more neurotic than realistic. The exploration of the behavior, the patient's view of it, and the clinician's response can serve as models for the way in which other "reality" issues are explored in the treatment. The cell phone is an ambassador from the outer world that the patient brings into the session and thus provides an opportunity for exploring the way in which the patient copes with real-world challenges.

An unusual example was provided by an affluent professional woman who apologized at the beginning of a session, explaining that she would have to make an important call during the hour. At the appointed time, she took out her phone and did so. It became apparent that the call was to her representative who was bidding for an art object at auction. The interviewer asked how she felt conducting this activity in front of him. The ensuing discussion opened an exploration of her conflict about displaying her wealth, collecting valuables, eliciting envy from others, and unsuccessfully trying to use these strategies to compensate for feelings of frustration and desperation in her personal relationships. She had been successful in her bidding, but more important, she came to understand why it was so important to her.

E-MAIL

Communication between the patient and the clinician via e-mail or texting, if the clinician has provided her cell phone number to the patient, presents interesting challenges for the clinician. The sending of an e-mail or text is itself a communication, as is the clinician's decision to respond or not respond via e-mail or text. The response is an action that nonverbally transmits a message to the patient regarding the therapist's attitude toward the enactment. Time is such a scare commodity that when the patient wants to ask the clinician, "I have the following symptoms 1 hour after the first dose of my new medication. Do you want me to continue taking it?" this can be viewed as an appropriate use of e-mail that warrants an e-mail response. The patient may have trouble getting the clinician on the telephone because he is occupied, or the patient may be in a meeting when the therapist is free, but the patient's laptop computer is on and he can pick up an e-mail response. If there are deeper meanings, they can be explored at the next appointment.

E-mail is different from the telephone because the tone of voice, the rhythm of conversation, its starting and stopping, its pregnant pauses, and so on are absent. The only information transmitted is lexical—words. A patient talking on the telephone may say, "I'm fine, I don't know why my wife thinks otherwise," but his hesitation, tone of voice, and phrasing may convey something quite different. The same message via e-mail would consist only of the words, and much would be lost. Nonetheless, like any literary text, e-mail messages can readily convey affect through the choice of words or the presence of sarcastic or hostile comments. Patients can use written phraseology that connotes conflict or ambivalence concerning what they are writing. The immediacy of communication and its interactive component are diminished in e-mail. The back and forth of e-mail may come to resemble a psychological chess game in which each participant considers his next move before making it, but an interaction is taking place, one generally slowed down in real time. The clinician may find himself in an ongoing therapeutic engagement via e-mail.

Perhaps the most common use of e-mail is seemingly "administrative"—canceling or changing an appointment, requesting a form for insurance reimbursement, and so on. However, to a dynamic clinician, nothing is purely administrative, and the meaning of administrative communications, particularly those that the patient tries to conduct outside regular sessions, may have great significance. What goes on between clinician and patient, including e-mail, is never without unconscious meaning. The therapist keeps this in mind when reading such e-mails, deciding whether and how to respond and whether to bring them up in the next session. In general, if a response is not required before the next session, one would not reply immediately but bring up the matter then, modeling the expectation that these issues belong in the treatment. If a more immediate response is indicated, the clinician may note whether it could have been discussed in the previous session and, if so, might inquire about this at the next meeting. Patients may include accompanying comments that are direct transference signals—"I'm sorry to bother you," "I know you are busy," "I forgot to ask you," "Something really important has come up," or even "Will you charge me if I have to cancel?" The simplest rule of thumb is that these kinds of comments are what treatment is about, and the clinician brings them into the treatment and also notices and brings into the treatment the patient's attempt to keep them out of it. Frequent communication via e-mail with family and friends is a common part of many people's lives. The clinician, because of the transference, can easily be incorporated into this group and be bombarded with e-mails. The clinician's policy about communication should be conveyed to the patient at the outset. Whenever possible the clinical interaction should be confined to the clinician's office, although with the understanding that urgent communications via either the telephone or e-mail may occur.

Less common, but more difficult to manage, is the patient who tries to terminate treatment via e-mail.

A 30-year-old woman with a borderline personality disorder was given to sudden eruptions of rage. One occurred at the end of a session when the therapist seemed unsympathetic in response to her distress and then interrupted her to end the session at the usual time. A few hours later he received an e-mail: "I hate you. I never want to see you again." Knowing her pattern in the past and believing that it was vital to bring this into the treatment while at the same time feeling that the patient had to experience some triumphant retaliation, he responded, "I didn't realize that you were so angry. Can we discuss this further on Thursday at our usual time?" He purposely allowed the ambiguity of whether that would be on the phone or in person. She came to the session, and the treatment resumed its rocky course.

Some patients will send, via e-mail, communications to the therapist—jokes, cartoons, articles from the newspaper, or messages they have received from someone else. These rarely require any direct response, but once again are important to discuss at the next session.

A man who was struggling with his discomfort with the asymmetry of the therapeutic relationship sent his therapist a cartoon showing a patient who had just gotten off a couch, taken out a gun, and shot his analyst. The caption read: "You've helped me a lot, but you know too much." The patient didn't mention it in the next meeting, and the therapist commented, "I got your message about how uncomfortable you feel telling me your secrets." The patient immediately denied this, saying that "it was only a joke," but then admitted that he hated the thought that the therapist knew so much about him while he knew nothing about the therapist. The clinician asked, "What are your fears about my possessing all this personal knowledge of you?" The patient replied; "You might use it against me." This opened up an exploration of a previously unrevealed paranoid aspect of the patient, who felt that revealing his fears and conflicts was potentially damaging because he doubted the clinician's adherence to strict confidentiality concerning the treatment.

An intermittently psychotic woman who was the mother of two would regularly e-mail her male therapist copies of her children's report cards. They were doing well, and the underlying message was that she was a good mother, but a subtext was that the therapist was unconsciously viewed as the father. The issue of being a good mother was particularly crucial because the patient was in the process of a divorce and feared that her psychiatric condition would be used against her in the determination of custody. The therapist commented on the children's performance, added that the patient must be very proud, and inquired if she might be concerned that her soon-to-be ex-husband planned to question her competence to care for them.

There are, of course, an infinite number of other ways in which e-mail can be used, and most people find it part of their daily routine. Sometimes e-mail has the advantage, because of its distancing from immediate emotional engagement, to allow the more constricted patient to give voice to feelings that he is uncomfortable expressing in the clinician's office because of his fear of his own aggression or of the clinician's response. These hidden issues are now out in the open and can be productively examined in the consulting room. Clinicians must keep in mind that although the text communicates, it allows a great deal to be concealed and also prevents the immediate interaction that is essential to the conduct of therapy. However, the way that the patient uses it, along with the therapist's response and understanding, provides another opportunity for the enhancement of the therapeutic process.

AFTERWORD

Canst thou not minister to a mind diseased,
Pluck from the memory a rooted sorrow,
Raze out the written troubles of the brain
And with some sweet oblivious antidote
Cleanse the stuff'd bosom of that perilous stuff
Which weighs upon the heart?

So implores Shakespeare's Macbeth to the clinician concerning his wife's descent into madness. The doctor replies pessimistically:

Therein the patient
Must minister to himself.

Today we can be more sanguine. We can indeed minister to "a mind diseased," and the patient no longer has to "minister to himself." An essential part of that ministration is the perceptive sensitive psychiatric interview. We hope the reader of this book acquires an awareness of the "music" involved in the dialogue between patient and clinician that is the therapeutic essence of the psychiatric interview.

BIBLIOGRAPHY

Preface

American Psychiatric Association: Diagnostic and Statistical Manual of Mental Disorders, 5th Edition. Arlington, VA, American Psychiatric Association, 2013

Buckley PJ, Michels R, Mackinnon RA: Changes in the psychiatric landscape. Am J Psychiatry 163:757–760, 2006

Freud A: The widening scope of indications for psychoanalysis: discussion. J Am Psychoanal Assoc 2:607–620, 1954

Gabbard GO: Mind, brain, and personality disorders. Am J Psychiatry 162:648–655, 2005

Shedler J, Beck A, Fonagy P, et al: Personality disorders in DSM-5. Am J Psychiatry 167:1025–1028, 2010

Chapter 1

American Psychiatric Association: Diagnostic and Statistical Manual of Mental Disorders, 4th Edition, Text Revision. Washington, DC, American Psychiatric Association, 2000

Brenner C: The Mind in Conflict. New York, International Universities Press, 1982

Buckley PJ (ed): Essential Papers on Object Relations. New York, New York University Press, 1986

Cooper AM: Changes in psychoanalytic ideas: transference interpretation. J Am Psychoanal Assoc 35:77–98, 1987

Fenichel O: The Psychoanalytic Theory of Neurosis, 50th Anniversary Edition. New York, WW Norton, 1996

Gabbard GO: Psychodynamic Psychiatry in Clinical Practice, 5th Edition. Washington, DC, American Psychiatric Publishing, 2014

Gill M, Newman R, Redlich F: The Initial Interview in Psychiatric Practice. New York, International Universities Press, 1954

Gill MM: Psychoanalysis in Transition: A Personal View. Hillsdale, NJ, Analytic Press, 1994

Greenson RR: The Technique and Practice of Psychoanalysis. New York, International Universities Press, 1967

Kohut H: The Analysis of the Self. New York, International Universities Press, 1971

Kohut H: The Restoration of the Self. New York, International Universities Press, 1977

Loewald HW: On the therapeutic action of psychoanalysis, in Papers on Psychoanalysis. New Haven, CT, Yale University Press, 1980, pp 221–256

MacKinnon RA, Yudofsky SC: Principles of the Psychiatric Evaluation. Baltimore, MD, Lippincott Williams & Wilkins, 1991

Margulies A, Havens LL: The initial encounter: what to do first? Am J Psychiatry 138:421–428, 1981

Michels R, Abensour L, Eizirik C, et al (eds): Key Papers on Countertransference. London, Karnac, 2002

Perry S, Cooper AM, Michels R: The psychodynamic formulation: its purpose, structure and clinical application. Am J Psychiatry 144:543–550, 1987

Person ES, Cooper AM, Gabbard GO (eds): The American Psychiatric Publishing Textbook of Psychoanalysis. Washington, DC, American Psychiatric Publishing, 2005

Rado S: Adaptational Psychodynamics. New York, Science House, 1969

Sandler J, Dare C, Holder A: The Patient and the Analyst: The Basis of the Psychoanalytic Process, 2nd Edition. Revised and expanded by Sandler J, Dreher AU. Madison, CT, International Universities Press, 1992

Schwaber E (ed): The Transference in Psychotherapy: Clinical Management. New York, International Universities Press, 1985

Sullivan HS: The Psychiatric Interview. New York, WW Norton, 1954

Wallerstein RS: The growth and transformation of American ego psychology. J Am Psychoanal Assoc 50:135–169, 2001

Chapter 2

Arlow JA: Unconscious fantasy and disturbances of mental experiences. Psychoanal Q 38:1–27, 1969

Arlow JA, Brenner C: Psychoanalytic Concepts and the Structural Theory. New York, International Universities Press, 1964

Brenner C: The Mind in Conflict. New York, International Universities Press, 1982

Buckley PJ (ed): Essential Papers on Object Relations. New York, New York University Press, 1986

Cooper AM: Changes in psychoanalytic ideas: transference interpretation. J Am Psychoanal Assoc 35:77–98, 1987

Erikson E: Childhood and Society. New York, WW Norton, 1950

Fenichel O: The Psychoanalytic Theory of Neurosis, 50th Anniversary Edition. New York, WW Norton, 1996

Freud A: The ego and the mechanisms of defense (1936), in The Writings of Anna Freud, Vol 2. New York, International Universities Press, 1966

Gabbard GO: Psychodynamic Psychiatry in Clinical Practice, 5th Edition. Washington, DC, American Psychiatric Publishing, 2014

Gill MM: Psychoanalysis in Transition: A Personal View. Hillsdale, NJ, Analytic Press, 1994

Greenberg J, Mitchell SA: Object Relations in Psychoanalytic Theory. Cambridge, MA, Harvard University Press, 1983

Greenson RR: The Technique and Practice of Psychoanalysis. New York, International Universities Press, 1967

Kernberg OF: Object Relations Theory and Clinical Psychoanalysis. New York, Jason Aronson, 1976

Kernberg OF: Internal World and External Reality: Object Relations Theory Applied. New York, Jason Aronson, 1980

Kohut H: The Analysis of the Self. New York, International Universities Press, 1971

Kohut H: The Restoration of the Self. New York, International Universities Press, 1977

Loewald HW: On the therapeutic action of psychoanalysis, in Papers on Psychoanalysis. New Haven, CT, Yale University Press, 1980, pp 221–256

Mahler MS, Pine F, Bergman A: The Psychological Birth of the Human Infant: Symbiosis and Individuation. New York, Basic Books, 1975

Michels R, Abensour L, Eizirik C, et al (eds): Key Papers on Countertransference. London, Karnac, 2002

Perry S, Cooper AM, Michels R: The psychodynamic formulation: its purpose, structure, and clinical application. Am J Psychiatry 144:543–550, 1987

Person ES, Cooper AM, Gabbard GO: The American Psychiatric Publishing Textbook of Psychoanalysis. Washington, DC, American Psychiatric Publishing, 2005

Pine F: Drive, Ego, Object, and Self: A Synthesis for Clinical Work. New York, Basic Books, 1990

Rado S: Adaptational Psychodynamics. New York, Science House, 1969

Sandler J, Dare C, Holder A: The Patient and the Analyst: The Basis of the Psychoanalytic Process, 2nd Edition. Revised and expanded by Sandler J, Dreher AU. Madison, CT, International Universities Press, 1992

Schwaber E (ed): The Transference in Psychotherapy: Clinical Management. New York, International Universities Press, 1985

Stern DN: The Interpersonal World of the Infant: A View from Psychoanalysis and Developmental Psychology. New York, Basic Books, 1985

Thomä H, Kächele H: Psychoanalytic Practice, Vol 1: Principles. Translated by Wilson M, Roseveare D. New York, Springer-Verlag, 1987

Wallerstein RS: Self psychology and "classical" psychoanalytic psychology: the nature of their relationship, in The Future of Psychoanalysis: Essays in Honor of Heinz Kohut. Edited by Goldberg A. New York, International Universities Press, 1983

Wallerstein RS: The growth and transformation of American ego psychology. J Am Psychoanal Assoc 50:135–169, 2001

Winnicott DW: The Child, the Family and the Outside World. Reading, MA, Addison-Wesley, 1987

Chapter 3

Abraham K: Contributions to the theory of anal character (1921), in Selected Papers of Karl Abraham. London, Hogarth Press, 1942, pp 370–392

American Psychiatric Association: Diagnostic and Statistical Manual of Mental Disorders, 4th Edition, Text Revision. Washington, DC, American Psychiatric Association, 2000

Diaferia G, Bianchi I, Bianchi ML, et al: Relationship between obsessive-compulsive personality disorder and obsessive-compulsive disorder. Compr Psychiatry 38:38–42, 1997

Esman AH: Psychoanalysis and general psychiatry: obsessive-compulsive disorder as paradigm. J Am Psychoanal Assoc 37:319–336, 1989

Freud S: Notes upon a case of obsessional neurosis (1909), in The Standard Edition of the Complete Psychological Works of Sigmund Freud, Vol 10. Translated and edited by Strachey J. London, Hogarth Press, 1955, pp 151–318

McCullough PK, Maltsberger JT: Obsessive-compulsive personality disorder, in Treatments of Psychiatric Disorders, 2nd Edition, Vol 2. Edited by Gabbard GO. Washington, DC, American Psychiatric Press, 1995, pp 2367–2376

Chapter 4

American Psychiatric Association: Diagnostic and Statistical Manual of Mental Disorders, 2nd Edition. Washington, DC, American Psychiatric Association, 1968

American Psychiatric Association: Diagnostic and Statistical Manual of Mental Disorders, 3rd Edition. Washington, DC, American Psychiatric Association, 1980

American Psychiatric Association: Diagnostic and Statistical Manual of Mental Disorders, 4th Edition, Text Revision. Washington, DC, American Psychiatric Association, 2000

Breuer J, Freud S: Studies on hysteria (1893–1895), in The Standard Edition of the Complete Psychological Works of Sigmund Freud, Vol 2. Translated and edited by Strachey J. London, Hogarth Press, 1955, pp 1–319

Chodoff P: The diagnosis of hysteria: an overview. Am J Psychiatry 131:1073–1078, 1974

Chodoff P, Lyons H: Hysteria, the hysterical personality and "hysterical" conversion. Am J Psychiatry 114:734–740, 1958

Easser BR, Lesser SR: Hysterical personality: a re-evaluation. Psycho-anal Q 34:390–405, 1965

Freud S: Fragment of an analysis of a case of hysteria (1905 [1901]), in The Standard Edition of the Complete Psychological Works of Sigmund Freud, Vol 7. Translated and edited by Strachey J. London, Hogarth Press, 1953, pp 1–122

Gabbard GO: Hysterical and histrionic personality disorders, in Psychodynamic Psychiatry in Clinical Practice, 5th Edition. Washington, DC, American Psychiatric Publishing, 2014, pp 545–576

Gunderson JG, Gabbard GO (eds): Psychotherapy for Personality Disorders (Review of Psychiatry Series, Vol 19, No 3; Oldham JO and Riba MB, series eds). Washington, DC, American Psychiatric Press, 2000

Kernberg OF: Borderline Conditions and Pathological Narcissism. New York, Jason Aronson, 1975

Veith I: Hysteria: The History of a Disease. Chicago, IL, University of Chicago Press, 1965

Zetzel ER: The so-called good hysteric. Int J Psychoanal 49:256–260, 1968

Chapter 5

Adler G: Psychotherapy of the narcissistic personality disorder patient: two contrasting approaches. Am J Psychiatry 143:430–436, 1986

Akhtar S: The shy narcissist. Paper presented at the 150th American Psychiatric Association Annual Meeting, San Diego, CA, May 1997

Akhtar S, Thompson JA: Overview: narcissistic personality disorder. Am J Psychiatry 139:12–19, 1982

American Psychiatric Association: Diagnostic and Statistical Manual of Mental Disorders, 2nd Edition. Washington, DC, American Psychiatric Association, 1968

American Psychiatric Association: Diagnostic and Statistical Manual of Mental Disorders, 4th Edition, Text Revision. Washington, DC, American Psychiatric Association, 2000

Bach S: Narcissistic States and the Therapeutic Process. New York, Jason Aronson, 1985

Cooper AM: Further developments of the diagnosis of narcissistic personality disorder, in Disorders of Narcissism: Diagnostic, Clinical, and Empirical Implications. Edited by Ronningstam EF. Washington, DC, American Psychiatric Press, 1998, pp 53–74

Gabbard GO: Two subtypes of narcissistic personality disorder. Bull Menninger Clin 53:527–532, 1989

Graves R: Narcissus, in The Greek Myths. New York, Penguin Books, 1957, pp 286–288

Gunderson J, Ronningstam EF, Bodkin A: The diagnostic interview for narcissistic patients. Arch Gen Psychiatry 47:676–680, 1990

Gunderson J, Ronningstam EF, Smith L: Narcissistic personality disorder, in DSM-IV Sourcebook, Vol 2. Edited by Widiger TA, Frances AJ, Pincus HA, et al. Washington, DC, American Psychiatric Association, 1996, pp 745–756

Hibbard S: Narcissism, shame, masochism, and object relations: an exploratory correlational study. Psychoanal Psychol 9:489–508, 1992

Kernberg OF: Borderline Conditions and Pathological Narcissism. New York, Jason Aronson, 1975

Kernberg OF: The narcissistic personality disorder and the differential diagnosis of antisocial behavior. Psychiatr Clin North Am 12:553–570, 1989

Kernberg OF: Pathological narcissism and narcissistic personality disorder: theoretical background and diagnostic classifications, in Disorders of Narcissism: Diagnostic, Clinical and Empirical Implications. Edited by Ronningstam EF. Washington, DC, American Psychiatric Press, 1998, pp 29–51

Kohut H: The Analysis of the Self. New York, International Universities Press, 1971

Kohut H: Thoughts on narcissism and narcissistic rage. Psychoanal Study Child 27:360–400, 1972

Kohut H: The Restoration of the Self. New York, International Universities Press, 1977

Kohut H, Wolf E: The disorders of the self and their treatment: an outline. Int J Psychoanal 59:413–425, 1978

Miller A: Depression and grandiosity as related forms of narcissistic disturbances, in Essential Papers on Narcissism. Edited by Morrison AP. New York, New York University Press, 1986, pp 323–347

Millon T: DSM narcissistic personality disorder: historical reflections and future directions, in Disorders of Narcissism: Diagnostic, Clinical and Empirical Implications. Edited by Ronningstam EF. Washington, DC, American Psychiatric Press, 1998, pp 75–101

Morrison AP: Shame, ideal self, and narcissism, in Essential Papers on Narcissism. Edited by Morrison AP. New York, New York University Press, 1986, pp 348–371

Pulver SE: Narcissism: the term and the concept. J Am Psychoanal Assoc 18:319–341, 1970

Reich A: Pathological forms of self-esteem regulation. Psychoanal Study Child 15:215–232, 1960

Ronningstam EF: Pathological narcissism and narcissistic personality disorder in Axis I disorders. Harv Rev Psychiatry 3:326–340, 1996

Ronningstam EF (ed): Disorders of Narcissism: Diagnostic, Clinical and Empirical Implications. Washington, DC, American Psychiatric Press, 1998

Ronningstam EF, Gunderson J: Identifying criteria for narcissistic personality disorder. Am J Psychiatry 147:918–922, 1990

Ronningstam EF, Gunderson J: Differentiating borderline personality disorder from narcissistic personality disorder. J Personal Disord 5:225–232, 1991

Ronningstam EF, Gunderson J: Descriptive studies on narcissistic personality disorder. Psychiatr Clin North Am 12:585–601, 1998

Stern DN: The Interpersonal World of the Infant. New York, Basic Books, 1985

Chapter 6

American Psychiatric Association: Diagnostic and Statistical Manual of Mental Disorders, 4th Edition, Text Revision. Washington, DC, American Psychiatric Association, 2000

Bach S: The Language of Perversion and the Language of Love. Northvale, NJ, Jason Aronson, 1994

Bach S, Schwartz L: A dream of the Marquis de Sade. J Am Psychoanal Assoc 20:451–475, 1972

Broucek F: Shame and the Self. New York, Guilford, 1991

Cooper AM: Narcissism and masochism: the narcissistic–masochistic character. Psychiatr Clin North Am 12:541–552, 1989

Cooper AM: Psychotherapeutic approaches to masochism. J Psychother Pract Res 2:51–63, 1993

Chused JF: The evocative power of enactments. J Am Psychoanal Assoc 39:615–639, 1991

Deleuze G: Sacher-Masoch: An Interpretation. Translated by McNeil JM. London, Faber & Faber, 1971

Fairbairn WRD: The repression and return of bad objects. British Journal of Medical Psychology 19:327–341, 1943

Freud S: The economic problem of masochism (1924), in The Standard Edition of the Complete Psychological Works of Sigmund Freud, Vol 19. Translated and edited by Strachey J. London, Hogarth Press, 1961, pp 155–170

Khan MM: Alienation in Perversions. New York, International Universities Press, 1979

Krafft-Ebing RF: Psychopathia Sexualis, With Special Reference to Contrary Sexual Instinct: A Medico-Legal Study. London, FA Davis, 1886

McLaughlin J: Clinical and theoretical aspects of enactment. J Am Psychoanal Assoc 39:595–614, 1991

Novick KK: The essence of masochism. Psychoanal Study Child 42:353–384, 1987

Novick KK, Novick J: Some comments on masochism and the delusion of omnipotence from a developmental perspective. J Am Psychoanal Assoc 39:307–331, 1991

Sade DAF: The Marquis de Sade: The 120 Days of Sodom and Other Writings. Compiled and translated by Seaver R, Wainhouse A. New York, Grove Press, 1986

Chapter 7

American Psychiatric Association: Diagnostic and Statistical Manual of Mental Disorders, 4th Edition, Text Revision. Washington, DC, American Psychiatric Association, 2000

American Psychiatric Association: Practice Guideline for the Treatment of Patients With Major Depressive Disorder, 2nd Edition. Washington, DC, American Psychiatric Press, 2000

Busch FN, Rudden M, Shapiro T: Psychodynamic Treatment of Depression. Washington, DC, American Psychiatric Publishing, 2004

Freud S: Mourning and melancholia (1917 [1915]), in The Standard Edition of the Complete Psychological Works of Sigmund Freud, Vol 14. Translated and edited by Strachey J. London, Hogarth Press, 1957, pp 237–260

Havens L: Recognition of suicidal risks through the psychological examination. N Engl J Med 276:210–215, 1967

Hirschfeld RMA, Russell JM: Assessment and treatment of suicidal patients. N Engl J Med 337:910–995, 1997

Kendler KS, Kessler RC, Walters EE, et al: Stressful life events, genetic liability and onset of an episode of major depression in women. Am J Psychiatry 150:833–842, 1999

Nemeroff CB: The neurobiology of depression. Sci Am 278:42–49, 1998

Parker G, Fink M, Shorter E, et al: Issues for DSM-5: whither melancholia? The case for its classification as a distinct mood disorder. Am J Psychiatry 167(7):745–747, 2010

Schatzberg AF, Nemeroff CB (eds): The American Psychiatric Publishing Textbook of Psychopharmacology, 3rd Edition. Washington, DC, American Psychiatric Publishing, 2004

Solomon A: The Noonday Demon: An Atlas of Depression. New York, Scribners, 2001

Chapter 8

American Psychiatric Association: Practice guideline for the treatment of patients with panic disorder. Work Group on Panic Disorder. Am J Psychiatry 155 (5, suppl):1–34, 1998

American Psychiatric Association: Diagnostic and Statistical Manual of Mental Disorders, 4th Edition, Text Revision. Washington, DC, American Psychiatric Association, 2000

Breuer J, Freud S: Studies on hysteria (1893–1895), in The Standard Edition of the Complete Psychological Works of Sigmund Freud, Vol 2. Translated and edited by Strachey J. London, Hogarth Press, 1955, pp 125–134

Brown TA, Barlow DH: Comorbidity among anxiety disorders: implications for treatment and DSM-IV. J Consult Clin Psychol 60:835–844, 1992

Freud S: Inhibitions, symptoms and anxiety (1926), in The Standard Edition of the Complete Psychological Works of Sigmund Freud, Vol 20. Translated and edited by Strachey J. London, Hogarth Press, 1959, pp 75–175

Fricchione G: Generalized anxiety disorder. N Engl J Med 351:675–682, 2004

Kagan J, Snidman N: The Long Shadow of Temperament. Cambridge, MA, Harvard University Press, 2004

Klein DF: Delineation of two drug-responsive anxiety syndromes. Psychopharmacology 5:397–408, 1964

Shear MK: Psychotherapeutic issues in long-term treatment of anxiety disorder patients. Psychiatr Clin North Am 18:885–894, 1995

Shear MK, Cooper AM, Klerman GL, et al: A psychodynamic model of panic disorder. Am J Psychiatry 150:859–866, 1993

Stein DJ (ed): Clinical Manual of Anxiety Disorders. Washington, DC, American Psychiatric Publishing, 2004

Stein DJ, Hollander E (eds): Textbook of Anxiety Disorders. Washington, DC, American Psychiatric Publishing, 2002

Chapter 9

American Psychiatric Association: Diagnostic and Statistical Manual of Mental Disorders, 3rd Edition. Washington, DC, American Psychiatric Association, 1980

American Psychiatric Association: Diagnostic and Statistical Manual of Mental Disorders, 4th Edition. Washington, DC, American Psychiatric Association, 1994

American Psychiatric Association: Diagnostic and Statistical Manual of Mental Disorders, 4th Edition, Text Revision. Washington, DC, American Psychiatric Association, 2000

Deutsch H: Some forms of emotional disturbance and their relationship to schizophrenia. Psychoanal Q 11:301–321, 1942

Falret J: Etudes Cliniques sur les Maladies Mentales. Paris, Bailliére, 1890

Frosch J: The psychotic character: clinical psychiatric considerations. Psychiatr Q 38:1–16, 1964

Gabbard GO: Mind, brain, and personality disorders. Am J Psychiatry 162:648–655, 2005

Gabbard GO, Wilkinson SM: Management of Countertransference With Borderline Patients. Washington, DC, American Psychiatric Press, 1994

Grinker RR Jr, Werble B, Drye RC: The Borderline Syndrome: A Behavioral Study of Ego Functions. New York, Basic Books, 1968

Gunderson JG: Borderline Personality Disorder: A Clinical Guide. Washington, DC, American Psychiatric Publishing, 2001

Hoch P, Polatin P: Pseudoneurotic forms of schizophrenia. Psychiatr Q 23:248–276, 1949

Kernberg OF: Borderline personality organization. J Am Psychoanal Assoc 15:641–685, 1967

Kernberg OF: Borderline Conditions and Pathological Narcissism. New York, Jason Aronson, 1975

Kernberg OF: Severe Personality Disorder. New Haven, CT, Yale University Press, 1984

Kernberg OF: The management of affect storms in the psychoanalytic psychotherapy of borderline patients. J Am Psychoanal Assoc 51:517–545, 2003

Knight RP: Borderline states. Bull Menninger Clin 17:1–12, 1953

Linehan MM: Cognitive-Behavioral Treatment of Borderline Personality Disorder. New York, Guilford, 1993

Practice guideline for the treatment of patients with borderline personality disorder. American Psychiatric Association. Am J Psychiatry 158 (10, suppl):1–52, 2001

Steiner J: Psychic Retreats: Pathological Organizations in Psychotic, Neurotic and Borderline Patients. London, Routledge, 1993

Stern A: Psychoanalytic investigation of and therapy in the borderline group of neuroses. Psychoanal Q 7:467–489, 1938

Stone MH: The borderline syndrome: evolution of the term, genetic aspects, and prognosis, in Essential Papers on Borderline Disorders. Edited by Stone MH. New York, New York University Press, 1986, pp 475–497

Stone MH (ed): Essential Papers on Borderline Disorders. New York, New York University Press, 1986

Zanarini MC, Frankenburg FR, Hennen J, et al: The longitudinal course of borderline psychopathology. Am J Psychiatry 160:274–283, 2003

Chapter 10

American Psychiatric Association: Diagnostic and Statistical Manual of Mental Disorders, 3rd Edition. Washington, DC, American Psychiatric Association, 1980

American Psychiatric Association: Diagnostic and Statistical Manual of Mental Disorders, 4th Edition, Text Revision. Washington, DC, American Psychiatric Association, 2000

American Psychiatric Association: Diagnostic and Statistical Manual of Mental Disorders, 5th Edition. Arlington, VA, American Psychiatric Association, 2013

Andreasen NC, Noyes R Jr, Hartford CE, et al: Management of emotional reactions in seriously burned adults. N Engl J Med 286:65–69, 1972

Bergmann MS, Jucovy ME (eds): Generations of the Holocaust. New York, Columbia University Press, 1982

Birmes P, Hatton L, Brunet A, et al: Early historical literature for post-traumatic symptomatology. Stress and Health 19:17–26, 2003

Breslau N, Davis GC, Andreski P: Risk factors for PTSD-related traumatic events: a prospective analysis. Am J Psychiatry 152:529–535, 1995

Breslau N, Peterson EL, Schultz LR: A second look at prior trauma and the posttraumatic stress disorder effects of subsequent trauma. Arch Gen Psychiatry 65:431–437, 2008

Breuer J, Freud S: Studies on hysteria (1893–1895), in Standard Edition of the Complete Psychological Works of Sigmund Freud, Vol 2. Translated and edited by Strachey J. London, Hogarth Press, 1955, pp 1–319

Brown PJ, Wolfe J: Substance abuse and post-traumatic stress disorder comorbidity. Drug Alcohol Depend 35:51–59, 1994

Burgess AW, Holstrom L: Rape trauma syndrome. Am J Psychiatry 131:981–986, 1974

Coleridge ST: The rime of the ancient mariner (1834), in Coleridge Poetry and Prose. New York, WW Norton, 2004

Freud A: Comments on psychic trauma, in The Writings of Anna Freud, Vol 5. New York, International Universities Press, 1967

Freud S: Beyond the pleasure principle (1920), in Standard Edition of the Complete Psychological Works of Sigmund Freud, Vol 18. Translated and edited by Strachey J. London, Hogarth Press, 1955, pp 1–64

Grinker RR, Spiegel JP: Men Under Stress. Philadelphia, PA, Blakiston, 1945

Herman JL (with Hirschman L): Father-Daughter Incest. Cambridge, MA, Harvard University Press, 1981

Herman JL: Trauma and Recovery. New York, Basic Books, 1997

Horowitz MJ: Stress Response Syndromes. New York, Jason Aronson, 1976

Kardiner A: The Traumatic Neurosis of War. New York, Hoeber, 1941

Kardiner A, Spiegel H: War Stress and Neurotic Illness. New York, Hoeber, 1947

Kempe RS, Kempe CH: Child Abuse. Cambridge, MA, Harvard University Press, 1978

Kessler RC, Berglund P, Demler O, et al: Lifetime prevalence and age of onset distribution of DSM IV disorders in the national comorbidity survey replication. Arch Gen Psychiatry 62:593–602, 2005

Krystal H (ed): Massive Psychic Trauma. New York, International University Press, 1968

Krystal H: Trauma and affect. Psychoanal Study Child 33:81–116, 1978

Krystal H: Trauma and the stimulus barrier. Psychoanalytic Inquiry 5:121–161, 1985

Lifton RJ: Death in Life: Survivors of Hiroshima. New York, Random House, 1967

Lifton RJ: Home From the War; Vietnam Veterans: Neither Victims nor Executioners. New York, Simon & Schuster, 1973

Myers CS: A contribution to the study of shell shock. Being an account of the cases of loss of memory, vision, smell, and taste admitted to the Duchess of Westminster's War Hospital, Le Touquet. Lancet 185:316–320, 1915

O'Donnell ML, Creamer M, Pattison P: Posttraumatic stress disorder and depression following trauma: understanding comorbidity. Am J Psychiatry 161:1390–1396, 2004

Putman FW: Pierre Janet and modern views on dissociation. J Trauma Stress 2:413–430, 1989

Rivers WHR: Instinct and the Unconscious: A Contribution to a Biological Theory of the Psychoneuroses. Cambridge, UK, Cambridge University Press, 1920

Roberts AL, Austin SB, Corliss HL, et al: Pervasive trauma exposure among US sexual orientation minority adults and risk of posttraumatic stress disorder. Am J Public Health 100:2433–2441, 2010

Roberts AL, Gilman SE, Breslau J, et al: Race/ethnic differences in exposure to traumatic events, development of posttraumatic stress disorder, and treatment seeking for posttraumatic stress disorder in the United States. Psychol Med 41:71–83, 2011

ShatanC: The Grief of Soldiers: Vietnam Combat Veterans' Self-Help Movement. Am J Orthopsychiatry 43:640–653, 1973

Solzhhenitsyn A: The Gulag Archipelago 1918–1956. London, Collins, 1974

Southwick SM, Charney DS: Resilience: The Science of Mastering Life's Greatest Challenges. Cambridge, UK, Cambridge University Press, 2012

van der Kolk BA, van der Hart O: Pierre Janet and the breakdown of adaptation in psychological trauma. Am J Psychiatry 146:1530–1540, 1989

Chapter 11

American Psychiatric Association: Diagnostic and Statistical Manual of Mental Disorders, 2nd Edition. Washington, DC, American Psychiatric Association, 1968

American Psychiatric Association: Diagnostic and Statistical Manual of Mental Disorders, 3rd Edition. Washington, DC, American Psychiatric Association, 1980

American Psychiatric Association: Diagnostic and Statistical Manual of Mental Disorders, Fifth Edition. Arlington, VA, American Psychiatric Association, 2013

Bentley GE: The Stranger From Paradise: A Biography of William Blake. New Haven, CT, Yale University Press, 2001

Bowlby J: Attachment and Loss, Vol 1: Attachment. London, Hogarth Press, 1969

Breuer J, Freud S: Studies on hysteria (1893–1895), in the Standard Edition of the Complete Psychological Works of Sigmund Freud, Vol. 2. Translated and edited by Strachey J. London, Hogarth Press, 1955, pp 1–319

Charcot J-M: Oeuvres Completes de J-M Charcot. Paris, Lecrosnier et Babe, 1980

Dell PF: Understanding dissociation, in Dissociation and the Dissociative Disorders: DSM-V and Beyond. Edited by Dell PF, O'Neil JA. New York, Routledge, 2009, pp 709–825

Dutra L, Bianchi I, Siegel D, et al: The relational context of dissociative phenomena, in Dissociation and the Dissociative Disorders: DSM-V and Beyond. Edited by Dell PF, O'Neil JA. New York, Routledge, 2009, pp 83–92

Ferenczi S: Confusion of tongues between adults and children: the language of tenderness and of passion (1933). Int J Psychoanal 30:225–230, 1949

Foote B: Dissociative identity disorder: epidemiology, pathogenesis, clinical manifestations, course, assessment, and diagnosis. UpToDate, May 2015. Available at: http://www.uptodate.com/contents/dissociative-identity-disorder-epidemiology-pathogenesis-clinical-manifestations-course-assessment-and-diagnosis. Accessed June 3, 2015.

Freud S: Five lectures on psycho-analysis (1910), in Standard Edition of the Complete Psychological Works of Sigmund Freud, Vol 11. Translated and edited by Strachey J. London, Hogarth Press, 1957, pp 9–55

Freud S: Observations on transference-love (1914), in Standard Edition of the Complete Psychological Works of Sigmund Freud, Vol 12. Translated and edited by Strachey J. London, Hogarth Press, 1958, pp 159–171

Greenberg J: Theoretical models and the analyst's neutrality. Contemp Psychoanal 22:87–106, 1986

Herman JL: Trauma and Recovery. New York, Basic Books, 1992

Jones E: The Life and Work of Sigmund Freud. New York, Basic Books, 1961

Kluft RP: Incest and subsequent revictimization: the case of therapist-patient sexual exploitation, with a description of the sitting duck syndrome, in Incest-Related Syndromes of Adult Psychopathology. Edited by Kluft RP. Washington, DC, American Psychiatric Press, 1990, pp 263–287

Kluft RP: Dealing with alters: a pragmatic clinical perspective. Psychiatr Clin North Am 29(1):281–304, xii, 2006 16530598

Knox RA: Enthusiasm: A Chapter in the History of Religion. New York, Oxford University Press, 1950

Kohut H: The two analyses of Mr. Z. Int J Psychoanal 60(1):3–27, 1979 457340

Kohut H: How Does Analysis Cure? Chicago, IL, University of Chicago Press, 1984

Lewis IM: Ecstatic Religion: A Study of Shamanism and Spirit Possession. New York, Routledge, 1989

Liotti G: Attachment and dissociation, in Dissociation and the Dissociative Disorders: DSM-V and Beyond. Edited by Dell PF, O'Neil JA. New York, Routledge, 2009, pp 53–66

Loewenstein RJ: Posttraumatic and dissociative aspects of transference and countertransference in the treatment of multiple personality disorder, in Clinical Perspectives on Multiple Personality Disorder. Edited by Kluft RP, Fine CG. Washington, DC, American Psychiatric Press, 1993, pp 51–85

Lyons-Ruth K, Dutra L, Schuder MR, et al: From infant attachment disorganization to adult dissociation: relational adaptations or traumatic experiences? Psychiatr Clin North Am 29(1):63–86, viii, 2006 16530587

O'Neil JA: Dissociative multiplicity and psychoanalysis, in Dissociation and the Dissociative Disorders: DSM-V and Beyond. Edited by Dell PF, O'Neil JA. New York, Routledge, 2009, pp 287–325

Putnam F: Diagnosis and Treatment of Multiple Personality Disorder. New York, Guilford, 1989

Shusta-Hochberg SR: Therapeutic hazards of treating child alters as real children in dissociative identity disorder. J Trauma Dissociation 5:13–27, 2004

Veith I: Hysteria: The History of a Disease. Chicago, IL, University of Chicago Press, 1965

Chapter 12

American Psychiatric Association: Diagnostic and Statistical Manual of Mental Disorders, 4th Edition, Text Revision. Washington, DC, American Psychiatric Association, 2000

Cleckley HM: The Mask of Sanity: An Attempt to Clarify Some Issues About the So-Called Psychopathic Personality, 5th Edition. St Louis, MO, CV Mosby, 1976

Gabbard GO, Coyne L: Predictors of response of antisocial patients to hospital treatment. Hosp Community Psychiatry 34:243–248, 1986

Galanter M, Kleber HD (eds): The American Psychiatric Publishing Textbook of Substance Abuse Treatment, 3rd Edition. Washington, DC, American Psychiatric Publishing, 2004

Hare RD: Diagnosis of antisocial personality disorder in two prison populations. Am J Psychiatry 140:887–890, 1983

Hare RD: Psychopathy: a clinical construct whose time has come. Crim Justice Behav 23:25–54, 1995

Kernberg OF: Severe Personality Disorders: Psychotherapeutic Strategies. New Haven, CT, Yale University Press, 1984

Kernberg OF: Pathological narcissism and narcissistic personality disorder: theoretical background and diagnostic classification, in Disorders of Narcissism. Edited by Ronningstam EF. Washington, DC, American Psychiatric Press, 1998, pp 29–51

Kraepelin E: Psychiatrie, 8th Edition. Leipzig, Barth, 1909

Luntz BX, Wisdom CS: Antisocial personality disorder in abused and neglected children grown up. Am J Psychiatry 151:493–498, 1994

Mannuzza S, Klein RG, Bessler A, et al: Adult psychiatric status of hyperactive boys grown up. Am J Psychiatry 155:493–498, 1998

Meloy JR: Antisocial personality disorder, in Treatments of Psychiatric Disorders, 2nd Edition, Vol 2. Edited by Gabbard GO. Washington, DC, American Psychiatric Press, 1995, pp 2273–2290

Stone MH: Gradations of antisociality and responsivity to psychosocial therapies, in Psychotherapy for Personality Disorders (Review of Psychiatry series Vol 19, No 3; Oldham JM and Riba MS, series eds). Edited by Gunderson JG, Gabbard GO. Washington, DC, American Psychiatric Press, 2000, pp 95–130

Chapter 13

Akhtar S: Paranoid personality disorder: a synthesis of developmental, dynamic and descriptive features. Am J Psychother 44:5–25, 1990

American Psychiatric Association: Diagnostic and Statistical Manual of Mental Disorders, 4th Edition, Text Revision. Washington, DC, American Psychiatric Association, 2000

Auchincloss EL, Weiss RW: Paranoid character and the intolerance of indifference. J Am Psychoanal Assoc 40:1013–1037, 1992

Bak R: Masochism in paranoia. Psychoanal Q 15:285–301, 1946

Blum HP: Object inconstancy and paranoid conspiracy. J Am Psychoanal Assoc 29:789–813, 1981

Cameron N: The development of paranoic thinking. Psychological Review 50:219–233, 1943

Freud S: Psycho-analytic notes on an autobiographical account of a case of paranoia (dementia paranoides) (1911), in The Standard Edition of the Complete Psychological Works of Sigmund Freud, Vol 12. Translated and edited by Strachey J. London, Hogarth Press, 1958, pp 1–82

Freud S: Some neurotic mechanisms in jealousy, paranoia and homosexuality (1922), in The Standard Edition of the Complete Psychological Works of Sigmund Freud, Vol 18. Translated and edited by Strachey J. London, Hogarth Press, 1955, pp 221–232

Klein M: Contributions to Psychoanalysis 1921–1945. London, Hogarth Press, 1948

Chapter 14

American Psychiatric Association: Diagnostic and Statistical Manual of Mental Disorders, 4th Edition, Text Revision. Washington, DC, American Psychiatric Association, 2000

American Psychiatric Association: Practice guideline for the treatment of patients with bipolar disorder (revision). Am J Psychiatry 159 (4, suppl):1–36, 2002

Bowers MB: Retreat From Sanity. Baltimore, MD, Penguin, 1974

Buckley PJ: Experiencing madness. Am J Psychother 68(3):273–276, 2014

Feinsilver D: Towards a Comprehensive Model of Schizophrenic Disorders. Hillsdale, NJ, Lawrence Erlbaum, 1986

Freud S: Psycho-analytic notes on an autobiographical account of a case of paranoia (dementia paranoides) (1911), in The Standard Edition of the Complete Psychological Works of Sigmund Freud, Vol 12. Translated and edited by Strachey J. London, Hogarth Press, 1958, pp 1–82

Fromm-Reichmann F: Psychoanalytic psychotherapy with psychotics. Psychiatry 6:277–279, 1943

Goodwin FK, Jamison KR: Manic-Depressive Illness. New York, Oxford University Press, 1990

Grotstein J: Deciphering the schizophrenic experience. Psychoanalytic Inquiry 3:37–69, 1983

Jamison KR: An Unquiet Mind. New York, Vintage Books, 1995

Lehman AF, Lieberman JA, Dixon LB, et al: Practice guideline for the treatment of patients with schizophrenia, 2nd edition. Am J Psychiatry 161 (2, suppl):1–56, 2004

Lewin BD: The Psychoanalysis of Elation. New York, WW Norton, 1950

Michels R: "The Relationship between Psychoanalysis and Schizophrenia" by R. Lucas: a commentary. Int J Psychoanal 84:9–12, 2003

Schatzberg AF, Nemeroff CB (eds): The American Psychiatric Publishing Textbook of Psychopharmacology, 3rd Edition. Washington, DC, American Psychiatric Publishing, 2004

Searles HF: Collected Papers on Schizophrenia and Related Subjects. London, Hogarth Press, 1965

Steiner J: Psychic Retreats: Pathological Organizations in Psychotic, Neurotic, and Borderline Patients. London, Routledge, 1993

Strauss JS, Carpenter WT Jr: Schizophrenia. New York, Plenum, 1981

Sullivan HS: Schizophrenia as a Human Process. New York, WW Norton, 1962

Volkan V: Identification with the therapist's functions and ego-building in the treatment of schizophrenia. Br J Psychiatry 23:77–82, 1994

Willick MS: Psychoanalytic concepts of the etiology of severe mental illness. J Am Psychoanal Assoc 38:1049–1081, 1990

Willick MS: Psychoanalysis and schizophrenia: a cautionary tale. J Am Psychoanal Assoc 49:27–56, 2001

Chapter 15

Asher R: Munchausen's syndrome. Lancet 1:339–341, 1951

Craig TJ, Boardman AP, Mills K, et al: The South London somatization study, I: longitudinal course and the influence of early life experiences. Br J Psychiatry 163:579–588, 1993

Dersh J, Polatin PB, Gatchel RJ: Chronic pain and psychopathology: research findings and theoretical considerations. Psychosom Med 64:773–786, 2002

Engel GL: "Psychogenic" pain and the pain-prone patient. Am J Med 26:899–918, 1959

Engel GL: The need for a new medical model: a challenge for biomedicine. Science 196:129–136, 1977

Feldman MD, Eisendrath SJ (eds): The Spectrum of Factitious Disorders. Washington, DC, American Psychiatric Press, 1996

Folks DG, Freeman AM 3rd: Munchausen's syndrome and other factitious illness. Psychiatr Clin North Am 8:263–278, 1985

Groves JE: Taking care of the hateful patient. N Engl J Med 298:883–887, 1978

Horowitz M: Stress Response Syndromes. New York, Jason Aronson, 1976

Massie MJ (ed): Pain: What Psychiatrists Need to Know. Washington, DC, American Psychiatric Press, 2000

Phillips KA (ed): Somatoform and Factitious Disorders (Review of Psychiatry Series, Vol 20, No 3; Oldham JO and Riba MB, series eds). Washington, DC, American Psychiatric Publishing, 2001

Pilowsky I: Dimensions of hypochondriasis. Br J Psychiatry 113:89–93, 1967

Stuart S, Noyes R: Attachment and interpersonal communication in somatization. Psychosomatics 40:34–43, 1999

Chapter 16

Alexopoulos GS, Borson S, Cuthbert BN, et al: Assessment of late life depression. Biol Psychiatry 52:164–174, 2002

Armstrong SC, Cozza KL, Watanabe KS: The misdiagnosis of delirium. Psychosomatics 38:433–439, 1997

Askin-Edgar S, White KE, Cummings JL: Neuropsychiatric aspects of Alzheimer's disease and other dementing illnesses, in The American Psychiatric Publishing Textbook of Neuropsychiatry and Clinical Neurosciences, 4th Edition. Edited by Yudofsky SC, Hales RE. Washington, DC, American Psychiatric Publishing, 2002, pp 953–988

Banerjee S, Smith SC, Lamping DL, et al: Quality of life in dementia: more than just cognition. An analysis of associations with quality of life in dementia. J Neurol Neurosurg Psychiatry 77:146–148, 2006

Breitbart W, Gibson C, Tremblay A: The delirium experience: delirium recall and delirium-related distress in hospitalized cancer patients. Psychosomatics 43:183–194, 2002

Cassem NH, Murray GB, Lafayette JM, et al: Delirious patients, in Massachusetts General Hospital Handbook of General Hospital Psychiatry. Edited by Stern TA, Fricchione GL, Cassem NH, et al. St Louis, MO, CV Mosby, 2004, pp 119–134

Cummings JL: Alzheimer's disease. N Engl J Med 351:56–67, 2004

Folstein MF, Folstein SE, McHugh PR: Mini-Mental State: A practical method for grading the cognitive state of patients for the clinician. J Psychiatr Res 12:189–195, 1975

Forrest DV: Psychotherapy for patients with neuropsychiatric disorders, in The American Psychiatric Publishing Textbook of Neuropsychiatry and Clinical Neurosciences, 4th Edition. Edited by Yudofsky SC, Hales RE. Washington, DC, American Psychiatric Publishing, 2002, pp 1199–1236

Inouye SK, Bogardus ST, Charpentier PA, et al: A multicomponent intervention to prevent delirium in hospitalized older patients. N Engl J Med 340:669–676, 1999

Levin M: Delirium: a gap in psychiatric teaching. Am J Psychiatry 107:689–694, 1951

Livingston G, Johnston K, Katona C, et al: Systematic review of psychological approaches to the management of neuropsychiatric symptoms of dementia. Old Age Task Force of the World Federation of Biological Psychiatry. Am J Psychiatry 162:1996–2021, 2005

Lockwood KA, Alexopoulos GS, van Gorp WG: Executive dysfunction in geriatric depression. Am J Psychiatry 159:1119–1126, 2002

Lyketsos CG, Olin J: Depression in Alzheimer's disease: overview and treatment. Biol Psychiatry 52:243–252, 2002

Lyketsos CG, Rosenblatt A, Rabins P: Forgotten frontal lobe syndrome or "executive dysfunction syndrome." Psychosomatics 45:247–255, 2004

Samton JB, Ferrando SJ, Sanelli P, et al: The Clock Drawing Test: diagnostic, functional, and neuroimaging correlates in older medically ill adults. J Neuropsychiatry Clin Neurosci 17:533–540, 2005

Trzepacz PT, Meagher DJ: Delirium, in The American Psychiatric Publishing Textbook of Psychosomatic Medicine. Edited by Levenson JL. Washington, DC, American Psychiatric Publishing, 2005, pp 91–130

Trzepacz PT, Baker RW, Greenhouse J: A symptom rating scale for delirium. Psychiatry Res 23:89–97, 1988

Chapter 17

Allen MH (ed): Emergency Psychiatry (Review of Psychiatry Series, Vol 21, No 3; Oldham JO and Riba MB, series eds). Washington, DC, American Psychiatric Publishing, 2002

Forster PL, Wu LH: Assessment and treatment of suicidal patients in an emergency setting, in Emergency Psychiatry. Edited by Allen MH. Washington, DC, American Psychiatric Publishing, 2002, pp 75–113

Lindenmayer JP, Crowner M, Cosgrove V: Emergency treatment of agitation and aggression, in Emergency Psychiatry. Edited by Allen MH. Washington, DC, American Psychiatric Publishing, 2002, pp 115–149

Chapter 18

Druss RG, Douglas CJ: Adaptive responses to illness and disability: healthy denial. Gen Hosp Psychiatry 10:163–168, 1988

Griffith JL, Gaby L: Brief psychotherapy at the bedside: countering demoralization from medical illness. Psychosomatics 46:109–116, 2005

Klausner EJ, Alexopoulos GS: The future of psychosocial treatments for elderly patients. Psychiatr Serv 50:1198–1204, 1999

Perry S, Cooper AM, Michels R: The psychodynamic formulation: its purpose, structure, and clinical application. Am J Psychiatry 144:543–550, 1987

Viederman M: Active engagement in the consultation process. Gen Hosp Psychiatry 24:93–100, 2002

Viederman M, Perry SW 3rd: Use of a psychodynamic life narrative in the treatment of depression in the physically ill. Gen Hosp Psychiatry 2:177–185, 1980

Chapter 19

Blazer DG: The psychiatric interview of older adults, in The American Psychiatric Publishing Textbook of Geriatric Psychiatry. Edited by Blazer DG, Steffens DC, Busse EW. Washington, DC, American Psychiatric Publishing, 2004, pp 165–177

Buckley PJ: Observing the other: reflections on anthropological fieldwork. J Am Psychoanal Assoc 42:613–634, 1994

Carter JH: Culture, race and ethnicity in psychiatric practice. Psychiatr Ann 34:500–504, 2004

Clifford J: The Predicament of Culture. Cambridge, MA, Harvard University Press, 1988

Evans-Pritchard EE: Social Anthropology and Other Essays. New York, Free Press, 1962

Fernando S: Mental Health, Race, and Culture. New York, St Martin's Press, 1991

Friedman RC, Downey JI: Homosexuality. N Engl J Med 331:923–930, 1994

Kleinman A: Culture and depression. N Engl J Med 351:951–953, 2004

Kracke W: Encounter with other cultures: psychological and epistemological aspects. Ethos 15:58–81, 1987

Ritter KY, Terndrup AI: Handbook of Affirmative Psychotherapy With Lesbians and Gay Men. New York, Guilford, 2002

Roughton RE: Four men in treatment: an evolving perspective on homosexuality and bisexuality, 1965 to 2000. J Am Psychoanal Assoc 49:1187–1217, 2001

Ruiz P: Addressing culture, race and ethnicity in psychiatric practice. Psychiatr Ann 34:527–532, 2004

Chapter 20

Arlow J: The supervisory situation. J Am Psychoanal Assoc 2:576–594, 1963

Jacobs D, David P, Meyer DJ: The Supervisory Encounter. New Haven, CT, Yale University Press, 1995

Perry S, Cooper AM, Michels R: The psychodynamic formulation: its purpose, structure, and clinical application. Am J Psychiatry 144:543–550, 1987

Chapter 21

Lester D (ed): Crisis Intervention and Counseling by Telephone. Springfield, IL, Charles C Thomas, 2002

MacKinnon R, Michels R: The role of the telephone in the psychiatric interview. Psychiatry 33:82–93, 1970

Peterson MR, Beck RL: E-mail as an adjunctive tool in psychotherapy: response and responsibility. Am J Psychother 57:167–181, 2003

Afterword

Shakespeare W: The Tragedy of Macbeth. The Pelican Shakespeare. Edited by Harbage A. Baltimore, MD, Penguin Books, 1956, Act 5, Scene 3

INDEX

Abandonment feelings or experiences, 50
  of antisocial patient, 419, 426
  of borderline patient, 313, 317, 319, 322, 329, 330
  of depressed patient, 241, 252, 254
  of histrionic patient, 153
  of hospitalized patient, 561, 567
  of masochistic patient, 208, 210
  of obsessive-compulsive patient, 132
  of psychotic patient, 494
  of traumatized patient, 341, 368
Abstract thinking, 80, 483, 516
"Acting in," 24–25
Acting out, 22–25
  by antisocial patient, 429–430
  by borderline patient, 331
  definition of, 22, 429
  by dissociative identity disorder patient, 401
  by histrionic patient, 140, 143, 168
  by masochistic patient, 206, 215, 218
Acute stress disorder (ASD), 349
  DSM-5 diagnostic criteria for, 350–352
"Adaptive regression in the service of the ego," 81
ADHD (attention-deficit/hyperactivity disorder), 406–407, 419
Adolescent development, 51
Adolescent patient, 590–591
Affect(s), 9, 21, 39, 82. *See also* Emotions of patient
  of antisocial patient, 410, 411, 412–413, 424

  of borderline patient, 313, 314–316
  of cognitively impaired patient, 524
    delirium, 516
    dementia, 517
  of conduct disorder patient, 409
  of depressed patient, 225, 228, 229–230, 261, 264
  of dissociative identity disorder patient, 375, 376, 377, 380, 381, 387
  of histrionic patient, 21, 133, 144, 145–146, 153
  of manic patient, 243, 477
  of narcissistic patient, 175
  object relations models of, 99–100
  of obsessive-compulsive patient, 21, 116, 119
  of psychotic patient, 477, 480–482, 489
  resistance and, 21
Affect storms, 316
Age of patient
  determining during telephone contact, 627
  differences between clinician's age and, 590–593
  transference and, 15
Aggression, 31, 78, 86, 96. *See also* Dangerousness; Violence
  of antisocial patient, 407, 412, 414
  of anxiety disorder patient, 278, 282, 284, 285, 293, 299, 300, 307
  of borderline patient, 212, 313, 316, 318, 322, 328, 332, 333
  as character trait, 89